Manual of Definitive Surgical Trauma Care: Incorporating Definitive Anaesthetic Trauma Care

Manual of Definitive Surgical Trauma Care: Incorporating Definitive Anaesthetic Trauma Care

FIFTH EDITION

Kenneth D Boffard

Professor Emeritus, Department of Surgery
Milpark Hospital and University of the Witwatersrand
South Africa

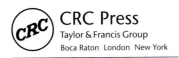

CRC Press
Taylor & Francis Group
Boca Raton London New York

CRC Press is an imprint of the
Taylor & Francis Group, an **informa** business

CRC Press
Taylor & Francis Group
6000 Broken Sound Parkway NW, Suite 300
Boca Raton, FL 33487-2742

© 2019 by Taylor & Francis Group, LLC
CRC Press is an imprint of Taylor & Francis Group, an Informa business

No claim to original U.S. Government works

Printed on acid-free paper by Ashford Colour Press Ltd

International Standard Book Number-13: 978-0-367-24468-2 (Hardback)
978-1-138-50011-2 (Paperback)

Visit the Taylor & Francis Web site at
http://www.taylorandfrancis.com

and the CRC Press Web site at
http://www.crcpress.com

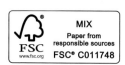

This manual is dedicated to the six surgeons who, in 1993, saw the need for a course in operative trauma surgery and surgical decision-making for those surgeons who would not routinely be involved in the care of the trauma patient, and from whose foresight the course has been developed.

Howard Champion, Bethesda, Maryland, United States

Stephen Deane, Sydney, Australia

Abe Fingerhut, Poissy, France

Stenn Lennquist, Linkoping, Sweden

David Mulder, Montreal, Canada

Donald Trunkey, Portland, Oregon, United States

Contents

Video Contents

A companion card is included with this copy of *Manual of Definitive Surgical Trauma Care, Fifth Edition*.

To use the card:

1. Insert.
2. Open from My Computer.
3. Click on Index.
4. If asked, 'allow blocked content.'
5. The welcome page will appear, together with a human skeleton.
6. Click on the '+' sign of each area to open files for procedures in that area.

Included on the card:

- Access to the neck
- Access to the anterior mediastinum
- Aorta
- Access to the axilla
- Bleeding control
- Craniotomy
- Fasciotomy
- Heart
- Heart and lung
- Iliac shunting
- Kidney
- Laparotomy
- Liver
- Pancreas
- Pelvic packing
- Small bowel
- Spleen
- Sternotomy
- Stomach
- Thoracic
- Ureteric repair

Additional Videos:

- Excision and grafting of major burns
- Application of the Vacuum Dressing

Preface

'He who desires to practice Surgery must go to war'
Corpus Hippocraticum
Hippocrates (460–377 BCE)

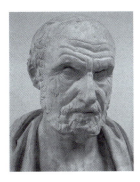

'Related to this is the surgery of wounds arising in military service, which concerns the extraction of missiles. In city practice experience of these is but little, for very rarely even in a whole lifetime are there civil or military combats. In fact such things occur most frequently and continuously in armies abroad. Thus, the person intending to practice this kind of surgery must serve in the army and accompany it on expeditions abroad; for in this way he would become experienced in this practice'.

Hippocrates – The Physician, 14, trans. by Paul Potter
Loeb Classical Library, *Hippocrates, Vol. VIII*

Unless dealing with major trauma on a frequent basis, few surgeons, anaesthesiologists or intensive care specialists can attain and sustain the level of skill necessary for decision-making in the care of a patient with multiple injuries. This includes both the intellectual decisions (mind-set), and the manual dexterity (skillset) required to perform all the manoeuvres for surgical care. These can be particularly challenging, may be infrequently required, yet rapid access to, and control of sites of haemorrhage following trauma can be a lifesaving intervention. The correct sequence of the decisions required is critical, and many situations require specialist trauma expertise, but often this is simply not available within the time frame or situation in which it is required.

In years past, many surgeons honed their skills in war, and translated them into the techniques required in peace. In the 21st century, this has changed, so that most surgeons work in an environment of peace, while a few serve in lower key conflicts. In many countries, the incidence of injury, particularly from vehicle-related trauma, has fallen below the numbers recorded since records were first kept. Many injuries are now treated non-operatively, so operative exposure and the skills required are reduced. Occasionally, for this reason, the decision *not* to operate is based on inexperience or insecurity, rather than on good clinical judgement.

It is not enough to be a good operator. The effective practitioner is part of a multidisciplinary team that plans for and is trained to provide the essential medical and surgical response required in the management of the injured patient.

Planning the response requires a clear understanding of:

- The causation including mechanism of injuries occurring within the local population.
- The initial, pre-hospital and emergency department care of the patient.
- The condition in which the patient is delivered to the hospital and subsequently to the operating theatre will be determined by the initial response, which itself may determine outcome.
- The resources, both physical and intellectual within the hospital, and the ability to anticipate and identify the specific problems associated with patients with multiple injuries.
- The limitations in providing specialist expertise within the time frame required.

In 1993, five surgeons (Don Trunkey and Howard Champion, USA; Stephen Deane, Australia; Abe Fingerhut, France; and David Mulder, Canada), all members of the International Society of Surgery – Société Internationale de Chirugie (ISS–SIC) and the International Association for Trauma Surgery and Intensive Care (IATSIC), met in San Francisco during the meeting of the American College of Surgeons. It was apparent that there was a specific need for further training in the technical aspects of surgical care of the trauma patient, and that routine surgical training was too organ specific or area specific to allow the development of appropriate judgement and decision-making skills in traumatized patients with multiple injuries.

They suggested that a short course focusing on the life-saving surgical techniques and surgical decision-making was required for surgeons, in order to further train the surgeon who dealt with major surgical trauma on an infrequent basis. This course would meet a world-wide need, and would supplement the well-recognized and accepted American College of Surgeon Advanced Trauma Life Support (ATLS®) course. The experience that Sten Lennquist, who joined the group, had gained offering five-day courses for surgeons in Sweden was integrated into the programme development, and prototype courses were offered in Paris, Washington, and Sydney.

At International Surgical Week in Vienna in 1999, IATSIC's members approved a core curriculum and a manual that forms the basis of the Definitive Surgical Trauma Care (DSTC™) course. The manual was first published in 2003 and subsequently in 2007, 2011, 2015, and this fifth edition in 2019. The manual is updated approximately every four years.

Initial Definitive Surgical Trauma Care (DSTC™) courses were then launched in Austria (Graz), Australia (Melbourne and Sydney), and South Africa (Johannesburg). The material presented in these courses has been refined, a system of training developed using professional education expertise, and the result forms the basis of the standardized DSTC™ course that now takes place. The course uses a mixture of education (to modify the 'mind-set' of the participating learners), and training (to modify the 'skill-set' of those learners). A unique feature of the course is that while the principles are standardized, once the course has been established nationally in a country, it can then be modified to suit the needs and circumstances of the environment in which the care takes place. The Education Committee of IATSIC oversees the quality and content of the courses. In addition to the initial 'founding' countries (Australia, Austria, and South Africa), courses have been delivered in more than 32 countries across the world, with the new

participants joining the IATSIC programme each year. The course and its manuals are presented in Japanese, French, Hebrew, Portuguese, and Spanish, as well as English. The requirements for the programme can be found in Appendix C of this manual.

By 2014, it was recognized that the indispensable contribution also made by anaesthetic and critical care colleagues has enhanced the approach to trauma, as has the concept of a fully multidisciplinary trauma team. Anaesthesiology, through the enthusiastic inputs of the Anaesthetic Faculty in the Netherlands, Scandinavia, Switzerland, the United Kingdom, and many other countries has in parallel with this course, developed the Definitive Anaesthetic Trauma Care (DATC™) course. We are delighted to incorporate these aspects of care into this manual, and many countries are now presenting a fully integrated course.

This fifth edition had been revised and updated, considering new evidence-based information. The increasing (and occasionally harmful) role of non-operative management (NOM) has been recognized. With the increased need for humanitarian intervention, as well as military peacekeeping, and modern asymmetrical conflicts, each carrying their own spectra of injury, the military module has been substantially updated and broadened to reflect recent conflict experience, and a new expanded section highlighting trauma management under austere conditions has been added.

The Board of Contributors, responsible for this manual, is made up of those who have contributed to global trauma care and the DSTC™ and DATC™ programme, and continues to support and update this manual. I would like to thank them for their very great efforts put into the preparation, editing, dissection, redissection, and assembly of the manual and the course. The keynote chapter (Chapter 1), written by Nigel Tai and Joe Dawson, sets the tone for the manual, and for trauma surgery today. Their efforts, and those of the entire board are greatly appreciated.

The book is divided into sections:

- Trauma system and crew resource management (CRM) communication principles.
- Physiology and the body's response to trauma:
  - Resuscitation physiology.
  - Transfusion.
  - Damage control.
- Chapters on each anatomical area or organ system, divided into both an overview of the problems and pitfalls specific to that system, and the surgical

techniques required to deal with major injury in that area including burns, brain injury, and extremes of age.

- Chapters on modern diagnostic and therapeutic technology:
  - The role of minimally invasive surgery.
  - Imaging.
- Additional modules which cover specific aspects of specialized care:
  - Trauma anaesthesia.
  - Trauma support services.

- Austere and military conditions.
- Critical care.
- A separate appendix for the use of operating room scrub nurses is included.
- As before, the manual contains all the resources for trauma scoring and injury assessment.

This manual is dedicated to those who care for the injured patient and whose passion is to do it well.

Kenneth D Boffard

Introduction

In both developed and developing countries, trauma continues to be a major public health problem and financial burden, both in the pre-hospital setting and within the hospital system, claiming 6 million lives every year. In addition to increasing political and social unrest in many countries, and an increasing use of firearms for interpersonal violence, the motor vehicle has become a substantial cause of trauma worldwide. These socio-economic determinants result in large numbers of injured patients. Injury prevention is a key element in limiting the societal impact of trauma but once injured, effective acute care and rehabilitation are essential for optimal patient outcomes. Improving all aspects of emergency care is important, however improved surgical and resuscitation skills have a particular role in saving lives and minimizing disability.

In most developed countries, there is a limited exposure to the full range of trauma presentations. This means it is difficult to develop and maintain experience in trauma resuscitation and trauma surgery. Standard surgical training is increasingly organ-specific, reducing even further the broad skills required for trauma management. Laparoscopic surgery, microsurgery, robotics, interventional radiographic procedures, and other sophisticated operating techniques may improve outcomes pertaining to elective surgery, but have a negative impact on acquisition of the complex skill-set needed to manage a severely injured trauma patient.

INJURY PREVENTION

Injury prevention can be divided into three parts:

- *Primary prevention*: Education and legislation are used to reduce the incidence of injury, for example, driving under the influence of alcohol.
- *Secondary prevention*: Minimizing the incidence of injury through design, for example, seatbelts, helmets, etc.

- *Tertiary prevention*: Once the injury has occurred, minimizing the effects of that injury by better and earlier care, preferably evidence-based.

Although primary and secondary prevention of injury will undoubtedly play the major role in reducing the incidence of trauma, it will not be eliminated, and therefore there is a need to maintain effective tertiary prevention. This requires training within complex multidisciplinary teams, and a focus on both the decision-making, and the medical and surgical procedures required, for the advanced management of patients with multiple injuries, and correction of any associated deranged physiology.

TRAINING IN THE INITIAL MANAGEMENT OF SEVERE TRAUMA

The Advanced Trauma Life Support® (ATLS®) Course

Promulgated by the American College of Surgeons, this is the most widely accepted trauma programme in the world. It has been in use for nearly 40 years, and with over 60 national programmes involved, more than 1 million physicians have been trained. Its focus is on the initial management of the severely injured patient and addresses those injuries and their consequences that can cause death within the first hour after injury.

The National Trauma Management Course (NTMC™)

IATSIC has developed the NTMC™ as part of an initiative towards improving trauma care in resource-challenged countries, where medical expertise may be available, but the area is resource poor. Based on the ATLS® course, modified for local conditions, and very cost effective, the course can be offered either as an isolated course organized by IATSIC, or under the banner of a local trauma organization. To date, some 7000 physicians have been trained under the aegis of organizations such as the Academy of Traumatology of India (www.indiatrauma.org), The College of Surgeons of Sri Lanka (www.lankasurgeons.org), and IATSIC itself, in some 12 countries worldwide.

Surgical Trauma Training Beyond Initial Care

Globally, injury is the third leading cause of death for all ages, and the leading cause of death from age 1 to 44 years. More than 50% of all deaths occur minutes after injury, and most immediate deaths are due to massive haemorrhage or neurological injury. Autopsy data demonstrate that central nervous system injuries account for 50%–70% of all injury deaths, and haemorrhage accounts for 15%–30%. It is within this latter group of haemorrhage-related deaths where prompt decision-making and effective use of surgical techniques has the greatest opportunity to save lives.

With improving pre-hospital care across the world, patients who would previously have died are reaching the hospital alive. In many situations, their airway and ventilation are controlled, but the deaths occur in hospital from uncontrollable bleeding. While there are surgical techniques for the control of bleeding, the timing and appropriateness of their use and a clear understanding of the physiology of trauma are essential for a successful outcome.

There is a further problem in caring for the injured in a military context. Modern conflicts are in general asymmetric (with only one side in uniform), are generally local and well-contained, and do not produce casualties in large numbers nor on a frequent basis. For this reason, it is difficult to maintain the number of military specialists required, who can be deployed immediately to perform highly technical surgical or resuscitative procedures in the battlefield arena or under austere conditions. It is also difficult for career military surgeons to gain adequate exposure to battlefield casualties, or indeed penetrating trauma in general, and many military training programmes are now looking to their civilian counterparts for assistance.

The statistics mandate that surgical teams responsible for the management of injured patients, whether military or civilian, are skilled in the assessment, diagnosis and operative and resuscitative management of life-threatening injuries. There remains a poorly developed appreciation of the potential impact that timely and appropriate surgical intervention can have on the outcome of a severely injured patient. Partly through lack of exposure, difficulty in time availability or release from hospital duties, and partly because of other interests, many specialists quite simply no longer have the expertise to deal with such life-threatening situations.

There is thus an increasing need to provide training in the skills and techniques necessary to resuscitate and manage seriously injured patients surgically, not only in the emergency department, but also during the period *after* initial care is complete. A course is needed and must be flexible so that it meets the local needs of the country in which it is being taught.

Surgical Training Courses in Trauma

THE ADVANCED TRAUMA OPERATIVE MANAGEMENT (ATOM®) COURSE

This American College of Surgeons course was originally developed by Lenworth M. Jacobs about 15 years ago and is a one-day course comprising a didactic lecture series followed by exercises on live, tissue models. It is an effective method of increasing surgical competence and confidence in the operative management of penetrating injuries to the chest and abdomen.

THE ADVANCED SURGICAL SKILLS FOR EXPOSURE IN TRAUMA (ASSET®) COURSE

Another programme developed by the American College of Surgeons. It is a one-day cadaver-based course designed to teach the anatomical exposures necessary for control of haemorrhage in the trunk, neck, extremities, and junctional areas.

THE DEFINITIVE SURGICAL TRAUMA CARE™ (DSTC) COURSE

This course was developed in 1993, through an international collaboration of six surgeons, and is controlled by the International Association for Trauma Surgery and Intensive Care (IATSIC), the Integrated Society of the International Society of Surgery – Société Internationale de Chirugie (ISS–SIC) in Zurich, Switzerland. It comprises a three-day course with short interactive presentations, group discussions, case discussions, and operative exercises on a live tissue model. The emphasis teaches learners both the critical decision-making processes required through advanced education (modification of mind-set), and training in the surgical techniques required (modification of skill-set) to choose the best method of management. Currently, the course has taken place in 32 countries, and in several languages (English, French, Hebrew, Japanese, Portuguese, and Spanish).

The Definitive Anaesthetic Trauma Care (DATC™) course was established in 2006 as pre-deployment training for military anaesthesiologists. It developed as an add-on to the DSTC™ course to enhance understanding of trauma management. In 2015, the DSTC™ was introduced into IATSIC as a subgroup of DSTC™. Cooperation between the two specialities allows the complex teamwork required in the management of a major trauma patient to be simulated and practised. The integration of DATC™ into the DSTC™ course programme and including the aspects of Critical Care required highlights the importance of modern-day trauma management techniques with the focus on the multidisciplinary nature of trauma care by a trauma team. The current DATC™/DSTC™ courses having participants from interventional radiology, medical and surgical specialities as well as nursing scrub staff, thus making the course unique in its team approach. Details of the course appear in Appendix C of this manual.

THE DSTC™ COURSE

Course Objectives

By the end of the course, the participant has:

- Enhanced knowledge of the surgical physiology of the trauma patient
- Enhanced resuscitation and surgical decision-making capabilities in trauma
- Enhanced surgical expertise in the techniques for the management of major trauma
- An improved awareness of the treatment possibilities in major trauma and their evidence base.

THE DATC™ COURSE

Course Objectives

By the end of the course, the participant has:

- An enhanced knowledge of trauma surgery decision-making and the procedures involved.

- An enhanced knowledge of the physiological abnormalities associate with trauma and the management before, during, and after surgery.
- An enhanced knowledge of trauma induced coagulopathy and its management.
- Enhanced technical skills needed to expedite the surgical and critical care process.

Description of the Course

A prerequisite of the DSTC™ and DATC™ courses is a complete understanding of all the principles outlined in a general surgical training, and the ATLS® course. For this reason, there are no presentations on the basic principles of trauma surgery, nor the initial resuscitation of the patient with major injuries.

The course consists of a core curriculum, designed to be an activity lasting at least two and one-half days. In addition to the core curriculum there are a variety of add-on modules that can be used to enhance the course, thereby adapting to local needs.

The course consists of several core components:

- Interactive presentations – designed to introduce and cover the key concepts of surgical resuscitation, the end points and an overview of the best access to organ systems.
- Cadaver sessions (optional session) – in which use is made of fresh or preserved human cadavers and dissected tissue. These are used to reinforce the vital knowledge of human anatomy related to access in major trauma. Other alternatives are available if local custom or legislation does not permit the use of such laboratories.
- Skills laboratories with use of live tissue. The instructor introduces various injuries. The objects of the exercise are to both improve psychomotor skills and teach new techniques for the preservation of organs and the control of haemorrhage. This creates the real-world scenario of managing a severely injured patient in the operating room.
- Case presentations – this component is a strategic thinking session illustrated by case presentations. Different cases are presented that allow free discussion between the students and the instructors. These cases are designed to put the didactic and psychomotor skills that have been learned into the context of real patient management scenarios.

SUMMARY

The course is designed to prepare the relatively fully-trained surgeon to manage difficult injuries that might present to a major trauma centre. The combined DSTC™/DATC™ courses provide a higher level of trauma understanding by focusing on the multidisciplinary nature of the decision-making processes and the core concepts of teamwork in managing patients with severely compromised physiology. The course fulfils the educational, cognitive, and psychomotor needs for surgeons and anaesthetists, be they mature or trainee, civilian or military, all of whom need to be comfortable in dealing with life-threatening penetrating and blunt injury, irrespective of whether it is in the military or the civilian arena.

Board of Contributors

AUTHOR

Kenneth D Boffard
Professor Emeritus
Department of Surgery
University of the Witwatersrand
Trauma Director
Milpark Academic Trauma Centre
Johannesburg
South Africa

BOARD OF CONTRIBUTORS

Philip Barker
Professor Emeritus
Royal College of Surgeons of England
Armed Forces UK
British Columbia
Canada

Chris Bleeker
Consultant Anaesthetist
Radboud University Medical Center
Nijmegen
Netherlands

Adam Brooks
Consultant Surgeon
Queens Medical Centre
Nottingham
United Kingdom

Ian Civil
Consultant Surgeon
Auckland Hospital
Auckland
New Zealand

Damian Clarke
Professor
Grey's Hospital
Pietermaritzburg
South Africa

Scott D'Amours
Consultant Surgeon
Liverpool Hospital
University of New South Wales
Sydney, NSW
Australia

Joe Dawson
Consultant Trauma and Vascular Surgeon
Clinical Senior Lecturer
Royal Adelaide Hospital
University of Adelaide
Adelaide
South Australia

Elias Degiannis
Professor Emeritus
Department of Surgery
University of the Witwatersrand
Milpark Academic Trauma Centre and Leratong
Hospital
Johannesburg
South Africa

Jesper Dirks
Consultant Anaesthetist
Department of Anaesthesia
Centre for Head and Orthopaedics
Rigshospitalet
Copenhagen University Hospital
Copenhagen
Denmark

Dietrich Doll
Head: Department of Procto-Surgery
St. Mary's Hospital Vechta
University of Saarland
Vechta
Germany

Abe Fingerhut
Associate Professor
University of Graz
Graz
Austria

Sache Flohé
Consultant Surgeon
Klinikum Solingen
Solingen
Germany

Tina Gaarder
Consultant Surgeon
Head: Department of Traumatology
Ulleval University Hospital
Oslo
Norway

Georgios Gemenetzis
Senior Clinical Fellow
Department of Surgery
Glasgow Royal Infirmary
Glasgow
Scotland

Lauri Handolin
Trauma Surgeon
Helsinki University Hospital
Helsinki
Finland

Timothy Hardcastle
Consultant Trauma Surgeon
Director: Trauma Service
Inkosi Albert Luthuli Hospital
University of KwaZuluNatal
Durban
South Africa

Catherine Heim Schoettker
Consultant Anaesthetist
University Hospital of Lausanne
Lausanne
Switzerland

Gareth Hide
Consultant Surgeon
Sunninghill Hospital
Johannesburg
South Africa

Anders Holtan
Consultant Anaesthesiologist
Oslo University Hospital
Oslo
Norway

Tal Hörer
Consultant Vascular Surgeon
Associate Professor of Surgery
Örebro University Hospital
Örebro University
Örebro
Sweden

Ilja Laesser
Senior Consultant in Thoracic Radiology
Sahlgrenska University Hospital
University of Gothenburg
Gothenburg
Sweden

Rifat Latifi
Director
Department of Surgery and Chief of Trauma and
General Surgery
Westchester Medical Center Health Network
New York Medical College
Valhalla, NY
United States of America

Ari Leppaniemi
Chief of Emergency Surgery
Meilahti Hospital
University of Helsinki
Helsinki
Finland

Gilberto Leung
Tsang Wing-Hing Professor in Clinical Neuroscience
Queen Mary Hospital
University of Hong Kong
Hong Kong
People's Republic of China

Graeme Pitcher
Clinical Professor of Paediatric Surgery
University of Iowa
Stead Family Children's Hospital
University of Iowa
Iowa City, IA
United States of America

Frank Plani
Consultant Trauma Surgeon
Adjunct Professor and Co-chair
Academic Division of Trauma Surgery
University of the Witwatersrand
Trauma Director
Chris Hani Baragwanath Academic Hospital
Consultant Trauma Surgeon
Milpark Union Hospital Trauma Centre
Johannesburg
South Africa

Tarek Razek
Chief of Trauma Surgery
Montreal General Hospital
McGill University Health Center
Montreal
Canada

Michael C Reade
Defence Professor of Military Medicine and Surgery
Joint Health Command
Australian Defence Force
Royal Brisbane and Women's Hospital
University of Queensland
Brisbane
Australia

Louis Riddez
Consultant Surgeon
Associate Professor
Karolinska University Hospital Department
of Emergency Surgery and Trauma
Karolinska Institute
Stockholm
Sweden

Jeffrey V Rosenfeld
Senior Neurosurgeon
Department of Neurosurgery
The Alfred Hospital
Monash University
Clayton
Melbourne
Australia

Patrick Schoettker
Professor and Head Physician Department
of Anesthesiology
CHUV Centre Hospitalier
Lausanne
Switzerland

C William Schwab
Professor of Surgery
Chief
Division of Traumatology & Surgical
Critical Care
Hospital of the University of Pennsylvania
Philadelphia, PA
United States of America

Jacob Steinmetz
Consultant Anaesthetist
Associate Professor
Trauma Centre & Department of Anaesthesia
Rigshospitalet
Copenhagen University Hospital
Copenhagen
Denmark

Jakob Stensballe
Consultant Anaesthetist
Department of Anaesthesiology
Centre for Head and Orthopaedics
Trauma Centre & Section for Transfusion Medicine
Capital Region Blood Bank
Rigshospitalet
Copenhagen University Hospital
Copenhagen
Denmark

Elmin Steyn
Associate Professor of Surgery
Head
Department of Surgery
Tygerburg Hospital
University of Stellenbosch
Cape Town
South Africa

Nigel Tai
Consultant Trauma Vascular Surgeon
UK Defence Medical Service
The Royal London Hospital
Barts NHS Trust
London
United Kingdom

Fernando Turegano
Head
Emergency Surgery
University General Hospital Gregorio Marañón
Complutense of Madrid
Madrid
Spain

Selman Uranues
Professor and Head
Section for Surgical Research
Centre for Minimally Invasive Surgery Graz
Austria

Pantelis Vassiliu
Assistant Professor of Surgery
4th Surgical Clinic
Attikon Hospital
National and Kapodistrian University
of Athens (NKUA)
Athens
Greece

Arie B van Vugt
Trauma and Military Surgeon
Medisch Spectrum Twente
Enschede
Netherlands

Jonathan White
Consultant ICU & Anaesthesiologist
Physician
Rigshospitalet
Copenhagen University Hospital
Copenhagen
Denmark

Adrian O Wilson
Visiting Professor of Medicine and Geriatrics
Mpilo Central Hospital
National University of Science & Technology
Bulawayo
Zimbabwe

Virginia S Wilson
Physical and Rehabilitation Medicine
Netcare Rehabilitation Hospital
Johannesburg
South Africa

David Zonies
Associate Professor
Oregon Health & Sciences University
Portland, OR
United States of America

Acknowledgements

The Board of Contributors, responsible for this manual, is made up of those who have contributed to global trauma care and the DSTC™ and DATC™ programme, and they continue to support and update this manual. I would like to thank them for their very great efforts put into the preparation, editing, dissection, re-dissection, and assembly of the manual and the course. Their efforts, and those of the entire board, are greatly appreciated.

I would also like to thank the following members of the Board of Contributors from the previous edition whose work continues to benefit readers:

Douglas Bowley
Consultant Surgeon
Centre for Defence Medicine
Birmingham
United Kingdom

Mark Bowyer
Consultant Surgeon
Mayo Clinic
Rochester, MN
USA

Megan Fisher
Consultant Urologist
Linksfield Hospital
Johannesburg
South Africa

Annette Holian
Consultant Orthopaedic Surgeon
National Critical Care and Trauma Response
Centre at Royal Darwin Hospital
Darwin
Australia

Lenworth M Jacobs
Professor of Surgery
University of Connecticut School of Medicine
Hartford, CT
USA

Peter F Mahoney
Defence Professor of Anaesthesia & Critical Care
Visiting Professor
Department of Bioengineering
Imperial College London
Birmingham
United Kingdom

Andrew Nunn
Instructor in Surgery
Division of Traumatology, Surgical Critical Care and
Emergency Surgery
Perelman School of Medicine
University of Pennsylvania
Philadelphia, PA
USA

James Ralph
Consultant Anaesthetist
Centre for Defence Medicine
Birmingham
United Kingdom

Noelle Sailliant
Instructor in Surgery Division of
Traumatology, Surgical Critical Care and
Emergency Surgery
Perelman School of Medicine
University of Pennsylvania
Philadelphia, PA
USA

About the Author

Professor Kenneth D Boffard is Professor of Surgery and Trauma Director at Milpark Hospital, Johannesburg, and until recently, Head of the Department of Surgery at Johannesburg Hospital and the University of the Witwatersrand. He was previously Head of the Johannesburg Hospital Trauma Unit. He qualified in Johannesburg, and trained in surgery at the Birmingham Accident Hospital and Guy's Hospital.

He is the Secretary-General, and a previous President of the International Society of Surgery (ISS), President of the International Association for Trauma Surgery and Intensive Care (IATSIC), and Chair of the IATSIC Education Committee. He is a fellow of five surgical colleges, and has received honorary fellowships from the American College of Surgeons, Royal College of Surgeons of Thailand, College of Surgeons of Sri Lanka, the Japanese Association for the Surgery of Trauma, and the Association of Surgeons of Great Britain and Ireland.

His passion is surgical education, and various aspects of trauma resuscitation, intensive care, and regional planning of trauma systems. His interests include flying (he is a licensed fixed wing and helicopter pilot), scuba diving, and aeromedical care. His research interests include coagulation, haemostasis, and critical bleeding.

He is a colonel in the South African Military Health Service.

He is a Freeman of the City of London by redemption, and an elected Liveryman of the Guild of Air Pilots of London.

He is married with two children.

Part 1

Trauma system and communication principles

Safe and Sustainable Trauma Care **1**

1.1 INTRODUCTION

In terms of hazard, the injured patient faces *'double jeopardy'*: the risks to their health owing to the traumatic insult to tissue and physiology; and the risk posed by the therapy required to restore health. Minimizing the potential for iatrogenic harm through the provision of safe care is especially challenging in trauma owing to the complexity and urgency of major trauma as a disease. Factors such as injury severity, acute physiological derangement, temporal urgency limiting diagnosis, or physiological stabilization, a multitude of definitive treatment options and interdisciplinary specialist interactions, can combine to compound the risk of something going wrong.

Despite this, safer and better trauma care is certainly achievable by focusing on reducing the risk of harm to an already injured patient from both the *injury* and the *treatment*. Reducing the risk that the original injury poses to the patient involves both technical and systematic elements. The technical aspects include pre-hospital and emergency care, imaging, surgery, interventional radiology, and post-operative critical care, and are considered in detail elsewhere in this manual.

Treatment of major trauma is a multifaceted endeavour, set within a complicated system that comprises an almost infinite range of interconnecting 'moving parts'. The difficult question of how to improve safety in trauma care may be simplified by taking a hierarchical approach, focusing initially on the individuals and teams that provide trauma care, and then adopting a more strategic perspective concerning hospital institutions, regional and national trauma networks and governance, and finally a consideration of trauma care on an international level.

The question of safe trauma care also requires an examination of the sustainability of trauma care within the workforce and training, and the role of innovative simulation models, research and innovation, translation from military experience as means to ensure that healthcare professionals working with trauma patients can continue to offer the very best care available, and the use of reliable existing data. The aim of this chapter is to iterate the minimal essential components of individual, hospital, and system practice in order to deliver safe care.

1.2 SAFE TRAUMA CARE

1.2.1 Individual Factors

It is accepted that in order to practise safe surgery in the trauma setting, the trauma surgeon and trauma anaesthesiologist must have undergone a validated general training pathway culminating in exposure to a period of specific trauma training. Domain knowledge and technical skills represent the foundational aspects, but by themselves are insufficient. Professionalism is also characterized by rigorous adherence to personal safety (personal protection, sharps, needle-stick, vaccinations), consistent use of the World Health Organisation Safe Surgery Checklist (see Section 1.2.6), and compliance with continuing medical education imperatives. However, the reality is that a significant amount of trauma care in the world is delivered by individuals who may not have had the requisite training nor resources required.

Over the past decade, the importance of non-technical skills (see also Chapter 2) has become increasingly well recognized. The nomenclature for such skills differs from sector to sector (e.g. medicine = *non-technical skills*; aviation = *crew resource management (CRM) skills;* social science = *interpersonal skills*; psychology = *emotional intelligence*; US Army = *soft skills*), but the competencies are broadly the same: teamwork, communication, leadership, decision-making, conflict resolution, assertiveness, management of stress and fatigue, workload management, prioritization of tasks, and situational awareness.[1]

Consistent delivery of non-technical skills is very important in minimizing error, as very few preventable trauma deaths are attributable to purely technical mistakes.

1.2.1.1 HEURISTICS AND COGNITIVE BIASES

Inherent bias in cognition affects perception; such biases are a universal feature of human decision-making and result from default to heuristics; numerous, unconscious mental shortcuts that allow the brain to arrive at quick, but approximate, conclusions with limited information. Such heuristics are advantageous (and thus highly conserved in evolutionary terms) when time or resource pressure demands a quick solution or judgment under conditions of uncertainty or limited knowledge in dynamic, complex or dangerous situations.[2] These cognitive short-cuts can help us manage:

- Information overload – quickly filter and skim data for importance.
- Lack of meaning – fill in the gaps if data is lacking and map it to existing mental model.
- The need for swift action – survival and success can depend on decisions without time for deep analysis.
- The need to remember – helps decide what new information to remember and what can be forgotten.[2]

However, heuristic processes are a double-edged sword. Filtering out information regarded as useless may also discard information that is important. Assessment without all available information may cause false assumptions to be made and false narratives to be laid down. Rapidity of decision-making increases risk of error and relying on experience does not always map on to the present, particularly if post-hoc processing leads to overly-optimistic interpretation of the success of previous strategy and thus reinforcement error.

There are numerous classes of cognitive bias, and some are highly relevant for trauma decision-makers to understand:

- *Confirmation bias*: This is the tendency to interpret data in a way that confirms pre-existing belief. It can act to combat information overload and fit data to pre-existing diagnoses. However, aspects of the case that contradict pre-existing beliefs are not acknowledged as meaningful or are dismissed.

- *Confabulation bias*: In attempting to deal with scarcity of data in order to combat lack of meaning, generalizations lead to false narratives and inappropriate assumptions.
- *Overconfidence effect*: Unreflective practice without objective review of performance leads to overly-optimistic assessment of capability.

1.2.1.2 INDIVIDUAL – LEADERSHIP

The leadership function within a trauma team encompasses prioritization of competing injuries; swift planning, coordination, and orchestration of clinical assessment and intervention mediated by effective communication; assessment of patient trajectory and dynamic appraisal of response to treatment and motivation/supervision of team members (such that individual/team performance is lifted). However, investing all these functions within one individual (i.e. The classical model of 'Leader-Follower') may not be ideal for trauma practice settings. Expertise is distributed among various members of the trauma team and the leadership function may flux between different team members according to the phase of trauma resuscitation and the need to respond dynamically to changes in patient condition (the 'Hierarchical-but-Fluid' Model).[3] Leadership demands accurate assessment of the situation and the ability to continually monitor progress and reappraise the array of options for each decision-node – a characteristic formulated as the '3D trauma surgeon' by Hirshberg and Mattox.[4] Elements that the 3D surgeon should be able to deliver include:

- Tactics – technical aspects of the operation.
- Strategy – the 'big picture' appreciation of the risks that the patient faces immediately and in the near- and medium-term elements of operation.
- Team – clear communication to coordinate efforts to ensure working towards same goals.

Mishandling the team dimension during a trauma operation is one of the worst mistakes you can make

1.2.1.3 TRAUMA TEAM

Trauma[3] and theatre teams[5] face several challenges in performing to a consistent level. Perhaps the greatest of these is that it is rarely the same team that manages the patient: shift work introduces different leaders, different specialists and different levels of expertise. Furthermore, beyond the effect of staff rotas there is staff turnover, with new team members assigned only while their rotation lasts. Given the fact that they may face the requirement to deliver critical resuscitative functions within moments of meeting each other, there is ample opportunity for error owing to inappropriate skill mix, unfamiliarity with each other's style or even names, with significant potential for excess morbidity and mortality.[5]

Dysfunctional teams are usually obvious to external observers but not necessarily so from within, when poor behaviours (lack of communication leading to failure to establish shared mental model) may become habitual and normalized. Sharing clinical information amongst trauma team members has been shown in two test scenarios to be as low as 27%,[6] and two-thirds of serious medical errors result from lapses in communication.[7]

Conversely, high performing teams talk to each other and are safer. They demonstrate the following behaviours:[5,7]

- Situational awareness (SA) – seeking behaviour.
- Clear leadership + followership with the facility to model adaptive behaviours when needed with appropriate distribution of workload and monitoring/support of team members.
- Closed-loop communication (seeking confirmation that intended messages are understood by recipient) with clear means of escalating urgency (standardized prompts), and facilitation of calm assertiveness.
- Low gradient or flat hierarchy of communication such that team members are empowered to speak up and relay concerns as they see fit.
- Readiness to participate in an open team debrief in order to review performance, learn why things went well or less well, and adopt change if required.

1.2.1.4 TEAM – TRAINING

Simulation training has been shown to improve teamwork behaviour and performance[5] including performance in the operating theatre[8,9] and that of Emergency Department (ED) trauma teams,[10] ATLS courses,[11] and amongst physicians and nurses rotating through a trauma centre,[12] with evidence supporting a significant reduction in surgical mortality following such team training.[13,14] Specific courses designed to deliver non-technical competencies (situational awareness, decision-making, communication, teamwork, and leadership) are increasingly available (e.g. The Non-Technical Skills for Surgeons (NOTSS) course[15] – see also Chapter 2), and contain lessons derived from other safety-critical industries such as in aviation,[16]

where failure may lead to catastrophe. These courses tend to provide maps of how errors occur (e.g. the well understood 'Swiss Cheese' Model[5]) whilst teaching communication skills, assertiveness, decision-making under pressure, and appropriate leadership. The Interpersonal Competence Training – run by the German Society for Orthopaedics and Trauma in conjunction with Lufthansa Flight Training[16] – teaches the edicts of crew resource management (CRM), as does the US Department of Defense 'TeamSTEPPS' programme.[17]

1.2.2 Institutional Factors

1.2.2.1 DEDICATED TRAUMA SERVICE

A dedicated trauma admitting team is responsible for the poly-trauma patient from admission to discharge. This involves acute and ongoing in-patient trauma care, daily ward rounds, and identification of ongoing care needs, liaison with other surgical and non-surgical services, safe discharge, and follow-up.

The extent to which a consultant's role is explicitly defined within this framework tends to be ill-defined with variable degrees of formal training and definition of the competencies required to lead such a team. Ongoing care does not automatically map to an individual surgical specialty, and could be any appropriately trained surgeon, emergency medicine consultant, or clinician from another acute specialty.[18] Where such roles and responsibilities are formalized, mortality and preventable death rates can be positively impacted. At the Royal London Hospital in the UK, the implementation of a dedicated trauma service (in-patient) team was associated with a reduction in mortality in severely injured patients by 48% and a reduction in preventable deaths from 9% to 2%.[19] At the same time, St George Hospital in Sydney Australia reported similar results with a reduction in deaths from 20% to 12%.[20]

1.2.3 Performance Improvement Activities

Institutional performance improvement or quality improvement activity encompasses:

i. The identification of preventable death and contributory factors.[1] (Such peer-review endeavour may be more effective than use of Trauma and Injury Severity Score (TRISS) for the identification of potentially-preventable death.[21])

ii. Tracking of trends via long-term mortality monitoring. (Which allows for institution of corrective action plans and is associated with improvement in patient outcome in level 1 trauma centres.[22,23])

iii. Improvement in patient pathways, development of evidence-based standard operating procedures designed to reduce variation of care, teamworking, decision-making, and inter-professional dynamics.[21]

One of the most effective methods to improve patient safety at a hospital level is a robust, respectful, and constructive mortality and morbidity meeting. These meetings should **never** be used to humiliate or apportion blame! The purpose of these meetings is to review and discuss all trauma management errors and to peer review all trauma deaths. Stratification of cause of death or severe complications into 'anticipated' (not-preventable), and 'unanticipated but without room for improvement' (potentially-preventable), and 'unanticipated with room for improvement' (preventable), allows further in-depth discussion where issues are discussed, action plans made, and most importantly, implemented and audited. Areas for improvement are often related to resuscitation issues,[1,21,22] airway management,[1] massive transfusion,[22] pelvic fracture management,[22] venous thrombo-embolism (VTE) prophylaxis[1], and missed injuries.[1] Other common themes included timely interventional radiology and surgical intervention, prompt spine clearance, reduced time to computerised tomography (CT) scan, reduced dwell time in the ED, and neurosurgery management.[21] Within this framework 'near-misses' are just as important to discuss, as deaths.[1,21,22] In the USA, this process is required for trauma centre verification, and in the English major trauma system such activity is required to be formally resourced and evidenced during major trauma centre (MTC) peer review in order to retain designated status.

1.2.4 Regional Activities

Safety propagates through, and is marked by, a collaborative approach between providers of trauma care within a set geographical area. Whilst severely injured patients are 15% to 20% less likely to die if admitted to a designated trauma centre,[24] not all trauma systems are the same. An 'inclusive' trauma system is one in which all trauma-care facilities (pre-hospital, local district hospitals, trauma centres, and rehabilitation hospitals) are incorporated at a regional level to provide continuity of care to the entire population by matching injured patients to appropriate facilities, thereby ensuring system-wide efficient use of available resources.[25] Inclusive trauma systems have been shown to reduce mortality across the world as the concentration of experience and expertise improves outcomes.

This contrasts with 'exclusive' trauma systems that are institution-based, focusing exclusively on designated trauma centres.

As previously discussed at an institutional level, ongoing audit and governance of processes ensures the highest possible outcomes and this is no different on the larger scale of trauma networks. Most trauma networks have in place governance frameworks such as those described within the NHS in London,[25] and Australian states such as South Australia.[26]

Remote and rural communities are particularly vulnerable as the risk of death from trauma in remote areas is four times higher than that in a major city.[27] Strong regional trauma systems can thus have additional benefits over and above expected impacts in rural communities. The unique healthcare requirements that these areas need has driven the introduction of sub-specialty surgical training in some countries that are characterized by vast areas and sparse populations, such as Australia (rural surgery) and Scotland (remote and rural surgery). Although such training is characteristically general, a significant component includes the initial management of trauma.

1.2.5 National Activities

The benefit of audit and quality improvement initiatives can be followed from the team level all the way up to the national level, for example, the NHS Major Trauma Review in which several recommendations were made at each level of the trauma system, including network improvements, pre-hospital care, reception and resuscitation, definitive care, and rehabilitation.[28]

National trauma registries such as the National Trauma Database (NTDB) of the American College of Surgeons, TARN (Trauma Audit and Research Network) in the UK, and the Australian Trauma Registry as part of AusTQIP (Australian Trauma Quality Improvement Program[29]) involve the collection of data of trauma patients including mechanism of injury, injuries sustained, including injury severity scores, treatments received, and outcomes. Such national registries are valuable for research, audit and peer-comparison, and institution of national quality improvement initiatives.

Surgical colleges have a vital role in trauma care by raising awareness, community advocacy, injury prevention, providing position papers, and delivering education. The three-point lap belt was invented in Sweden in 1958, by Nils Bohlin, a Swedish engineer and inventor working for Volvo, and a year later was fitted in all Volvo cars from. The 1970s saw the first car seat belt legislation introduced in Victoria, Australia and Sweden. Other initiatives include cycle helmet and drink-driving counter measures. Courses such as ATLS®, and DSTC™ enable healthcare workers involved in trauma care to develop and practice skills in a safe environment.

Several non-government, non-profit organizations exist to audit, research, educate, and implement national initiatives in injury prevention. As road traffic collisions comprise the majority of trauma in Australasia and Western Europe, the majority are based on road safety. These include the Australasian College of Road Safety, the Australian Road Safety Conference, and Sweden's impressive 'Vision Zero' campaign, which led to a drop in traffic fatalities of 30% since its inception in 1997, despite a significant increase in traffic volume during the same period.[30] The Vision Zero initiative has since spread globally, including the USA and Canada.

1.2.6 **Global Activities**

A massive disparity exists in the likelihood of survival of a person sustaining a life-threatening but salvageable injury in a low-income country (36% mortality) compared to a high-income country (6%).[31] Consequently, 90% of trauma deaths occur in low- and middle-income countries and are the leading cause of death globally, killing more people than HIV, malaria, and TB combined. Road traffic accidents are the eighth leading cause of death globally, and international meetings such as the World Innovation Summit for Health (WISH) Forum for Road Traffic and Trauma Care focus on the global impact of such trauma, a large majority of which occur in low- and middle-income countries.[32] The excess burden of trauma mortality shouldered by the developing world is a stark fact that has been recognized for decades; in 2004, following the Essential Trauma Care (EsTC) Project, the world Health Organisation (WHO) produced *Guidelines for Essential Trauma Care*, a set of minimum standards for worldwide trauma care.[31] These were based on low-cost improvements that are achievable in

virtually every setting across the globe. In 2008, WHO produced the Safe Surgery Checklist, and whilst not specific to trauma, certainly has application and utility. Initial uncontrolled studies demonstrated reduced mortality associated with its use in both low- and high-income countries.[33] Further rigorous studies (randomized with controls) replicated these initial findings with mortality odds ratios dropping from 1.16 without the checklist to 0.4 with the checklist.[33] In addition, there is evidence that this low-fidelity process can also reduce complications with a relative risk reduction of 0.42 associated with the checklist and a number needed to treat of 12 to prevent major morbidity.[33]

With the success of the standard WHO checklist now firmly embedded into routine surgical practice, WHO produced a Trauma Care Checklist which has subsequently been tested in 11 centres around the world, nine of these in low- and middle-income countries.[34] The 18-point checklist covers history, examination, investigations, and monitoring, and improved the processes measured and may improve outcomes.[34]

Charitable organizations can play an important global role, particularly in trauma education. 'ATLS-like' courses in developing countries. Examples include the University of Maryland running the Sequential Trauma Education Programme (STEPS) course in Egypt,[35] and the largest programme for developing countries is the IATSIC National Trauma Management Course (NTMC™), across India, Sri Lanka, and 12 other developing countries (see also Introduction: Management of severe Trauma). Safe Surgery 2020 is a collaboration of foundations, non-profit organizations, educational institutions, and local governments with the aim of making surgery safe, affordable, and accessible across the world. Currently working in Ethiopia and Tanzania they are developing local surgical leaders and scaling programs that directly address local challenges.[36]

Delivery of safe trauma care in the model generated by high-income countries is typified by complexity and expense. In developing countries with more limited resources, the focus needs to be on strengthening local processes preferentially, by using existing resources to ensure solutions are locally relevant. For example, one study in the most landmine-infested province of Northwest Cambodia looked at the result of systemically training local, non-graduate care providers (non-doctors) in trauma care. They found that 150-hours of training over a 4-year training period improved the quality of trauma surgery in rural hospitals.

1.3 SUSTAINABLE TRAUMA CARE

1.3.1 Workforce Development

Safe delivery of trauma care requires a trained healthcare workforce, but in many countries, trauma surgery is not recognized as a surgical specialty within its own right, with a lack of formalized training pathways to produce trauma consultants. As such, the delivery of trauma surgery in many countries relies on small groups of enthusiasts. In addition, in many high-income countries, there is a reduction in trauma surgery exposure due in part to increasing elective sub-specialization, increasing non-operative management, and interventional radiology management, associated with a reduction in working hours. In this environment, where previously the general surgeon had usually acted as a holistic provider of trauma care, this role is eroding, again in part due to a rise in super-specialist training in elective disciplines.[37,38] Recently the 'acute care surgeon' has emerged, a general surgeon dedicated to the management of acute surgical illness, including trauma. This role has developed for different reasons in different countries, including the need to recover a generalist approach to emergency surgical care, dispossession of such territory by super specialists, and the move to increase surgical operating time by trauma surgeons deprived of suitable case loads owing to the rise of non-operative management. Advocates of the acute care surgeon model argue that such training programmes can deliver the knowledge base, technical skills, and scope of practice required to deliver major trauma care,[39] and evidence from the USA supports the model.[40]

For trainee surgeons there are several opportunities that can be pursued in order to address deficiencies in standard training programmes. These include informal fellowships at high volume centres (typically USA and South Africa), dedicated Trauma/Critical Care Fellowships in the USA and the Resuscitative Trauma Surgeon pilot scheme in the UK,[38] military deployment, simulation training, and specific trauma courses. Development of specific technical competence can be facilitated through simulation and advanced human patient simulators have been developed to allow simulation training in trauma skills ranging from low-fidelity rigs to highly sophisticated mannequins. Examples include 'Trauma Man' and 'Synman' (intercostal drain insertion, pericardiocentesis, peritoneal lavage, cricothyroidotomy, and tracheostomy), 'Air-Man' (airway complications), 'VIRGIL' (chest trauma), and 'UltraSim' (FAST scan training).[7] The novel use of cadavers, such

as a pulsatile cadaveric model (perfused cadaver), allows very realistic training in cardiac penetrating injuries, lung lacerations, liver and retrohepatic vena cava injuries, cricothyroidotomy, tracheostomy, open fractures, and carotid and extremity vessel injuries.[41] Simulation is a key component of the burgeoning suite of courses that exist to develop trauma surgery skills and teamwork utilizing mannequins, simulators, cadavers, and animals. Simulation can also be used to evaluate competency, to refine leadership and teamwork skills, and may enhance patient safety through facilitation of insight and rapid feedback and reinforcement of correct skills. Simulation training appears effective, although the long-term retention of skills acquired through simulation is unproven.[7] However, simulation is still inadequate when it comes to mimicking physiological dynamic changes, coagulation, haemostasis, packing, and anatomical reconstruction. The mere fact that it is a simulation removes some credibility. The more sophisticated a simulator, often the more expensive it is, making expensive courses even more expensive, and sometimes unaffordable.

1.4 CONCLUSION

There are numerous opportunities for safer trauma care at every level. At the individual and team level, this is predominantly in the reduction of human error by understanding cognitive biases and improving communication and teamwork. At the institutional level, scrupulous audit and peer review identifies not only individual and team errors, but more importantly institutional systemic failures and ensures constant performance improvement. At a regional level, the implementation and governance of trauma networks ensures the best trauma care to a whole population or geographical area, taking into consideration its individual requirements and needs. Injury prevention initiatives at a national level have been shown to have tremendous impact on mortality, and finally, to redress the imbalance of trauma outcomes between low- and high-income countries, numerous initiatives are in place.

REFERENCES

1. Ivatury RR. Patient Safety in Trauma: Maximal Impact Management Errors at a Level I Trauma Center. *J Trauma.* 2008 Feb;**64(2)**:265–70; discussion 270-2. doi: 10.1097/ TA.0b013e318163359d.

2. Benson B. Heuristics and cognitive biases. Available from: https://betterhumans.coach.me/cognitive-bias-cheat-sheet-55a472476b18 (accessed online Dec 2018).

3. Klein KJ, Ziegert JC, Knight A, Xiao Y. A Leadership System for Emergency Action Teams: Rigid Hierarchy and Dynamic Flexibility. *Team Leadership System*. University of Pennsylvania and University of Maryland, Baltimore. Available from: http://d1c25a6gwz7q5e.cloudfront.net/papers/1282.pdf (accessed online Dec 2018).

4. Hirschberg A, Mattox K. Top Knife – The Art & Craft of Trauma Surgery. Hirshberg & Mattox. tfm Publishing Ltd, 2005 (Reprinted 2018).

5. Hunt EA, Shilkofski NA, Stavroudis TA, Nelson KL. Simulation: Translation to Improved Team Performance. *Anesthesiology Clin*. 2007 Jun;**25(2)**:301–19. Review.

6. Blum RH, Raemer DB, Carroll JS, Dufresne RL, Cooper JB. A method for measuring the effectiveness of simulation-based team training for improving communication skills. *Anesth Analg*. 2005 May;**100(5)**:1375–80.

7. Cherry RA and Ali J. Current Concepts in Simulation-Based Trauma Education. *Trauma*. 2008 Nov;**65(5)**:1186–93. doi: 10.1097/TA.0b013e318170a75e.

8. Hansen KS, Uggen PE, Brattebø G, Wisborg T. Team-oriented training for damage control surgery in rural trauma: a new paradigm. *J Trauma*. 2008 Apr;**64(4)**:949–53; discussion 953-4. doi: 10.1097/TA.0b013e31816a243c.

9. Armour Forse R, Bramble JD, McQuillan R. Team training can improve operating room performance. *Surgery*. 2011; **150**:771–8. doi: 10.1016/j.surg.2011.07.076.

10. Marshall RL, Smith JS, Gorman PJ, Krummel TM, Haluck RS, Cooney RN. Simulation based team work training for emergency department staff: Does it improve clinical team performance when added to an existing didactic teamwork curriculum? *Qual Saf Health Care*. 2004;**13(6)**:417–21.

11. Marshall RL, Smith JS, Gorman PJ, Krummel TM, Haluck RS, Cooney RN. Use of a human patient simulator in the development of resident trauma management skills. *J Trauma*. 2001 Jul;**51(1)**:17–21.

12. Holcomb JB, Dumire RD, Crommett JW, Stamateris CE, Fagert MA, Cleveland JA, et al. Evaluation of trauma team performance using an advanced human patient simulator for resuscitation training. *J Trauma*. 2002 Jun;**52(6)**:1078–85; discussion 1085-6.

13. Dunn EJ, Mills PD, Neily J, Crittenden MD, Carmack AL, Bagian JP. Medical team training: Applying crew resource management in the Veterans Health Administration. *Jt Comm J Qual Patient Saf*. 2007;**33(6)**:317–25.

14. Neily J, Mills PD, Young-Xu Y, Carney BT, West P, Berger DH, Mazzia LM, et al. Association between implementation of a medical team training program and surgical mortality. *JAMA*. 2010 Oct 20;**304(15)**:1693–700. doi: 10.1001/jama.2010.1506.

15. The Non-Technical Skills for Surgeons (NOTSS) System Handbook V1.2. University of Aberdeen and Royal College of Surgeons of Edinburgh, Scotland. 2012. Available from https://www.iscp.ac.uk/static/help/NOTSS_Handbook_2012.pdf (accessed online Dec 2018).

16. Physicians will learn assertiveness. Human Resources. Healthcare-in-Europe.com. 2016; Available from: https://healthcare-in-europe.com/en/news/physicians-will-learn-assertiveness.html (accessed online Dec 2018).

17. King HB, Battles J, Baker DP, Alonso A, Salas E, Webster J, et al. In: Henriksen K, Battles JB, Keyes MA, Grady ML, editors. Source Advances in Patient Safety: New Directions and Alternative Approaches (Vol. 3: Performance and Tools). Rockville (MD): Agency for Healthcare Research and Quality (US); 2008 Aug.

18. Major Trauma Workforce Sustainability. *Outcomes of the RCS Major Trauma Workgroup*. The Royal College of Surgeons of England, London. 2016.

19. Davenport RA, Tai N, West A, Bouamra O, Aylwin C, Woodford M, McGinley A, et al. A major trauma centre is a specialty hospital not a hospital of specialists. *BJS*. 2010 Jan;**97(1)**:109–17. doi: 10.1002/bjs.6806.

20. Ursic C, Curtis K, Zou Y, Black D. Improved trauma patient outcomes after implementation of a dedicated trauma admitting service. *Injury*. 2009 Jan;**40(1)**:99–103. doi: 10.1016/j.injury.2008.06.034.

21. Fallon WF Jr, Barnoski AL, Mancuso CL, Tinnell CA, Malangoni MA. Benchmarking the quality-monitoring process: a comparison of outcomes analysis by trauma and injury severity score (TRISS) methodology with the peer-review process. *J Trauma*. 1997 May;**42(5)**:810–5; discussion 815-7.

22. Sarkar B, Brunsvold ME, Cherry-Bukoweic JR, Hemmila MR, Park PK, Raghavendran K, et al. American College of Surgeons' Committee on Trauma Performance Improvement and Patient Safety Program: Maximal Impact in a Mature Trauma Center. *J Trauma*. 2011 Nov;**71(5)**:1447–53; discussion 1453-4. doi: 10.1097/TA.0b013e3182325d32.

23. Hoyt DB, Coimbra R, Potenza B, Doucet J, Fortlage D, Holingsworth-Fridlund P A twelve-year analysis of disease and provider complications on an organized Level I trauma service: as good as it gets? *J Trauma*. 2003 Jan;**54(1)**:26–36; discussion 36-7.

24. Celso B, Tepas J, Langland-Orban B, Pracht E, Papa L, Lottenberg, et al. A Systematic Review and Meta-Analysis Comparing Outcome of Severely Injured Patients Treated in Trauma Centers Following the Establishment of Trauma Systems. *J Trauma*. 2006 Feb;**60(2)**:371–8; discussion 378. Review.

25. The London Trauma System: A review of trauma systems and the effect of the London Trauma Network on outcomes in an established major trauma centre. Dawson J. University of Edinburgh, Scotland (Dissertation). 2018.

26. Trauma Governance Framework and State-wide Model of Care. Transforming Health. SA Health. Government of South Australia. 19 January 2017.

27. Fatovich DM, Jacobs IG. The relationship between remoteness and trauma deaths in Western Australia. *J Trauma*. 2009 Nov;**67(5)**:910–4. doi: 10.1097/TA.0b013e3181815a26.

28. Major Trauma 2015 - National Peer Review Report. An overview of the findings from the 2015 National Review of Trauma Networks, Centres and Units in England. NHS England.

29. Caring for the severely injured in Australia. Inaugural report of the Australian Trauma Registry. Australian Trauma Quality Improvement Program. 2010-2012.

30. Vision Zero Initiative Sweden. 1997. Available from: https://visionzeroai.com/resource/vision-zero-initiative (accessed online Dec 2018).

31. Guidelines for Essential Trauma Care. World Health Organisation, International Society of Surgery, (ISS) and International Association for the Surgery of Trauma and Surgical Intensive Care (IATSIC) 2004. Available from: http://www.who.int/violence_injury_prevention/publications/services/guidelines_traumacare/en/ (accessed online Dec 2018).

32. Hyder AA, Puvanachandra P, Allen KA. Road Traffic Injury and Trauma Care: Innovations for Policy (Road Trip). Report of the Road Traffic Injury and Trauma Care Working Group 2013. Available from http://www.wish.org.qa/wp-content/uploads/2018/01/27425_WISH_Road_Injuries_Report_web.pdf (accessed January 2019).

33. Haynes AB, Berry WR, Gawande AA. What Do We Know About the Safe Surgery Checklist Now? *Annals of Surgery*. 2015 May;**261(5)**:829–30. doi: 10.1097/SLA.0000000000001144.

34. Lashoher A, Schneider EB, Juillard C, Stevens K, Colantuoni E, Berry WR, et al. Implementation of the World Health Organisation Trauma Care Checklist Programme in 11 Centres Across Multiple Economic Strata: Effect on Care Process Measures. *World J Surg*. 2017 Apr;**41(4)**:954–62. doi: 10.1007/s00268-016-3759-8.

35. El-Shinawi M, McCunn M, Sisley AC, El-Setouhy M, Hirshon JM. Developing Sustainable Trauma Care Education in Egypt: Sequential Trauma Education Program (STEPS) to Success. *J Surg Educ*. 2015;**72(4)**:e29–32. doi: 10.1016/j.jsurg.2014.12.001.

36. Safe Surgery 2020. Available from: http://safesurgery2020.org (accessed online Dec 2018).

37. Tai NR, Ryan JM, Brooks AJ. The neglect of trauma surgery. To improve outcomes, general trauma surgeons need training and recognition. *BMJ*. 2006;**332(7545)**:805–6.

38. Tai NRM. *Delivering a sustainable major trauma workforce*. Royal College of Surgeons of England, London. 2016.

39. Roettger RH, Taylor SM, Youkey JR, Blackhurst DW. The general surgery model: a more appealing and sustainable alternative for the care of trauma patients. *Am Surg*. 2005;**71(8)**:633–8; discussion 638-9.

40. Søreide K. Trauma and the acute care surgery model – should it embrace or replace general surgery? *Scand J Trauma Resusc Emerg Med* 2009;**17**:4.e-pub. doi: 10.1186/1757-7241-17-4.

41. Aboud ET, Krisht AF, O'Keeffe T, Nader R, Hassan M, Stevens CM, et al. Novel Simulation for Training Trauma Surgeons. *J Trauma*. 2011 Dec;**71(6)**:1484–90. doi: 10.1097/TA.0b013e3182396337.

Communication and Non-Technical Skills for Surgeons (NOTSS) in Major Trauma: The Role of Crew Resource Management (CRM)

2.1 OVERVIEW

The recognition that human factors, and not mechanical failure, were a recurring theme in many aviation disasters led to an increased focus on non-technical skill training in the training programme of pilots, referred to in aviation as crew resource management (CRM).

Other high-risk industries subsequently followed suit and 30 years ago the medical community adopted CRM as a component in the training of critical clinical situations. The subsequent years have seen implementation of CRM in numerous surgical and medical subspecialties, of which the setting of traumatology has been no exception. Trauma team training based upon the principles of CRM has become an integral part of the daily practice in trauma centres all over the world.

The principles of CRM are built upon a concept of training in human factors with the aim of optimizing communication dynamics in the setting of the multidisciplinary team. The goal is to reduce medical errors, and improve decision-making and outcomes in trauma care.

The most important aspects of CRM include:

- Situational awareness.
- Preparation and planning.
- Calling for help early.
- Effective leadership.
- Allocating attention wisely and use of all available resources.
- Prioritizing and distributing the workload.
- Communicating effectively.

The complex task of managing a severely injured trauma patient requires both highly specialized surgical and medical skills, as well as an ability to master the core concepts of CRM. It is mandatory for the entire trauma team to participate in training on the CRM principles.

2.1.1 The 'Swiss Cheese' Theory

Described initially in 2001, by James T. Reason, a British psychologist at the University of Manchester, the model has become the standard for assessing patient security in order to expose the failure of system such as medical mishap. and has been used by the healthcare industry, emergency services organizations, aviation industry, and safety industry since it was developed. It is also known as the cumulative act effect.[1,2] Reason's Swiss cheese model has become the dominant paradigm for analyzing medical errors and patient safety incidents.

In a complicated system, prevention of hazards is done by analysis of a chain of barriers. All barriers contain unplanned holes or weaknesses; hence the likeness to Swiss cheese. The holes in the Swiss cheese model randomly close and open owing to inconsistent weaknesses. The defence of an organization against the failure are represented like barriers in slices of Swiss cheese, and individual weaknesses are shown by the holes in the slices as part of the system; all holes are different in position and size in those slices. The hazard reaches the patient only when all the holes simultaneously align.

In most of the cases, there can be four levels of failure for an accident:

- Unsafe supervision.
- Unsafe act.
- Organizational influence.
- Preconditions for unsafe acts.

The failure of the system occurs when holes in slices simultaneously align in aggregate, giving permission, as James Reason called 'a trajectory of accident opportunity', so that in all the defences, jeopardy passes through all the holes, which causes failure.

2.2 COMMUNICATION IN THE TRAUMA SETTING

For trauma care to be effective, there needs to be open communication between all members of the trauma team. At the centre of this process are the surgeon and the anaesthetist, who in collaboration have the responsibility of prioritizing interventions and management. The team leader, be it the surgeon or anaesthetist, must keep the entire team constantly orientated regarding the management of a patient whose physiology and subsequent treatment plans are under constant evolution. The delivery of optimal care in a trauma patient undergoing damage control surgery is a complex process whereby a group of individuals need to function as one unit with all members being heard (listened to) and their individual skills utilized to deliver the most appropriate medical care.

Human factors are vital to the timely assessment and treatment of the complex trauma patient.[3] In the stressful and sometimes highly charged environment of the trauma bay or in the theatre, surgeons and anaesthetists can be tempted to focus on immediate individual tasks with the potential of developing what is commonly termed 'tunnel vision'. This can lead to a situation where management and focus on single problems is prioritized instead of addressing other life-threatening issues, thereby leading to loss of control of the situation. The loss of situational awareness described and the evolution of fixation errors may prove fatal to the outcome of the severely injured trauma patient. In trauma care, as in other disciplines, inadequate communication, poor teamwork, and lack of leadership have been shown to have a profound impact on patient outcomes.

2.2.1 Initial Handover

The handover is a critical phase during patient management; many medical errors arise here and thus it has been the focus of intense evaluation as to which strategies should be optimized. It is important that the handover is conducted in silence, unless there is an imminent threat to the patient's survival. The most commonly-used acronym, MIST, is used to describe in a short and concise manner the salient aspects of a traumatized patient:

- **M**echanism of injury.
- **I**njuries sustained.
- **S**igns and symptoms.
- **T**reatment.

2.2.2 Resuscitation and Ongoing Management

Communication during the resuscitation and ongoing management of the unstable trauma patient, from an operational perspective, can be described in four phases:

- Initial decision-making process prior to resuscitation in the emergency department.
- Before commencement of surgery.
- Re-evaluation during surgery.
- Completion of surgery, and transfer to the critical care environment.

Prior to patient arrival, it is pertinent to establish what has been termed 'zero-point survey' (Cliff Reid, unpublished 2017). This enables the team to survey and optimize their clinical environment and assign roles prior to engaging in clinical/non-clinical care. The information gleaned from the incoming pre-hospital services form the backbone for this survey.

The critical decision-making process is typically started in the emergency department/trauma bay and the surgeon together with the anaesthetist agree on a management plan for resuscitation, damage control surgery, and critical care.[4] At this early stage, evaluation of futility of care is also a legitimate consideration.

In the operating room, or shortly before the commencement of surgery, the surgeon states the surgical plan based on the clinical, laboratory, and imaging findings (if present). The anaesthesiologist summarizes the physiological status of the patient including blood volume/transfusion status, the presence of coagulopathy

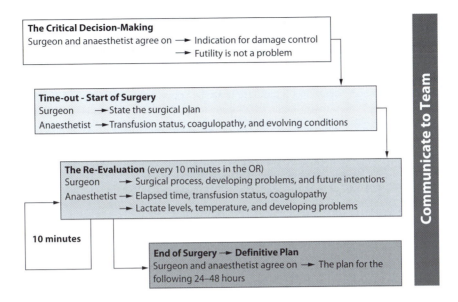

Figure 2.1 Communication in trauma.

and any other evolving conditions that will affect immediate management.

During damage control surgery and resuscitation, re-evaluation is performed around every 10 minutes in order to maintain team situational awareness and allow effective anticipation and planning of all aspects of the care of the patient. During the re-evaluation, the surgeon states the surgical progress, developing problems, and future intentions while the anaesthetist reports the elapsed time, transfusion status, developing coagulopathy, lactate levels, temperature, and other relevant developing problems.

Upon completion of surgery, the anaesthetist and surgeon recapitulate the patient's condition and the procedures performed and agree on the plan for the following 24–48 hours. They are responsible for ensuring the transfer of relevant information internally in the team and externally with collaborators such as the ICU, the blood bank, etc. The trauma leader plans the tertiary survey within the following 24 hours. The process is summarised in Figure 2.1.

2.3 LEADERSHIP IN TRAUMA CARE

Leadership is key to the management of trauma. A good team leader should possess the ability to make quick decisions under pressure based on all available information, maintain an overview, plan and execute treatment strategies in cooperation with team members, and perform regular reviews of the patient's response to treatment. Communication should be performed concisely and be unambiguous, but at the same time the team leader should be open and responsive to input from all team members. There are several ways of describing successful leadership; one is the Non-Technical Skills for

Table 2.1 Non-Technical Skills for Surgeons (NOTSS) Taxonomy

Category	Element
Situation awareness	Gathering information Understanding information Projecting and anticipating future state
Decision-making	Considering options Selecting and communicating options Implementing and reviewing decisions
Task management	Planning and preparation Flexibility/responding to change
Leadership	Setting and maintaining standards Supporting others Coping with pressure
Communication and teamwork	Exchanging information Establishing a shared understanding Coordinating team activities

Table 2.2 Potential Errors Related to Each Behavioural Theme

Themes	Potential Errors
Cognitive Skills – Situational Awareness	
Mechanism	• Failure to obtain data from the pre-hospital setting • Failure to incorporate knowledge of mechanism into understanding of potential forces patient has been subjected to, or which structures may potentially have been injured
Physiological burden	• Failure to obtain vital signs from pre-hospital setting • Failure to evaluate for neurological status • Failure to assess need for airway control • Failure to evaluate for respiratory status • Failure to evaluate for haemodynamic status • Failure to take into consideration trend in physiological parameters • Failure to take into consideration timing of physiological parameters
Injury and pattern recognition	• Failure to recognize a critical/unstable patient and lacking awareness of the overall trauma burden • Failure to pick up on the subtle cues that suggest severe injury
Active and confirmatory reconciliation	• Failure to evaluate response to treatment • Failure to consistently reassess diagnoses and management plans
Data processing and metacognition	• Losing sight of the bigger picture by focusing too much on irrelevant details (inattentional blindness/tunnel vision) • Allowing non-empirical data and biases to influence judgment
Environmental limitations	• Lacking awareness of the resources of the institution, thereby leading to delays • Failure to call for additional resources and personnel when necessary • Transferring the patient without rendering the patient safe for transfer
Self-limitations	• Failure to recognize when a given situation surpasses one's abilities (e.g. skill-set, experience, comfort level, and fatigue) • Failure to call for additional personnel when help is needed
Cognitive Skills – Decision-Making	
Forward planning	• Minimizing severity of injuries • Failure to mobilize the proper resources in a timely fashion • Failure to plan for worst-case scenarios and potential patient deterioration
Managing the injury	• Failure to follow ATLS protocols • Failure to follow best-practice guidelines and established management algorithms • Failure to investigate all body cavities to determine site of injury
Prioritizing	• Under-triaging patients • Failure to address life-threatening injuries before non-urgent injuries
Escalation of aggressiveness	• Devising and implementing a management plan that is not aggressive enough • Devising and implementing a management plan that is inappropriately aggressive

(Continued)

Table 2.2 (Continued) Potential Errors Related to Each Behavioural Theme

Themes	Potential Errors
Interpersonal Skills – Leadership	
	• Failure to introduce yourself as team leader • Ineffective coordination of team members (e.g. losing control of team members) • Overly micromanaging specific tasks instead of acting as the leader • Inability to cope under pressure in a chaotic environment • Failure to provide feedback to team members on performance
Interpersonal Skills – Teamwork and Communication	
	• Failure to establish team member roles ahead of time • Failure to listen to other team members • Failure to obtain confirmation of task delegation (closed loop communication) • Failure to effectively share management plan with other team members • Failure to limit the physical environment to necessary personnel only

Source: Reproduced with permission: Madani A et al. *J Surg Educ.* 2018;75(2):365.

Surgeons (NOTSS) taxonomy identified by the University of Aberdeen Industrial Psychology Research, Scotland, and the Royal College of Surgeons of Edinburgh, UK.[5] NOTSS can also be used for behavioural scoring and research. A multilevel assessment, which is simulation based, has been described (Table 2.1).[6–9]

These non-technical skills are not learnt from a textbook; they are acquired and reinforced through training in simulated environments with professional instructors who have expertise in both the principles of CRM as well as briefing and debriefing. These skills should then be used in daily practice.

2.4 POTENTIAL ERRORS RELATED TO EACH BEHAVIOURAL THEME

Errors will occur. By understanding the potential pitfalls, and with a mind-set like that in the aviation environment, they can be minimized (Table 2.2).[10]

Error is normal.
Therefore do not blame error:
Anticipate and prevent it.

2.5 SUMMARY

Trauma care is particularly challenging, in that the decision-making processes and interventions must be executed in a very condensed time period, for example,

minutes or even seconds compared to hours and even days/weeks in other less urgent forms of medical practice. Factors such as injury severity, physiology, and interdisciplinary specialist interactions, combine to compound the risk of error in high-stress situations, and elicits the same responses as in the aviation environment. Advance planning, good leadership and teamwork, and the timely anticipation of problems where possible will minimize risks to the patient.

REFERENCES AND RECOMMENDED READING

References

1. Reason JT, Carthey J, de Leval MR. Diagnosing "vulnerable system syndrome": an essential prerequisite to effective risk management. *Qual Health Care.* 2001 Dec;**10**: Suppl 2: ii21–5.
2. 'James Reason's Swiss Cheese Theory', Available from: http://www.researchomatic.com/James-Reasons-Swiss-Cheese-Theory-129350.html > 2012 (accessed online Dec 2018).
3. Catchpole K, Ley E, Wiegmann D, Blaha J, Shouhed D, Gangi A, et al. A Human Factors Subsystems Approach to Trauma Care. *JAMA Surg.* 2014 Sept;**149(9)**:962–98.
4. Arul GS, Pugh HE, Mercer SJ, Midwinter MJ. Optimising communication in the damage control resuscitation: Damage Control Surgery sequence in major trauma management. *J Roy Army Med Corps.* 2012 Jun;**158(2)**:82–4.

5. Non-Technical Skills for Surgeons (NOTSS). The Royal College of Surgeons of Edinburgh. 2018. Available from: https://www.rcsed.ac.uk/professional-support-development-resources/learning-resources/non-technical-skills-for-surgeons-notss (accessed online Dec 2018).

6. Doumouras AG, Keshet I, Nathens AB, Ahmed N, Hicks CM. Trauma Non-Technical Training (TNT-2): the development, piloting and multilevel assessment of a simulation-based, interprofessional curriculum for team-based trauma resuscitation. *Can J Surg*. 2014 Oct;**57(5)**:354–5. Review.

7. Hicks C, Petrosoniak A. The Human Factor: Optimizing Trauma Team Performance in Dynamic Clinical Environments. *Emerg Med Clin North Am*. 2018 Feb;**36(1)**:1–17. doi: 10.1016/j.emc.2017.08.003. Review.

8. Hughes KM, Benenson RS, Kritchten AE, Clancy KD, Ryan JP, Hammond C. A Crew Resource Management Program Tailored to Trauma Resuscitation Improves Team Behaviour and Communication. *J Am Coll Surg*. 2014 Sept;**219(3)**:545–51. doi: 10.1016/j.jamcollsurg.2014.03.049.

9. McCulloch P, Rathbone J, Catchpole K. Interventions to improve teamwork and communications among health care staff. *Br J Surg*. 2011 Apr;**98(4)**:469–79. doi: 10.1002/bjs.7434.

10. Madani A, Gips A, Razek T, Deckelbaum DL, Mulder DS, Grushka JR. Defining and Measuring Decision-Making for the Management of Trauma Patients. *J Surg Educ*. 2018 Mar–Apr;**75(2)**:358–69. doi: 10.1016/j.jsurg.2017.07.012.

Recommended Reading

NOTSS Handbook

The Non-Technical Skills for Surgeons (NOTSS) System Handbook V1.2. University of Aberdeen and Royal College of Surgeons of Edinburgh, Scotland. 2012. Available from https://www.iscp.ac.uk/static/help/NOTSS_Handbook_2012.pdf (accessed online Dec 2018).

Pre-Hospital and Emergency **3**
Trauma Care

3.1 RESUSCITATION IN THE EMERGENCY DEPARTMENT AND PRE-HOSPITAL SETTING

Patients with life-threatening injuries represent approximately 10%–15% of all patients hospitalized for injuries.[1] Some authors have defined severe trauma as a patient who has an Injury Severity Score (ISS) greater than 15.[2–4] For triage purposes, information available in the pre-hospital phase and primary survey should be used.

A standardized approach, utilizing the 'MIST' (also known as the '((AT)MIST') handover, should be used (Table 3.1).

3.2 MANAGEMENT OF MAJOR TRAUMA

The principles of management for patients suffering major trauma are:

- Simultaneous assessment and resuscitation.
- Life-saving surgery.
- A complete physical examination.
- Diagnostic studies if the patient becomes haemodynamically stable.

The first physician to treat a severely injured patient must start the resuscitation immediately and collect as much information as possible. In addition to patient symptoms, necessary information includes mechanism of injury and the presence of pre-existing medical conditions that may influence the critical decisions to be made. Time is working against the patient: 62% of all trauma patients who die in hospital do so within the first 4 hours of hospitalization.[5] The majority either bleed to death or die from primary or secondary injuries to the central nervous system. In order to reduce this mortality, prompt restoration of adequate tissue oxygenation and perfusion, and control of haemorrhage is critical; however this requires time, which is usually not available, and the work-up of the critically injured patient often must be rushed. To maximize resuscitative efforts and to avoid missing life-threatening injuries, various protocols for resuscitation have been developed, of which the Advanced Trauma Life Support Course® (ATLS)[6] is a model.

Guideline times for the length of stay in the emergency department (ED) should be as follows:

- **For the unstable patient, time in the ED should be no longer than 30 minutes (unless surgery is performed in the ED), and the unstable patient should either be in the operating room or the intensive care unit (ICU) within 30 minutes.**
- **For the stable patient, time in the ED should be no longer than 30–60 minutes.**
- **The *stable* patient should be in the computed tomography (CT) scanner or ICU within 60 minutes.**

3.2.1 Resuscitation

Resuscitation is traditionally performed in the (C) ABCDE format, where (C) is for controlling bleeding. Where there is extremity bleeding including traumatic amputation, the use of pre-hospital tourniquets has found a place, initially used in the military setting, and subsequently in the civilian setting.

Table 3.1 The MIST Handover

		Trauma/Medical Handover
(AT)	**Age**	Name, age, sex
(AT)	**Time**	Time of incident
M	**Mechanism of injury** **Medical complaint**	Speed, mass, height, restraints, number and type of collisions, helmet use and damage, weapon type. Medical onset, duration, history.
I	**Injuries sustained** **Illness**	Pain, deformity, injuries, injury patterns STEMI/stroke
S	**Signs and symptoms**	Vitals: Initial/current/worst RR, SPO$_2$, ETCO$_2$, blood gases HR, BP GCS: Eyes ____ Motor ____ Verbal ____ Total ____/15
T	**Treatment**	Tubes, lines (location and size), fluids Medications and response Immobilization and dressings

3.2.1.1 CIVILIAN PRE-HOSPITAL TOURNIQUET USE

Although underused, civilian pre-hospital tourniquet application was independently associated with a six-fold mortality reduction in patients with peripheral vascular injuries. More aggressive pre-hospital application of extremity tourniquets in civilian trauma patients with extremity haemorrhage and traumatic amputation is warranted.[7]

Pitfall

It is essential to document the time of application of the tourniquet (there is usually a tag on the tourniquet itself to write this down). It is very easy to miss this and then ischaemic damage to tissue occurs instead of exsanguination!

Resuscitation itself is divided into two components:

- The primary survey and initial resuscitation.
- The secondary survey and continuing resuscitation.

All patients undergo the primary survey of airway, breathing, and circulation. Only those patients who become haemodynamically stable will progress to the secondary survey, which focuses on a complete physical examination that directs further diagnostic studies. The great majority of patients who remain haemodynamically unstable require immediate operative intervention.

3.2.1.2 PRIMARY SURVEY

The priorities of the primary survey are:

- Establishing a patent airway with cervical spine control.
- Adequate ventilation.
- Maintaining circulation (including intravascular volume and cardiac function).
- Assessing the global neurological status.

3.2.1.2.1 Airway

Patients with extensive trauma who are unconscious or in shock benefit from immediate endotracheal intubation,[8,9] which may often happen pre-hospital. To prevent spinal cord injury, the cervical spine must be protected during intubation. Intubation via the oral route is successful in most injured patients. On rare occasions, bleeding, deformity, or oedema from maxillofacial injury will require emergency cricothyroidotomy or planned tracheostomy. Patients who may require a surgical airway include those with a laryngeal fracture and those with a penetrating injury of the neck or throat. The airway priorities are to clear the upper airway, to establish high-flow oxygen initially with a bag mask, and to proceed immediately to a definitive airway (cuffed tube in the trachea) – an endotracheal tube in most cases and to a surgical airway on a few occasions.

3.2.1.2.2 Breathing

Patients with respiratory compromise are not always easy to detect. Simple parameters such as the respiratory rate (RR) and adequacy of breathing should be examined within the first minute after arrival. One of the most important things is to detect a tension pneumothorax, necessitating direct drainage by needle thoracostomy followed by the insertion of a chest tube. Intubated patients are usually on positive-pressure ventilation, and in time critical conditions such as in the pre-hospital setting, a thoracostomy incision alone with an occlusive dressing sealed in three of the four sides can often be enough. The chest tube could be inserted upon arrival at the hospital. Other major threats to life, for example, massive haemothorax, flail chest and pulmonary contusion, cardiac tamponade, and tracheal-bronchial injury must be identified and treatment instituted urgently.

3.2.1.2.3 Circulation

Simultaneous with airway management, a quick assessment of the patient will determine the degree of shock present. Shock is a clinical diagnosis and should be apparent. A quick first step is to feel an extremity. If shock is present, the extremities will be cool and pale, lack venous filling, and have poor capillary refill. The pulse will be thready and consciousness will be diminished. As a guideline, major clinical shock results from bleeding into only five sites:

'Blood on the floor, and four more...'

- External bleeding ('blood on the floor').
  ... and four more:
- Bleeding into the chest (exclude by chest x-ray).
- Bleeding into the abdomen.
- Bleeding into the pelvis (exclude by clinical examination and pelvic x-ray).
- Bleeding into the extremities (exclude by clinical examination and long bone x-ray).

At the same time, the status of the neck veins must be noted. A patient who is in shock with flat neck veins is assumed to have hypovolaemic shock until proven otherwise. If the neck veins are distended, the most likely possibilities are:

- Tension pneumothorax.
- Pericardial tamponade.
- Myocardial contusion (cardiogenic shock).
- Myocardial infarction (cardiogenic shock).
- Air embolism.

Pitfall

Note that the absence of distended neck veins does not exclude these diagnoses because the circulating volume may be so depleted that the circulation is empty.

Tension pneumothorax should always be the number one diagnosis in the physician's differential diagnosis of shock since it is the life-threatening injury that is easiest to treat in the ED. A simple tube thoracostomy is the definitive management.

Pericardial tamponade is most commonly encountered in patients with penetrating injuries to the torso. Approximately 25% of all patients with cardiac injuries will reach the ED alive. The diagnosis is often obvious. The patient has distended neck veins and poor peripheral perfusion, and a few will have pulsus paradoxus. Ultrasonography may establish the diagnosis in those few patients with equivocal findings. Pericardiocentesis is of doubtful diagnostic or therapeutic use; ultrasound is a more reliable diagnostic modality, and a subxiphoid pericardial window is preferable therapeutically. However, proper treatment is immediate thoracotomy, preferably in the operating room, although ED thoracotomy can be life-saving.[10]

Myocardial contusion is a rare cause of cardiac failure in the trauma patient.

Myocardial infarction from coronary occlusion is not uncommon in the elderly. It may be the cause of the initial crash.

Air embolism[11,12] is a syndrome that has relatively recently been appreciated as important in injured patients; it represents air in the systemic circulation caused by a bronchopulmonary venous fistula. Air embolism occurs in 4% of all major thoracic injuries. Thirty-five per cent of the time it is due to blunt trauma, usually a laceration of the pulmonary parenchyma by a fractured rib. In 65% of patients, it is due to gunshot wounds or stab wounds. The surgeon must be vigilant when pulmonary injury has occurred. Any patient who has no obvious head injury but has focal or lateralizing neurological signs may have air bubbles occluding the cerebral circulation. The observation of air in the retinal vessels on fundoscopic examination confirms cerebral air embolism. Any intubated patient on positive-pressure ventilation who has a sudden cardiovascular collapse is presumed to have either tension pneumothorax or air embolism to the coronary circulation. Doppler monitoring of an artery can be a useful aid in detecting air embolism. Definitive treatment requires immediate thoracotomy followed by clamping of the hilum of the injured lung to prevent further embolism, followed by expansion of the intravascular volume. Open cardiac massage, intravenous adrenaline (epinephrine) and venting the left heart and aorta with a needle to remove residual air may be required. The pulmonary injury is treated definitively by oversewing the laceration or resecting a lobe.

If the patient's primary problem in shock is blood loss, the intention is to stop the bleeding. If this is not possible, the priorities are:

- To gain venous access to the circulation.
- To obtain a blood sample from the patient.
- To determine where the volume loss is occurring.
- To give appropriate resuscitation fluids.
- To prevent and treat coagulopathy.
- To prevent hypothermia.

Access is preferably central, via the subclavian route, and an 8.5 French Gauge (FG) introducer, more commonly used for passing a pulmonary artery catheter, can be used. Alternative routes are the jugular or femoral veins, or venous cut-down.

As soon as the first intravenous line has been established, baseline blood work is obtained that includes haematocrit, toxicology, blood type and cross match, and a screening battery of laboratory tests if the patient is older and has premorbid conditions. Blood gas determinations should be obtained early during resuscitation.

The third priority is to determine where the patient may have occult blood loss. Three sources for hidden blood loss are the pleural cavities, which can be eliminated as a diagnosis by rapid chest x-ray or ultrasound, the thigh and the abdomen, inclusive of the retroperitoneum and pelvis. A fractured femur should be clinically obvious. However, assessment of the abdomen by physical findings can be extremely misleading. Fifty per cent of patients with significant haemoperitoneum have no clinical signs.[13] Common sense dictates that if the patient's chest x-ray is normal, the femur is not fractured, and there is no external bleeding, the patient who remains in shock must be suspected of having ongoing haemorrhage in the abdomen or pelvis. Most of these unstable patients require immediate laparotomy to avoid death from haemorrhage. An important caveat is not to delay mandated therapeutic interventions to obtain non-critical diagnostic tests.

The fourth priority for the resuscitating physician is to consider activation of the massive bleeding protocol and order resuscitation fluids, starting with crystalloids and adding type-specific whole blood or blood components as soon as possible. Although whole blood is preferred, especially in the military situation, it is commonly difficult to obtain whole blood from modern blood banks, forcing the use of blood components. Loss of more than 2 units of blood and ongoing bleeding that requires blood transfusion should invoke a predefined massive bleeding protocol (most current massive transfusion protocols – MTPs, aim at predefined ratios of packed red blood cells:fresh frozen plasma:platelets, mimicking whole blood), and monitored by frequent coagulation tests, conventional laboratory tests, clotting studies, and more functional goal-directed haemostasis using thrombo-elastography (TEG) or rotary thromboelastomerography (RoTEM) when available. Use pharmacological haemostatic adjuncts (topical and systemic) such as tranexamic acid when indicated (see also Chapter 5). Blood components such as red blood cells, liquid plasma, or cryoprecipitate are now used in several systems, including Helicopter Emergency Medical Systems.

The use of crystalloids should be restrictive, and permissive hypotension is preferable in unstable bleeding patients both pre-hospitally and initially in the ED until haemorrhage control (see also Chapter 6).

The criteria for adequate resuscitation are simple and straightforward:

- Keep the atrial filling pressure at normal levels.
- Give enough fluid to achieve adequate urinary output (0.5 mL/kg per hour in the adult, 1.0 mL/kg per hour in the child).
- Maintain peripheral perfusion.

In elderly patients with extensive traumatic injuries, utilizing a cardiac computer may be prudent because it will be used to direct a sophisticated multifactorial resuscitation in the operating room or ICU. Resuscitation should be directed to achieve adequate oxygen delivery and oxygen consumption. An important caveat is not to delay mandated therapeutic interventions to obtain non-critical diagnostic test results.

3.2.1.2.4 Neurological Status (Disability)

The next priority during the primary survey is to quickly assess neurological status and to initiate diagnostic and treatment priorities. The key components of a rapid neurological evaluation are:

- Determine the level of consciousness.
- Observe the size and reactivity of the pupils.
- Check eye movements and oculovestibular responses.
- Document skeletal muscle motor responses and spontaneous movement of extremities.
- Determine the pattern of breathing.
- Perform a peripheral sensory examination.

3.2.1.2.5 Neurological Status is Often Described Using the Glasgow Coma Scale (3–15/15)

A decreasing level of consciousness is the single most reliable indication that the patient may have a serious head injury or secondary insult (usually hypoxic or hypotensive) to the brain. Consciousness has two components: awareness and arousal. Awareness is manifested by goal-directed or purposeful behaviour. The use of language is an indication of functioning cerebral hemispheres. If the patient attempts to protect himself from a painful insult, this also implies cortical function. Arousal is a crude function that is simple wakefulness. Eye-opening, either spontaneous or in response to stimuli, is indicative of arousal and is a brainstem function. Coma is a pathological state in which both awareness and arousal are absent. Eye-opening does not occur, there is no comprehensible speech detected, and the extremities move neither to command nor appropriately to noxious stimuli. By assessing all components and making sure the primary reflexes (pupillary, ankle, knee, biceps, and triceps) are assessed, and repeating this examination at frequent intervals, it is possible to both diagnose and monitor the neurological status in the ED. An improving neurological status reassures the physician that resuscitation is improving cerebral blood flow. Neurological deterioration is strong presumptive evidence of either a mass lesion or significant neurological injury. A CT scan (including the cervical spine) should be done as soon as possible.

3.2.1.2.6 Environment

The clothes are to be removed in order to examine the whole patient. A logroll must be performed, especially after penetrating injuries, in order to identify all wounds. The patient is at risk of hypothermia, and warming measures should be promptly instituted.

The body temperature of trauma patients decreases rapidly, and if the 'on-scene time' has been prolonged, for example by entrapment, patients arrive in the resuscitation room hypothermic. This is aggravated by the administration of cold fluid, the presence of abdominal or chest wounds, and the removal of clothing.

Patients can be expected to drop their core temperature by 1°–2°C per hour.

All fluids need to be at body temperature or above, and there are rapid infusor devices available that will warm fluids at high flow rates prior to infusion. Patients can be placed on warming mattresses and their environment kept warm using warm air blankets. Early measurement of the core temperature is important to prevent heat loss that will predispose to problems with coagulation. Hypothermia will shift the oxygen dissociation curve to the left, reduce oxygen delivery, reduce the liver's ability to metabolize citrate and lactic acid, and may produce arrhythmias.

The minimum diagnostic studies that should be considered in the haemodynamically unstable patient as part of the primary survey include:

- FAST ultrasound.
- Chest x-ray.
- Plain film of the pelvis.

Focused assessment with sonography in trauma (FAST) examination may be helpful:

- To assess whether there is blood in the abdomen or chest (extended FAST).
- To exclude cardiac tamponade.
- Extended FAST will assess for pneumothorax as well.

It must be emphasized that resuscitation should not cease during these films, and the resuscitating team must wear protective lead aprons. Optimally, the x-ray facilities, and especially the CT scanner, are juxtaposed to the ED, but the essential x-rays can all be obtained with a portable machine.

3.2.1.3 SECONDARY SURVEY

Finally, if the patient stabilizes, a secondary survey and diagnostic studies are carried out. However, if the patient remains unstable, he or she should be taken immediately to the operating room in order to achieve surgical haemostasis, or to the surgical ICU.

The patient must have a full 'top-to-toe' and 'front-to-back' examination. If the patient has been haemodynamically unstable, the site of the bleeding is traditionally:

'Blood on the floor, and four more'.

3.2.1.3.1 The Haemodynamically Normal Patient

There is ample time for a full evaluation of the patient, and a decision can be made regarding surgery or non-operative management. CT scanning is currently the modality of choice.

3.2.1.3.2 The Haemodynamically Stable Patient

The stable patient, who is not haemodynamically normal, but who is maintaining blood pressure, and other parameters with resuscitation, will benefit from investigations aimed at establishing:

- Whether the patient has bled into the abdomen?
- Whether the bleeding has stopped?

Thus, serial investigations of a quantitative nature will allow the best assessment of these patients. CT scan is the modality of choice, provided awareness of the fact that the patient may decompensate.

3.2.1.3.3 The Haemodynamically Unstable Patient

Efforts must be made to try to define the cavity where bleeding is taking place, for example, chest, pelvis, or abdominal cavity. Negative chest and pelvic x-rays leave the abdomen as the most likely source. Diagnostic modalities are of necessity limited. FAST is effective for detecting free fluid in the abdomen and pericardium, but is operator dependent – haemodynamic instability caused by intraperitoneal haemorrhage is likely to be readily found, but a negative FAST does not exclude intra-abdominal bleeding. FAST can be performed without moving the patient from the resuscitation area, since an unstable patient should not have a CT scan, even if it were to be readily available. Diagnostic peritoneal lavage (DPL) can also be used in mass casualty incidents when there is a lack of CT scanners due to a larger number of patients.

3.2.2 Management of Penetrating Trauma

Many forces can act on the torso to cause injury to the outer protective layers or the contained viscera.

Penetrating trauma is most often due to knives, missiles, and impalement. Knife wounds and impalement usually involve low-velocity penetration, and mortality is directly related to the organ injured. Secondary effects such as infection are due to the nature of the weapon and the material (i.e. clothing and other foreign material) that the missile carries into the body tissue. Infection is also influenced by spillage of contents from an injury to a hollow viscus organ.

An equally important component of the physical examination is to describe the penetrating wound. It is imperative that surgeons do not label the entrance or exit wounds unless common sense dictates it – an example is a patient with a single penetrating missile injury with no exit. However, in general, it is best to describe whether the wound is circular or ovoid and whether there is surrounding stippling (powder burn) or bruising from the muzzle of a weapon. Similarly, stab wounds should be described as longitudinal, triangular-shaped (hunting knives), or circular depending on the instrument used. Experience has shown that surgeons who describe wounds as entrance or exit may be wrong as often as 50% of the time. Experience with forensic pathology is required to be more accurate.

It is good practice to place metallic objects such as paper clips on the skin pointing to the various wounds on the chest wall, which aid in determining the missile track. It is recommended that an 'unfolded' paper clip be placed on any anterior penetrating injury, and a 'folded' one on any posterior injury (Figure 3.1).[14] This also can be useful for stab wounds. Tracking the missile helps to determine which visceral organs may be injured and

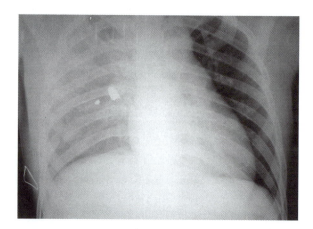

Figure 3.1 Chest x-ray showing the use of markers to show the wound track.

whether there is potential transgression of the diaphragm and/or mediastinum.

In the pre-hospital setting patients with penetrating torso trauma should be treated with a 'scoop and run' modality where on-scene time is minimized. Procedures should rather be performed en route to the hospital instead of at the scene of the incident.

3.3 EMERGENCY DEPARTMENT SURGERY

The emergency management of a critically injured trauma patient continues to be a substantial challenge. It is essential to have a very simple, effective plan that can be put into place to meet the challenges presented by resuscitating the moribund patient. ATLS® principles apply throughout.

As a basic consideration, for all major trauma victims with a systolic blood pressure of less than 90 mm Hg, there is a 50% likelihood of death, which, in one-third of cases, will occur within the next 30 minutes if the bleeding has not been controlled. If death is likely to occur in the next 5 minutes, it is essential to determine in which body cavity the lethal event will occur, as the only chance of survival will be the immediate control of haemorrhage.

If death is likely to occur in the next hour, there is time to proceed with an orderly series of investigations and, time permitting, radiographic or other diagnostic aids, to determine precisely what is injured, and to effect an operative plan for the management for this life-threatening event.

3.3.1 Head Trauma

In the event of severe facial, (and often associated severe neck injuries) surgical control of the airway may be necessary, using ATLS® described techniques.

It is unusual but possible to exsanguinate from a massive scalp laceration – ('Blood on the floor...'). For this reason, it is essential to gain control of the vascular scalp laceration with rapidly placed surgical clips or primary pressure and immediate suturing, using deep sutures rather than staples, and a pressure dressing.

The more common cause of death is from intracranial mass lesions. Extradural haematomas and subdural haematomas can be rapidly lethal. A rapid diagnosis of an ipsilateral dilated pupil with contralateral hemiplegia is diagnostic of mass lesion with significant enough intracranial pressure to induce coning. This requires immediate decompression. Moderate hyperventilation to produce mild hypocapnia, and vasoconstriction is only used immediately prior to neurosurgical intervention. The use of mannitol or hypertonic saline is useful as a temporizing adjunct only.

Attention should be paid to monitoring the end-tidal carbon dioxide, as a proxy for $PaCO_2$, which should not be allowed to fall below 30 mm Hg (4 kPa). This should decrease intracranial volume, and therefore intracranial pressure. There should be an immediate positive effect that usually lasts long enough to obtain a three-cut CT scan to determine a specific site of the mass lesion and the type of haematoma. This will direct the surgeon specifically to the location of the craniotomy for removal of the haematoma.

Intravenous mannitol should be administered as a bolus injection in a dose of 0.5–1.0 g/kg or hypertonic (7.5%) saline as a dosage of 1 mmol/kg. This should not delay any other diagnostic or therapeutic procedures.

3.3.2 Chest Trauma

Lethal injuries to the chest include tension pneumothorax, cardiac tamponade, and transected aorta.

Tension pneumothorax is diagnosed clinically with deviation of the trachea away from the lesion (a late sign), hypertympany on the side of the lesion, and decreased breath sounds on the affected side. There is usually associated elevated jugular venous pressure in the neck veins, unless the patient is hypovolaemic. This is a clinical diagnosis, and once made, an immediate needle thoracostomy or tube thoracostomy should be performed to relieve the tension pneumothorax. The tube should then be placed to underwater seal.

It is far better to perform a thoracotomy in the operating room, either through an anterolateral approach or a median sternotomy, with good light and assistance and the potential for autotransfusion and potential bypass, than it is to attempt heroic emergency surgery in the resuscitation suite. However, if the patient is in extremis with blood pressure in the 40 mm Hg or lower range despite volume resuscitation, there is no choice but to proceed immediately with a left anterior thoracotomy to relieve the tamponade and control the penetrating injury to the heart. If there is an obvious penetrating injury to either the left or the right ventricle, a Foley catheter can be introduced into the hole and the balloon distended to create a tamponade. The end of the Foley should be clamped.

Pitfalls

Great care should be taken to apply minimal traction on the Foley – just enough to allow sealing. Excessive traction will pull the catheter out and extend the wound by tearing the muscle. Once the bleeding is controlled, the wound can be easily sutured with pledgetted sutures.

- *The chance of survival after emergency thoracotomy is better after a penetrating rather than a blunt trauma mechanism.*

Massive haemorrhage from intercostal vessels secondary to multiple rib fractures will frequently stop without operative intervention. This is also true for most bleeding from the lung. It is helpful to collect the shed blood from the hemithorax into an autotransfusion collecting device and return it to the patient.

Aortic transection is usually diagnosed with a widened mediastinum and confirmed with an arteriogram or a CT scan (see also Chapter 8). Once the diagnosis has been made, it is useful to maintain control of hypotension in the 100 mm Hg range so as not to precipitate free rupture from the transection, until stenting or operative repair can take place.

NB: Abdominal injury generally takes priority over thoracic aortic injury.

3.3.3 Abdominal Trauma

Significant intra-abdominal or retroperitoneal haemorrhage can be a reason to go rapidly to the operating room. The abdomen may be distended and dull to percussion. Ultrasound (FAST) is a useful tool as it is specific for blood in the peritoneum, but it is operator-dependent. A positive FAST result in an unstable patient is an indication for laparotomy. Conversely, a negative FAST result does not exclude intra-abdominal bleeding and repeat FAST or other investigations need to be considered. A definitive diagnosis can be made with FAST, a grossly positive DPL, or CT scan. The decision to operate for bleeding should be based on the haemodynamic status.

Non-operative management has become the treatment of choice in haemodynamically stable patients with liver and spleen injuries regardless of injury grade. (See Sections 9.4: Liver and 9.5: Spleen.)

The CT scanner is highly sensitive and very specific for the type, character and severity of injury to a specific organ. However, patients whose condition is unstable should NOT be considered.

3.3.4 Pelvic Trauma

Pelvic fractures can be a significant cause of haemorrhage and death. It is essential to return the pelvis to its original configuration as swiftly as possible. As an emergency procedure, a compressing sheet, or commercially available pelvic binders can be used. There are also external fixation devices such as the C-clamp and the external fixator, which can be placed in the resuscitation suite, and return the pelvis to its normal anatomy. However, their fixation may be time-consuming, requires skill, and may not present advantages over the non-invasive binders for initial management. As the pelvis is realigned, it helps to compress the haematoma in the pelvis. Since approximately 85% of pelvic bleeding is venous, compressing the haematoma usually stops most pelvic bleeding.

If the patient continues to be hypotensive, resuscitation should continue, and an angiogram should be considered. This will identify the presence of significant arterial bleeding in the pelvis, which then can be embolized immediately. If the patient is exsanguinating from the pelvic injury or is haemodynamically unstable, damage control surgery should be performed with extraperitoneal packing of the pelvis combined with a laparotomy, on occasion surgical central vascular control, before angiography. Resuscitative endovascular balloon occlusion of the aorta (REBOA) (see also Section 15.3) has recently been introduced as an alternative to surgery in several EDs (and even a few pre-hospital settings), but the benefit over surgery remains largely unproven.

3.3.5 Long Bone Fractures

Lone bone fractures, particularly of the femur, can bleed significantly. The damage control approach to fractures is external fixation. The immediate treatment for a patient who is hypotensive from haemorrhage from a femoral fracture is to put traction on the distal limb, pulling the femur into alignment. This not only realigns the bones but also reconfigures the cylindrical nature of the thigh. This has an immediate tamponading effect on the bleeding in the muscles of the thigh. It is frequently necessary to maintain traction with a Thomas or Hare traction splint. Attention should be paid to the distal pulses to be sure that there is continued arterial inflow. If the pulses are absent, an arteriogram should be performed to determine whether there are any injuries to major vascular structures. A determination is then made as to the timing of arterial repair and bony fixation. Re-establishing perfusion to the limb takes priority over fracture treatment.

3.3.6 **Peripheral Vascular Injuries**

Peripheral vascular injuries are not in themselves life-threatening providing that the bleeding is controlled. However, it is critical to assess whether ischaemia and vascular continuity are present, since this will influence the overall planning.

Every ED should have access to a simple flow Doppler monitor to assess pressures and flow. If there is any doubt over whether the vessel is patent, the ankle–brachial index should be measured, and if it is less than 0.9, an arteriogram is mandatory. Time and availability decide whether the patient can be transported to an angiography suite or should have an angiogram performed in the operating room or ED. Although it is desirable to do this in the angiography suite, it is not always possible, and the necessary equipment may not be available. If there is any doubt, consideration should be given to the use of the ED angiogram.[15]

3.4 **SUMMARY**

The decision of whether to operate in the ED or in the operating room should be made based on an overview of the urgency and the predicted outcome.

It is useful to have a well-thought-out plan for dealing with the critically injured trauma patient so that both clinical diagnosis and relevant investigations can be performed immediately, and an operative or non-operative therapeutic approach implemented.

> **There is no future in altering only the geographical site of death.**

REFERENCES AND RECOMMENDED READING

References

1. *Resources for Optimal Care of the Injured Patient* 6th Edn (Red Book) *2014*. Committee on Trauma. American College of Surgeons. Chicago, IL, USA:2014. Available from www.facs.org (accessed online Dec 2018).
2. Ciesla DJ, Kerwin AJ, Tepas III, J. Trauma systems, Triage, and Transport. In: Moore EE, Feliciano DV, Mattox KL. eds. *Trauma*, 8th Edn. McGraw-Hill Education, New York, NY, USA. 2017:54–76.
3. Baker SP, O'Neill B, Haddon W, Long WB. The Injury Severity Score: a method for describing patients with multiple injuries and evaluating emergency care. *J Trauma*. 1974 Mar;**14**:187–96.
4. American Association for the Advancement of Automotive Medicine. *The Abbreviated Injury Scale: 2015 Revision*. Barrington, IL: American Association for the Advancement of Automotive Medicine, 2015. Available from: https://www.aaam.org/abbreviated-injury-scale-ais/ (accessed online Dec 2018).
5. Trunkey DD. Trauma. *Sci Am*. 1983;**249**:28–35.
6. American College of Surgeons. *Advanced Trauma Life Support®: Student Course Manual*, 10th edn. American College of Surgeons, Chicago IL, USA. 2018.
7. Teixera GR, Brown CVR, Emigh B, Long M, Foreman M, Eastridge B, Gale S, et al. Civilian prehospital tourniquet use is associated with improved survival in patients with peripheral vascular injury. *J Am Coll Surg*. 2018 May;**226(5)**:769–76.e1. doi: 10.1016/j.jamcollsurg.2018.01.047.
8. Jacobs LM, Berrizbeitia LD, Bennett B, Madigan C. Endotracheal intubation in the prehospital phase of emergency medical care. *JAMA*. 1983;**250**:2175–7.
9. Taryle DA, Chandler JE, Good JT, Potts DE, Sahn SA. Emergency room intubations – complications and survival. *Chest* 1979 May;**75**:541–3.
10. Baker CC, Thomas AN, Trunkey DD. The role of emergency room thoracotomy in trauma. *J Trauma*. 1980 Oct; **20(10)**:848–55.
11. Thomas AN, Stephens BG. Air embolism: a cause of morbidity and death after penetrating chest trauma. *J Trauma*. 1974 Aug;**14(8)**:633–8.
12. Yee ES, Verrier ED, Thomas AN. Management of air embolism in blunt and penetrating trauma. *J Thor Cardiovasc Surg*. 1983 May;**85(5)**:661–8.

13. Bivens BA, Sachatello CR, Daugherty ME, Ernst CB, Griffen WD. Diagnostic peritoneal lavage is superior to clinical evaluation in blunt abdominal trauma. *Am Surg.* 1978 Oct; **44(1)**:637–41.

14. Brooks A, Bowley DMG, Boffard KD. Bullet markers – a simple technique to assist in the evaluation of penetrating trauma. *J R Army Med Corps.* 2002 Sep;**148(3)**: 259–61.

15. MacFarlane C, Saadia R, Boffard KD. Emergency room arteriography: a useful technique in the assessment of peripheral vascular injuries. *J Roy Coll Surg Edin.* 1989 Dec; **34(6)**:310–13.

Recommended Reading

American College of Surgeons. *Advanced Trauma Life Support Course for Doctors: Student Course Manual*, 10th edn. Chicago: American College of Surgeons, 2018.

Committee on Trauma. Resources for Optimal Care of the Injured Patient 2014. Chicago: American College of Surgeons, (Red Book) 2014. Sixth Edition. www.facs.org (accessed online Dec 2018).

Jacobs LM, ed. *Advanced Trauma Operative Management.* Chicago/Woodbury, CT: American College of Surgeons/ Ciné-Med Publishing, 2010.

Part 2

Physiology and the body's response to trauma

Resuscitation Physiology **4**

4.1 METABOLIC RESPONSE TO TRAUMA

4.1.1 Definition of Trauma

Physical injury is accompanied by systemic as well as local effects. Following trauma, the body responds locally by inflammation and by a general response which is often protective and which conserves fluid and provides energy for repair. Proper resuscitation may attenuate the response but will not abolish it.

The response is characterized by an acute catabolic reaction, which precedes the metabolic process of recovery and repair. This metabolic response to trauma traditionally was divided into an ebb and flow phase by Cuthbertson in 1932.[1]

The ebb phase is relatively short lived and corresponds to the period of severe shock characterized by depression of enzymatic activity and oxygen consumption.

After effective resuscitation has been accomplished with restoration of adequate oxygen transport, the flow phase comes into play. The flow phase can be divided into:

- A catabolic phase with fat and protein mobilization associated with increased urinary nitrogen excretion and weight loss.
- An anabolic phase with restoration of fat and protein stores, and weight gain.

The appropriate protective flow phase is characterized by:

- A normal or slightly elevated blood glucose level.
- Increased glucose production.
- Normal or slightly elevated free fatty acid levels, with increased flux.
- A normal or elevated insulin concentration.
- High normal or elevated levels of catecholamine and an elevated glucagon level.
- A normal blood lactate level.

- Elevated oxygen consumption.
- Increased cardiac output.
- Elevated core temperature.

These responses are marked by hyperdynamic circulatory changes, signs of inflammation, glucose intolerance, and muscle wasting.

4.1.2 Initiating Factors

The magnitude of the metabolic response depends on the degree of trauma and concomitant contributory factors such as infection, tissue necrosis, and pre-existing systemic disease. The response will also depend on the age and sex of the patient, the genetic composition, the underlying nutritional state, and the timing of treatment and its effectiveness. In general, the more severe the injury (i.e. the greater the degree of tissue damage), the greater the metabolic response.

The metabolic response alterations seem to be less aggressive in children and the elderly and in the premenopausal female. Starvation and nutritional depletion also modify the response. Patients with poor nutritional or immunological status (e.g. those with human immunodeficiency virus – HIV) have a reduced metabolic response to trauma compared to healthy well-nourished patients, while burns and severe traumatic brain injury cause a relatively greater response than other mechanical injuries.

Wherever possible, efforts should be made to reduce the magnitude and duration of the initial insult, since by doing so it may be possible to reduce the extent of the metabolic changes. Thus, aggressive resuscitation, control of pain and temperature, limiting acidosis, adequate devitalized tissue debridement, avoidance of unnecessary blood component administration with coagulopathy, and nutritional (preferably enteral) support are critical.

The precipitating factors can be broadly divided into:

4.1.2.1 HYPOVOLAEMIA

- Decrease in circulating blood volume.
- Increase in alimentary loss of fluid.
- Loss of interstitial volume.
- Extracellular fluid shift.

4.1.2.2 AFFERENT IMPULSES

- Somatic.
- Autonomic.
- Sympathetic ↑.
- Cholinergic ↓.

4.1.2.3 WOUND FACTORS: INFLAMMATORY AND CELLULAR

- Platelets – PF4.
- Neutrophils – superoxide, elastase.
- Macrophages/dendritic cells.
- Endothelial cells.
- Cytokines – interleukins IL1, IL2, IL6, IL10, IL-17, TNF.
- Chemokines – IL8.
- Eicosanoids – LTB4, LTC4, TXA_2, PGE_2.
- Damage associated molecular patterns (DAMPs) $HMGB_1$, HSP_{70}.

4.1.2.4 TOXINS/SEPSIS

- Endotoxins.
- Exotoxins.

4.1.2.5 FREE RADICALS

- Superoxide and derivatives.
- Nitrogen radicals.

4.1.2.6 HYPOVOLAEMIA

Hypovolaemia, specifically tissue hypoperfusion, is the most potent precipitator of the metabolic response. Hypovolaemia can be due to external losses, internal shifts of extracellular fluids, and changes in plasma osmolality. However, the most common cause is blood loss (see also Section 4.2).

The hypovolaemia will stimulate release of catecholamines, which in turn trigger the neuroendocrine response. This plays an important role in volume and electrolyte conservation and protein, fat, and carbohydrate catabolism.

4.1.2.7 AFFERENT IMPULSES

Hormonal responses are initiated by pain and anxiety. The metabolic response may be modified by administration of adequate analgesia, which may be parenteral, enteral, regional, or local. Somatic blockade may need to be accompanied by autonomic blockade, in order to minimize or abolish the metabolic response.

4.1.2.8 WOUND FACTORS

Endogenous factors may prolong or even exacerbate the systemic trauma insult, even though the primary cause is treated well. Tissue injury activates a diverse response via release of DAMPs activating toll-like receptors (TLR), and by release of multiple inflammatory mediators locally at the site of injury and/or infection through two predominant pathways:

- Humoral pathway.
- Cellular pathway.

Uncontrolled activation of endogenous inflammatory mediators and cells may contribute to a syndrome called the systemic inflammatory response syndrome (SIRS). The result of an excessive SIRS response is diffuse bystander organ injury.

Both humoral and cell derived activation products play a role in the pathophysiology of organ dysfunction.[2] It is important, therefore, to monitor post-traumatic biochemical and immunological abnormalities whenever possible, as a guide to direct and confirm the appropriateness of resuscitative interventions.

4.1.3 Immune Response

The immune response is complex and consists of an early enhanced upregulation of the primarily proinflammatory innate system and a concomitant prolonged suppression of the adaptive immune system. The magnitude of these responses is modified by the depth and duration of insult caused by the injury, as well as the patient's genetic composition and preexisting comorbidities.

4.1.3.1 THE INFLAMMATORY PATHWAY

The inflammatory mediators of injury have been implicated in the induction of numerous cellular dysfunctions.

While neutrophils have been invoked as primary mediators of inflammatory processes for more than 100 years, we now recognize that these initial responses involve numerous cellular mediators including platelets, macrophages, endothelium, and epithelium.

4.1.3.1.1 Cytokines

The term cytokine refers to a diverse group of polypeptides and glycoproteins that are important mediators of inflammation. They are produced by a variety of cell types, but predominantly by leucocytes. Cytokines are generally divided into pro-inflammatory, and anti-inflammatory, but some have both properties, for example IL-6.

4.1.3.1.2 Pro-Inflammatory Cytokines

Certain cytokines, particularly TNF, IL-1, and IL-8 promote the inflammatory response by up-regulating expression of genes that generate the pro-inflammatory mediators. Pro-inflammatory cytokines also mediate inflammation by activating neutrophils, endothelium, and epithelium – all of which lead to tissue damage.

The TNF and IL-1 act synergistically to produce the acute innate immune response to ischaemia/reperfusion in many organs. TNF causes neutrophils to be attracted to injured epithelium, thereby helping to regulate the inflammatory response. It also stimulates endothelial cells to produce a cytokine subset known as chemokines (e.g. IL-8), which produce leukocyte migration into the tissues and IL-1 production. Like TNF, IL-1 is a primary responder in the inflammatory cascade, and its actions are similar to TNF, but it does not induce apoptosis or programmed cell death.

Interferon gamma (IFN-γ) is produced in response to antigens processed by macrophages, an event enhanced by IL-12. The IL-12 is produced by mononuclear phagocytes, and dendritic cells in response to intracellular microbes. IL-6 is produced by mononuclear phagocytes, endothelial cells, and fibroblasts, and acts in a pro-inflammatory manner by providing a potent stimulus for hepatocyte synthesis of acute phase proteins.

The IL-2, unlike the above cytokines which exert most of their influence via the innate immune system, stimulates acquired immunity, and has other immunomodulatory functions as well.

4.1.3.1.3 Anti-inflammatory Cytokines

The anti-inflammatory cytokines exert their effects by inhibiting the production of pro-inflammatory cytokines or countering their action. They reduce gene expression and mitigate or prevent numerous inflammatory effects.

The IL-10 is important in the control of innate immunity. It can prevent fever, pro-inflammatory cytokine release, and clotting cascade activation during endotoxin challenge. Other potent anti-inflammatory modulators include IL-4, IL-13, and transforming growth factor beta (TGF-β).

4.1.3.1.4 Modulation of Cytokine Activity in Sepsis, Systemic Inflammatory Response Syndrome (SIRS), and Compensatory Inflammatory Response Syndrome (CIRS)

Systemic inflammatory activity, which occurs in response to infectious or non-infectious stimuli, is the fundamental overall clinical phenomenon that can provoke whole body SIRS and can lead ultimately to multiple organ dysfunction syndrome (MODS) and multiple organ failure (MOF), which is associated with a mortality of up to 50%. It was initially suggested that SIRS and sepsis were attributable to an overwhelming pro-inflammatory innate immune response, mediated by TNF and numerous other cytokines. However, simultaneously, the body also mounts an endogenous counter- or anti-inflammatory reaction to restore homeostasis, which can then lead to CARS. Early, after severe injury or sepsis, the pro-inflammatory response predominates and SIRS and shock result. If the counter-inflammatory response leads to homeostasis the patient does well and recovers. However, if the suppressive response is excessive, it leads to immunosuppression, and greatly increased susceptibility to nosocomial infections that are frequently seen in the severely injured and critically ill patients.. The modern view is that, following injury, SIRS and CARS activate simultaneously.

The role of cytokines in sepsis is critical to outcomes and is very complex, with both pro-inflammatory and anti-inflammatory factors playing a role and determining clinical outcome.

4.1.3.1.5 Activated Protein C

Pro-inflammatory mediators have a role in triggering the clotting cascade by stimulating the release of tissue factor from monocytes and the vascular endothelium leading to thrombin formation and a fibrin clot. At the same time, thrombin stimulates many inflammatory pathways and suppresses natural anticoagulant responses by activating thrombin-activatable fibrinolysis inhibitor (TAFI). This overall procoagulant response leads to microvascular thrombosis and is implicated in the multiple organ failure associated with sepsis. On the other hand, thrombin binding to endothelial thrombomodulin, generates activated protein C (APC), which is an endogenous anticoagulant. However, previous reports of benefit to providing exogenous APC in the setting of sepsis have subsequently been shown to provide no improvement in survival. While the concepts involved are no doubt important, our ability to appropriately modify their activity to benefit the critically ill patient remains elusive.

4.1.3.1.6 Eicosanoids

These compounds, derived from eicosapolyenoic fatty acids, are subdivided into prostanoids (the precursors of the prostaglandins), and leucotrienes (LT). Eicosanoids are synthesized from arachidonic acid (AA), which has been synthesized from phospholipids of cell walls, by the action of phospholipase A2 (in part, released by activated neutrophils). Cyclo-oxygenase converts arachidonic acid to prostanoids, the precursors of prostaglandins (PG), prostacyclins (PGI), and thromboxanes (TX). The term prostaglandins is used loosely to include all prostanoids. The leucotrienes are produced by the action of 5-lipoxygenase on AA with subsequent by-products produced by LTA4 hydrolase (i.e. LTB4 and LTC4 synthase). Eicosanoids modulate blood flow to organs and tissues by altering local balances between vasodilators and vasoconstricting mediators, and, in addition, directly stimulate certain immune cells.

The prostanoids (prostaglandins of the E and F series), PGI_2, and TX not only cause vasoconstriction (TXA_2 and PGF_1), but also vasodilatation (PGI_2, PGE_1 and PGE_2). TXA_2 activates and aggregates platelets and white cells, and PGI_2 and PGE_1 inhibit white cells and platelets. The leucotriene LTB4 is a very potent polymorphonucleocyte (PMN) chemo-attractant and activator, while LTC4 causes vasoconstriction, increased capillary permeability and bronchoconstriction.

4.1.3.2 **THE CELLULAR PATHWAY**

The classical pathway of complement activation involves an interaction between the specific antibody and the initial trimer of complement components C^1, C^4, and C^2. In the classical pathway, this interaction then cleaves the complement products C^3 and C^5, via proteolysis to produce the very powerful chemotactic factors C^{3a} and C^{5a}.

The so-called alternative pathway appears to be primarily involved following trauma. It is activated by properdin, and proteins D or B, to activate C^3 convertase, which generates the anaphylotoxins C^{3a} and C^{5a}. Its activation appears to be the earliest trigger for activating the innate immune cellular system and is responsible for aggregation of neutrophils and activation of basophils, mast cells, and platelets to secrete histamine and serotonin, which alter vascular permeability and are vasoactive. In trauma patients, the serum C^3 level is inversely correlated with the Injury Severity Score (ISS).[3] Measurement of C^{3a} is the most useful because the other products are more rapidly cleared from the circulation.

The short-lived fragments of the complement cascade, C^{3a} and C^{5a}, stimulate macrophages to secrete interleukin-l (IL-1) and proteolysis inducing factor (PIF), an active circulating cleavage product. These mediators cause proteolysis and lipolysis along with fever. The IL-1 activates T_4 helper cells to produce IL-2, which enhances the adaptive cell-mediated immunity. The IL-1 and PIF are also potent stimulators of the liver, bone marrow, spleen, and lymph nodes to produce acute-phase proteins, including complement, fibrinogen, α2-macroglobulin, and other proteins required for immune defence mechanisms.

There is also considerable cross-talk between the clotting cascade and inflammation. For example, activation of factor XII (Hageman factor A) stimulates kallikrein to produce bradykinin from bradykininogen, which affects capillary permeability and vaso-reactivity. Overall, the overlapping combination of these reactions causes the systemic inflammatory response. Kalligren can activate plasmin to promote fibrinolysis

4.1.3.3 **TOXINS**

Endotoxin is a lipopolysaccharide component of bacterial cell walls. Endotoxin and other bacterial and viral cell wall components are known to activate many immune cells, along with hepatocytes and myocardiocytes primarily via the TLR receptors. Activated cells release tumour necrosis factor (TNF) and a broad spectrum of potent mediators from macrophages. neutrophils, endothelial cells, and many others. Endotoxins cause vascular margination and sequestration of leukocytes, particularly in the capillary bed. At high doses, direct granulocyte destruction is seen.

4.1.3.4 **PAMPS AND DAMPS**

Injury causes a SIRS clinically much like sepsis. Multicellular animals detect pathogens via a set of pattern recognition receptors (TLRs), which recognize pathogen-associated molecular patterns (PAMPs), which in turn activate innate immunocytes. Evidence is accumulating that trauma and its associated tissue damage are recognized at the cell level by a similar cell receptor-mediated detection of intracellular products released by injured and dying cells. The term 'alarmin' has been used to categorize these endogenous DAMPs that signal tissue and cell damage.[4] A major source of DAMPs is injury-induced release of mitochondrial products, including mitochondrial DNA, coined the 'enemies within'. Endogenous DAMPs and exogenous PAMPS therefore convey a similar message and elicit similar responses.[5] Surgical source control, whether for infection or necrotic tissue, is an attempt to minimize the host exposure to these toxic moieties.

4.1.3.5 FREE RADICALS

Oxygen radical (O_2^-) formation by white cells is a normal host defence mechanism. Diffuse activation after severe injury, however, may lead to excessive production by neutrophils and macrophages, with deleterious cellular effects on diffuse organ function. Nitric oxide (NO) is released by macrophages and endothelial cells, causing vasodilatation and decreased systemic vascular resistance. NO also combines with O_2^- to form a potent oxidizing agent. Toxic hydroxyl ion (OH^-) and hydrogen peroxide are also increased following sepsis or stress. Protective endogenous anti-oxidants are rapidly depleted following injury or sepsis leading to an even more enhanced cellular bystander injury.

4.1.4 Hormonal Mediators

In response to trauma, many circulatory hormones are altered. Adrenaline (epinephrine), noradrenaline (norepinephrine), cortisol, and glucagon are increased, while certain others are decreased. The sympathetic-adrenal axis is a major system by which the body's response to injury is activated.

4.1.4.1 HYPOTHALAMUS/PITUITARY

The hypothalamus is the highest level of integration of the stress response. The major efferent pathways of the hypothalamus are endocrine via the pituitary, and the efferent sympathetic and parasympathetic systems. In contrast, the cholinergic system is now recognized to have a variety of anti-inflammatory effects. The pituitary gland responds to trauma with increased levels of adrenocorticotrophic hormone (ACTH), prolactin, and growth hormone, while the remaining hormones are relatively unchanged.

Pain receptors, osmoreceptors, baroreceptors, and chemoreceptors stimulate or inhibit ganglia in the hypothalamus to induce sympathetic nerve activity. The neural endplates and adrenal medulla secrete catecholamines. Pain stimuli via the pain receptors also stimulate secretion of endogenous opiates, β-endorphin, and pro-opiomelanocortin (precursor of the ACTH molecule), which modifies the response to pain and reinforces the catecholamine effects. The β-endorphin has little effect but serves as a marker for anterior pituitary secretion.

Hypotension, hypovolaemia in the form of a decrease in left ventricular pressure, and hyponatraemia stimulate secretion of vasopressin, antidiuretic hormone (ADH) from the supra-optic nuclei in the anterior hypothalamus, aldosterone from the adrenal cortex, and renin from the juxtaglomerular apparatus of the kidney. The increase in aldosterone secretion results in conservation of sodium, and, thereby, water. As osmolality increases, the secretion of ADH increases, and more water is reabsorbed, thereby decreasing the serum osmolality (negative feedback control system).

Hypovolaemia stimulates receptors in the right atrium and hypotension stimulates receptors in the carotid artery. This results in activation of paraventricular hypothalamic nuclei, which secrete pituitary releasing hormone from the median eminence into capillary blood, which stimulates the anterior pituitary to ACTH. ACTH stimulates the adrenal cortex to secrete cortisol and aldosterone. Changes in glucose concentration influence the release of insulin from the β cells of the pancreas, and high amino-acid levels, the release of glucagon from the α cells.

4.1.4.2 ADRENAL HORMONES

Plasma cortisol and glucagon levels rise following trauma. The degree is related to the severity of injury. The function of glucocorticoid secretion in the initial metabolic response is uncertain, since the hormones have little direct action, and primarily they seem to augment the effects of other hormones such as the catecholamines.

4.1.4.3 PANCREATIC HORMONES

There is a rise in the blood sugar following trauma. The insulin response to glucose is reduced substantially with alpha-adrenergic stimulation and enhanced with beta-adrenergic stimulation.[6]

4.1.4.4 RENAL HORMONES

Aldosterone secretion is increased by several mechanisms. The renin-angiotensin mechanism is the most important. When the glomerular arteriolar inflow pressure falls, the juxtaglomerular apparatus of the kidney secretes renin, which acts with angiotensinogen to form angiotensin I. This is converted to angiotensin II, a substance that stimulates production of aldosterone by the adrenal cortex. Reduction in sodium concentration stimulates the macula densa, a specialized area in the tubular epithelium adjacent to the juxtaglomerular apparatus, to activate renin release. An increase in plasma potassium concentration also stimulates aldosterone release. Volume losses and a fall in arterial pressure stimulate release of ACTH via receptors in the right atrium and the carotid artery.

4.1.4.5 OTHER HORMONES

Atrial natriuretic factor (ANF) or peptide (ANP) is a hormone produced by the atria, along with brain or B-type natriuretic peptide (BNP) produced by the ventricular muscle cells, in response to an increase in vascular volume and thus distension and pressure.[7] ANF and BNP produce similar increases in glomerular filtration and pronounced natriuresis and diuresis to decrease intravascular volume by inhibition of aldosterone which also minimizes kaliuresis.

ANF and BNP also emphasize the heart's function as an endocrine organ.

4.1.5 Effects of the Various Mediators

4.1.5.1 HYPERDYNAMIC STATE

Following illness or injury, the systemic inflammatory response occurs, in which there is an increase in activity of the cardiovascular system, reflected as tachycardia, widened pulse pressure, and a greater cardiac output. There is an increase in the metabolic rate, with an increase in oxygen consumption, increased protein catabolism, and hyperglycaemia.

The cardiac index may exceed 4.5 L/min/m² after severe trauma in those patients able to respond. Ideally, decreases in vascular resistance accompany this increased cardiac output and there is an increase in oxygen delivery to the microcirculation. This hyperdynamic state elevates the resting energy expenditure to more than 20% above normal, total body oxygen consumption (VO_2) is increased and, due to the increase in metabolism, core temperature is increased. With an inadequate response, and a cardiac index of less than 2.5 L/min/m², oxygen consumption may fall to values of less than 100 mL/min/m² (normal = 120–160 mL/min/m²). Endotoxins and anoxia may injure cells and limit their ability to utilize oxygen for oxidative phosphorylation.

The amount of adenosine triphosphate (ATP) synthesized by an adult is considerable. However, there is no reservoir of ATP or creatinine phosphate, and therefore, cellular injury and lack of oxygen results in rapid deterioration of processes requiring energy, and lactate is produced. Because of anaerobic glycolysis, only two ATP equivalents instead of 34 are produced from one mol of glucose in the Krebs cycle. Lactate is formed from pyruvate, which is the end-product of glycolysis. It is normally reconverted to glucose in the Cori cycle in the liver. However, in shock, the oxidation reduction (redox) potential declines and conversion of pyruvate to acetyl co-enzyme A for entry into the Krebs cycle is inhibited. Lactate therefore accumulates because of impaired hepatic gluconeogenesis, causing a metabolic acidosis.

Lactic acidosis after injury correlates with the ISS, and is an early and important clinical sign of acute blood loss, reflecting tissue hypoperfusion. Persistent lactic acidosis is indicative of inadequate resuscitation and predictive of the development of MOF and adult respiratory distress syndrome (ARDS).[8]

4.1.5.2 WATER AND SALT RETENTION

Secretion of ADH from the supra-optic nuclei in the anterior hypothalamus is stimulated by volume reduction and increased osmolality of the circulation. The latter is due mainly to increased sodium content of the extracellular fluid. Volume receptors are in the atria and pulmonary arteries, and osmoreceptors are located near ADH neurones in the hypothalamus. ADH acts mainly on the connecting tubules of the kidney but also on the distal tubules to promote reabsorption of water.

Aldosterone acts mainly on the distal renal tubules to promote reabsorption of sodium and bicarbonate and increased excretion of potassium and hydrogen ions.

Aldosterone also modifies the effects of catecholamines on cells, thus affecting the exchange of sodium and potassium across all cell membranes. The release of large quantities of intracellular potassium into the extracellular fluid may cause a significant rise in serum potassium especially if renal function is impaired. Retention of sodium and bicarbonate may produce metabolic alkalosis with impairment of the delivery of oxygen to the tissues. After injury, urinary sodium excretion may fall to 10–25 mmol/24 hours and potassium excretion may rise to 100–200 mmol/24 hours.

4.1.5.3 EFFECTS ON SUBSTRATE METABOLISM

4.1.5.3.1 Carbohydrates

Critically ill patients develop a glucose intolerance, which resembles that found in diabetic patients. This is a result of both increased mobilization and decreased uptake of glucose by the tissues. The turnover of glucose is increased, and the serum glucose is higher than normal.

As blood glucose rises during the phase of hepatic gluconeogenesis, blood insulin concentration rises, sometimes to very high levels. Provided that the liver circulation is maintained, gluconeogenesis will not be suppressed by hyperinsulinaemia or hyperglycaemia, because the accelerated rate of glucose production in the liver is required for clearance of lactate and amino acids, which are not able to be used for protein synthesis. This period of breakdown of muscle protein for gluconeogenesis and the resultant hyperglycaemia characterizes the catabolic phase of the metabolic response to trauma.

The glucose level following trauma should be monitored carefully in the intensive care unit (ICU). The optimum blood glucose level remains controversial, but the maximum level should be 10 mmol/L (see also Chapter 15). Excessive levels of glucose correlate directly with infectious complications, particularly in surgical or injury wounds. Control of the blood glucose is best achieved by titration with intravenous insulin, based on a sliding scale. However, because of the degree of insulin resistance associated with trauma, the quantities required may be considerably higher than normal. Nevertheless, over-aggressive control of blood glucose increases the risk of hypoglycaemia and must be avoided.

Enteral nutrition is preferred but parenteral nutrition may be required, and this will exacerbate the problem. However, glucose remains the safest energy substrate following major trauma: 60%–75% of the caloric requirements should be supplied by glucose, with the remainder being supplied as a fat emulsion.

4.1.5.3.2 Fat

A major source of energy following trauma is adipose tissue. Lipids stored as triglycerides in adipose tissue are mobilized when insulin falls below 25 units/mL. Initially, because of the suppression of insulin release by the catecholamine spike after trauma, as much as 200–500 g of fat may be broken down early after severe trauma.[9]

Catecholamines and glucagon activate adenyl cyclase in the fat cells to produce cyclic adenosine monophosphate (cyclic AMP). This activates lipase, which promptly hydrolyses triglycerides to release glycerol and fatty acids. Growth hormone and cortisol play a minor role in this process as well. Glycerol provides substrate for gluconeogenesis in the liver, which derives energy by β-oxidation of fatty acids, a process inhibited by hyperinsulinaemia.

The free fatty acids provide energy for all tissues and for hepatic gluconeogenesis.

4.1.5.3.3 Amino Acids

The intake of protein by a healthy adult is between 80 and 120 g of protein: 1 to 2 g protein/kg/day. This is equivalent to 13–20 g of nitrogen per day. In the absence of an exogenous source of protein, amino acids are principally derived from the breakdown of skeletal muscle protein. Following trauma or sepsis, the release rate of amino acids increases by three to four times. The process manifests as marked muscle wasting.

Cortisol, glucagon, and catecholamines play a role in this reaction. The mobilized amino acids are utilized for gluconeogenesis or oxidation in the liver and other tissues, but also for synthesis of acute-phase proteins required for immuno-competence, clotting, wound healing, and maintenance of cellular function.

After severe trauma or sepsis, as much as 20 g/day of urea nitrogen is excreted in the urine. Since 1 g urea nitrogen is derived from 6.25 g degraded amino acids, this protein wastage is up to 125 g/day.

One gram of muscle protein represents 5 g wet muscle mass. The patient in this example, would be losing 625 g of muscle mass per day. A loss of 40% of body protein is usually fatal, because failing immunocompetence leads to overwhelming infection. Nitrogen excretion usually peaks several days after injury, returning to normal after several weeks. This is a characteristic feature of the metabolic response to illness. The most profound alterations in metabolic rate and nitrogen loss occur after burns and may persist for months.

4.1.5.3.4 The Gut

The intestinal mucosa requires rapid synthesis of amino acids. Depletion of amino acids results in atrophy of the mucosa causing failure of the mucosal barrier. This may lead to bacterial translocation from the gut to the portal system. The extent of bacterial translocation in trauma has not been defined.[10] The presence of food in the gut lumen is a major stimulus for mucosal cell growth. Food intake is invariably interrupted after major trauma, and the supply of glutamine may be insufficient for mucosal cell growth. Early nutrition (within 24–48 hours), and early enteral rather than parenteral feeding may prevent or reduce these events.

4.1.6 **The Anabolic Phase**

During this phase the patient is in positive nitrogen balance, regains weight, and restores fat deposits. The hormones, which contribute to anabolism, are growth hormones, androgens, and 17 beta-ketosteroids. The utility of growth hormone, and more recently, of insulin-like growth factor (IGF-1), in reversing catabolism following injury is critically dependent on adequate caloric intake.

4.1.7 **Clinical and Therapeutic Relevance**

Survival after injury depends on a balance between the extent of cellular damage, the efficacy of the metabolic response, and the effectiveness of treatment.

Tissue injury, hypoxia, pain, and toxins from invasive infection add to the initiating factor of hypovolaemia. The degree to which the body can compensate for injury is astonishing, although sometimes the compensatory mechanisms may work to the patient's disadvantage. Adequate resuscitation to shut off the hypovolaemic stimulus is important. However, once hormonal changes have been initiated, the effects of the hormones will not cease merely because hormonal secretion has been turned off by replacement of blood volume.

Mobilization and storage of the energy fuel substrates, carbohydrate, fats, and protein is regulated by insulin, balanced against catecholamines, cortisol, and glucagon. However, infusion of hormones has failed to cause more

than a modest response. Rapid resuscitation, maintenance of oxygen delivery to the tissues, removal of devitalized tissue or pus, and control of infection are the cornerstones. The best metabolic therapy is excellent surgical care.

4.2 **SHOCK**

4.2.1 **Definition of Shock**

Shock is defined as inadequate delivery of oxygenated blood to the tissues, resulting in cellular hypoxia. This at first leads to reversible ischaemic-induced cellular injury. If the process is sufficiently severe or protracted, it ultimately results in irreversible cellular and organ injury and dysfunction. The precise mechanisms responsible for the transition from reversible to irreversible injury and death of cells are not clearly understood, although the biochemical/morphological sequence in the progression of ischaemic cellular injury has been well elucidated.[11] By understanding the events leading to cell injury and death, we may be able to intervene therapeutically in shock by protecting sub-lethally injured cells from irreversible injury and death.

4.2.2 **Classification of Shock**

The classification of shock is of practical importance if the pathophysiology is understood in terms that make a fundamental difference in treatment. Although the basic definition of shock, 'insufficient nutrient flow', remains inviolate, six types of shock, based on a distinction not only in the pathophysiology, but also in the management of the patients, are recognized:

1. Hypovolaemic.
2. Cardiogenic.
3. Cardiac compressive (e.g. cardiac tamponade).
4. Distributive (previously inflammatory) (e.g. septic shock).
5. Neurogenic.
6. Obstructive (e.g. mediastinal compression).

In principle, the physiological basis of shock is based on the following:

$$\text{Cardiac Output} = \text{Stroke Volume} \times \text{Heart Rate}$$

$$\text{Blood Pressure} \propto \text{Cardiac Output}$$
$$\times \text{TotalPeripheral Resistance}$$

Table 4.1 Classes of Hypovalaemic Shock

Class	% Blood Loss	Volume	Pulse Rate	Blood Press.	Pulse Press.	Resp. Rate
Class I	15	<750 mL	<100	Normal	Normal	14–20
Class II	30	750–1500 mL	>100	Normal	Increased	20–30
Class III	40	2000 mL	>120	Decreased	Narrowed	30–40
Class IV	>40	>2000 mL	>140	Decreased	Narrowed	>35

Stroke volume is determined by the pre-load, the contractility of the myocardium, and by the afterload.

4.2.2.1 HYPOVOLAEMIC SHOCK

Hypovolaemic shock is caused by a decrease in the intravascular volume. This results in significant degeneration of both pressure and flow. It is characterized by significant decreases in filling pressures with a consequent decrease in stroke volume. Cardiac output is temporarily maintained by a compensatory tachycardia. With continuing hypovolaemia, the blood pressure is maintained by reflex increases in peripheral and, importantly, splanchnic vascular resistance and myocardial contractility mediated by neurohumoral mechanisms.

Hypovolaemic shock is divided into four classes (see Table 4.1).

Initially, the body compensates for shock, and Class I and Class II shock is compensated shock. When the blood volume loss exceeds 30% (Class III and Class IV shock), the compensatory mechanisms are no longer effective and the decrease in cardiac output causes a decreased oxygen transport to peripheral tissues. These tissues attempt to maintain their oxygen consumption by increasing oxygen extraction. Eventually, this compensatory mechanism also fails, and tissue hypoxia leads to lactic acidosis, hyperglycaemia, and failure of the sodium pump with swelling of the cells from water influx.

4.2.2.1.1 Clinical Presentation

The classic features of hypovolaemic shock are hypotension, tachycardia, pallor secondary to vasoconstriction, sweating, cyanosis, hyperventilation, confusion, and an oliguria. Cardiac function can be depressed without gross clinical haemodynamic manifestations. The heart shares in the total body ischaemic insult. Systemic arterial hypotension increases coronary ischaemia, causing rhythm disturbances and decreased myocardial performance. As the heart fails, left ventricular end-diastolic pressure rises, ultimately causing pulmonary oedema. Hyperventilation may maintain arterial PaO$_2$ at near normal levels but the PaCO$_2$ falls to 20–30 mm Hg (2.7–4 kPa). Later, pulmonary insufficiency may supervene from alveolar collapse and pulmonary oedema, resulting from damaged pulmonary capillaries, cardiac failure, or inappropriate fluid therapy.

Renal function is also critically dependent on renal perfusion. Oliguria is an inevitable feature of hypovolaemia. During volume loss, renal blood flow falls correspondingly with the blood pressure. Anuria sets in when the systolic blood pressure falls to around 50 mm Hg. Thus, urine output is a good indicator of peripheral perfusion. Oliguria in the hypovolaemic patient is a sign of renal success not failure.

4.2.2.2 CARDIOGENIC SHOCK

When the heart fails to produce an adequate cardiac output, even though the end diastolic volume is normal, cardiogenic shock is said to be present. Intravascular obstructive shock results when intravascular obstruction, excessive stiffness of the arterial walls, or obstruction of the microvasculature imposes an undue burden on the heart. The obstruction to flow can be on either the right or the left side of the heart. Causes include pulmonary embolism, air embolism, ARDS, aortic stenosis, calcification of the systemic arteries, thickening or stiffening of the arterial walls as a result of the loss of elastin and its replacement with collagen (as occurs in old age), and obstruction of the systemic microcirculation as a result of chronic hypertension or the arteriolar disease of diabetes.

Cardiac function is often impaired in shocked patients even if myocardial damage is not the primary cause. Reduced myocardial function in shock includes dysrhythmias, myocardial ischaemia from systemic hypotension and variations in blood flow, and myocardial lesions from high circulatory levels of catecholamines, angiotensin, and other myocardial depressant factors, such as DAMPs and other inflammatory mediators.

The reduced cardiac output can be a result of:

- Reduced stroke volume.
- Impaired myocardial contractility due to ischaemia, reperfusion induced oedema, infarction, cardiomyopathy or direct trauma.
- Altered ejection fraction.
- Coronary air embolism.
- Mechanical complications of acute myocardial infarction – acute mitral valvular regurgitation, ventricular septal rupture, or trauma.
- Arrhythmias.
- Conduction system disturbances (bradydysrhythmias and tachydysrhythmias).

Other forms of cardiogenic shock include those clinical examples in which the patient may have a nearly normal resting cardiac output but cannot raise the cardiac output under circumstances of stress because of poor myocardial reserves or an inability to mobilize those myocardial reserves due to pharmacologic beta-adrenergic blockade, for example propanolol for hypertension. Heart failure and dysrhythmias are discussed in depth elsewhere in this book.

4.2.2.2.1 Clinical Presentation

The clinical picture will depend on the underlying cause. Clinical signs of peripheral vasoconstriction are prominent, pulmonary congestion is frequent, and oliguria is almost always present. Pulmonary oedema may cause severe dyspnoea, central cyanosis, and crepitations, audible over the lung fields and lung oedema visible on x-rays. A systolic murmur appearing after myocardial infarction suggests mitral regurgitation or septal perforation.

Haemodynamic findings consist of a systolic arterial pressure less than 90 mm Hg, decreased cardiac output, usually less than 1.8 L/min/m², and a pulmonary arterial wedge pressure (PAWP) of greater than 20 mm Hg. However, cardiogenic shock can occur without the PAWP being elevated. This may be a result of excess diuretic therapy, plasma volume depletion by fluid lost into tissues (i.e. third spacing), or blood loss. Patients with relative hypovolaemia below the levels where there is a risk of pulmonary oedema, and, patients with significant right ventricular failure will also not have elevated PAWP. These patients, although their shock is cardiogenic, will respond dramatically to plasma volume expansion and will deteriorate if diuresis is attempted.

4.2.2.3 CARDIAC COMPRESSIVE SHOCK

The pathophysiology of cardiac compressive shock is very different from cardiogenic shock. External forces compress the thin-walled chambers of the heart (the atria and the right ventricle), the great veins (systemic or pulmonary), or any combination of these. Impaired diastolic filling will result. Clinical conditions capable of causing compressive shock include pericardial tamponade, tension pneumothorax, positive pressure ventilation with large tidal volumes or high airway pressures (especially in a hypovolaemic patient), an elevated diaphragm (as in pregnancy), displacement of abdominal viscera through a ruptured diaphragm, and the abdominal compartment syndrome (e.g. from ascites, abdominal distension, abdominal or retroperitoneal bleeding, or a stiff abdominal wall, as in a patient with deep burns to the torso).

The consequence of this compression is an increase in right atrial pressure, without an increase in volume, impeding venous return and reducing end diastolic volumes and provoking hypotension.

4.2.2.3.1 Clinical Presentation

Cardiac tamponade follows blunt or penetrating trauma and is a classic example of compressive cardiac shock. As a result of the presence of blood in the pericardial sac, the atria are compressed and cannot fill adequately. The systolic blood pressure is less than 90 mm Hg, there is a narrowed pulse pressure and a pulsus paradoxus exceeding 10 mm Hg. Distended neck veins may be present, unless the patient is hypovolaemic as well. Heart sounds are muffled. The limited compliance of the pericardial sac means that a very small amount (<25 mL blood) may be enough to cause decompensation. Similarly, tension pneumothorax can also produce compressive heart failure. In the patient with chest trauma and hypotension, the problem usually can be identified immediately, from decreased breath sounds, hyper-resonance of the affected side, and displacement of the trachea to the opposite side. Neck veins also may be distended. Immediate release of the tension, prior to waiting for an x-ray is required to prevent cardiac arrest.

4.2.2.4 DISTRIBUTIVE (INFLAMMATORY) SHOCK

Dilatation of the capacitance reservoirs in the body occurs with endotoxic shock, or prolonged hypovolaemic shock. Endotoxin can have a major effect on this form of peripheral pooling and even though the blood volume is normal, the distribution of that volume is changed so that there is insufficient nutrient flow to meet aerobic metabolism needs.

Ultimately, all shock leads to cellular defect shock. Aerobic metabolism takes place in the cytochrome system in the cristae of the mitochondria. Oxidative phosphorylation in the cytochrome system produces high-energy phosphate bonds by coupling oxygen and glucose, forming the freely diffusable by-products carbon dioxide and water. Several poisons uncouple oxidative phosphorylation but the most common in clinical practice is endotoxin. Sepsis is frequent in hospitalized patients and endotoxic shock is distressingly common. There is fever; tachycardia may or may not be present, the mean blood pressure is usually below 60 mm Hg, yet the cardiac output varies between 3 and 6 L/m²/min. This haemodynamic state is indicative of low peripheral vascular resistance.

In addition to maldistribution of blood volume due to increase in capacitance and low peripheral resistance as causes of hypotension in septic shock, other causes inhibiting the cardiovascular system maintenance of cardiac output at a level enough to maintain normal blood pressure in sepsis include:

- Hypovolaemia due to fluid translocation from the blood into interstitial spaces.
- Elevated pulmonary vascular resistance owing to ARDS.
- Bioventricular myocardial depression manifested by reduced contractility and an inability to increase stroke-work.

The ultimate cause of death in septic shock is failure of energy production at the cellular level as reflected by a decline in oxygen consumption. It is not only the circulatory insufficiency that is responsible for this, but also the impairment of cellular oxidative phosphorylation by endotoxin or endogenously produced superoxides. There is a narrowing of arterial-mixed venous oxygen difference as an indication of reduced oxygen extraction, which often precedes the fall of cardiac output. Inadequate oxidative phosphorylation leads to anaerobic glycogenolysis and a severe metabolic acidosis owing to lactate.

4.2.2.5 NEUROGENIC SHOCK

Neurogenic shock is a hypotensive syndrome in which there is loss of α-adrenergic tone and dilatation of the arterial and venous vessels. The cardiac output is normal, or may even be elevated, but because the total peripheral resistance is reduced, the patient is hypotensive. The consequence is a reduced perfusion pressure. In trauma it often occurs owing to spinal cord injury.

A simple example of this type of shock is syncope ('vaso-vagal syncope'). It is caused by a strong vagal discharge resulting in dilatation of the small vessels of the splanchnic bed. The next cycle of the heart has less venous return so that the ventricle will not fill, and the next stroke volume does not adequately perfuse the cerebrum, causing a faint. No blood is lost, but there is a sudden increase in the amount of blood trapped in one part of the circulation where it is no longer available for perfusion to an obligate aerobic glycolytic metabolic bed – the central nervous system.

4.2.2.5.1 Clinical Presentation

Commonly seen with high spinal cord injury, the patient usually has weakly palpable peripheral pulses, warm extremities, brisk capillary filling, and may be anxious. The pulse pressure is wide, with both systolic and diastolic blood pressure being low. Heart rate is below 100 beats per minute, and there may even be a bradycardia. However, the diagnosis of neurogenic shock should only be made once other causes of shock have been ruled out, since the common cause is injury, and there may be other injuries present causing a hypovolaemic shock in parallel.

4.2.2.6 OBSTRUCTIVE SHOCK

Intravascular obstructive shock results when intravascular obstruction, excessive stiffness of the arterial walls, or obstruction of the microvasculature imposes an undue burden on the heart. Because of the decreased venous return, the atrial filling is reduced with consequent hypotension. The obstruction to flow can be on either the right or the left side of the heart. Causes include pulmonary embolism, air embolism, ARDS, aortic stenosis, calcification of the systemic arteries, thickening or stiffening of the arterial walls as a result of the loss of elastin and its replacement with collagen (as occurs in old age), and obstruction of the systemic microcirculation as a result of chronic hypertension or the arteriolar disease of diabetes. The blood pressure in the pulmonary artery or the aorta will be high; the cardiac output will be low.

4.2.3 **Measurements in Shock**

In physics, flow is directly related to pressure and inversely related to resistance. This universal flow formula is not dependent on the type of fluid and is applied to the flow of electrons. In electricity, it is expressed as Ohm's law. This law applies just as appropriately to blood flow.

$$Flow = \frac{Pressure}{Peripheral\ resistance}$$

From this law it can be deduced that shock is just as much a state of elevated resistance as it is a state of low blood pressure. However, the focus should remain on flow rather than simply on pressure, since most drugs that result in a rise in pressure do so by raising the resistance, which in turn decreases flow while simultaneously increasing work and oxygen consumption by the myocardium.

4.2.3.1 CARDIAC OUTPUT

Blood flow is dependent on cardiac output. Three factors determine cardiac output:

- Pre-load or the volume entering the heart.
- Contractility of the heart.
- After-load or the resistance against which the heart must function to deliver the nutrient flow.

These three factors are interrelated to produce the systolic ejection from the heart. Up to a point, the greater the pre-load, the greater the cardiac output. As myocardial fibres are stretched by the pre-load the contractility increases according to the Frank-Starling principle. However, an excessive increase in pre-load leads to symptoms of pulmonary/systemic venous congestion without further improvement in cardiac performance. The pre-load is a positive factor in cardiac performance up the slope of the Frank-Starling curve, but not beyond the point of cardiac decompensation.

Contractility of the heart is improved by inotropic agents. The product of the stroke volume and the heart rate equals the cardiac output. Cardiac output acting against the peripheral resistance generates the blood pressure. Diminished cardiac output in patients with pump failure is associated with a fall in blood pressure. To maintain coronary and cranial blood flow there is a reflex increase in systemic vascular resistance to raise blood pressure. An exaggerated rise in systemic vascular resistance can lead to further depression of cardiac function by increasing ventricular after-load. After-load is defined as the wall tension during left ventricular ejection and is determined by systolic pressure and the radius of the left ventricle. Left ventricular radius is related to end-diastolic volume, and systolic pressure to the impedance to blood flow in the aorta, or total peripheral vascular resistance.

However, the critical emphasis in the definition of shock is on flow, we need to find improved methods to measure flow.

4.2.3.2 INDIRECT MEASUREMENT OF FLOW

In many patients in shock, simply laying a hand upon their extremities will help to determine flow by the cold clammy appearance of hypoperfusion owing to increased resistance. Probably the most important clinical observation to indirectly determine adequate nutrient flow to a visceral organ will be the urine output.

The kidney responds to decreased nutrient flow with several compensatory changes to protect its own perfusion. Over a range of blood pressure, the kidneys maintain a nearly constant blood flow. If the blood pressure decreases, the kidney's autoregulation of resistance results in dilatation of the vascular bed. It keeps nutrient flow constant by lowering the resistance even though the pressure has decreased. This allows selective shunting of blood to the renal bed.

For practical purposes, if a patient is producing a normal quantity of normal quality urine, then they are not in shock.

Another vital perfusion bed that reflects the adequacy of nutrient flow is the brain itself. Since adequate nutrient flow is a necessary, but not the only requirement for cerebration, normal consciousness also can be used to evaluate the adequacy of nutrient flow in the patient with shock.

4.2.3.3 DIRECT MEASUREMENTS

4.2.3.3.1 Central Venous Pressure

Placement of a central venous line that will allow accurate measurement of the hydrostatic pressure of the right atrium following fluid boluses can help differentiate between the different shock states. The actual measurement, except at the extremes, is frequently inaccurate in determining intravascular volume and less important than the change in value, especially in the acute resuscitation of a patient. Normal is 4–12 cm water. A value below 4 cm indicates that the venous system is empty, and thus the pre-load is reduced, usually as a result of dehydration or hypovolaemia (blood loss), while a high value indicates that the pre-load is increased, either as a result of a full circulation or due to pump failure (e.g. cardiogenic shock due to aetiologies such as tension pneumothorax, cardiac tamponade, or myocardial contusion).

Generally, if a patient in shock has both systemic arterial hypotension and central venous hypotension, the shock is due to volume depletion. On the other hand, if central venous pressure is high though arterial pressure is low, shock is not due to volume depletion and is more likely due to pump failure.

4.2.3.3.2 Routes

Cannulation of the central venous system is generally achieved using the subclavian, jugular, or femoral route.

4.2.3.3.2.1 *Subclavian Access*

The subclavian route is preferred in the trauma patient, particularly when the status of the cervical spine is unclear. Ultrasonic guidance is not required, as visualization of the anatomy may be difficult. It is ideal for the intensive care setting, where occlusion of the access site against infection is required. Lines are easy to secure, and the incidence of line sepsis is lower than any other route. Pitfalls include arterial puncture and pneumothorax.

4.2.3.3.2.2 *Internal Jugular Access*

The internal jugular route or, occasionally, the external jugular route is the one most commonly utilized by anaesthesiologists, preferably under ultrasonic guidance. It provides ease of access, especially under operative conditions. However, there are significant dangers in the trauma patient, especially where the cervical spine has not yet been cleared, and other routes may be preferable. The ability to occlude the jugular site, especially in the awake patient in the ICU, is however, more limited, and there is greater discomfort for the patient.

4.2.3.3.2.3 *Femoral Access*

The femoral route is easy to access, especially when the line also will be used for venous transfusion. However, the incidence of femoral vein thrombosis is high, and the line should not be left beyond 48 hours because of the risk of infection. Pitfalls include placing the cannula inside the abdominal cavity. This can be particularly misleading if blood is present inside the abdominal cavity, since aspiration of the cannula will yield blood, and a false sense of security! The use of ultrasound can reduce catheter insertion complications.

4.2.3.3.3 Systemic Arterial Pressure

Systemic arterial pressure reflects the product of the peripheral resistance and the cardiac output. Measurement can be indirect or direct.

Indirect measurement involves the use of a blood pressure cuff with auscultation of the artery to determine systolic and diastolic blood pressure.

Direct measurement involves placement of a catheter into the lumen of the artery, with direct measurement of the pressure.

In patients in shock, with an elevated systemic vascular resistance, there is often a significant difference obtained between the two measurements. In patients with increased vascular resistance, low cuff pressure does not necessarily indicate hypotension. Failure to recognize this may lead to dangerous errors in therapy.

Cannulation of the brachial artery is not recommended because of the potential for thrombosis and for ischaemia of the lower arm and hand.

4.2.3.3.4 Pulmonary Arterial Pressure

The right-sided circulation is a valveless system through which flows the entire cardiac output from the right side of the heart. It is rarely used in the initial resuscitation phase.

4.2.3.3.5 Cardiac Output

Cardiac output can be measured with the thermodilution technique.[12] A thermodilution pulmonary artery catheter has a thermistor at the distal tip. When a given volume of a solution that is cooler than the body temperature is injected into the right atrium, it is carried by the blood past the thermistor, resulting in a transient fall in temperature. The temperature curve so created is analyzed, and the rate of blood flow past the thermistor (i.e. cardiac output) can be calculated. By measuring the mixed oxygen saturation in the pulmonary artery, blood oxygen extraction across the circulation can be determined.

4.2.4 **Endpoints in Shock Resuscitation**[13]

The ultimate measurement of the impact of shock must be at the cellular level. The most convenient measurement is a determination of the blood gases.

Measurement of PaO_2, $PaCO_2$, pH, base deficit (BD), and arterial lactate will supply information on oxygen delivery and utilization of energy substrates. Both PaO_2 and $PaCO_2$ are concentrations – partial pressure of oxygen and carbon dioxide in arterial blood. If the $PaCO_2$ is normal, there is adequate alveolar ventilation. CO_2 is one of the most freely diffusable gases in the body and is not overproduced or under-diffused. Consequently, its partial pressure in the blood is a measure of its excretion through the lung, which is a direct result of alveolar ventilation. The PaO_2 is a similar concentration but it is the partial pressure of oxygen in the blood and not the oxygen content. A concentration measure in the blood does not tell us the delivery rate of oxygen to the tissues per unit of time without knowing something of the blood flow that carries this concentration.

For evaluation of oxygen utilization, however, data are obtainable from arterial blood gases that can indicate what the cells are doing metabolically, which is the most important reflection of the adequacy of their nutrient flow. The pH is the hydrogen ion concentration, which can be determined easily and quickly. Loss of buffering by base excess also mirrors excess acid load. Nevertheless, the pH, BD, and the two carbon fragment metabolites are very important indicators of cellular function in shock.

In shock, there is a fundamental shift in metabolism. When there is adequate nutrient flow, glucose and oxygen are coupled to produce in glycolysis the high-energy phosphate bonds necessary for energy exchange. This process of aerobic metabolism also produces two freely diffusable by-products – carbon dioxide and water – both of which leave the body by excretion through the lungs and the kidneys. Aerobic metabolism is efficient, therefore, there is no accumulation of any products of this catabolism, and a high yield of ATP is obtained from this complete combustion of metabolites.

When there is inadequate delivery of nutrients and oxygen, as occurs in shock, the cells shift to anaerobic metabolism within 3–5 minutes. There are immediate consequences of anaerobic metabolism in addition to its inefficient yield of energy. In the absence of aerobic metabolism, energy extraction takes place at the expense of accumulating hydrogen ion, lactate, and pyruvate, which have toxic effects on normal physiology. These products of anaerobic metabolism can be seen as the 'oxygen debt'. There is some buffer capacity in the body that allows this debt to accumulate within limits, but it must ultimately be shut off by adequate oxygen and nutrient delivery.

Acidosis has significant consequences in compensatory physiology. Oxyhaemoglobin dissociates more readily as hydrogen ions increase; however, there is a significant toxicity of hydrogen ions as well. Despite the salutary effect on oxyhaemoglobin dissociation, the hydrogen ion has a negative effect on oxygen delivery. Catecholamines speed up the heart's rate and increase its contractile force, and the product of this inotropic and chronotropic effect is an increase in cardiac output. Catecholamines, however, are physiologically effective at alkaline or neutral pH. Therefore, an acid pH inactivates this catecholamine method of compensation for decreased nutrient flow. Lactate acidosis in the best single predictor of blood loss initially, and inadequate restoration of homeostasis after several hours in the ICU.

4.2.5 Post-Shock and Multiple Organ Failure Syndromes

Although the primary consequences of sepsis following trauma and shock is the development of multiple organ failure as discussed elsewhere in this book, it is important to briefly reiterate the usual sequence of events following shock to enable logical discussion of the management of shock.

The ultimate cause of death in shock is failure of energy production as reflected by a decline in oxygen consumption (VO_2) to less than 100 mL/min/m². Circulatory insufficiency is responsible for this fall in energy, compounded by impairment of cellular oxidative phosphorylation by endotoxin and endogenously produced substances, such as toxic oxides.

In shock, whether hypovolaemic or septic, energy production is insufficient to satisfy cellular requirements. In the presence of oxygen deprivation and cellular injury, the conversion of pyruvate to Acetyl Co-enzyme A (Acetyl CoA) for entry into the Krebs cycle is inhibited. Lactic acid accumulates and the oxidation reduction potential falls. Although lactate is normally used by the liver via the Cori cycle to synthesize glucose, hepatic gluconeogenesis may fail in hypovolaemic or septic shock because of hepatocyte injury and inadequate circulation. Terminally, the lactic acidosis cannot necessarily be corrected by improvement of circulation and oxygen delivery once the cells are irreparably damaged.

In the low-output shock-state, plasma concentrations of free fatty acids and triglycerides rise to high levels because ketone production by beta-oxidation of fatty acids in the liver is reduced, suppressing the acetoacetate-to-betahydroxybutarate ratio in the plasma.

The post-shock sequel of inadequate nutrient flow, therefore, is progressive loss of function. The rate at which this loss occurs depends upon the cell's ability to switch metabolism, to convert alternate fuels to energy, the increased extraction of oxygen from haemoglobin, and the compensatory collaboration of failing cells and organs whereby nutrients may be shunted selectively to more critical systems. Not all cells are equally sensitive to shock nor similarly refractory to restoration of function when adequate nutrient flow is restored. As cells lose function, the reserves of the organ composed of those cells are depleted until impaired function of the organ results. These organs function in systems and a 'system failure' results. Multiple systems failure occurring in sequence leads to the collapse of the organism.

4.2.6 **Management of the Shocked Patient**

The primary goal of shock resuscitation is the early establishment of adequate oxygen delivery (DO_2). The calculated variable of DO_2 is the product of cardiac output, and arterial oxygen content (CaO_2).

By convention, CO is indexed to body surface area and expressed as a cardiac index (CI), and when multiplied by CaO_2, yields an oxygen delivery index (DO_2I). Normal DO_2I is roughly 450 mL/min/m^2.

CaO_2 and DO_2I are calculated as follows:

$$CaO_2(mL \cdot O_2/dL = [Hb](g/dL.) \times 1.38\,mL \cdot O_2/g\,Hb$$
$$\times SaO_2(\%) + [PaO_2(mm\,Hg) \times 0.003\,mL \cdot O_2/mm\,Hg]$$

$$DO_2I(mL/min/m^2) = CI(L/min/m^2)$$
$$\times CaO_2(mL/dL) \times 10dL/L$$

where
Hb   haemoglobin concentration
SaO_2 haemoglobin oxygen saturation
PaO_2 arterial oxygen tension
0.003   solubility of O_2 in blood.

Early work demonstrated that the 'survivor' response to traumatic stress is to become hyperdynamic. Supranormal resuscitation based on the DO_2I was therefore proposed. Subsequent randomized controlled trials have failed to demonstrate improved outcomes with goal

directed supranormal therapy, and, in fact, this strategy increased ACS, MOF, and death.

Best practice guidelines for shock resuscitation are summarized by the large-scale collaborative project called 'Glue Grant' that provides standard operating procedures for clinical care. The 'Glue Grant' study for shock resuscitation suggests using a CI >3.8 L/min/m^2 as the resuscitation goal.[14]

The purpose for distinguishing the different pathophysiologic mechanisms of shock becomes important when treatment must be initiated. The final aim of treatment is to restore aerobic cellular metabolism. This requires restoration of adequate flow of oxygenated blood (which is dependent on optimal oxygenation of sufficient red blood cells, i.e. haematocrit and adequate cardiac output). The initial focus is securing a patent airway and controlling ventilation to prevent inadequate alveolar ventilation and oxygenation.

Restoration of optimal circulating blood volume, enhancing cardiac output using inotropic agents and/or mean arterial pressure (MAP) through vasopressors, the correction of acid-base disturbances and metabolic deficits, and the combating of sepsis, are all vital in the management of the shocked patient.

4.2.6.1 OXYGENATION

The severely traumatized, hypovolaemic, or septic patient has an oxygen demand that may exceed twice the normal. However, the traumatized shocked patient usually cannot generate the additional respiratory effort required, and therefore often develops respiratory failure followed by a lactic acidosis owing to tissue hypoxaemia.

In some patients, an oxygen mask may be enough to maintain oxygen delivery to the lungs. In more severe cases, endotracheal intubation and ventilatory assistance may be necessary. It is important to distinguish between the need for *intubation*, and the need for *ventilation*. Early intubation is preferable to cardiac collapse.

4.2.6.1.1 Airway Indications for Intubation

- Obstructed airway.
- Inadequate gag reflex.

4.2.6.1.2 Breathing Indications for *Intubation*

- Inability to breathe. (e.g. paralysis, either spinal or drug induced).
- Tidal volume less than 5 mL/kg.

4.2.6.1.3 Breathing Indications for *Ventilation*

- Inability to oxygenate adequately.
- PaO$_2$ less than 60 mm Hg (7.9 kPa) on 40% O$_2$ or SpO$_2$ of less than 90% on oxygen.
- A respiration rate of 30 breaths or more per minute and excessive ventilatory effort.
- A PaCO$_2$ of greater than 45 (6 kPa) mm Hg with metabolic acidosis, or greater than 50 mm Hg (6.6 kPa) with normal bicarbonate levels.

4.2.6.1.4 Circulation Indication for Intubation

- Systolic blood pressure less than 75 mm Hg despite resuscitation.

4.2.6.1.5 Disability Indications for Intubation

- High spinal injury with inability to breathe.
- Coma (GCS <9/15).

4.2.6.1.6 Environmental Indication for Intubation

- Core temperature of <32°C.

If ventilatory support is instituted the goals are relatively specific.

The respiratory rate should be adjusted to ensure a PaCO$_2$ of between 35 and 40 mm Hg (4.6–5.3 kPa). This will avoid respiratory alkalosis and a consequential shift of the oxyhaemoglobin dissociation curve to the left, which results in an increased haemoglobin affinity for oxygen, and significantly decreases oxygen availability to tissues, which will require increased cardiac output to maintain tissue oxygenation. Respiratory alkalosis also causes vasoconstriction of cerebral vessels and a further decrease in oxygen delivery to the CNS. For this reason, hyperventilation and hypocapnoea are no longer seen as appropriate for the management of brain injury.

The arterial PaO$_2$ should be maintained between 80–100 mm Hg (10.6–13.2 kPa) with the lowest possible inspired oxygen concentration.

It has also been shown that increased respiratory effort requires a disproportionate share of the total cardiac output for the respiratory muscles and, therefore, other organs are deprived of necessary blood flow and lactic acidosis is potentiated. Mechanical ventilation tends to reverse this lactic acidosis.

4.2.6.2 **FLUID THERAPY FOR VOLUME EXPANSION**

The preferred in hospital strategy is balanced blood component therapy. In the pre-hospital setting this strategy is also implemented in some countries (primarily Helicopter Emergency Services (HEMS) operations). Crystalloid, that is, Ringer lactate should be discouraged in the initial treatment of trauma patients, if balanced blood component therapy is available.

4.2.6.2.1 Hypotensive Resuscitation

In 1994, Bickell et al.[15] concluded that patients with penetrating torso trauma in hypovolaemic shock who were not given intravenous (i.v.) fluids during transport and emergency department evaluation had a better chance of survival than those who received conventional volume resuscitation. However, the only difference in survival was in the subgroup with pericardial tamponade. In animal studies, intravenous fluids have been shown to inhibit platelet aggregation, dilute clotting factors, modulate the physical properties of thrombus, and cause increases in blood pressure that can mechanically disrupt clots. Thus, the benefit of restricted resuscitation volumes was possibly because the reduced blood pressure limited the amount of blood loss. However, in the typical civilian trauma centre, blunt trauma is the most common form of injury and inadequate resuscitation leads to further organ injury due to inadequate oxygen delivery, particularly with traumatic brain injury (TBI). Thus, while the ideal approach is not known, the optimum systolic blood pressure for a patient with uncontrolled haemorrhage appears to be approximately 90 mm Hg, MAP should be approximately 70 mm Hg, for both the military environment, and, likely, the civilian setting also. However, a pre-hospital study by Schreiber et al. suggests the benefit of an even lower systolic blood pressure of 70 mm Hg.[16] Care must be exercised in cardiac patients and the elderly.

4.2.6.3 **ROUTE OF ADMINISTRATION**

4.2.6.3.1 Intravenous devices

In principle, with all intravenous lines, the shorter the line and the wider the diameter of the cannula, the faster will be the flow. For the same bore of line, flow rates are reduced:

14 G via peripheral cannula	Full flow
14 G via 20 cm central line	33% reduction in flow
14 G via 70 cm central line	50% reduction in flow

A minimum of two lines are required in the severely injured or hypotensive patient. In all cases of hypovolaemic shock, two large bore peripheral lines are essential. A central line is most useful for monitoring but can be used for transfusion as well. The monitoring line should be a central venous line, inserted ideally via the subclavian route. The subclavian route is preferable, since this approach avoids any movement of the head in a patient whose neck has not yet been cleared. The jugular and femoral routes are less preferable because of issues in securing the lines, and earlier sepsis at the insertion site owing to movement.

4.2.6.3.1.1 *Intraosseous Devices*

Intraosseous infusion is the process of injecting directly into the marrow of a bone to provide a non-collapsible entry point into the venous system. This technique is used in emergency and military situations to provide fluids and medication when intravenous access is not feasible. A comparison of intravenous, intramuscular, and intraosseous routes of administration concluded that in children, the intraosseous route is demonstrably superior to the intramuscular route, and comparable to the intravenous route.[17]

Insertion in adults requires less than a minute, and flow rates of up to 125 mL/min have been achieved. The devices are for emergency resuscitation and should be removed within 24 hours.

Suitable devices include the B.I.G.® gun (WaisMed, Houston, TX, USA) and the EZ-IO® (Vidacare Corp., San Antonio, TX, USA).

4.2.6.4 PHARMACOLOGIC SUPPORT OF BLOOD PRESSURE

Stroke volume is controlled by ventricular preload, after-load, and contractility. Ventricular preload is influenced primarily by the volume of circulating blood, but after-load and contractility can be enhanced by pharmacological agents. Reducing the systemic vascular resistance with vasodilators can be a very effective means of improving cardiac output when systemic pressures or cardiac filling pressures are normal or elevated, but is not currently recommended for acute trauma.

4.2.6.4.1 Noradrenaline (Norepinephrine)

The preferred inotropic agent for acute trauma is noradrenaline (norepinephrine). It is a sympathetic neurotransmitter with potent inotropic effects. It activates myocardial β-adrenergic receptors and vascular α-adrenergic receptors. It is used in the treatment of shock and hypotension characterized by low systemic vascular resistance and is unresponsive to fluid resuscitation.

4.2.6.4.2 Adrenaline (Epinephrine)

Adrenaline is a natural catecholamine with both α- and β-adrenergic agonist activity. The pharmacological actions are complex, and it can produce the following cardiovascular responses:

- Increased systemic vascular resistance.
- Increased systolic and diastolic blood pressure.
- Increased electrical activity in the myocardium.
- Increased coronary and cerebral blood flow.
- Increased strength of myocardial contraction.
- Increased myocardial oxygen requirement.

The primary beneficial effect of adrenaline is peripheral vasoconstriction, with improved coronary and cerebral blood flow. It works as a chronotropic and inotropic agent. The initial dose is 0.03 μg/kg/min, titrated upwards until the desired effect is achieved.

4.2.6.4.3 Dopamine

Dopamine hydrochloride is a chemical precursor, of noradrenaline, that stimulates dopaminergic, β_1-adrenergic and α-adrenergic receptors in a dose dependent fashion. Low doses of dopamine (<3 μg/kg/min) produce cerebral, renal, and mesenteric vasodilatation, and venous tone is increased. Urine output is increased, but there is no evidence to show that this is in any way protective to the kidneys.

At doses above 10 μg/kg/min, however, the α-adrenergic effects predominate. This results in marked increases in systemic vascular resistance, pulmonary resistance, and increases in preload due to marked arterial, splanchnic, and venous constriction. It increases systolic blood pressure without increasing diastolic blood pressure or heart rate.

Dopamine is used for haemodynamically significant hypotension in the absence of hypovolaemia.

4.2.6.4.4 Dobutamine

Dobutamine is a synthetic sympathomimetic amine that has potent inotropic effects by stimulating β_1- and α_1-adrenergic receptors in the myocardium. Dobutamine mediated increases in cardiac output also lead to a decrease in peripheral vascular resistance. At a dose of 10 μg/kg/min, dobutamine is less likely to induce tachycardia than either adrenaline or isoproterenol. Higher doses may produce a tachycardia. Dobutamine increases cardiac output and its lack of induction of noradrenaline release means that there is a minimal effect on myocardial oxygen demand. There is also increased coronary blood flow. Dobutamine in low doses has also been used as a renal protective agent. There is little evidence to support its use on its own, but it may be helpful in improving renal perfusion as an adjunct to the administration of high dose adrenaline

Dobutamine and dopamine have been used together. The combination of moderate doses of both (7.5 μg/kg/min) maintains arterial pressure with less increase in pulmonary wedge pressure than dopamine alone.

4.2.7 Prognosis in Shock

The prognosis of the shocked patient depends on the duration of the shock, the underlying cause, and the pre-existing vital organ function. The prognosis is best when the duration is kept short by early recognition and aggressive correction of the circulatory disturbance and when the underlying cause is known and corrected.

Occasionally, shock does not respond to standard therapeutic measures. Unresponsive shock requires an understanding of the potential occult causes of persistent physiologic disturbances.

These correctable causes include:

- Under-appreciated volume losses with inadequate fluid resuscitation and a failure to assess the response to a fluid challenge.
- Erroneous presumption of overload when cardiac disease is also present.
- Hypoxia caused by inadequate ventilation, barotrauma to the lung, pneumothorax, or cardiac tamponade.
- Undiagnosed or inadequately treated sepsis.
- Uncorrected acid-base or electrolyte abnormalities.
- Endocrine failure like adrenal insufficiency or hypothyroidism.
- Drug toxicity.

4.2.8 Recommended Protocol for Shock

4.2.8.1 MILITARY EXPERIENCE

Recent military experience from the Iraq war has shown the value of 'damage control resuscitation.'[18] (See also

Chapter 6: Damage Control.) This implies that damage control techniques are used from the time of injury, minimizing the time between injury and care, controlling the bleeding and contamination through use of minimal clear fluids, early fresh whole blood, early resuscitation, and early damage control surgery. The military use of whole blood has minimized some of the risks of component therapy and has also shown that survival is improved. From this philosophy has come the change in protocol in civilian practice towards minimizing crystalloid resuscitation (restrictive or limited resuscitation; not hypotensive) and early use of blood and blood products to maintain the normal coagulation profile as much as possible.

4.2.8.2 INITIAL RESUSCITATION

A. Major trauma patients arriving in shock (SBP <90 mm Hg and/or HR >130 bpm) are initially considered to be in haemorrhagic shock. Correction should be aimed at damage control through surgical control of bleeding, and damage control resuscitation (see also Chapter 6).

B. Patients with major torso trauma requiring ongoing resuscitation should have a central venous line placed in the emergency department when time allows for it.

C. Early CVP >15 mm Hg (before extensive volume loading) suggests cardiogenic or cardiac compressive shock.

D. CVP <10 mm Hg despite volume loading suggests ongoing bleeding. Endpoints are currently vague. At present the rational compromise is volume limited resuscitation (SBP = 90 mm Hg and HR <130 bpm) with moderate volume loading until haemorrhage is controlled.

E. Patients at risk for trauma induced coagulopathy (TIC) should have a massive transfusion protocol initiated (see also Section 5.7).

REFERENCES AND RECOMMENDED READING

References

1. Cuthbertson D. Observations on disturbance of metabolism produced by injury of the limbs. *Q J Med.* 1932;**25**:233–6.
2. Lilly MP, Gann DS. The hypothalamic-pituitary-adrenal immune axis. *Arch Surg.* 1992;**127(12)**:1463–74.

3. Kapur MM, Jain P, Gidh M. The effect of trauma on serum C3 activation, and its correlation with Injury Severity Score in man. *J Trauma*. 1986;**26(5)**:464–6.

4. Bianchi ME. DAMPS, PAMPS and alarmins: all we need to know about danger. *Journal of Leukocyte Biology* 2007;**81**:1–5.

5. Zhang Q, Raoof M, Chen Y, Sumi Y, Sursal T, Junger W, Brohi K, Itagaki K, Hauser CJ. Circulating mitochondrial DAMPS cause inflammatory responses to injury. *Nature* 2010;**464**:104–7.

6. Porte D, Robertson RP. Control of insulin by catecholamines, stress, and the sympathetic nervous system. *Federal Proceedings* 1973;**32**:1792–6.

7. Needleman P, Greenwald JF. Atriopeptin: a cardiac hormone intimately involved in fluid, electrolyte and blood pressure homeostasis. *New Engl J Med*. 1986;**314**:828–34.

8. Roumen RMH, Redl H, Schlag G, et al. Scoring systems and blood lactate concentrations in relationship to the development of adult respiratory distress syndrome and multiple organ failure in severely traumatized patients. *J Trauma*. 1993;**35**:3349–55.

9. Shaw JHF, Wolfe RR. An integrated analysis of glucose, fat and protein metabolism in severely traumatized patients: Studies in the basal state and the response to total parenteral nutrition. *Ann Surg*. 1989;**209(1)**:63–72.

10. Moore FA, Moore EE, Poggetti R, McAnena OJ, Peterson VM, Abernathy CM, et al. Gut bacterial translocation via the portal vein: A clinical perspective with major torso trauma. *J Trauma*. 1991 May;**31(5)**:629–36; discussion 636-8.

11. Teplitz C. The pathology, ultrastructure of cellular injury, inflammation in the progression, outcome of trauma sepsis, shock. In: Clowes GHA Ed. *Trauma Sepsis and Shock*. New York: Marcel Dekker Inc. 1988;71–120.

12. Elkayam U, Berkley R, Asen S, et al. Cardiac output by thermodilution technique. *Chest* 1983;**84**:418–22.

13. Gump FE. Whole body metabolism. In: Altura BM, Lefer AM, Shumer W. (eds), *Handbook of shock and trauma*. Vol I. Basic sciences. New York Raven Press, 1983;89–113.

14. Moore FA, McKinley BA, Moore EE, Nathens AB, West M, Shapiro M et al. Inflammation and the Host Response to Injury Large Scale Collaborative Research Program III. Guidelines for shock resuscitation. *Journal of Trauma* 2006;**61(1)**:82–9.

15. Bickell WH, Wall MJ, Pepe PE. Immediate versus delayed resuscitation for hypotensive patients with penetrating torso injuries. *New England Journal of Medicine* 1994;**331**:1105–7.

16. Schreiber MA, Meier EN, Tisherman SA, Kerby JD, Newgard CD, Brasel K, et al. ROC Investigators. A controlled resuscitation strategy is feasible and safe in hypotensive trauma patients: results of a prospective randomized pilot trial. *J Trauma Acute Care Surg*. 2015 Apr;**78(4)**:687–95;3.2.9.2.

17. Moore GP, Pace SA, Busby W. Comparison of intraosseus, intramuscular, and intravenous administration of succinyl choline. *Pediatric Emergency Care* 1989;**5(4)**:209–10.

18. Holcomb JB, Jenkins D, Rhee P, Johannigman J, Mahoney P, Mehta S, et al. Damage control resuscitation: directly addressing the early coagulopathy of trauma. *J Trauma*. 2007;**62(2)**:307–10.

Recommended Reading

Advanced Cardiovascular Life Support Provider manual. American Heart Association. Dallas, Texas. 2010.

Marino PL. *The ICU Book*. Wolters Kluver Hearlt / Lippincott Williams and Wilkins. Philadelphi PA, USA. 2014.

Rhodes A, Evans LE, Alhazzani W, Levy MM, Antonelli M, Ferrer R, et al. Surviving Sepsis Campaign: International Guidelines for Management of Sepsis and Septic Shock: 2016. *Intensive Care Med*. 2017 Mar;**43(3)**:304–77. doi: 10.1007/s00134-017-4683-6. Epub 2017 Jan 18.

Transfusion of blood and blood components is a fundamental part of trauma management and approximately 40% of the 13 million units of blood transfused in the United States each year are used in emergency resuscitation. Despite this, there is limited evidence to provide a rationale for administration of packed red blood cells (pRBCs) to trauma patients.

5.1 INDICATIONS FOR TRANSFUSION

5.1.1 Oxygen-Carrying Capacity

Anaemia is a decrease in the O_2-carrying capacity of blood, defined by a decrease in circulating red cell mass (to below 24 mL/kg in females and 26 mL/kg in males). Anaemia will result in an increase in cardiac output at a haemoglobin (Hb) level of <7 g/dL (4.0 mmol/L). Oxygen extraction increases as O_2 delivery falls, ensuring a constant O_2 uptake by the tissues. Normal humans can survive an 80% loss of red cell mass if they are normovolaemic and normothermic. The threshold for O_2 delivery to maintain adequate tissue oxygenation, is at a haematocrit of 10% and a Hb level of 3 g/dL (1.8 mmol/L) when breathing 100% O_2 and with a normal metabolic rate.

Volume-dependent markers (such as haematocrit and Hb) are poor indicators of anaemia because of the effect of dilution after fluid transfusion on their values, that is, they are relative values.

5.2 TRANSFUSION FLUIDS

5.2.1 Colloids

5.2.1.1 STARCHES

The use of starches is contraindicated in the actively bleeding patient, since starches deplete the von Willebrand/factor VIII complex, and may make the actively bleeding patient more coagulopathic from both factor depletion and dilution coagulopathy. Hydroxyethyl starch is an independent risk factor for acute kidney injury and death after blunt trauma.

5.2.1.2 ALBUMIN

Human albumin has not been evaluated for acute resuscitation, although animal experimentation suggests it may be appropriate. The Saline versus Albumin Fluid Evaluation (SAFE) study in 2007, tested saline versus albumin in the intensive care unit (ICU) and suggested an increased mortality in trauma patients and particularly in patients with traumatic brain injury (TBI). Albumin is not routinely used in trauma resuscitation.[1]

5.2.2 Blood

5.2.2.1 FRESH WHOLE BLOOD (FWB)

Humans are O_2-dependent organisms, and O_2 depletion causes major damage within minutes. Thus, in the exsanguinating patient, red blood cells (RBCs) are transfused in order to improve O_2 transport, although older blood does not carry oxygen well. Evidence from military and civilian trauma studies has suggested the advantage of fresh whole blood (FWB) in the resuscitation and survival of the exsanguinating patient.[2] The rationale is that fresh whole blood has more function than purely that of an O_2 transport medium and provides:

- Oncotic pressure (from plasma).
- Clotting factors and platelets (PLT).
- Temperature homeostasis (from warm circulating fluid).
- Fresh whole blood offers blood at close to 37°C, RBCs, plasma, and platelets in natural proportions,

to cover the need of the exsanguinating patient for O_2 and oncotic pressure. A 500 mL unit of FWB has:

- A haematocrit of 38%–50%.
- 50,000–400,000/mm³ fully functional platelets.
- 100% activity of clotting factors diluted only by the anticoagulant.
- Excellent oxygen carrying ability.

In addition, the viability and flow characteristics of fresh RBCs are better than their stored counterparts that have metabolic depletion and membrane dysfunction. However, FWB, unless in a military environment with availability of large numbers of healthy, pre-screened, young blood carriers, is generally not available. The levels of clotting factors V and VIII in FWB decline quickly for 24 hours after collection. The rate of decline then slows until clinically subnormal levels are reached within 7–14 days. It is because FWB contains these factors and is so effective in the correction of coagulopathy, that it is recommended for massive transfusion. The other clotting factors remain stable in stored blood. Fresh whole blood has lost most of its platelets after 3 days of storage. Fresh whole blood can, if warmed, be transfused within 24 hours, and considered still fresh if stored at 4°C for 48 hours.

5.2.2.2 PACKED RED BLOOD CELLS

Previous haemorrhage management transfused excessive amounts of crystalloids, which diluted native clotting factors, causing hypocoagulation.[3] This additional fluid aggravated the coagulopathy initiated from the moment of injury due to:

- Loss of warm blood and replacement with cooler fluid, resulting in decreased body temperature.
- Hypoperfusion, resulting in anaerobic metabolism, increased lactic acid production, and a decrease in pH.

Biochemical reactions within the body require a specific and narrow temperature and pH range to proceed. The coagulation cascade does not proceed, even in the presence of all the clotting factors, when the tissue pH is below 7.2 and temperature below 34°C. These factors are called trauma induced coagulopathy (TIC),[4] and differs from disseminated intravascular coagulopathy, which may develop after hours or days, when the septic component adds its consequences to trauma.

5.2.3 Component Therapy (Platelets, Fresh Frozen Plasma, Cryoprecipitate)

5.2.3.1 PLATELETS

A fall in platelet count occurs somewhat later than the loss of clotting factors. Hypothermia affects platelet adhesion more than enzymes, above 34°C, while hypothermia affects all aspects of coagulation below 34°C. There is general agreement that the indications for platelet transfusion are:

- *Prophylaxis*: If the platelet count <15,000/mm.
- *Pre-surgery*: Platelet count <50,000/mm³.
- *Active bleeding*: Platelet count <100,000/mm³.
- 1 unit increases the platelet count by 10,000/mm³ platelets.

1 (5 units) mega-unit of apheresis platelets increases the platelet count by 50,000/mm³.

5.2.3.2 FRESH FROZEN PLASMA

Massively bleeding trauma patients will need fresh frozen plasma (FFP) early. This is different from most recommendations, which are based on more controlled circumstances, and is founded on computer simulation of the amount of FFP required to avoid excessive plasma dilution compromising haemostasis.

Current evidence suggests that most patients will require 1 unit of FFP for every unit of blood transfused. A unit of FFP also contains most of the citrate anticoagulant from the unit of blood from which it was originally derived. It contains about 0.5 g fibrinogen, and normal levels of pro- and anticoagulants. Solvent-detergent-related/freeze-dried plasma carries about 20% less of the above per unit given. Potential advantages are:

- It contains all coagulation factors, but not all in equal concentration.
- It is preferred to cryoprecipitate, which contains 50% content of most normal coagulation factors, with the exception of fibrinogen, factor VIII and von Willebrand factor.

5.2.3.3 CRYOPRECIPITATE

Cryoprecipitate contains fibrinogen, von Willebrand factor/factor VIII complex, and fibrin stabilizing factor XIII. Cryoprecipitate may not be required in all cases of trauma. One unit (250 mL) of FFP contains 0.5 g fibrinogen; 1 unit of cryoprecipitate contains 0.25 g fibrinogen, but in 10 mL (rather than 250 mL). Therefore, in most cases, FFP will meet the needs required. However, if a rapid increase in the amount of fibrinogen is required, cryoprecipitate is a useful adjunct.

The CRYOSTAT trials are currently in progress: CRYOSTAT-1 was a feasibility study, which suggested that early cryoprecipitate therapy maintained acceptable blood fibrinogen levels during active bleeding, with a signal for reduced mortality in the treatment arm of the study. CRYOSTAT-2 will test the effect of early cryoprecipitate (within 90 minutes of admission) compared to standard blood transfusion therapy and is due for completion in 2020.

5.2.3.4 FIBRINOGEN CONCENTRATE

Fibrinogen concentrate can be used to correct acquired hypofibrinogenaemia in trauma. There are several guidelines, but evidence is lacking regarding treatment efficacy and safety in trauma.

5.3 EFFECTS OF TRANSFUSING BLOOD AND BLOOD PRODUCTS

Stored pRBCs (stored for a maximum of 42 days with current US Food and Drug Administration approved storage solutions) develop defects proportionate to the duration of storage that assume greater clinical significance when transfused rapidly, or in large quantities, such as in critically ill patients.

5.3.1 Metabolic Effects

- There is a storage related decreased ATP which precedes red blood cell membrane deformability and its survival during storage.
- Degradation of 2,3-diphosphoglycerate (2,3-DPG) has occurs after 7–10 days in storage. 2,3-DPG is an enzyme affecting the affinity of Hb for O_2. After 7 days of storage, the O_2-transporting ability of Hb drops by two-thirds. Adenine added to pRBCs may restore levels of 2,3-DPG *in vivo* after transfusion.
- Increased ammonia release occurs owing to the release of intracellular protein after disruption of the red cell membrane during storage.

5.3.2 Effects of Microaggregates

This remains controversial; however, microfilters are no longer used during transfusion to remove microaggregates or red cell debris after membrane rupture. Microaggregates are created from:

- Red cell membrane instability which leads to cell rupture.
- Increased amounts of microaggregates (platelets/leukocytes/fibrin debris) in the buffy coat.
- Impaired pulmonary gas exchange and adult respiratory distress syndrome (ARDS) and transfusion-related lung injury (TRALI) can occur.
- Reticulo-endothelial system (RES) depression.
- Activation of complement and coagulation cascades.
- Production of vasoactive substances.
- Antigenic stimulation.
- Acute-phase response.

5.3.3 Hyperkalaemia

Serum potassium levels rise in stored blood as the efficiency of the Na^+/K^+ pump decreases. Transfused blood may have a potassium concentration of >40 mmol/L. Transient hyperkalaemia may occur as a result, but often does not need correction.

5.3.4 Coagulation Abnormalities

Fresh frozen plasma contains all the clotting factors of the coagulation cascade. Thawed plasma is FFP brought to 4°C and stored for 5 days, this timeline being based on the lifetime of factors V and VIII. Recent studies have shown that thawed plasma stored at this temperature retains significant clotting function for up to 14 days.

- Thrombocytopenia and a loss of factors V and VIII in stored blood may contribute to the coagulopathy. Platelets have a short half-life, and their functioning is usually minimal after 3–5 days of storage.
- Levels of clotting factors V and VIII decline quickly for 24 hours after collection. The rate of decline slows until clinically subnormal levels are reached at 7–14 days.
- Packed red cells do not contain platelets as these are generally spun off, and whole blood has lost most of its platelets after 3 days of storage. Spontaneous bleeding rarely occurs if the platelet count is greater

than 30,000/mm³. Levels as low as this are seen after the replacement of one to two times the total blood volume and may result from dilution. Despite this, the body has large reserves of platelets, sequestrated in the spleen, liver, and endothelium that are mobilized when there is a need.

- In whole blood, platelets may contribute to microaggregates that find their way to the lungs. Their presence is less evident in packed red cells. Transfusion of pooled platelets carries a greater risk of infection, as several donors have contributed to a single pack of platelets.

It is important to detect trauma induced coagulopathy as early as possible, and coagulation tests, such as prothrombin time/international ratio (PT/INR), activated partial thromboplastin time (APTT), fibrinogen concentration, and platelet counts have traditionally been used. However, there is a striking lack of evidence to support the use of conventional coagulation tests (CCTs) to monitor blood component use in trauma. Increasingly, the transfusion of blood components is guided by viscoelastic haemostatic assays (VHA) such as thrombo-elastography (TEG or RoTEM). This is most relevant where surgical bleeding is controlled; however, in the face of continued bleeding, despite surgical control, blood products may need to be given empirically. VHA may be performed at point of care and provide results within minutes.

5.3.5 Other Risks of Transfusion

5.3.5.1 TRANSFUSION-TRANSMITTED INFECTIONS

- Hepatitis A, B, C, and D.
- Human immunodeficiency virus 'window period'.
- Cytomegalovirus.
- Atypical mononucleosis and a swinging temperature that can be present for 7–10 days post-transfusion.
- Malaria.
- Brucellosis.
- Yersinia.
- Syphilis.

5.3.5.2 HAEMOLYTIC TRANSFUSION REACTIONS

- Incompatibility: ABO, rhesus (blood type), and 26 other surface antigens (screen for these).
- To very cold blood, overheated blood, or pressurized blood.
- Immediate generalized reaction (plasma).

5.3.5.3 IMMUNOLOGICAL COMPLICATIONS

- Major incompatibility reaction (usually caused by 'wrong blood' owing to administrative errors).
- Graft-versus-host disease: TRALI.
- Immunomodulation: reports on transplant and oncology patients have provided evidence that transfusion induces a regulatory immune response in the recipient that increases the ratio of suppressor to helper T cells. These changes may render the trauma patient more susceptible to infection.

5.3.5.4 FACTORS IMPLICATED IN HAEMOSTATIC FAILURE

- *Hypothermia*: Blood is stored at 4°C, but body temperature is 37°C, so the body needs to provide 1255 kJ of energy to heat each unit of blood to body temperature.
- Acidosis (from citrate and lactate).
- Dilution, depletion, and decreased production of red cells and platelets.
- *Diffuse intravascular coagulation*: There is a consumption of clotting factors and platelets within the circulation, which are trapped in the microvascular thrombi created due to fibrin disposition.
- *Extrinsic*: Tissue thromboplastins, for example, blunt trauma and surgery, and burns.
- *Intrinsic*: Endothelial injury, endotoxin, hypothermia, hypoxia, acidosis, and platelet activation.
- Fibrinolysis.
- Consumption of red cells and platelets.
- Protein C activation.

Despite the extensive list quoted above, there is limited evidence regarding the risks of pRBC transfusion, although pRBC transfusion is an independent risk factor for:

- Increased nosocomial infections (wound infection, pneumonia, sepsis).
- Multiple organ failure and systemic inflammatory response syndrome.
- Longer ICU and hospital length of stay, increased complications, and increased mortality.
- Pre-storage leukocyte depletion of RBC transfusion reduces complication rates, some studies showing a reduction in infectious complications.
- There is a relationship between transfusion and TRALI and ARDS.
- Transfusion and pRBC and FFP increase the risk for DVT in trauma patients.

Blood has effects and side effects, some of which are 'bad', and we should use it in a rational and restrictive way in most patients. In trauma haemorrhage, there is no good alternative so far and prioritizing balanced transfusion as part of haemostatic resuscitation secures clotting and oxygenation. The less 'bad' blood may be FWB, and its surrogate components transfusion (which amounts to a reconstitution of whole blood). However, FWB is not generally available outside the military context, and may be logistically difficult to obtain in civilian practice.

5.4 CURRENT BEST TRANSFUSION PRACTICE

5.4.1 Initial Response

1. Aggressively pursue the diagnosis and treatment of haemorrhage.
2. Titrate administered fluids to maintain a lower than normal blood pressure (hypotensive resuscitation), until control of haemorrhage is achieved (see also Chapter 6).
3. Measure and closely follow serum lactate and arterial pH as indicators of the state of systemic perfusion.
   - If normal, attempt to maintain perfusion.
   - If abnormal, attempt a gradual improvement without elevating the blood pressure and aggravating the haemorrhage.
4. Maintain normothermia.
5. Control ventilation to achieve O_2 saturation of 99%–100% and a normal end-tidal carbon dioxide level.
6. Aim for a target Hb of 7–9 g/dL (4–5.5 mmol/L) and a normal prothrombin time at the time that haemorrhage is controlled. Consider maintaining a higher Hb concentration in older patients and in those with known ischaemic disease.
7. If massive transfusion is likely, attempt from the outset to maintain the composition of whole blood. Use early RBC, plasma, and platelet transfusion.

Blood pressure and heart rate are the current standard-of-care monitors of shock resuscitation in the field, and in the emergency department when associated with serum lactate or base excess (base deficit). Both are, however, insensitive markers of early compensated shock; alternative monitors are needed for assessing the adequacy of tissue perfusion, with a view to avoiding both under-resuscitation and over-resuscitation. The challenge is to identify as early as possible those patients who are not responding to early interventions. Blind and aggressive volume loading in the hope of normalizing blood pressure and heart rate, without appropriate emphasis on the control of haemorrhage, sets the stage for the so-called bloody vicious cycle, the abdominal compartment syndrome, or multiple organ failure (MOF).

5.4.2 Reduction in the Need for Transfusion

Blood is a scarce (and expensive) resource and is also not universally safe. Reducing the need for transfusion is the best way to limit complications:

- Treat the cause, that is, stop bleeding, and avoid hypothermia and acidosis.
- Treat deficiencies and complications as they arise. There is no evidence to support prophylactic therapy with FFP, platelets, etc.;[5] however, replacement of components becomes of great importance in massive transfusion.
- Follow a restrictive transfusion policy in ICU. One large multicentre trial documented a significantly lower mortality rate for critically ill patients managed with a restrictive transfusion strategy and a transfusion threshold of 7 g/dL (5 mmol/L) Hb.[6] However, this assumes normovolaemia, absence of ongoing bleeding, and an absence of pre-existing cardiovascular disease or severe brain injury.
- Develop a capacity for cell salvage.

5.4.3 Transfusion Thresholds

There is no level I evidence indicating the ideal trigger for transfusion in trauma patients. In general, the following guidelines apply:[7]

1. Identify the critically ill patient with a Hb less than 7 g/dL (5 mmol/L) or a haematocrit below 21%.
2. If the Hb is less than 7 g/dL, transfusion with pRBCs is appropriate.[8] For patients with severe cardiovascular disease, and trauma patients with ongoing bleeding or haemodynamic instability, a higher threshold of 8–10 g/dL (6–7 mmol/L) is appropriate, although this remains a non-evidence-based extrapolation of the TRICC study where they specifically excluded actively bleeding patients.
3. If the Hb is less than 7 g/dL, assess the patient for hypovolaemia. If this is found, administer

intravenous fluids to achieve normovolaemia, and reassess the Hb level.

4. If the patient is not hypovolaemic, determine whether there is evidence of impaired O_2 delivery.
5. If impaired O_2 delivery is present, consider cardiac output monitoring, using a Vigileo® (Edwards Life Sciences, Irvine, CA), or a similar monitor.
6. If impaired O_2 delivery is not present, monitor Hb as appropriate.

5.4.4 Transfusion Ratios

While principle largely favours FWB, blood component transfusion is the best feasible alternative in most civilian situations.

Military trauma[9] studies suggest transfusing pRBC:FFP:platelets in a proportion of 1:1:1, with life threatening bleeding, but the only randomized clinical trial failed to establish improved survival at 2 hours or 30 days.

The optimal ratio of RBCs to FFP remains, however, controversial. Currently, a ratio of 1:1:1/RBC:FFP: platelets appears to be reasonable.[10,11] If apheresis platelets (usually containing 5 or 6 units of platelets) are supplied, this ratio will become 5:5:1 or 6:6:1.

5.4.5 Adjuncts to Enhance Clotting

There has been extensive interest in the provision of adjuncts to enhance clotting as part of the resuscitation of the trauma patient. These include:

5.4.5.1 RECOMBINANT ACTIVATED FACTOR VII (rFVIIa)

Interest has focused on recombinant activated factor VIIa (rVIIa®) (NovoSeven). This was initially developed as an adjunct for the treatment of haemophilia. However, following its successful use in controlling the bleeding in a trauma patient, there was considerable interest in its use. A large multi-centre trial in 2005[12] showed a reduction in red cell transfusion requirements in blunt trauma patients, and the drug has been used extensively 'off-label'. A further large trial in 2008 showed a reduction in blood product usage of 3.6 units in blunt injury, but the study sample was too small to show significance on mortality, or for penetrating injury.[13] Consequently, rFVIIa is not widely used, but it is still utilized in certain countries, and in some military situations. A suitable protocol appears in Table 5.1.

5.4.5.2 TRANEXAMIC ACID (TXA)

Tranexamic acid is indicated for prolonged bleeding (empirically) or when there is evidence of hyperfibrinolysis (measured using TEG or RoTEM – see below).

The CRASH-2 trial showed a significant reduction in mortality with the use of tranexamic acid;[14] however, although the trial involved very large numbers of subjects, fewer than half the patients required red cell transfusion, in those who were transfused, the two arms utilized the same amount of blood, and the mortality rate in both arms did not correlate with that in other studies. In addition, no injury severity comparisons were included. Study of the use of TXA in the military context showed improved coagulation and survival, especially in those patients requiring massive transfusion (The MATTERs Study).[15]

However, a recent study indicated that most severely injured patients have a fibrinolysis shutdown (i.e. become hypercoagulable), so that TXA may have no effect.[16] No clear benefit has been shown when used in an urban environment, with access to major trauma centres.[17] The association between TXA treatment and an increased risk of vascular occlusive events is still unknown.

Current recommendations suggest administration of TXA:

- Within 3 hours from time of injury.
- At a dose of 1 gram intravenously administered over 10 minutes, then 1 gram intravenously administered over 8 hours.
- In adult trauma patients with severe haemorrhagic shock (SBP <75 mm Hg), with known predictors of fibrinolysis, or verified fibrinolysis by TEG (LY30).[18]

5.4.5.3 DESMOPRESSIN (DDAVP)

Desmopressin potentiates the function of platelets and is indicated only for functional platelet disorders, secondary to platelet inhibitors such as aspirin, clopidogrel, ticegrelor, prasugerl, etc., renal or hepatic failure, haemophilia-A and von Willebrand's disease.

5.4.6 Monitoring the Coagulation Status: Traditional and VHA

Ideally, the use of blood components should be guided by laboratory tests of clotting function. This is part of the concept of personalized medicine, or in trauma as

Table 5.1 Guidelines for the Use of Recombinant Activated Factor VII (rFVIIa) in Trauma

Definition

This guideline describes the use of rFVIIa as an *adjunct* in the management of coagulopathy following trauma with massive bleeding or the need to enter the massive transfusion protocol.

Issue

The blood bank will issue the required rFVIIa for administration immediately **after completion** of the 6th and 12th units of transfused blood.

Limitation

rFVIIa should **only** be used:

- **If all *surgical* bleeding has been controlled.**
- **In the presence of active bleeding.**
- **Where possible, its use should be backed up with a thromboelastogram (TEG).**
- Increased R (reaction) time despite fresh frozen plasma.
- After transfusion of >6 units of blood.
- If the platelet count is >50,000/mm³.
- If the pH is >7.2.
- If the temperature is >34°C.

Blood specimens

Disseminated intravascular coagulopathy screen:

- Full blood count and platelets.
- Fibrinogen.
- TEG or RoTEM or if not available.
- Prothrombin time, activated partial thromboplastin time, thrombin time, international normalized ratio, D-dimer.

Dose

The dose of rFVIIa should be 90 μg/kg, but may be as high as 120 μg/kg:

- Round UP to the nearest 1.2 mg.
  (Example: a 75 kg male receives 75 × 90 μg/kg = 6.75 mg rFVIIa. Round up to 7.2 mg.)

If the patient continues to bleed:

- Repeat the dose after 1 hour and after 3 hours from first dose.
- Repeat the dose after completion of the **12th** unit of transfused blood.

End points of administration

The first of:

- Cessation of bleeding;
  or
- Three doses.

part of the concept of goal-directed therapy, giving the patient only what is needed and avoiding transfusions that are not needed. Haemostasis, according to the cell-based model, is described in the phases of initiation, amplification, and propagation, from clot formation to clot lysis, with participation of all circulating plasmatic and cellular components. Thrombin generation is central for clot development and strength. It primarily occurs on the surface of activated platelets and, hence, platelets and thrombin generation are closely related to the development of coagulopathy.

5.4.6.1 TRADITIONAL ASSAYS

- International normalized ratio (INR) – extrinsic.
- Partial thromboplastin time (PTT) – intrinsic.
- D-dimer values (fibrinolysis).

All the above are cost effective if frequently done, but specimens are heated to the normal *in vivo* temperature of 37°C. All are time consuming. Therefore, the conventional approach is inappropriate for the hypothermic trauma patient, whose coagulation status changes rapidly with alterations in pH and temperature. Therefore, TEG/ROTEM is more effective at covering the assessment need in the trauma patient and providing an adjunct to goal-directed haemostasis.

5.4.6.2 VISCOELASTIC HAEMOSTATIC ASSAYS (VHA): THROMBOELASTOGRAPHY (TEG)/ROTARY THROMBOELASTOMEROGRAPHY (ROTEM)[19,20]

The VHA technology results in a visual profile, or trace, and variables with a reference value, see Figure 5.1a,b. Briefly, the collected whole blood sample is placed in a special designed small cup (approximately 1 cc). Inside

the cup is suspended a pin connected to a detector system (a torsion wire in TEG, an optical detector in ROTEM), and the cup and pin are oscillated relative to each other with movement initiated from either the cup (TEG) or the pin (ROTEM). As fibrin strings form between the cup and pin, the transmitted rotation from the cup to pin (TEG) or the impedance of the rotation of the pin (ROTEM) are detected at the pin and a trace is generated as seen in Figure 5.2. The standard assays are with kaolin activation in TEG, kaolin + tissue factor in RapidTEG® and tissue factor or kaolin activation, respectively, in the ExTEM and InTEM assays in ROTEM, and several other dedicated assays are available from both technologies.

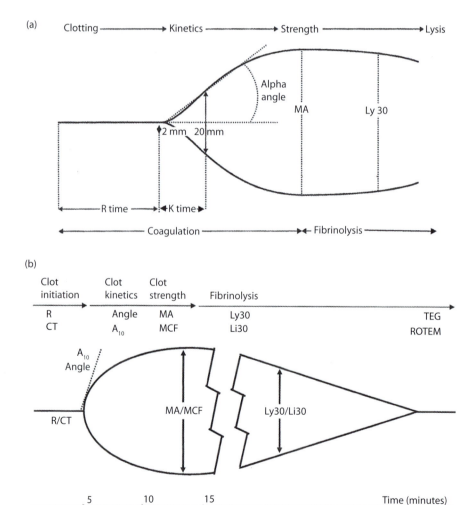

Figure 5.1 (a) Thromboelastogram. (b) RoTEM appearance. Abbreviations: α (alpha) angle, clot strength; A10, amplitude after 10 minutes; CT, clotting time; K time, kinetic time; Ly30/Li30, fibrinolysis after 30 minutes; MA, maximum amplitude – maximum clot strength; MCF, maximum clot firmness; R time, reaction time.

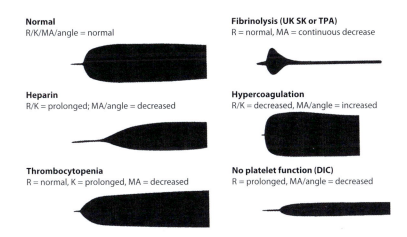

Normal
R/K/MA/angle = normal

Fibrinolysis (UK SK or TPA)
R = normal, MA = continuous decrease

Heparin
R/K = prolonged; MA/angle = decreased

Hypercoagulation
R/K = decreased, MA/angle = increased

Thrombocytopenia
R = normal, K = prolonged, MA = decreased

No platelet function (DIC)
R = prolonged, MA/angle = decreased

Figure 5.2 Abnormal appearances of the thromboelastogram. Abbreviations: DIC, disseminated intravascular coagulopathy; K, kinetic time; MA, maximum amplitude; R, reaction time; SK, streptokinase; TPA, tissue plasminogen activator; UK, urokinase.

The contribution of fibrinogen to clot strength can be evaluated in the functional fibrinogen assay in TEG and the FibTEM assay in ROTEM. VHAs are portable bedside devices but these are several advantages in running these in a standardized lab by skilled technicians.

The result is available within 3–10 minutes, in the form of a curve (Figure 5.1a or b). Several parameters can be measured (Table 5.2):

- K time (kinetic time) – the K time starts where the R time ends and ends when the curve is at 20 mm amplitude.
- MA (maximum amplitude) – the maximal clot strength.
- Ly30 – Amount of thrombolysis after 30 minutes, expressed as percent of the MA.

Table 5.2 Interpretation of the Parameters of the TEG and RoTEM

Measurement	TEG Parameter (Normal Range)	ROTEM Parameter (Normal Range)
Clotting factor activity	R time (3–8 minutes)	CT_{EXTEM} (38–79 seconds) CT_{INTEM} (100–240 seconds)
Kinetics to maximum clot strength	K time (1–3 mm)	
Rate of increase in clot strength	α (alpha) angle (55–69 degrees)	$A10_{EXTEM}$ (43–65 mm)
Maximum strength of the clot	MA (51–69 mm)	MCF_{EXTEM} (50–72 mm)
Fibrinolysis at 30 minutes	Ly30 (<4%)	LI30 (94%–100%)
Fibrinogen activity (level)	FF_{MA} (14–24 mm)	FibTEM MCF (9–16 mm)

Abbreviations: Thrombelastography (TEG) – α, alpha angle; FF_{MA}, functional fibrinogen; K, K time; Ly30, fibrinolysis after 30 minutes; MA, maximum amplitude; R, reaction time. Rotational thromboelastometry (ROTEM) – A10, amplitude after 10 minutes; Fib, fibrinogen; LI30, fibrinolysis after 30 minutes; MCF, maximum clot firmness.

- R time (reaction time)/clotting time – the latency from the time at which the blood is placed in the cup until the clot begins to form.
- The α (alpha) angle – the progressive increase in clot strength.

The VHAs allow for goal-directed haemostatic therapy, thereby only treating with what is needed. See Table 5.3 for one of several international validated algorithms. Furthermore, it is possible to decide if the bleeding is surgical or coagulopathic/pathological, which

Table 5.3 Goal-Directed Administration of Haemostatic Products and Medication, Based on TEG and ROTEM

TEG	RoTEM	Coagulopathy	Treatment Options
R 10–14 minutes	ExTEM CT 80–100 seconds InTEM CT 200–240 seconds	Coagulation factors ↓	FFP 20 mL/kg
R >14 minutes	ExTEM CT >100 seconds InTEM CT >240 seconds	Coagulation factors ↓↓	FFP 30 mL/kg rFVIIA (see Table 5.1)
FF_{MA} 7–14 mm	FibTEM MCF 6–9 mm	Fibrinogen ↓	FFP 20 mL/kg or cryoprecipitate 3 mL/kg or fibrinogen concentrate 20 mg/kg
FF_{MA} 0–7 mm	FibTEM MCF 0–6 mm	Fibrinogen ↓↓	FFP 30 mL/kg or cryoprecipitate 5 mL/kg or fibrinogen concentrate 30 g/kg
K (kinetic) time	>4 minutes		Cryoprecipitate 5 mL/kg or fibrinogen concentrate 30 mg/kg or rFVIIA (see Table 5.1)
α angle	<65°		Cryoprecipitate 5 mL/kg or fibrinogen concentrate 30 mg/kg or DDAVP
MA 45–49 mm and FF_{MA} >14 mm	ExTEM A_{10} 35–42 mm and FibTEM ≥10 mm ExTEM MCF <50 mm and FibTEM ≥10 mm	Platelets ↓	Platelets 5 mL/kg
MA <45 mm and FF_{MA} >14 mm	ExTEM A_{10} <35 mm and FibTEM ≥10 mm	Platelets ↓↓	Platelets 10 mL/kg
Ly30 >3 (−8) %	ExTEM Li 30 <94%	Hyperfibrinolysis	TXA 10 Gm or 10–20 mg/kg
Difference in R Hep TEG versus standard TEG R >2 minutes	InTEM CT/HepTEM CT > 1,25	Heparinization	Protamine 50–100 mg or FFP 10–20 mL/kg

Abbreviations: TXA, tranexamic acid; FFP, fresh frozen plasma; rFVIIA, recombinant factor VIIa.

clotting factors are missing, the function of platelets, and whether fibrinolysis is evolving normally. Transfusion of blood components, coagulation factors and additional medication can be administered rationally, based on the results.

The TEG offers substantial support to decision-making during the resuscitation, as it gives real-time accurate information on the coagulation status of the trauma patient, and facilitates the differentiation between pathological abnormality, and surgically correctable bleeding.

5.5 **AUTOTRANSFUSION**

Intra-operative and post-operative blood salvage and alternative methods for decreasing transfusion may lead to a significant reduction in allogenic blood usage.

Autotransfusion eliminates the risk of incompatibility and the need for crossmatching; the risk of transmission of disease from the donor is also eliminated. Autotransfusion is a safe and cost-effective method of sustaining RBC mass while decreasing demands on the blood bank. However, cell salvage in trauma patients is logistically challenging as, in the trauma patient, autotransfusion typically involves the collection of blood shed into wounds, body cavities – especially the chest, and drains.

Modern autotransfusion devices are basically of two types:

* Collection of blood that is collected, anticoagulated with heparin or citrate, and then run through a system in which it is washed and centrifuged, before being re-transfused.

 Reinfusion after filtration is less labour intensive and provides blood for transfusion quickly. Whole blood is returned to the patient with platelets and proteins intact, but free Hb and procoagulants are also reinfused. A high proportion of the salvaged blood is returned to the patient, and the most recent devices do not require mixing of the blood with an anticoagulant solution. In-line filters are essential when autotransfusion devices are used. These filters remove gross particles and macroaggregates during collection and reinfusion, thus minimizing microembolization.[21]

* Cell-washing and centrifugation techniques require a machine and (usually) a technician to be the sole operator. This latter requirement can limit the utility of the devices in everyday practice. The cell washing

cycle produces red cells suspended in saline with a haematocrit of 55%–60%. This solution is relatively free of free Hb, procoagulants and bacteria. However, bacteria have been shown to adhere to the iron in the Hb molecule and washing therefore does not eliminate the risk of infection.

To a degree, the simpler the system, the less likely it is that problems will occur. In elective situations, nurses, technicians or anaesthesia personnel can participate in the autotransfusion process. In emergency situations without additional personnel, such participation may not be possible. Systems that process reclaimed RBCs may require trained technicians, particularly if the procedure is used infrequently.

In practical terms, bleeding from the chest seems ideal for immediate autotransfusion as the contents of thoracic cavity are sterile, in contrast with abdominal bleeding, where visceral injury and contamination may coexist. The simplest effective method is to use the sterile chest drain container. Use saline to create the fluid valve at the end of a chest drainage tube, to which is added 1000 IU fractionated heparin. The contents of the bottle may be hung and (using a microfilter to collect microaggregates) immediately reintroduced intravenously.

Autotransfusion is generally contraindicated in the presence of bacterial or malignant cell contamination (e.g. open bowel, infected vascular prostheses, etc.), unless no other RBC source is available, and the patient is in a life-threatening situation. However, there are several studies showing the practice may not be as unreasonable as previously thought.[22]

Cell salvage techniques have been shown to be cost-effective and useful in some trauma patients (e.g. in splenic trauma with significant blood loss), but further studies are indicated to clarify the indications.

5.6 **RED BLOOD CELL SUBSTITUTES**[23]

The ideal pRBC substitute is cheap, has a long shelf-life, is universally compatible and well tolerated, and has an O_2 delivery profile identical to that of blood. Significant effort has been made to find a suitable substitute that could, essentially, be treated as an artificial O_2 carrier.

Artificial O_2 carriers can be grouped into perfluorocarbon (PFC) emulsions and modified Hb solutions. The native Hb molecule needs to be modified in order to decrease its O_2 affinity and to prevent rapid dissociation of the native $alpha_2$–$beta_2$ tetramer into $alpha_2$–$beta_2$ dimers.

5.6.1 **Perfluorocarbons**

Perfluorocarbons are carbon–fluorine compounds that are completely inert and have low viscosity but dissolve large amounts of gas. They do not mix with water and therefore need to be produced as emulsions. Unlike the sigmoid relationship of Hb, they exhibit a linear relationship with O_2; therefore, their efficacy relies on maintaining a high PaO_2; however, PFCs unload O_2 well. They do not expand the intravascular volume and can only be given in small volumes as they overload the reticulo-endothelial system. Once thought to hold potential, they have so far not been found to confer additional benefit compared with crystalloid solutions, especially as there is a significant incidence of side effects.

5.6.2 **Haemoglobin Solutions**

Although free haemoglobin can transport O_2 outside of the red cell membrane, it is too toxic to be clinically useful. Techniques have been developed to remove the need for the red cell membrane and create haemoglobin-based oxygen carriers (HBOCs).

5.6.2.1 LIPOSOMAL HAEMOGLOBIN SOLUTIONS

These are based on the encapsulation of Hb in liposomes. The mixing of phospholipid and cholesterol in the presence of Hb yields a sphere with Hb at its centre. These liposomes have O_2 dissociation curves similar to red cells, with low viscosity and their administration can transiently produce high circulating levels of Hb.

Problems associated with HBOCs relate to effects on vasomotor tone, which appears to be modulated by the carriers' interaction with nitric oxide, causing significant vasoconstriction.

5.6.2.2 POLYMERIZED HAEMOGLOBIN SOLUTIONS (HUMAN-OUTDATED/BOVINE RBCS)

Techniques have been developed for crosslinking the haemoglobin molecules, initially with a di-aspirin crosslink and recently as a haemoglobin polymer. Both human and bovine Hb have been used.

Considerable research has taken place in the past decade with regard to the development of synthesized Hb solutions. Bovine-derived Hb (Hemopure) is approved

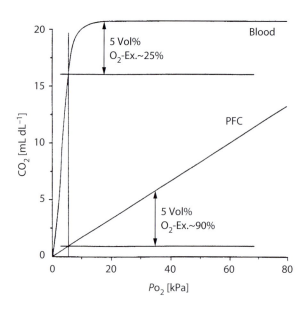

Figure 5.3 Oxygen transport characteristics of haemoglobin and perfluorocarbons.

for clinical use in South Africa. Currently, the products have not been licensed for use in the trauma patient.

The O_2 transport characteristics of modified Hb solutions and PFC solutions are fundamentally different (Table 5.3). The Hb solutions exhibit a sigmoid O_2 dissociation curve similar to that of blood, while PFC emulsions are characterized by a linear relationship between the partial pressure and the content of O_2. Haemoglobin solutions therefore provide O_2 transport and unloading characteristics similar to blood. This means that at a relatively low arterial O_2 pressure, substantial amounts of O_2 are being transported. In contrast, relatively high arterial O_2 partial pressures are necessary to maximize the O_2 transport of PFC emulsions (Figure 5.2).

Note that 5% O_2 can be offloaded by both blood and PFCs, PFC O_2 being more completely offloaded than blood-transported O_2 (Figure 5.3 and Table 5.4).

5.6.3 **Future Evolution**

The last few years' research on the use of the oxygen nanobubbles gives promising results on the reversal of tumour hypoxia that potentiates the effectiveness of therapy. Nano-engineering may open up new currently inconceivable ways to transfer oxygen to the hypoxic tissue.

Table 5.4 Advantages and Disadvantages of Haemoglobin-Based Solutions Compared with Hydrocarbons

Haemoglobin-Based Solutions	PFC-Based solutions
Advantages	**Advantages**
• Carries and unloads O_2	• Carries and unloads O_2
• Few and mild side effects	• Sigmoidal O_2 dissociation curve
• No known organ toxicity	• 100% FiO_2 not mandatory for maximum potency
	• Easy to measure
Disadvantages	**Disadvantages**
• 100% FiO_2 *is* mandatory for maximum potency	• Side effects
• Additional colloid is often necessary with potential side effects	• Vasoconstriction
	• Interference with laboratory methods (colourimetric)

5.7 MASSIVE HAEMORRHAGE/ MASSIVE TRANSFUSION[24]

5.7.1 Definition

Blood volume is approximately 70 mL/kg. Massive transfusion is defined as:

- The replacement of 100% of the patient's blood volume in less than 6 hours.
- The administration of 50% of the patient's blood volume in 1 hour.

There is a danger of death when blood loss is more than 150 mL per minute or 50% of blood volume in 20 minutes. Each trauma unit should have a policy for massive transfusion, which should be activated as soon as a potential candidate is admitted.

Also germane to the initial period of massive blood transfusion are the potential complications of acidosis, hypothermia, and hypocalcaemia. Hypothermia (<34°C) causes platelet sequestration and inhibits the release of platelet factors that are important in the intrinsic clotting pathway. In addition, it has consistently been associated with a poor outcome in trauma patients. Core temperature often falls insidiously because of exposure at the scene and in the emergency department, and because of the administration of resuscitation fluids stored at ambient temperature.

The use of bicarbonate in the treatment of systemic acidosis remains controversial. Administration of sodium bicarbonate may cause a leftward shift of the oxyhaemoglobin dissociation curve, reducing tissue O_2 extraction, and may worsen intracellular acidosis caused by carbon dioxide production. Use of sodium bicarbonate in the acidotic trauma patient is associated with an increase in mortality.[25]

Hypocalcaemia caused by citrate binding of ionized calcium does not occur until the blood transfusion rate exceeds 100 mL per minute (equivalent to 1 unit every 5 minutes). Decreased serum levels of ionized calcium depress myocardial function before impairing coagulation. Calcium gluconate or calcium chloride should be reserved for cases in which there is electrocardiographic (ECG) evidence of QT interval prolongation or, in rare instances, for cases of unexplained hypotension during massive transfusion. or where the active (ionized) fraction is >1 mmol/L on a blood-gas result.

5.7.2 Massive Transfusion Protocol (MTP)

An algorithm of coordinated action incorporating many hospital departments (surgery, blood bank, ICU, anaesthesiology) is activated upon the arrival of a trauma patient with massive haemorrhage. The protocol provides roles for the personnel, actions to be taken, and medications and blood products to be transfused. The target is the increase of survival of these patients. The basis of these protocols has been the knowledge recently acquired from modern battlefields, which has dramatically changed the way we manage these patients (Table 5.5).

5.8 HAEMOSTATIC ADJUNCTS IN TRAUMA

5.8.1 Overview

Haemostatic substances can be used after surgical haemostasis in trauma surgery to secure the surface of the

Table 5.5 Guidelines for Massive Transfusion

Definition
- The replacement of 100% of the patient's blood volume in less than 6 hours.
- The administration of 50% of the patient's blood volume in 1 hour.

Activation

The protocol will be activated **automatically by the blood bank** after 2 units of packed red blood cells (pRBCs) have been issued to a patient, *and* a request for a further four (4) units of blood or more is subsequently requested within any 24-hour period. A prospective tool utilizing PR >120 bpm and BP <90 *and* free blood in the abdomen can be used.[19]

Activation can also be done at the discretion of the treating physician.

It is essential the protocol activation to be based on criteria available on admission and not on parameters calculated after hours (e.g. blood loss) since by that time the salvation potential is zeroed.

Blood specimens

Group and crossmatch:
- Leukodepleted blood should be used wherever it is available.
- Crossmatched blood if available.
- Uncrossmatched group O blood.

The following **baseline blood specimens** are required
- Full blood count including platelets.
- Prothrombin time (PT), activated partial thromboplastin time (aPTT), thrombin time, International Normalized Ratio (INR), fibrinogen, D-dimer, thromboelastogram (TEG) or RoTEM.

The following are required **after every 6 units of transfused blood:**
- Repeat baseline blood samples.
- Full TEG or RoTEM.

Avoid hypothermia (patient and transfused fluid)
- Use an appropriate blood warmer.
- Keep the patient warm using an appropriate patient-warming device.
- Maintain a warm environment.

Blood and blood products

The blood bank will issue the following products (as part of a 2 or 6 unit 'massive transfusion pack'):

NB: Multiple '**2-unit packs**' are preferable as they can be returned if the 'cold chain' is intact
- Two units or 6 units of pRBCs using the *freshest blood available*.
- Two units or 6 units of **thawed** fresh frozen plasma (FFP).
- Two units or 5/6 units of platelets (apheresis unit – individual laboratory dependent).
  or
- For every 5 or 6 units of blood issued.
- One apheresis unit of platelets ('platelet mega-unit'). NB: may be 5 or 6 units of pooled platelets.

Administration

Microaggregate filters are **not** advised

Once administration of the 'massive transfusion pack' blood is begun, administer all the above in a **1:1:1 ratio,** (blood:FFP:platelets) or **6:6:1 / 5:5:1 / 4.4.1,** (blood:FFP:apheresis mega-platelet unit – depends on local interpretation of a megaplatelet unit). After every 6 units of red cells, if ongoing bleeding or need for transfusion is present:
- Give a further 4 units of FFP if PT or APTT is >1.5 times mid-normal or according to TEG/RoTEM.
- Give 10 units of cryoprecipitate if fibrinogen <1 g/L or according to TEG/RoTEM.
- Give 10 mL 10% calcium chloride **only** if the above additional doses are given.
- Give at least 1 Megaunit of pooled platelets if the platelet count is <75,000/mm³.
  Return all unused 'massive transfusion packs' to the blood bank as soon as possible.

(Continued)

Table 5.5 (Continued) Guidelines for Massive Transfusion

End points of transfusion
- Any active surgical bleeding has been controlled.
- No further need for red cells.
- Temperature >35°C.
- pH >7.3.
- Fibrinogen >1.5 g/L.
- INR better than 1.5, PT less than 16 seconds, aPTT less than 42 seconds.
- Haemoglobin 8–10 g/dL (4–6 mmol/L).

wound. Tissue adhesives are used alone or in combination with other haemostatic measures.

The main indications for using adhesives are:

- To arrest minor oozing of blood.
- To secure the wound area to prevent subsequent bleeding.

Various forms of fibrin sealing are available and are suitable for treating injuries, especially of the parenchymatous organs. The different presentations make some suitable for superficial bleeding surfaces, and others easier to apply in deep lacerations. Some are readily available, while preparation is time-consuming in others. It is important that the surgeon knows what haemostatic agents are available and how and where they can be used.

5.8.2 Tissue Adhesives

5.8.2.1 FIBRIN

Of the adhesives currently available, fibrin glue is the most suitable for treating injuries to the parenchymatous organs and retroperitoneum. It is also possible to make autologous fibrin from the patient's own blood (Vivostat system; Vivolution A/S Birkeroed, Denmark); the fibrin is applied with a sprayer. The necessary volume of blood (125 mL) can already be drawn in the emergency room, and the autologous adhesive is ready within 30 minutes.

Fibrin sealing is based on the transformation of fibrinogen to fibrin. Fibrin promotes clotting, tissue adhesion, and wound healing through interaction with the fibroblasts. The reaction is the same as in the last phase of blood clotting. One such heterologous fibrin is Tisseel/Tissucol (Baxter Hyland Immuno, Vienna, Austria). Heterologous fibrin is a biological two-component adhesive and has high concentrations of fibrinogen and factor XIII, which, together with thrombin and calcium, result in clotting. Resorption time and resistance to tearing

depend on the size and thickness of the glue layer, and on the proportion by volume of the two components. The fibrin sealant is best applied with a sprayer or syringe injection system such as the Tissomat sprayer (Baxter Hyland Immun, Rochester, MN, USA).

5.8.2.2 TACHOSIL®

TachoSil® (Baxter Corporation, Deerfield, IL, USA), is a fixed, ready-to-use combination of a collagen sponge coated with a dry layer of the human coagulation factors fibrinogen and thrombin, making it easy to employ. It is most suitable for oozing from the raw surfaces of solid organs or to seal air leaks from lung injuries. It is available in most countries in Europe and Australasia.

5.8.2.3 HEMOPATCH®

Similarily, HemoPatch® (Baxter Hyland Immuno, Vienna) has recently become available.

HemoPatch® is a soft, thin, and flexible patch consisting of a porous collagen matrix, which facilitates clotting, coated on one side with a thin protein-binding layer (pentaerythritol polyethylene glycol ether tetrasuccinimidyl glutarate (NHS-PEG)) which allows rapid adhesion (within 2 minutes) via electrophilic crosslinking. The patch consequently has a dual-method mechanism of action, in which the two components interact to achieve hemostasis by sealing off the bleeding surface and initiating the body's own clotting mechanisms. The patch is resorbed within 6–8 weeks.

5.8.2.4 COLLAGEN FLEECE

Even after surgical haemostasis, deep parenchymal injuries can require a resorbable tamponade; here, collagen fleece (e.g. TissoFleece, Baxter, Vienna) is suitable. Collagen fleece is composed of heterologous collagen fibrils obtained from devitalized connective tissue and is fully resorbable. Collagen fleece promotes the aggregation of thrombocytes when in contact with blood. The platelets degenerate and liberate clotting factors, which in turn activate haemostasis. The spongy structure of the collagen stabilizes and strengthens the coagulate. Another alternative for deep parenchymal injuries is FloSeal (Baxter Corporation, Deerfield, IL, USA).

Fibrin glue and collagen fleece are used preferentially to treat slight oozing of blood. Before application, the bleeding surface should be tamponaded and compressed with a warm pad for a few minutes. Immediately after removal of the pad, air alone is first sprayed, followed by short bursts of fibrin. This creates a surface that is free from blood and nearly dry when the fibrin glue is sprayed onto it. A dry field is essential for most fibrin sprays in order to secure adequate haemostasis.

If collagen fleece is to be applied, a thin layer of fibrin is sprayed onto the fleece, which, in turn, is pressed onto the wound. After a few moments compression, the fleece is sprayed with fibrin glue. The thickness of the fibrin layer will depend on the size and depth of the injury.

5.8.3 Other Haemostatic Adjuncts

5.8.3.1 CHITOSAN (CELOX (MEDITRADE LTD., CREWE, UK)/ HEMCON (HEMCON MEDICAL TECHNOLOGIES, PORTLAND, OR, USA))

Chitosan is a granular product made from a natural polysaccharide derived from chitin from shellfish. Chitosan is the deacetylated form of chitin. In the form of an acid salt, chitosan demonstrates mucoadhesive activity. Chitosan stops bleeding by bonding with red blood cells and gelling with fluids to produce a sticky pseudoclot. This reaction is not exothermic and has been used successfully within body cavities. Chitosan is broken down by enzymatic action within the body to produce glucosamine. The dressing is sold as pads or bandages.

5.8.3.2 MINERAL ZEOLYTE (QUIKCLOT® (Z-MEDICAL CORPORATION, WALLINGFORD CT, USA))

Mineral zeolyte, when made moist, produces an exothermic reaction that seals blood vessels and results in haemostasis. The initial preparation was in the form of granules and was very exothermic, resulting in significant tissue damage. The current preparation is presented in bags ('tea-bags') that are packed into the wound and may cause less damage.

REFERENCES AND RECOMMENDED READING

References

1. Allen CJ, Valle EJ, Jouria JM, Schulman CI, Namias N, Livingstone AS, et al. Differences between blunt and penetrating trauma after resuscitation with hydroxyethyl starch. *J Trauma.* 2014 Dec;**77(6)**:859–64; discussion 864. doi: 10.1097/TA.0000000000000422.

2. Kauvar DS, Holcomb JB, Norris GC, Hess JR. Fresh whole blood transfusion: a controversial military practice. *J Trauma.* 2006;**61**:181–4.

3. Spinella PC, Holcomb JB. Resuscitation and transfusion principles for traumatic hemorrhagic shock. *Blood Rev.* 2009;**23**:231–40.

4. Hess JR, Brohi K, Dutton RP, Hauser CJ, Holcomb JB, Kluger Y, et al. The coagulopathy of trauma: a review of mechanisms. *J Trauma.* 2008 Oct;**65(4)**:748–54. doi: 10.1097/TA.0b013e3181877a9c. Review.

5. Pandit TN, Sarode R. Blood component support inin acquired coagulopathic conditions: Is there a method to the madness? *Am J Hematol.* 2012 May;87 Suppl 1:S56–62. doi: 10.1002/ajh.23179. Epub 2012 Mar 31.

6. Dutton RP, Carson JL. Indications for early red blood cell transfusion. *J Trauma.* 2006;**60(6)**:Suppl. S35–40.

7. Napolitano LM, Kurek S, Luchette FA, Anderson GL, Bard MR, Bromberg W, et al. Clinical practice guideline: red blood cell transfusion in adult trauma and critical care. *J Trauma.* 2009 Dec;**67(6)**:1439–42. doi: 10.1097/TA.0b013e3181ba7074.

8. Hébert PC, Wells G, Tweeddale M, Martin C, Marshall J, Pham B, et al. Does transfusion practice affect mortality in critically ill patients? Transfusion Requirements in Critical Care (TRICC) Investigators and the Canadian Critical Care Trials Group. *Am J Respir Crit Care Med.* 1997 May;**155(5)**: 1618–23.

9. Holcomb JB, Tilley BC, Baraniuk S, Fox EE, Wade CE, Podbielski JM, et al. Transfusion of plasma, platelets, and red blood cells in a 1:1:1 vs a 1:1:2 ratio and mortality in patients with severe trauma: the PROPPR randomized clinical trial. *JAMA.* 2015 Feb 3;**313(5)**:471–82. doi: 10.1001/jama.2015.12.

10. Holcomb JB, del Junco DJ, Fox EE, Wade CE, Cohen MJ, Schreiber MA, et al. The Prospective, Observational, Multicenter, Major Trauma Transfusion (PROMMTT) study. *J Trauma Acute Care Surg.* 2013 Jul;**75**(1 Suppl 1):S1–2. doi: 10.1097/TA.0b013e3182983876.

11. Ishikura H, Kitamura T. Trauma-induced coagulopathy and critical bleeding: the role of plasma and platelet transfusion. *Journal of Intensive Care.* 2017;**5(2)**. doi: 10.1186/s40560-016-0203-y

12. Boffard KD, Riou B, Warren B, Choong PI, Rizoli S, Rossaint R, et al. NovoSeven Trauma Study Group. Recombinant factor VIIa as adjunctive therapy for bleeding control in severely injured trauma patients: two parallel randomized, placebo-controlled, double-blind clinical trials. *J Trauma.* 2005;**59(1)**:8–15; discussion 15-8.

13. Hauser CJ, Boffard K, Dutton R, Bernard GR, Croce MA, Holcomb JB, et al., for the CONTROL Study Group. Results of the CONTROL Trial: efficacy and safety of recombinant activated factor VII in the management of refractory traumatic hemorrhage. *J Trauma.* 2010;**69**:489–500. doi: 10.1097/TA.0b013e3181edf36e.

14. CRASH-2 Trial Collaborators. Effects of tranexamic acid on death, vascular occlusive events, and blood transfusion in trauma patients with significant haemorrhage (CRASH-2): a randomised, placebo-controlled trial. *Lancet* 2010;**376**: 27–32.

15. Morrison JJ, Dubose JJ, Rasmussen TE, Midwinter MJ. Military Application of Tranexamic Acid in Trauma Emergency Resuscitation (MATTERs) Study. *Arch Surg.* 2012 Feb;**147(2)**:113–9. doi: 10.1001/archsurg.2011.287. Epub 2011 Oct 17.

16. Moore HB, Moore EE, Gonzalez E, Chapman MP, Chin TL, Silliman CC, et al. Hyprinofibrinolysis, physiologic fibrinolysis, and fibrinolysis shutdown: The spectrum of post injury fibrinolysis and relevance to antifibrinolytic therapy. *J Trauma Acute Care Surg.* 2014 Dec;**77(6)**:811–7; discussion 817. doi: 10.1097/TA.0000000000000341.

17. Napolitano LM, Cohen MJ, Cotton BA, Schreiber MA, Moore EE. Tranexamic acid in trauma: How should we use it? *J Trauma Acute Care Surg.* 2013 Jun;**74(6)**:1575–86. doi: 10.1097/TA.0b013e318292cc54.

18. Napolitano LM. Prehospital tranexamic acid: what is the current evidence? *Trauma Surg Acute Care Open.* 2017 Jan 13;**2(1)**:e000056. doi: 10.1136/tsaco-2016-000056. eCollection 2017.

19. Stensballe J, Ostrowski SR, Johansson PI. Viscoelastic guidance of resuscitation. *Curr Opin Anaesthesiol.* 2014;**27(2)**: 212–8.

20. TEG/ROTEM. Available from www.surgicalcriticalcare.net/Guidelines (accessed online Dec 2018).

21. Hughes LG, Thomas DW, Wareham K, Jones JE, John A, Rees M. Intra-operative blood salvage in abdominal trauma: a review of 5 years' experience. *Anaesthesia* 2001; **56**:217–20.

22. Bowley DM, Barker P, Boffard KD. Intraoperative blood salvage in penetrating abdominal trauma: a randomised controlled trial. *World J Surg.* 2006;**30(6)**:1074–80.

23. Moradi S, Jahanian-Najafabadi A, Roudkenar MH. Artificial Blood Substitutes: First Steps on the Long Route to Clinical Utility. *Clin Med Insights Blood Disorders* 2016 Oct;**27(9)**: 33–41. eCollection 2016. Review.

24. Nunez TC, Young PP, Holcomb JB, Cotton BA. Creation, implementation, and maturation of a massive transfusion protocol for the exsanguinating trauma patient. *J Trauma.* 2010 Jun;**68(6)**:1498–505. doi: 10.1097/TA.0b013e3181d3cc25.

25. Wilson RF, Spencer AR, Tyburski JG, Dolman H, Zimmerman LH. Bicarbonate therapy in severely acidotic trauma patients increases mortality. *J Trauma Acute Care Surg.* 2013 Jan;**74(1)**:45–50; discussion 50. doi: 10.1097/TA.0b013e3182788fc4.

Recommended Reading

1. Hess JR, Holcomb JB, Hoyt DB. Damage control resuscitation: the need for specific blood products to treat the coagulopathy of trauma. *Transfusion* 2006;**46(5)**: 685–6.

2. https://lifeinthefastlane.com/ccc/thromboelastogram-teg/ (accessed online Dec 2108).

3. https://only4medical.wordpress.com/2017/05/20/teg-interpretation-made-easy-with-wine-glasses/ (accessed online Dec 2018).

4. Johansson PI, Ostrowsky SR, Secher NH. Management of major blood loss: an update. *Acta Anaesthesiol Scand.* 2010;**54**:1039–49.

5. Malone DL, Hess JR, Fingerhut A. Massive transfusion practices around the globe and a suggestion for a common massive transfusion protocol. *J Trauma.* 2006;**60**(6, Suppl.):S91–6.

6. Marino PL. Blood components. In: *The ICU Book*, 4th edn. Wolters Kluwer Health / Lippincott Williams & Wilkins, 2014. Philadelphia PA, USA.

7. Moore EE, Moore HB, Chapman MP, Gonzalez E, Sauia A. Goal-directed hemostatic resuscitation for trauma induced coagulopathy: Maintaining homeostasis. *J Trauma Acute Care Surg.* 2018 Jun;**84**(6 Suppl 1):S35–40. doi: 10.1097/TA.0000000000001797.

Damage Control **6**

6.1 **INTRODUCTION**

Damage control has as its objective, delay in imposition of additional surgical stress at a moment of physiological frailty.[1] The goal is to focus on the body physiology, and align the objectives of the surgical intervention (specifically to stop bleeding and control contamination), with the resuscitation objectives as an overarching damage control principle.

Damage control resuscitation (DCR), damage control surgery (DCS), and damage control orthopaedics (DCO) are a deliberate and pre-emptive set of non-traditional manoeuvres used to reverse the pre-terminal effect of exsanguination, massive injury, and shock. The primary goal is to temporize management of major injuries with directed resuscitation and staged surgery, to allow for resuscitation and restoration of normal physiology.

The concept of damage control is not new, and livers were packed more than 100 years ago by Pringle. However, with the failure to understand the underlying physiological rationale, the results were disastrous. Over time, the concept has evolved into the modern technique of better resuscitation (DCR), a staged laparotomy (DCS), with establishment of intra-abdominal pack tamponade, control of contamination, delayed definitive management, and the restoration of normal physiological parameters and coagulation. The use of adjuncts, such as angiography and embolization, has been beneficial where packing of the viscera has failed (e.g. as in uncontrolled pelvic bleeding or soft tissue destruction).

Damage control concepts are not restricted to the abdomen and extend to every cavity in the body as well as vascular damage control. The need for damage control in children is much less common; however, they are much more prone to hypothermia given larger surface area relative to their smaller blood volume. Although the physiological parameters are very different, the principles are the same. At the other end of the spectrum, the application of damage control to the elderly who have decreased physiological reserve and a high morbidity and mortality has also been successful, with survival of greater than 50% when damage control is applied to this group.[2] Damage control surgery may be performed in smaller hospitals before transfer to a larger centre. Damage control surgery procedures, on properly selected patients, can be life-saving, and may have to be performed in any hospital admitting trauma cases.

Damage control can also be applied to the general surgery population in patients with intra-abdominal catastrophes such as perforated viscous pancreatitis, ischemia, or gastrointestinal haemorrhage. DCS allows for rapid source control with the ability to re-evaluate the source easily. It also allows for frequent re-evaluation of bowel viability in the setting of ischaemia. Finally, and possibly most importantly, DCS decreases (but does not eliminate) the incidence of abdominal compartment syndrome (see also Section 17.10). This patient population often receives a massive amount of intravenous volume during the initial resuscitation, which results in bowel oedema and increased intra-abdominal pressure. A temporary abdominal closure lowers the risk of this potentially devastating process.

The application of damage control principles has influenced military care and disaster planning. The need to triage mass casualty scenarios makes an abbreviated surgical and damage control approach advantageous in maximizing the use of limited resources to many patients in a restricted time span or space. A recent prospective observational military study reported that damage control was utilized in 77% abdominal operations performed in Afghanistan and was safe.[3] The study concluded that DCR and DCS was the optimal approach to abdominal war injury and should be considered in logistical planning for future military operations. Events such as the Boston Marathon bombing showed that the critical patient surge placed on hospitals within minutes of an incident was well handled with good outcomes when the abbreviated DCS strategy was used to manage all patients.[4]

6.2 DAMAGE CONTROL RESUSCITATION

The optimal strategy for the management of the haemorrhaging patient is now termed DCR and is a critical adjunct to the application of DCS, with which it occurs in parallel.[5] During World War II, it was noted that there were improved outcomes with slightly lower blood pressures (owing to the reduction in blood loss). Permissive hypotension reduces blood loss, the need for additional fluids which might cause a dilutional coagulopathy, and avoids the associated acidosis, hypothermia, and clotting derangements.

DCR is the proactive, anticipatory treatment of the coagulopathy, hypothermia, and acidosis that presents with critical injury and shock. DCR priorities include the following:[6-8]

- Permissive hypertension with resuscitation only to a pressure that allows organ *perfusion* ('hypotensive resuscitation'), rather than achieving *normotension*.

  Permissive hypotension is a strategy to reduce blood loss by limiting systolic pressure to the minimum necessary to maintain perfusion of vital organs. In massively bleeding patients, raising blood pressure to normal levels before achieving surgical haemostasis has been shown to enhance bleeding by displacing clots formed during the body's attempt at primary haemostasis ('popping the clot'). The strategy is not new, and was reported during the World War I, when it was stated that 'if the pressure is raised before the surgeon is ready to check any bleeding that may take place, blood that is sorely needed may be lost'. Although safe limits of blood pressure in terms of preservation of organ perfusion are unknown, a systolic blood pressure of 80 mm Hg, and in case of concomitant severe brain trauma, a mean arterial pressure (MAP) of over 80 mm Hg are recommended. While there is no hard evidence for these limits, it is very clear that such low pressures should be maintained for the shortest possible time in order to limit vital organ ischaemia. The importance of early surgical haemostasis and the need for the DCR concept being applied must be emphasized.

- Minimizing the use of crystalloid and early use of blood products during resuscitation – facilitated by use of a massive transfusion protocol (see also Section 5.7).

- Blood product administration with liberal use of fresh frozen plasma (FFP) and platelets.

  The optimal ratio of blood component therapy has yet to be determined, but a ratio approaching 1:1:1 has been suggested. In certain environments properly cross-matched whole blood may also be used.

  Early and aggressive administration of blood and blood products has shown to improve survival after trauma-related haemorrhagic shock. Lost blood volume should be replaced by blood products aiming at near equal ratios of packed red blood cell (pRBC):FFP:platelets.[9,10] Such regimens have demonstrated improved outcomes. Data suggest that plasma-based resuscitation when compared to crystalloids is better at preserving endothelial integrity. FFP administration after haemorrhagic shock has anti-inflammatory properties and a potential glycocalyx-restoring capacity.[11]

- Targeting coagulopathy with goal-directed haemostasis, using viscoelastic assays such as TEG or RoTEM, if available, may be used to guide product therapy.

- Restoration of normothermia.

  Hypothermia below 35°C has a profound impact on surgical site infection rates after trauma laparotomy. Hypothermia also adversely affects coagulation as well as cardiac output and function in most bodily organs.

The recent EAST guidelines on DCR[12] addressed the requirements (Table 6.1).

The implementation of a massive transfusion protocol (MTP) is recommended, which will allow the ready availability of blood products (see also Chapter 5). Availability of an MTP has shown to be associated with a reduction of organ failure and improved 30-day survival after severe trauma.[13]

6.3 DAMAGE CONTROL SURGERY

DCS is a technique whereby the surgeon minimizes operative time and surgical intervention in the grossly unstable patient. The primary reason for this is to minimize hypothermia, metabolic acidosis, and coagulopathy ('the lethal triad'), which are often apparent after the patient has sustained massive tissue destruction, or significant blood volume loss. The focus is exclusively on

Table 6.1 Evidence-Based Guidelines for Aspects of DCR

	Question	Guidelines
1	In adult patients with severe trauma, should a massive transfusion protocol (MT)/damage control resuscitation (DCR) versus no MT/DCR be used to decrease mortality or total blood products used?	In adult patients with severe trauma we *recommend* the use of a massive transfusion/damage control resuscitation protocol in comparison to no protocol to reduce mortality.
2	In adult patients with severe trauma, should a high ratio of plasma to red blood cells (PLAS:RBC) and platelet to red blood cells (PLT:RBC) versus a low ratio be administered to decrease mortality or total blood products used?	In adult patients with severe trauma we *recommend* targeting a high ratio of plasma and platelets to red blood cells as compared to a low ratio to reduce mortality. This is best achieved by transfusion equal amounts of red blood cells, plasma, and platelets, during the early empirical phase of resuscitation.
3	In adult patients with severe trauma, should the haemostatic adjunct recombinant factor VIIa (rVIIa) versus no rVIIa be administered to decrease mortality, total blood products used, or MT? Does the use of rVIIa increase venous thromboembolism (VTE) rates?	In adult patients with severe trauma we *cannot recommend* for or against the use of rVIIa as a haemostatic adjunct in comparison to no rVIIa. We feel that the use rVIIa needs further study with particular attention to optimal doses and the timing of administration, relative to blood product administration. As with other haemostatic agents, the VTE rates need to be more carefully evaluated with the use of a defined surveillance protocol.
4	In adult patients with severe trauma, should the hemostatic adjunct tranexamic acid (TXA) versus no TXA be administered to decrease mortality, total blood products used, or MT? Does the use of TXA increase VTE rates?	There is no clear universal mortality benefit to TXA. In adult patients with severe trauma we *conditionally recommend* the use of TXA as an in-hospital haemostatic adjunct in comparison to no TXA. These recommendations only apply to the use of TXA in a hospital setting pending the results of pre-hospital trials. As with other haemostatic agents, the VTE rates need to be more carefully evaluated with the use of a defined surveillance protocol.

life-saving surgical procedures (bleeding and contamination control), thus permitting more successful resuscitation and normalization of the patient's physiology. After a post-operative intensive care resuscitation and stabilization period, the patient is returned to the operating room as soon as physiologically possible, for definitive surgical care (e.g. restoration of bowel continuity). Although the principles are sound, extreme care needs to be exercised to avoid over-utilization of the concept, causing secondary insults to viscera. Furthermore, surgery must be appropriate, to minimize activation of the inflammatory cascade and the consequences of systemic inflammatory response syndrome (SIRS) and organ dysfunction.

Damage control can be divided into five distinct stages: this begins with patient selection (Stage 1) and continues through potential late abdominal wall reconstruction (Stage 5).

6.3.1 **Stage 1: Patient Selection**

Proper patient selection is crucial to optimize outcomes following damage control surgery. All patients should undergo a very rapid trauma evaluation, and appropriate DCR. The duration of this stage is dictated by the patient's physiological stability as well as the underlying pathology. Delays to the operating room must be avoided. Rapid manoeuvres to control external bleeding (tourniquets, digital control of bleeding, etc.), are indicated as transition to the operating room occurs.

> **'The treatment of bleeding is to stop the bleeding...'**

In any hospital managing trauma or a high number of emergency surgical cases, protocols for massive transfusion supporting haemostatic resuscitation should be in place and supported by anaesthesia, blood bank, and intensive care staff (see also Chapter 5). The surgeon is well advised to call for an additional surgeon to assist, if available.

The indications to consider in selecting a patient for damage control are:

- Haemodynamic instability:
  - Systolic blood pressure <90 mm Hg and not responding to resuscitation.
- Temperature <35°C.
- Metabolic instability:
  - Temperature <35°C.
  - pH <7.2.
  - Base excess ≥–5 and worsening.
  - Serum lactate ≥5 mmol/L.
- Coagulopathy:
  - Abnormal viscoelastic haemostatic assays (VHA): TEG or RoTEM.
  - Prothrombin time (PT) >16 seconds.
  - Partial thromboplastin time (PTT) >60 seconds.
- Surgical anatomy:
  - Complex life-threatening injuries (e.g. major vascular injury or moderate vascular injury with complex hollow viscus injuries, complex liver injury, exsanguinating retroperitoneal pelvis, multi-cavitary exsanguination etc.).
  - Anticipated need for a time-consuming surgical procedure in a patient with a suboptimal response to resuscitation.
  - Inability to perform the definitive repair in a timely fashion.
  - Demand for non-operative control of other injuries, for example a fractured pelvis.
  - Inability to approximate the abdominal incision
- Environment and/or resource demands
  - Blood requirement requiring an MTP.
  - Operating time greater than 60 minutes.

- Logistics:
  - Multiple patients/mass casualty situation.
- Minimal resources:
  - (e.g. personnel, medical equipment, safety concerns).

It is critical to identify these potential scenarios before the patient becomes metabolically unsalvageable. The decision to deploy a damage control physiological-based approach should be done to PREVENT this metabolic deterioration from occurring in the first place. It can often be a decision that is made at the very beginning of the surgical intervention.

If resources allow, the use of a hybrid operating room expedites definitive haemorrhage control and can complement damage control therapy in the exsanguinating patient.

Irrespective of the setting, a coagulopathy is the single most common reason for abortion of a planned procedure or curtailment of definitive surgery. It is important to abort the surgery *before* the coagulopathy becomes obvious.

The technical aspects of the surgery are dictated by the injury pattern.

6.3.2 **Stage 2: Operative Haemorrhage and Contamination Control**

See also: The Trauma Laparotomy (Chapter 9.1).

6.3.2.1 INITIAL INCISION

A very large midline laparotomy incision is necessary to allow for wide retraction of the abdominal wall and rapid visualization of the liver, abdominal great vessels, and all other retroperitoneal structures. Two experienced surgeons are recommended. Rapid control of the largest source of blood loss is critical and in those cases with several sources of bleeding and manual pressure, packing, and temporary ligation may be necessary. Each case is unique in presentation; however, the principle is to control active large blood loss first.

6.3.2.2 HAEMORRHAGE CONTROL

The operative process works through the following (see also Section 9.1):

- Arrest arterial and major venous bleeding. Failure to control ongoing bleeding will lead to the patient's demise:

- Major arterial bleeding must be controlled at the index procedure. A temporary intravascular shunt is preferred for named vessels; however, ligation may be required to save an exsanguinating patient.
- Resuscitative endovascular balloon occlusion of the aorta (REBOA) may be effective in controlling arterial haemorrhage in difficult access areas such as the pelvis, the retroperitoneum, or the kidney (see also Section 15.3).
- Temporary intravascular shunting (see Figure 6.1)
  - Use tubing approximately 50% of the diameter of the vessel being shunted.
  - Allow 3–4 cm of the tube in each end of the vessel.
  - The shunt can either be a straight (linear) shunt (Figure 6.1a), for example, for iliac vessels, portal vein, etc., or a 'pig-tail' shunt (Figure 6.1b) where access is difficult (e.g. superior mesenteric artery, or some temporary mobility is expected (e.g. shunting a superficial popliteal or distal femoral artery prior to orthopaedic repair.
- Tamponade using wraps or packs.
- Occlusion of inflow into the bleeding organ (e.g. Pringle's manoeuvre for bleeding liver).
- Repair or ligation of accessible blood vessels.
- Intra-operative or post-operative catheter directed embolization.

6.3.2.3 CONTROL OF CONTAMINATION (HOLLOW VISCUS ORGANS)

- Defects in the bowel or hollow viscous organs can be controlled with simple suturing or stapler applications.
- Damaged segments can be resected with clamps or staples.
- Biliary and genitourinary injuries can be temporized with external drainage (T-tube, ureterostomy, etc.).
- Pancreatic injuries should be widely drained and packed.

Avoid definitive repair, restoration of intestinal continuity, stoma formation, and creation of feeding access at this stage.

6.3.2.4 COPIOUS WASHOUT

At the end of the procedure, before temporary closure, the abdominal cavity must be washed out with copious (several litres of normal saline, especially if there has been contaminations by faeces, for example). After washing out, suck out all fluid. Leave the cavity as dry as possible.

6.3.2.5 TEMPORARY ABDOMINAL CLOSURE (TAC)

The abdominal cavity should be closed to prevent heat and moisture loss, and to protect the viscera.

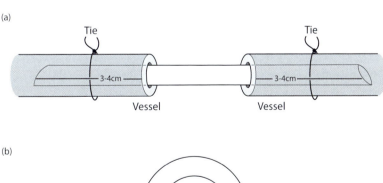

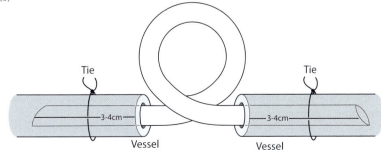

Figure 6.1 Diagram of an intravascular shunt. (a) Straight shunt; (b) 'pig-tail' shunt.

Delayed closure is required when any combination of the factors listed above under damage control, or re-look surgery, exists. Patients with multiple injuries who have undergone protracted surgery with massive volume resuscitation to maintain haemodynamic stability will often develop tissue interstitial oedema. This may predispose to the development of abdominal compartment syndrome (ACS) or may simply make primary closure of the sheath impracticable. In addition, significant enteric or other contamination will raise the risk of intra-abdominal sepsis, or the extent of tissue damage may raise doubt over the viability of any repair; these conditions usually mandate planned re-laparotomy and thus a temporary closure.

In these circumstances, a temporary abdominal closure is required. The needs of such a closure can be summarized as:

- Quick to do.
- Cheap.
- Keeps the abdominal contents inside the abdominal cavity.
- Allows drainage of fluid.
- Minimizes sepsis.
- Facilitates delayed primary fascial closure.

Vacuum-based closure is recommended for the management of the open abdomen. A review of the literature available suggests that negative-pressure wound vacuum therapy may have improved facial closure rates and may be associated with improved outcomes over alternative abdominal closure techniques (mesh, Velcro, bag-type dressings).

Many temporary closure systems are available, of which the most cost effective is the 'sandwich technique' first described by Schein in 1986[14] and was popularized by Rotundo and Schwab.[1]

A sheet of self-adhesive incise drape (Opsite® – Smith and Nephew, London, UK, Steri-Drape® or Ioban® – 3M Corporation, St Paul, MN, USA) is placed flat, sticky side up, and an abdominal swab is placed upon it. The objective is to create a non-stick membrane on one side of the abdominal swab to place against the visceral organs. The size should be large enough that, when inserted, the sheet will extend laterally to the paracolic gutters, and 10 cm cranial and caudal to the incision. The edges are folded over to produce a composite sheet with a membrane (i.e. the drape) on one side, and an abdominal swab on the other. The membrane is utilized as an on-lay with the margins 'tucked in' under the edges of the open sheath as far the paracolic gutters, with only the membrane in contact with the bowel.

Pitfalls

Table 6.2 Dos and Don'ts

DO

- Cover only one side of the swab. Covering both sides impedes drainage by preventing capillary wicking through the weave of the swab.
- Insert the sandwich, plastic side against the bowel.
- Insert the sandwich as a 'diamond', with the points tucked in at top and bottom of the incision, and laterally.

DO NOT

- Make any holes (slits) in the membrane. Holes would allow the suction to be transmitted directly to the serosa of the bowel, with possible risk of fistula formation.
- Have a vacuum above a maximum of 25 mm Hg. Higher suction pressures, especially in a cold hypotensive patient, transmitted directly on to the bowel may exceed capillary pressure.
- Preferably avoid the commercial equivalents (e.g. VAC® – Kinetic Concepts Incorporated (KCI), San Antonio, TX, USA or Renasys® – Smith and Nephew, London UK), currently. These should be reserved for the definitive closure of a wound, both for cost reasons, and the higher vacuum suction pressure often present.

The appreciable drainage of serosanguinous fluid that occurs is best dealt with by placing a pair of drainage tubes (e.g. sump-type nasogastric tubes or closed-system suction drains) through separate stab incisions, with the tips placed in the caudal end of the incision. The tubes lie on either side of the incision, under the edge of the anterior abdominal peritoneum, and the gauze of the swab., and utilizing continuous low-vacuum suction.

This arrangement is covered by an occlusive incise drape applied to the skin, thus providing a closed system (the 'sandwich'; Figures 6.2 and 6.3).

The 'Bogota bag' and towel clips, etc. are no longer used, and for temporary abdominal closure, no sutures should be placed in the sheath, nor skin.

The timing of transfer of the patient from the operating theatre to the intensive care unit (ICU) is critical. Prompt transfer is cost-effective; premature transfer is counter-productive. Control of bleeding and

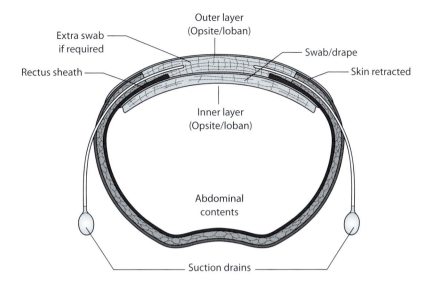

Figure 6.2 Diagrammatic representation of the sandwich technique for temporary abdominal closure.

contamination must be achieved. On the other hand, once haemostasis has been properly achieved, it may not be necessary to abort the procedure in the same fashion.

In the operating room, efforts must be started to reverse all the associated adjuncts, such as acidosis, hypothermia, and hypoxia, and it may be possible to improve the coagulation status through these methods alone. Adequate time should still be allowed for this, following which reassessment of the abdominal injuries should take place, as it is not infrequent to discover further injuries or ongoing bleeding.

6.3.3 **Stage 3: Physiological Restoration in the ICU**

Priorities in the ICU are as follows.

6.3.3.1 RESTORATION OF BODY TEMPERATURE

- Passive rewarming using warming blankets, convection blankets, warmed fluids, heat lamps, elevation of the ambient room temperature, etc.
- Active rewarming with lavage of the chest or abdomen.

6.3.3.2 OPTIMIZATION OF OXYGEN DELIVERY

- Volume loading to restore circulating blood volume.
- Haemoglobin optimization to a haemoglobin level of 8–10 g/dL (80–100 g/L), (4–6 mmol/L).

- Monitoring of cardiac output.
  - Ultrasonic cardiac output devices.
  - Cardiac arterial output monitors.
  - Correction of acidosis to a pH >7.3.
- Measurement and correction of lactic acidosis to less than 2.5 mmol/L.
- Inotropic support as required, but not prioritized over *adequate* blood product resuscitation.

6.3.3.3 CORRECTION OF CLOTTING PROFILES

- Blood component repletion.
- Assessment and normalization of any coagulopathy.
  - Coagulation studies.
- Thromboelastography (TEG) or rotational thromboelastometry (RoTEM).

6.3.3.4 IMPROVEMENT OF PHYSIOLOGICAL ENDPOINTS: AS EVIDENCED BY

- Lactate clearance.
- SvO_2.
- Urine output.
- Haemodynamics.
- Resolution of acidaemia.
- Inotropic support decreased once intravascular volume has been repleted.

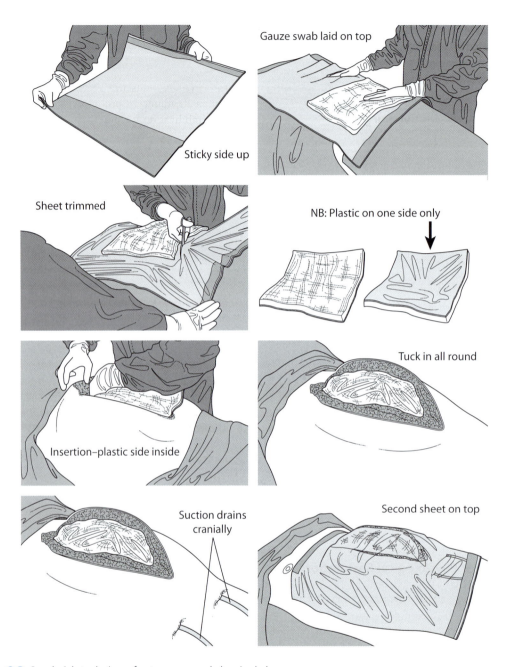

Figure 6.3 Sandwich technique for temporary abdominal closure.

6.3.3.5 MONITORING FOR AND MINIMIZING THE INCIDENCE OF INTRA-ABDOMINAL HYPERTENSION (AH) AND ABDOMINAL COMPARTMENT SYNDROME (ACS) (SEE ALSO SECTION 17.10)

- Measurement of intra-abdominal pressure (IAP).
  - Foley (bladder) catheter.
  - Intragastric catheter.

6.3.3.6 RECOGNITION OF ADDITIONAL INJURIES

- Review of injury mechanism, presentation, and those steps in the standard trauma resuscitation, along with diagnostics and therapies that were not completed to facilitate damage control.

- Tertiary survey.
- Additional imaging as needed.
- Review of history, co-morbid conditions, and medications.

6.3.4 Stage 4: Definitive Surgery

The patient is returned to the operating theatre as soon as physiological stability has been achieved. Ideally this would be within 24–48 hours, as delaying beyond 48 hours can be detrimental; however, the timing for this is determined by:

- The indication for damage control in the first place.
- The pattern of injury.
- The physiological response to resuscitation, warming, and evaluation as above.

Patients with ongoing bleeding despite correction of the other parameters require immediate return to the operating theatre or angiography suite.

Patients who develop major abdominal compartment syndrome must undergo re-look surgery early, and any further underlying causes must be corrected. This can and does occur even in the patient with a temporary abdominal closure.

Every effort must be made to return *all* patients to the operating theatre within 24–36 hours of their initial surgery. By leaving matters longer, other problems such as acute respiratory distress syndrome, SIRS, and sepsis may intervene (cause or effect) and may preclude further surgery.

6.3.4.1 THE 'RE-LOOK LAPAROTOMY'

The re-look laparotomy may be:

- *Planned*, that is, decided upon at the time of the initial procedure and usually for reasons of contamination, doubtful tissue viability, for retrieval of intra-abdominal packs or for further definitive surgery after a damage control exercise.
- *On demand*, that is, when evidence of intra-abdominal complication develops. In these cases, the principle applies of re-operation 'when the patient fails to progress according to expectation'. Failure to act in these circumstances may have dire consequences in terms of morbidity and mortality.

Re-exploration should be thorough, with careful evaluation for previously undiagnosed injuries. If the patient's physiological parameters deteriorate again, then the damage control philosophy should be reapplied with aggressive resuscitation, abbreviated laparotomy, and possible adjunctive procedures such as angiography, pelvic stabilization, or evaluation of extra abdominal injury. In many cases, repacking combined with aggressive correction of physiological endpoints including coagulopathy, along with further warming and coagulopathy, are necessary.

If a stoma (colostomy or ileostomy) is needed, the stoma is positioned more laterally, between the musculature of the anterior and mid axillary lines. The rectus fascia and musculature are thereby spared for future reconstruction, and the stoma is positioned well away from the midline wound, thus minimizing contamination. As the abdominal wall is reapproximated the stoma will move toward the anterior midline.

6.3.5 Stage 5: Abdominal Wall Closure

Once the patient has completed definitive surgery and no further operations are contemplated, the abdominal wall can be closed. In most series most patients had the fascia closed after the first re-look, or within 7 to 8 days from injury. This varies greatly depending on patient size and body habitus, time to achieve physiological stabilization, volume of fluid used to resuscitate, and injuries sustained.

6.3.5.1 DELAYED PRIMARY ABDOMINAL CLOSURE

Delayed closure will be required once the reasons for the temporary surgery have been removed or treated. This is usually possible after an interval of 24–48 hours (or longer). Usually, the abdominal wall can be closed in layers using normal closure techniques. However, this should only be performed when no further surgery is contemplated and should be accomplished without any fascial tension.

If abdominal viscera are protruding above the fascia in the supine anaesthetized patient, further management with temporary closure (vacuum assisted) is recommended. Return to the operating room after another 24–48 hours of intensive care and fluid mobilization in most cases will then allow primary fascial closure. Both surgeon and anaesthetist must be aware of the danger of causing ACS as a result of the closure, and intra-abdominal or respiratory pressures must be closely monitored.

6.3.5.2 SECONDARY ABDOMINAL CLOSURE

If, for various reasons, a delayed primary closure is not possible, then it will be necessary to accept (but minimize) the defect that results. The skin of the abdominal wall and the underlying fascia retract, and thus prevent a primary closure from being achieved. During the period of the open abdomen, in this situation, several techniques are usually combined to get to a point where the fascia can be closed without tension and safely. The goal is to achieve fascial closure, and subsequent skin closure.

Methods involved which will minimize or reduce the eventual defect include:

- Vacuum-assisted closure:
  - Commercial closures have been shown to reduce the defect and assist in closure of the sheath. These include V.A.C. (Kinetic Concepts Inc., San Antonio, TX, USA), and Renasys (Smith and Nephew, London, UK).[15]
- Skin-only closure:
  - Grafts using Vicryl® mesh (Johnson and Johnson, New Brunswick, NJ, USA) or Gore-Tex® sheets (W L Gore and Associates Inc., Flagstaff, AZ, USA) or other synthetic sheets.
  - Biologic meshes – human dermal matrix (AlloDerm® – LifeCell, Bridgewater, NJ, USA) or porcine dermal matrix (Permacol – Covidien, Mansfield, MA, USA).
  - Split-thickness skin grafts directly on granulated bowel or mesh.

6.3.5.3 SECONDARY CLOSURE

If delayed primary closure is not possible after several days or a week, there are several options:

- Closure of skin only, allowing the formation of a hernia.
- Biological material such as human (AlloDerm) or porcine (Permacol) dermal matrix used as mesh early to prevent hernia formation, providing skin coverage.
- Continued vacuum-assisted temporary abdominal closure such as V.A.C.® (Kinetic Concepts Inc.,

KCI. San Antonio, TX, USA) and Renasys® (Smith and Nephew, London, UK) until granulation over bowel occurs, for subsequent split-thickness skin grafting.
- If a synthetic mesh is left *in situ*, skin coverage of the resulting defect by split-grafting or flap transfer – *never use a polypropylene only mesh.*
- For large hernias, often the need for later reconstruction using different techniques such as component separation and flap construction.
- A Wittmann patch.
- A multitude of tension assist devices that are now available.

An absorbable mesh of polyglycolic acid such as Vicryl® (Johnson and Johnson, New Brunswick, NJ, USA) elicits minimal tissue reaction and in-growth. Thus, it has a low risk of infection or fistula formation.

Membranes such as polytetrafluoroethylene (PTFE) (Gore-Tex® – W L Gore and Associates, Flagstaff, AZ, USA), which elicit minimal tissue reaction and in-growth and thus minimize risk of infection or fistula formation, can be used, but this is considerably costlier. Recently, composite meshes have shown promise. The mesh can then have a skin graft placed upon it (or even directly on bowel), and definitive abdominal wall reconstruction can take place at a later stage.

Should any mesh be used and left *in situ*, however, the resulting defect will require skin coverage by split-grafting or flap transfer.

6.3.5.4 PLANNED HERNIA

A planned hernia approach aims at skin coverage with subsequent delayed abdominal wall reconstruction. Conditions favouring a planned hernia strategy include the inability to reapproximate the retracted abdominal wall edges, sizeable tissue deficit, risk of tertiary abdominal compartment syndrome, inadequate infection source control, anterior enteric fistula, and poor nutritional status of the patient. Various techniques have been applied. Autologous split-thickness skin grafting over the visceral content of the abdomen allows coverage of the exposed bowel. Maturation of the skin graft requires about 6–12 months, after which the grafted skin can be easily removed from the bowel surface for reconstruction.

Bridging mesh is often employed, and absorbable mesh is preferred. Non-absorbable (polypropylene mesh, etc.) has been abandoned because of infection and high rates of fistula formation.

More commonly a component separation is performed. A large relaxing incision is placed in the exterior oblique muscle component of the anterior rectus muscle bilaterally. This can be combined with mobilization of the rectus muscle from the posterior fascial sheath to provide local advancement across the hernia defect. Modification of this technique has been described with division of the internal oblique to the arcuate line. Large abdominal wall defects can be reconstructed with pedicular or microvascular flaps. The most commonly used is the tensor fascia lata (TFL) flap.

6.3.6 **Outcomes**

In a recent study of 88 damage control patients with a mean injury severity score of 34, Brenner et al. reported of the 63 survivors, 81% had gone back to work and resumed normal daily activities.[16]

6.4 **DAMAGE CONTROL ORTHOPAEDICS**[17]

It used to be orthopaedic standard of care that patients who were too sick, should have their surgery delayed for up to two weeks. However, with the arrival of DCS techniques, even in the critically ill, it became apparent that morbidity, post-operative complications, lengths of stay, and outcomes were improved by a damage control approach, with early (even temporary) fixation. Fracture care (possibly because of the large energy required to break the bone in the first place), plays a large part in minimizing the body's systemic inflammatory response to trauma.

The goals of damage control orthopaedics are to limit ongoing haemorrhage and soft tissue through efficient fracture stabilization, while minimizing additional physiological insult. Care is to follow normal damage control principles, such as avoiding the triad of hypothermia, coagulopathy, and acidosis, and minimizing secondary injury to organ systems (kidney, brain, etc.). External fixation is employed for long-bone fractures and pelvic injuries. In addition to wound toilet and removal of devitalized tissues, surgical management of haemorrhage and fasciotomies for potential or actual compartment syndrome are performed.

REFERENCES AND RECOMMENDED READING

References

1. Rotondo MF, Schwab CW, McGonigal MD, Phillips GR, Fruchterman TM, Kauder DR, et al. Damage control: an approach for improved survival in exsanguinating penetrating abdominal injury. *J Trauma*. 1993 Sep;**35(3)**:375–82; discussion 382-3.

2. Newell MA, Schlitzkus LL, Waibel BH, White MA, Schenarts PJ, Rotondo MF. "Damage control" in the elderly: futile endeavour or fruitful enterprise? *J Trauma*. 2010 Nov; **69(5)**:1049–53. doi: 10.1097/TA.0b013e3181ed4e7a.3.

3. Smith IM, Beech ZKM, Lundy JB, Bowley DM. A prospective observational study of abdominal injury management in the contemporary military operations: Damage control laparotomy is associated with high survivability and low rates of fecal diversion. *Ann Surg*. 2015 Apr;**261(4)**:765–73. doi: 10.1097/SLA.0000000000000657.

4. Gastes J, Arabian S, Biddinger P, Blansfield J, Burke P, Chung S, et al. The initial response to the Boston Marathon Bombing: Lessons to prepare for the next disaster. *Ann Surg*. 2014 Dec;**260(6)**:960–6. doi: 10.1097/SLA.00000000000009145.

5. Holcomb JB, Jenkins D, Rhee P, Johannigman J, Mahoney P, Mehta S, et al. Damage control resuscitation: directly addressing the early coagulopathy of trauma. *J Trauma*. 2007 Feb;**62(2)**:307–10.

6. Hess JR, Holcomb JB, Hoyt DB. Damage control resuscitation: the need for specific blood products to treat the coagulopathy of trauma. *Transfusion* 2006 May;**46(5)**:685–6.

7. Lamb CM, MacGoey P, Navarro AP, Brooks AJ. Damage control surgery in the era of damage control resuscitation. *Br J Anaes*. 2014 Aug;**113(2)**:242–9. doi: 10.1093/bja/aeu233.

8. Schreiber MA, Meier EN, Tisherman SA, Kerby JD, Newgard CD, Brasel K, et al. ROC Investigators. A controlled resuscitation strategy is feasible and safe in hypotensive trauma patients: results of a prospective randomized pilot trial. *J Trauma Acute Care Surg*. 2015 Apr;**78(4)**:687–95; discussion 695–7. doi: 10.1097/TA.0000000000000600.

9. Gunter OL, Jr., Au BK, Isbell JM, Mowery NT, Young PP, Cotton BA. Optimising outcomes in damage control resuscitation: identifying blood product ratios associated with improved survival. *J Trauma*. 2008 Sep;**65(3)**:527–34. doi: 10.1097/TA.0b013e3181826ddf.

10. Holcomb JB, Wade CE, Michalek JE, Chisholm GB, Zarzabal LA, Schreiber MA, et al. Increased plasma and platelet to red blood cell ratios improves outcome in 466 massively

transfused civilian trauma patients. *Ann Surg.* 2008 Sep; **248(3)**:447–58. doi: 10.1097/SLA.0b013e318185a9ad.

11. Kozar RA, Peng Z, Zhang R, Holcomb JB, Pati S, Park P, et al. Plasma restoration of endothelial glycocalyx in a rodent model of hemorrhagic shock. *Anesthesia & Analgesia.* 2011 Jun;**112(6)**:1289–95. doi: 10.1213/ANE.0b013e318210385c.

12. Cannon JW, Khan MA, Raja AS, Cohen MJ, Como JJ, Cotton BA, et al. Damage control resuscitation in patients with severe traumatic hemorrhage: A practice management guideline from the Eastern Association for the Surgery of Trauma. *J Trauma Acute Care Surg.* 2017 Mar; **82(3)**:605–617. doi: 10.1097/TA.0000000000001333.

13. Cotton BA, Au BK, Nunez TC, Gunter OL, Robertson AM, Young PP. Predefined massive transfusion protocols are associated with a reduction in organ failure and postinjury complications. *J Trauma.* 2009 Jan;**66(1)**:41–8; discussion 48–9. doi: 10.1097/TA.0b013e31819313bb.

14. Schein M, Saadia R, Jamieson JR, Decker GA. The 'sandwich technique' in the management of the open abdomen. *Br J Surg.* 1986;**73**:369–70.

15. Roberts DJ, Zygun DA, Grendar J, Ball CG, Robertson HL, Ouellet JF, Cheatham ML, Kirkpatrick AW. Negative-pressure wound therapy for critically ill adults with open abdominal wounds: a systematic review. *J Trauma Acute Care Surg.* 2012 Mar;**73(3)**:629–39. Review.

16. Brenner M, Bochicchio G, Bocchicchio K, Ilahi O, Rodriguez E, Henry S, et al. Long-term impact of damage control laparotomy: a prospective study. *Arch Surg.* 2011 Apr;146(4):395–9. doi: 10.1001/archsurg.2010.284.

17. Boulton CL. Damage Control Orthopaedics. Orth Knowledge Online J. 2013 11(2): https://www.aaos.org/periodicalissue/?issue=OKOJ/vol11/issue2 (accessed online Dec 2018).

Recommended Reading

Chovanes J, Cannon JW, Nunez TC. The evolution of damage control surgery. *Surg Clin North Am.* 2012 Aug;**92(4)**:859–75, vii-viii. doi: 10.1016/j.suc.2012.04.002.

Cirocchi R, Abraha I, Montedori A, Farinella E, Bonacini I, Tagliabue L, et al. Damage control surgery for abdominal trauma. *Cochrane Database Syst Rev.* 2010;**(1)**:CD007438.

Godat L, Kobayashi L, Costantini T, Coimbra R. Abdominal damage control surgery and reconstruction: World Society of Emergency Surgery position paper. *World J Emerg Surg.* 2013 Dec;**17(8)**:53. doi: 10.1186/1749-7922-8-53.

Holcomb JB, Jenkins D, Rhee P, Johannigman J, Mahoney P, Mehta S, et al. Damage control resuscitation: directly addressing the early coagulopathy of trauma. *J Trauma.* 2007 Feb;**62(2)**:307–10.

O'Connor JV, DuBose JJ, Scalea TM. Damage-control thoracic surgery: Management and outcomes. *J Trauma Acute Care Surg.* 2014 Nov;**77(5)**:660–665.

Rossaint R, Bouillon B, Cerny V, Coats TJ, Duranteau J, Fernández-Mondéjar E, et al. The European guideline on management of major bleeding and coagulopathy following trauma: fourth edition. *Crit Care.* 2016 Apr 12;**20**:100. doi: 10.1186/s13054-016-1265-x.

Part 3

Anatomical and organ system injury

The Neck 7

7.1 OVERVIEW

The high density of critical vascular, aerodigestive, and neurological structures within the neck makes the management of penetrating injuries difficult and contributes to the morbidity and mortality seen in these patients.

Before World War II, non-operative management of penetrating neck trauma resulted in mortality rates of up to 15%. Therefore, the exploration of all neck wounds penetrating the platysma muscle became mandatory. However, in recent years, numerous centres have challenged this principle of mandatory exploration, since up to 50% of neck explorations may be negative for significant injury.

7.2 MANAGEMENT PRINCIPLES: PENETRATING CERVICAL INJURY

7.2.1 Initial Assessment and Definitive Airway

Patients with signs of significant neck injury with active bleeding or an expanding haematoma, will require prompt exploration. However, initial assessment and management of the patient should be carried out according to Advanced Trauma Life Support® principles.

The major initial concern in any patient with a penetrating neck wound is early control of the airway. Supplemental oxygen is critical. Oxygenate the patient with simple measures first (i.e. basic airway opening techniques).

Intubation in these patients is complicated by the possibility of associated cervical spine injury, laryngeal trauma, and large haematomas in the neck. Appropriate protective measures for possible cervical spine injury

must be implemented. While it is important to protect the unstable/potentially unstable cervical spine with immobilization, a rapid risk/benefit assessment must be done in the presence of a deteriorating airway. Cervical spine immobilization techniques make endotracheal intubation more difficult.

The route of intubation must be carefully considered in these patients since it may be complicated by distortion of anatomy, haematoma, dislodging of clots, laryngeal trauma, and cervical spinal injury. It may be possible to place an endotracheal tube over a bronchoscope, enter the trachea under direct vision, and then slide the endotracheal tube into place. Use of the fibre-optic portable video laryngoscope (Glidescope Go®, Verathon, Bothell, WA, USA) may prove useful.

Recent UK military experience in Afghanistan is that most patients can be managed with a rapid sequence induction of anaesthesia followed by endotracheal intubation with a relatively small tube (e.g. size 6.5 mm or 7.0 mm in an adult male) aided by a gum-elastic bougie or stylet. The caveat is that a surgeon is scrubbed and ready to perform a cricothyroidotomy if it becomes immediately obvious that the trachea cannot be intubated following rapid sequence induction (RSI).

Patients have also been managed by a gas induction of anaesthesia (supplemented with small boluses of ketamine – 10 mg IV), laryngoscopy while still breathing, then endotracheal intubation.

Patients with signs of significant neck injury, and those whose condition is unstable, should be explored urgently in the operating room with good light, good instruments, and good assistance, once rapid initial assessment has been completed and the airway has been secured. Tracheostomy has no place in the emergency department. Cricothyroidotomies should be converted to formal tracheostomies within about 48 hours.

Pitfalls

- Be aware that bleeding into the airway will rapidly obscure the view of the cords.
- Laryngeal mask airways (LMAs) do NOT provide a definitive airway in the presence of complex neck injuries, but can be used to attempt oxygenation prior to endotracheal tube intubation or surgical airway.
- Endotracheal intubation should be considered at a very early stage in the presence of a large or expanding haematoma, before the anatomy is lost. Subsequent cricothyroidotomy or emergency percutaneous tracheostomy (only to be considered if the enabling environment, with extensive experience in the technique, is available), can be technically difficult as by entering the haematoma planes, torrential bleeding via the skin incision may result.
- *NB: The use of paralysing agents in these patients should be used as a last resort, and with extreme caution, since the airway may be held open only by the patient's own use of muscles.* Abolishing the use of muscles in such patients may result in the immediate and total obstruction of the airway and, with no visibility owing to the presence of blood, may result in catastrophe. Ideally, local anaesthetic spray should be used with sedation, and a cricothyroidotomy (below the injury) should be considered when necessary.

Managing complicated airway injuries should be rehearsed along with back-up plans for alternate techniques to secure the airway if the initial plan fails. The decision as to what technique is the most appropriate should be made rapidly and jointly by the surgeon, anaesthetist, and trauma team leader.

There should be no hesitation in performing an emergency cricothyroidotomy should circumstances warrant it.

7.2.2 Control of Haemorrhage

Control of haemorrhage should be done by direct pressure where possible. If the neck wound is *not* bleeding, do not probe or finger the wound, as the clot may be dislodged. If the wound is actively bleeding, the bleeding should be controlled by digital pressure or if ineffective, a Foley catheter may be inserted into the wound and the balloon inflated. This is often useful for stopping haemorrhage deep in the neck. Occasionally, the wound may

need to be sutured around the catheter to produce the required tamponade.

Pitfall

This may result in converting external haemorrhage into concealed bleeding deep within the neck if tamponade is not achieved and will further compromise an already compressed airway. Hence the importance of securing an early definitive airway. More than one Foley catheter is sometimes needed.

7.2.3 Injury Location

Division of the neck into anatomical zones (Figure 7.1) helps the categorization and management of neck wounds:

- *Zone I* extends from the level of the sternal notch to the lower border of the cricoid cartilage. Within zone I lie the great vessels, the trachea, the oesophagus, the thoracic duct, and the upper mediastinum and lung apices.
- *Zone II* includes the area between the cricoid cartilage and the angle of the mandible. Enclosed within its region are the carotid and vertebral arteries, jugular veins, pharynx, larynx, oesophagus, and trachea.
- *Zone III* includes the area above the angle of the mandible to the base of the skull, the pharynx, and the distal extracranial carotid and vertebral arteries, as well as segments of the jugular veins.

Injuries in zone II are readily evaluated and exposed operatively. In trauma centres with a high volume of penetrating trauma, a decision on immediate surgery can be reached on clinical grounds without any pre-operative investigations. Zones I and III are difficult to assess clinically and to access operatively. Therefore, in those two zones it is important in the physiologically stable patient

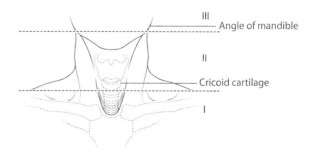

Figure 7.1 Anterior view showing zones of the neck.

to proceed with diagnostic work-up so that the presence or absence of injury is established, the possibility of dealing with it without an operative procedure is decided (e.g. embolization of bleeding artery), as should operation be necessary, this will be facilitated by knowing the type of injury and its topography.

Pitfall

Assuming that a wound in one zone means an injury in that zone. Not infrequently, a wound in one zone is associated with the injury in quite another area. For example, a long knife may penetrate the skin in zones I or II, but the injury may lie in the superior mediastinum. Similarly, bullets and missile fragments often transgress zone boundaries. Either may cross the midline, giving rise to contralateral injured structures.

7.2.4 Mechanism

Gunshot wounds carry a higher risk of major injury than stab wounds, because of their tendency to penetrate more deeply and their ability to damage tissue outside the tract of the missile owing to cavitation, or a percussion wave injury.

7.2.5 Frequency of Injury

The carotid artery and internal jugular vein are the most frequently injured vessels. Owing to its relatively protected position, the vertebral artery is involved less frequently. The larynx and trachea, and pharynx and oesophagus are frequently injured. The spinal cord is damaged less often, but injury should not be ruled out until examination has confirmed its integrity.

7.2.6 Use of Diagnostic Studies

In the stable patient without indications for immediate neck exploration, additional studies are often obtained, including computed tomography (CT) angiography, endoscopy, contrast radiography, and bronchoscopy.

7.2.6.1 COMPUTED TOMOGRAPHY SCANNING WITH CONTRAST/COMPUTED TOMOGRAPHY ANGIOGRAPHY

Modern CT scanners have provided a means of creating a three-dimensional (3D) images of high quality, and CT scanning is now the investigation of choice for penetrating injury in the stable patient. Angiography has been largely replaced by CT-angiography and should include both internal and external carotid arteries on both sides (four vessel CT angiography), as well as the vertebral arteries, preferably with 3D reconstruction. All patients with zone I and III neck injuries should undergo CT angiography provided their vital signs are stable.

7.2.6.2 ANGIOGRAPHY

Especially in zone I or zone III injuries, where surgical exposure can be difficult, open angiography allows arterial embolization, as well as stenting of a particular vessel.

Using a selective approach to the management of zone II wounds, angiography is useful in excluding carotid injuries, especially with soft signs of injury, including stable haematoma and history of significant bleeding, or when the wound is near the major vessels.

7.2.6.3 OTHER DIAGNOSTIC STUDIES

The selective management of penetrating neck wounds involves evaluation of the oesophagus, larynx, and trachea. Modern fluoroscopy machines with water-soluble contrast of an iso-oncotic nature (e.g. Omnipaque) will detect 99% of clinically relevant oesophageal injuries.[1] Flexible endoscopy may increase the yield even further. Laryngoscopy and bronchoscopy are useful adjuncts in localizing or excluding injury to the hypopharynx or trachea. A recent development is 3D CT reconstruction of the trachea and bronchi can replace endoscopy in suspected injuries of these anatomical structures.

7.3 MANAGEMENT

7.3.1 Mandatory versus Selective Neck Exploration

Recommendations for the management of patients with penetrating cervical trauma depend on the zone of injury and the patient's clinical status. If the platysma is not penetrated, the patient may be observed. Mandatory exploration for penetrating neck injury in patients with hard signs of vascular or aerodigestive tract injury is still appropriate.

Missed injuries are associated with a high morbidity and mortality due to missed visceral injuries, and the negligible morbidity caused by negative exploration are important; however, exploration of all stab wounds of the neck may yield a high rate of non-therapeutic procedures. Thus, the selective management of penetrating neck wounds based on CT evaluation has been recommended.

7.3.2 Management Based on Anatomical Zones

- Zone I injuries require angiography because of the increased association of vascular injuries with penetrating trauma to the thoracic outlet. Angiography helps the surgeon plan the surgical approach.
- Zone II injuries may require angiography if the vertebral vessels are thought to be injured. Venous phasing should be requested.
- Zone III injuries require angiography because of the relationship of the blood vessels to the base of the skull. Often these injuries can be best managed by either non-operative techniques or manoeuvres remote from the injury site such as balloon tamponade or embolization.

Pitfall

Angiography will *not* rule out significant injury to the trachea or oesophagus.

7.4 ACCESS TO THE NECK

The operative approach selected to explore neck injuries is determined by the structures known or suspected to be injured. Surgical exploration should be done formally and systematically in a fully equipped operating room under general anaesthesia with endotracheal intubation. Blind probing of wounds or mini-explorations in the emergency department should **never** be attempted.

7.4.1 Position

Active bleeding from a penetrating wound should be controlled digitally. Penetrating wounds to the neck should not be probed, cannulated or locally explored because these procedures may dislodge a clot and cause uncontrollable bleeding or air embolism. Skin preparation should include the entire chest and shoulder, extending above the angle of the mandible. The face, neck, and anterior chest should be prepped and widely draped. The patient is placed in the supine position on the operating table with the arms tucked at the sides. If possible, the head should be extended and rotated to the contralateral side. A sandbag may be placed between the shoulder blades, and the neck extended and rotated away from the side of injury – provided that the cervical spine has been cleared pre-operatively (Figure 7.2).

7.4.2 Incision

Always expect the worst! Plan the incision to provide optimal access for early vascular source control or immediate access to the airway. The most universally applicable approach is via an incision along the anterior border of sternomastoid, which can be lengthened proximally and distally, extended to a median sternotomy or augmented with lateral extensions (Figure 7.3).

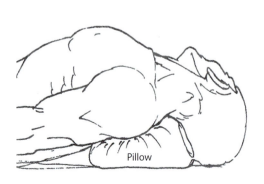
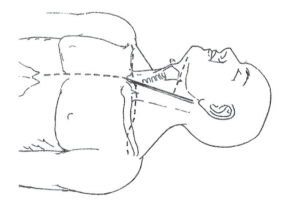

Figure 7.2 Approach to the left side of the neck – patient positioning.

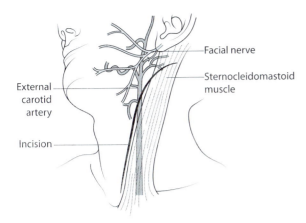

Figure 7.3 Approach to the left side of the neck – initial incision.

Having made the sternocleidomastoid muscle incision, platysma is divided, and the sternomastoid is retracted laterally to expose the fascial sheath covering the internal jugular vein. The vein cannot be mobilized until the common facial vein is divided. Omohyoid muscle is the only strap muscle that crosses the carotid sheath obliquely, and acts as a landmark for the common carotid artery. Lateral retraction of the jugular vein and underlying carotid artery allows access to the trachea, oesophagus, and thyroid, and medial retraction of the carotid sheath and its contents will allow the dissection to proceed posteriorly to the prevertebral fascia and vertebral arteries. Posterior to the carotid sheath, the sympathetic chain lies

on longus colli, which separates it from the transverse processes of the cervical vertebrae (Figure 7.4).

7.4.3 **Surgical Access**

7.4.3.1 ZONE I

Zone I vascular injuries at the base of the neck require aggressive management. Frequently, uncontrollable haemorrhage will require immediate thoracotomy for initial proximal control. In an unstable patient, quick exposure often may be achieved via a median sternotomy and a supraclavicular extension.

The location of the vascular injury will dictate the definitive exposure. For right-sided great vessel injuries, a median sternotomy with a supraclavicular extension allows optimal access. On the left side, a left anterolateral thoracotomy may provide initial proximal control. Further operation for definitive repair may require a sternotomy, or extension into the right side of the chest or up into the neck. 'Trapdoor' or 'clamshell' incisions are **not** recommended. They are often difficult to perform, do not significantly improve the exposure, but significantly increase the morbidity postoperative disability. Avoid injury to the phrenic and vagus nerves as they enter the thorax. In the stable patient in whom the vascular injury has been confirmed by CT, the right subclavian artery or the distal two-thirds of the left subclavian artery can be exposed through an incision immediately superior to the medial third of the clavicle. Injuries to the vessels behind

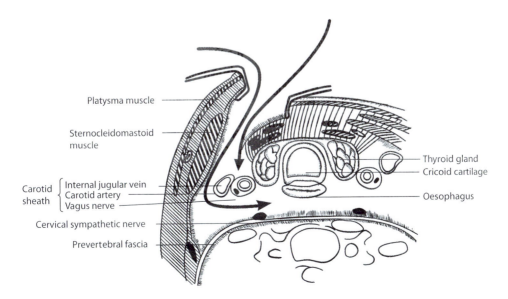

Figure 7.4 Approach to the left side of the neck showing retraction of the platysma and sternomastoid muscles.

the clavicle can be controlled by combining supra- and infra-clavicular incisions. The clavicle does *not* need to be divided or resected. Grafts can easily be tunnelled underneath the bone, avoiding risk to the subclavian vein.

- Injuries to the internal jugular vein should be repaired if possible. In severe injuries that require extensive debridement, ligation is preferred. Venous interposition grafts should not be performed.
- Vertebral artery injuries are generally found to have been injured only on angiographic study. These rarely require surgical repair, as they are best dealt with by angioembolization. Operative exposure may be difficult, and it may be easier to ligate it at its origin off the subclavian artery, or passage of a size 3 or 4 Fogarty catheter into the lumen and inflation of the balloon to provide tamponade. This may be left permanently if required, with very small incidence of neurological damage. Venous bleeding can be stopped by packing around the area of injury.

Many carotid artery injuries can be managed with intraluminal stenting. This approach is now used most frequently in situations where arterial lesions are not surgically accessible or when anticoagulation is contraindicated.

7.4.3.2 ZONE II

Zone II injuries are explored by an incision made along the anterior border of the sternocleidomastoid muscle, as for carotid endarterectomy. An extended collar incision or bilateral incisions along the anterior edge of the sternocleidomastoid muscles may be used for wounds that traverse both sides of the neck. Proximal and distal control of the blood vessel is obtained. If the vessel is actively bleeding, direct pressure is applied to the bleeding site while control is obtained. Use of anticoagulation is optional. If there are no injuries that preclude its use, heparin may be given in the management of carotid injuries. Vascular shunts are rarely needed in patients with carotid injuries, especially if the distal clamp is applied proximal to the bifurcation of the internal and external carotid arteries. Repair techniques for cervical trauma do not differ significantly from those used for other vascular injuries.

7.4.3.3 ZONE III

Zone III injuries, at the very base of the skull, are complex and should be explored with great care. Access is often extremely difficult, and on rare occasions, it may not be

possible to control the distal stump of a high internal carotid artery injury. Bleeding from this injury can be controlled either temporarily or permanently by inserting a Fogarty catheter into the distal segment and inflating the balloon. The catheter is secured, transected, and left in place. It may be necessary to control the internal carotid artery from within the cranial cavity (usually the realm of the neurosurgeon).

7.4.4 Priorities

- The first concern in the patient with a penetrating injury of the neck is early control of the airway.
- The next concern is to stop bleeding, either by digital pressure or using a Foley catheter.
- The stability of the patient decides the appropriate diagnostic and treatment priorities. Never make the operation more difficult than necessary by inadequate exposure. Adequate exposure of the area involved is critical.
- The intra-operative decisions are influenced by the patient's preoperative neurological status. If the patient has no neurological deficit preoperatively, the injured vessel should he repaired. (The one exception may be if a complete obstruction of blood flow is found at the time of surgery, because restoration of flow may cause distal remobilization or haemorrhagic infarction.)
- Operative management of the patient with a carotid injury and a preoperative neurological deficit is controversial. Vascular reconstruction should be performed in patients with mild-to-moderate deficits in whom retrograde flow is present. Ligation is recommended for patients with severe preoperative neurological deficits greater than 48 hours old, and without evidence of retrograde flow at the time of operation.

7.4.4.1 VASCULAR INJURIES

If associated injuries allow, 5000–10,000 units of heparin as a bolus should be given before any of the arteries in the neck are occluded. Because they have no branches, the common and internal carotid arteries can be safely mobilized for some distance from the injury to ensure a tension-free repair.

7.4.4.2 CAROTID ARTERY

For exposure of the proximal carotid artery in zone I, the artery is exposed by division of the omohyoid muscle between the superior and inferior bellies. More proximal control may require a midline sternotomy.

Exposure of the carotid artery in zone III is obtained by ligating the middle thyroid and common facial veins and retracting the internal jugular laterally together with the sternocleidomastoid. The vagus, nerve lying posteriorly within the carotid sheath, must be preserved. The occipital artery and inferior branches of the *ansa cervicalis* may be divided. To expose the carotid bifurcation, the dissection is carried upwards to the posterior belly of the digastric muscle, which is divided behind the angle of the jaw. Care must be taken to find and preserve the hypoglossal nerve, which runs forward across both internal and external carotid artery to enter the floor of the mouth. It usually is found either at the lower border of the posterior belly of digastric, or just deep to that muscle (Figure 7.5).

For distal zone III carotid injuries, consider angiographic stenting. However, if surgical intervention is required:

- Use nasotracheal intubation, not orotracheal. The tube between the teeth opens the mouth and reduces the space behind the ramus.
- Access to the internal carotid can be improved by dividing the sternocleidomastoid muscle near its origin at the mastoid. Care must be taken not to injure the accessory nerve where it enters the sternomastoid muscle 3 cm below the mastoid, or the glossopharyngeal nerve crossing anteriorly over the internal carotid artery.

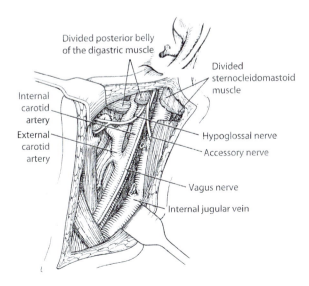

Figure 7.5 Approach to the left side of the neck with divided sternomastoid and digastric muscles.

- More distal exploration of the internal carotid artery may require unilateral mandibular subluxation, division of the ascending ramus.
- A Langenbeck retractor can be used to pull the upper pole of the mandibular ramus forward, increasing access to the internal carotid artery in zone III.
- The styloid process may be excised after division of the stylohyoid ligament and styloglossus and stylopharyngeus muscles. The facial nerve lies superficial to these muscles and must be preserved.
- To reach the internal carotid artery where it enters the carotid canal, part of the mastoid bone can be removed. Fortunately, this is rarely required.

7.4.4.3 TRACHEAL INJURIES

Injuries to the trachea should be closed in a single layer with absorbable sutures. Larger defects may require a fascia flap. These injuries should be drained.

7.4.4.4 PHARYNGEAL AND OESOPHAGEAL INJURIES

Oesophageal injuries are often missed at neck exploration. Injuries to the hypopharynx and cervical oesophagus may also be difficult to diagnose preoperatively. Perforations of the hypopharynx or oesophagus should be closed in two layers if possible, though the mucosal layer is the key to leak-proof repair. The site should be widely drained. Identification may be aided by the passage of a nasogastric tube. For devastating oesophageal injuries requiring extensive resection and debridement, a cutaneous oesophagostomy for feeding, and pharyngostomy for diversion, may be necessary.

7.4.5 **Midline Visceral Structures**

The trachea, oesophagus, and thyroid are approached by retracting the carotid sheath laterally. The inferior thyroid artery should be divided laterally near the carotid artery, and the thyroid lobe is lifted anteriorly to expose the trachea and oesophagus posteriorly. Oesophageal identification is aided by passing a large dilator or nasogastric tube. The recurrent laryngeal nerves should be carefully preserved: the left nerve runs vertically in the tracheo-oesophageal groove, but the right nerve runs obliquely across the oesophagus and trachea from inferolateral to superomedial. Both nerves are at risk of injury with circumferential mobilization of the oesophagus.

Bilateral exposure of the midline structures may require transverse extension of the standard incision.

7.4.6 **Root of the Neck**

The structures at the root of the neck can be approached by extending the incision laterally above the clavicle. The clavicular head of the sternocleidomastoid is divided, and the supraclavicular fat pad is cleared by blunt dissection. This fat pad is a constant feature, even in the thinnest of individuals. It is complicated in its removal by containing many small blood vessels, lymph nodes, and the thoracic duct. Removal reveals the scalenus anterior muscle, with the phrenic nerve crossing it from the lateral side. Division of the scalenus anterior, with preservation of the phrenic nerve, allows access to the second part of the subclavian artery. The distal subclavian artery can be exposed by a further infra-clavicular incision and obtaining control of the proximal axillary artery, or dividing the clavicle at its mid-point, and dissecting away the subclavius muscle and fascia. The clavicle should not be resected as this leads to considerable morbidity. To fix the divided bone, the periosteum should be approximated with strong polyfilament absorbable sutures, or a mini-plate can be inserted.

7.4.7 **Collar Incisions**

These are rarely used unless there is absolute certainty that the injury is limited to the area about to be exposed. In trauma in general, it is wiser to make incisions that can be extended both proximally and distally. It may be preferable to utilize bilateral sternomastoid incisions that can be joined for bilateral injuries in the form of a 'U'.

Some surgeons adopt the collar incisions. Horizontal or 'collar' incisions placed either over the thyroid or higher up over the thyroid cartilage can sometimes useful to expose bilateral injuries or injuries limited to the larynx or trachea. The transverse incision is carried through the platysma, and subplatysmal flaps are then developed: superiorly up to the thyroid cartilage notch, and inferiorly to the sternal notch. The strap muscles are divided vertically in the midline and retracted laterally to expose the fascia covering the thyroid. The thyroid isthmus can be divided to expose the trachea. A high collar incision, placed over the larynx, is useful for repairing isolated laryngeal injuries.

7.4.8 **Vertebral Arteries**

The proximal part of the vertebral artery is approached via the anterior sternomastoid incision, with division of the clavicular head of the sternomastoid. The internal jugular vein and common carotid artery are mobilized, the vein is retracted medially, and the artery and nerve are retracted laterally. The proximal vertebral artery lies deeply between these structures. The vertebral artery is crossed by branches of the cervical sympathetic chain and on the left side by the thoracic duct. The inferior thyroid artery crosses in a more superficial plane just before the vertebral artery enters its bony canal.

Access to the distal vertebral artery is challenging and rarely needed. The contents of the carotid sheath are retracted anteromedially, and the prevertebral muscles are longitudinally split over a transverse process above the level of the injury. The anterior surface of the transverse process can be removed with a small rongeur, or a J-shaped needle may be used to snare the artery in the space between the transverse processes.

The most distal portion of the vertebral artery can be approached between the atlas and the axis after division of the sternocleidomastoid near its origin at the mastoid process. The prevertebral fascia is divided over the transverse process of the atlas. With preservation of the C2 nerve root, the levator scapulae and splenius cervicus muscles are divided close to the transverse process of the atlas. The vertebral artery can now be visualized between the two vertebrae and may be ligated with a J-shaped needle. This area of dissection is more commonly the in province of a neurosurgeon if available.

Neck exploration wounds are closed in layers after acquiring homeostasis. Drainage is usually indicated, mainly to prevent haematomas and sepsis.

REFERENCES AND RECOMMENDED READING

References

1. Nel L, Whitfield Jones L, Hardcastle TC. Imaging the Oesophagus After Penetrating Cervical Trauma Using Water Soluble Contrast Alone: Simple, Cost Effective And Accurate. *Emerg Med J*. 2009 Feb;**26(2)**:106–8. doi: 10.1136/emj.2008.063958.

Recommended Reading

Demetriades D, Asensio JA, Velmahos G, Thal E. Complex problems in penetrating neck trauma. *Surg Clin North Am.* 1996 Aug;**76**:661–83.

Fabian TC, George SM Jr, Croce MA, Mangiante EC, Voeller GR, Kusdk KA. Carotid artery trauma: management based on mechanism of injury. *J Trauma.* 1990 Aug;**30(8)**:953–61; discussion 961-3.

Osborn TM, Bell RB, Qaisi W, Long WB. Computed angiography as an aid to clinical decision making in the selective management of penetrating injuries of the neck: A reduction in the need for operative exploration. *J Trauma.* 2008 Jun;**64(6)**:1466–71. doi: 10.1097/TA.0b013e3181271b32.

The Chest 8

8.1 OVERVIEW

Thoracic injury constitutes a significant problem in terms of mortality and morbidity. Somewhat less clearly defined is the extent of appreciable morbidity following chest injury, most usually the long-term consequences of hypoxic brain damage.

A significant proportion of deaths occur virtually immediately (i.e. at the time of injury), for example, rapid exsanguination following traumatic rupture of the aorta in blunt injury or major vascular disruption after penetrating injury.

Of survivors with thoracic injury who reach hospital, some die in hospital as the result of mis-assessment or delay in treatment. These deaths occur *early*, owing to blood loss, or *late* as the result of respiratory failure, multiple organ failure, and sepsis. Most life-threatening thoracic injuries can be simply and promptly treated after identification with simple and effective techniques that can be performed by any trained physician.

Emergency department thoracotomy (EDT) has specific indications, usually related to patients in extremis with penetrating injury. Indiscriminate use of EDT, however, especially in blunt trauma, will not alter patient outcomes, but will increase the risk of communicable disease transmission to health workers.

Injuries to the chest wall and thoracic viscera can directly impair oxygen transport mechanisms. Hypoxia and hypovolaemia resulting because of thoracic injury, may cause secondary injury to patients with brain injury or may directly cause cerebral oedema.

Conversely, shock and/or brain injury can secondarily aggravate thoracic injuries and hypoxaemia by disrupting normal ventilatory patterns or by causing loss of protective airway reflexes and aspiration.

The lung is a target organ for secondary injury following shock and remote tissue injury. Microemboli formed in the peripheral microcirculation embolize to the lung, causing ventilation – perfusion mismatch and right heart failure. Tissue injury and shock can activate the inflammatory cascade, which can contribute to pulmonary injury (reperfusion).

8.2 THE SPECTRUM OF THORACIC INJURY

Thoracic injuries are grouped into two types, as described below.

8.2.1 Immediately Life-Threatening Injuries

- Airway obstruction due to any cause, including laryngeal or tracheal disruption with obstruction or extensive facial bony and soft tissue injuries.
- Impaired ventilation owing to tension pneumothorax, major bronchial disruptions, open pneumothorax, or flail chest.
- Impaired circulation owing to massive haemothorax or pericardial tamponade.
- Air embolism.

8.2.2 Potentially Life-Threatening Injuries

- Blunt cardiac injury.
- Pulmonary contusion.
- Pneumothorax.
- Haemothorax.
- Flail chest (multiple fractured ribs with paradoxical chest wall movement).
- Traumatic rupture of the aorta.
- Traumatic diaphragmatic herniation.
- Tracheobronchial tree disruption.
- Oesophageal disruption.

Penetrating wounds traversing the mediastinum frequently damage several mediastinal structures and are thus more complex in their evaluation and management.

8.3 PATHOPHYSIOLOGY OF THORACIC INJURIES

The well-recognized pathophysiological changes occurring in patients with thoracic injuries are essentially the result of:

- Impairment of ventilation.
- Impairment of gas exchange at the alveolar level.
- Impairment of circulation due to haemodynamic changes.
- Impairment of cardiac function due to tamponade or air embolus.

The approach to the patient with thoracic injury must therefore take all these elements into account. Specifically, hypoxia at a cellular or tissue level results from inadequate delivery of oxygen to the tissues, with development of acidosis and associated hypercapnia. The late complications resulting from mis-assessment of thoracic injuries are directly attributable to these processes.

Penetrating chest injuries should be obvious. Exceptions include small puncture wounds such as those caused by ice picks, or ballistic fragments. Bleeding is generally minimal secondary to the low pressure within the pulmonary system. Exceptions to these management principles include wounds to the great vessels as they exit over the apex of the chest wall to the upper extremities, or injury to any systemic vessel that may be injured in the chest wall, such as the internal mammary or intercostal vessels.

Penetrating injuries to the mid-torso generate more controversy. These will require an aggressive approach, particularly with anterior wounds. If the wound is between one posterior axillary line and the other and obviously penetrates the abdominal wall, laparotomy is indicated. If the wound does not obviously penetrate, an option is to explore the wound under local anaesthesia to determine whether it has penetrated the peritoneum or the diaphragm. If peritoneal penetration has occurred, laparotomy is indicated. Other options include laparoscopy or thoracoscopy to determine whether the diaphragm has been injured, and for evacuation of clots (see Section 9.3: Diaphragm).[1]

In the haemodynamically unstable patient with penetrating injury to the upper torso whose bleeding is occurring into the chest cavity, it is important to insert a chest tube as soon as possible during the initial assessment and resuscitation. In the patient in extremis who has chest injuries or in whom there may be suspicion of a transmediastinal injury, bilateral chest tubes may be indicated. X-ray is *not* required to insert a chest tube, but it *is* useful after the chest tubes have been inserted to confirm proper placement.

In haemodynamically stable patients, the widespread use, free availability, and training in performing eFAST (extended Focused Assessment with Sonography in Trauma) and other clinician performed modalities, has further reduced the need for plain x-rays in thoracic trauma. However, chest x-ray performed in the emergency department (ED) remains the gold standard for diagnosis of a pneumothorax or haemothorax. In these patients, it is preferable to have the x-ray completed before placement of a chest tube. The decrease in air entry may not be due to a pneumothorax, and especially following blunt injury may be due to a ruptured diaphragm with bowel or stomach occupying the thoracic cavity, or simply pulmonary contusion (which will be missed on eFAST).

When it comes to the removal of chest tubes, bedside thoracic ultrasonography of the fourth intercostal space can reliably determine safe removal of tube thoracostomy after traumatic injury, by excluding the presence of an ongoing pneumothorax, and ensuring a new pneumothorax has not redeveloped by repeating the examination in 4–6 hours.[2]

8.3.1 Paediatric Considerations

There are several important considerations in the assessment and management of paediatric and adolescent chest trauma.[3]

- In children, the ribs are more flexible, so the presence of rib fractures implies a high energy injury, a higher incidence of associated head, thoracic, and abdominal solid organ injuries.[4]
- Penetrating cardiac wounds in the paediatric age have a poorer prognosis than in adults and are associated with a low in-hospital survival (<30%).[5]
- In children, the thymus may be very large, and care should be taken to avoid damage to it.

- The sternum is relatively soft and can be divided using a pair of heavy scissors.
- Intercostal drains should be *tunnelled subcutaneously over at least one rib space* to facilitate later removal without air leaks. The child may not cooperate with a Valsalva manoeuvre, and pressure on the extended tract may prevent iatrogenic pneumothorax on removal.

Paediatric patients with and pneumothoraces after blunt torso trauma, are uncommon, and most are not identified on the ED chest x-ray. Nearly half of pneumothoraces, and most occult pneumothoraces, can be managed without tube thoracostomy.[6] An important issue in dealing with severe paediatric chest trauma is the unavailability and unsuitability of adult-sized aortic stent grafts for the very rare occasions of traumatic aortic injuries in this age group.

8.4 APPLIED SURGICAL ANATOMY OF THE CHEST

It is useful to broadly view the thorax as a container with an inlet, walls, a floor and contents.

8.4.1 The Chest Wall

This is the bony 'cage' constituted by the ribs, thoracic vertebral column, and sternum with the clavicles anteriorly and the scapula posteriorly. The associated muscle groups and vascular structures (specifically the intercostal vessels and the internal thoracic vessels) are further components.

Remember the 'safe area' of the chest. This triangular area is the thinnest region of the chest wall in terms of musculature. This is the area of choice for tube thoracostomy insertion. In this area, there are no significant structures within the walls that may be damaged; however, note that there is a need to avoid the intercostal vascular and nerve bundle on the under surface of the rib (Figure 8.1).

8.4.2 The Chest Floor

This is formed by the diaphragm with its various openings. This broad sheet of muscle with its large, trefoil-shaped central tendon has hiatuses through which pass

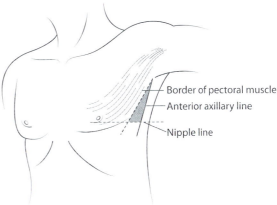

The 'triangle of safety'

Border of pectoral muscle
Anterior axillary line
Nipple line

Figure 8.1 Anatomy of the chest wall for placement of a chest drain.

the aorta, the oesophagus and the inferior vena cava, and is it innervated by the phrenic nerves. The oesophageal hiatus also contains both vagus nerves. The aortic hiatus contains the azygos vein and the thoracic duct.

During normal breathing, the diaphragm moves about 2 cm, but it can move up to 10 cm in deep breathing. During maximum expiration, the diaphragm may rise as high as the fifth intercostal space. Thus, any injury below the fifth intercostal space may involve the abdominal cavity.

8.4.3 The Chest Contents

- The left and right pleural spaces containing the lungs, lined by the parietal and visceral pleurae, respectively.
- The mediastinum and its viscera are in the centre of the chest. The mediastinum itself has anterior, middle, posterior and superior divisions (Figure 8.2). The superior mediastinum is contiguous with the thoracic inlet and zone I of the neck.
- From a functional and practical point of view, it is useful to regard the chest in terms of a 'hemithorax and its content', both in evaluation of the injury and in choosing the option for access. Figures 8.3 and 8.4 illustrate the hemithoraces and their respective contents.

8.4.3.1 TRACHEOBRONCHIAL TREE

The trachea extends from the cricoid cartilage at the level of the fifth cervical vertebra, to the carina at the

The mediastinum

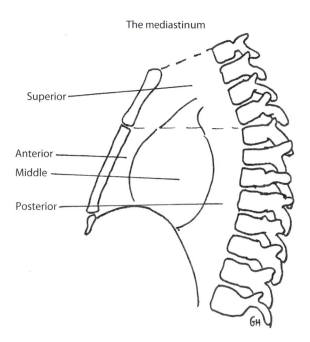

Figure 8.2 Chest contents.

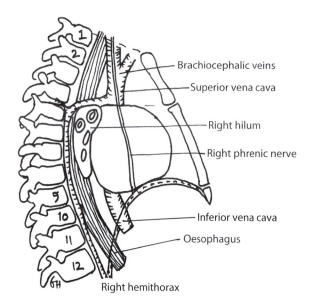

Figure 8.3 Right hemithorax and mediastinum.

level of the upper border of the sixth thoracic vertebra, where it bifurcates. The right main bronchus is shorter, straighter and at less of an angle compared with that on the left side. It lies just below the junction between the azygos vein and the superior vena cava, and behind the right pulmonary artery.

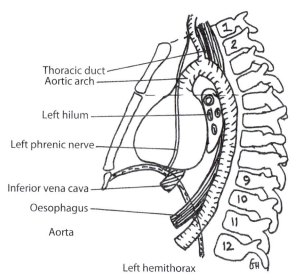

Figure 8.4 Left hemithorax and mediastinum.

8.4.3.2 LUNGS AND PLEURAE

The right lung constitutes about 55% of the total lung mass and has oblique and transverse fissures that divide it into three lobes. The left lung is divided into upper and lower lobes by the oblique fissure. Both lungs are divided into bronchopulmonary segments corresponding to the branches of the lesser bronchi and are supplied by branches of the pulmonary arteries. The right and left pulmonary arteries pass superiorly in the hilum, anterior to each respective bronchus. There are superior and inferior pulmonary veins on each side, the middle lobe usually being drained by the superior vein.

The pleural cavities are lined by parietal and visceral pleura. The parietal pleura lines the inner wall of the thoracic cage. The visceral pleura is intimately applied to the surface of the lungs and is reflected onto the mediastinum to join the parietal pleura at the hilum.

8.4.3.3 HEART AND PERICARDIUM

The heart lies in the middle mediastinum, extending from the level of the third costal cartilage to the xiphisternal junction. Most of the anterior surface of the heart is represented by the right atrium and its auricular appendage superiorly, and the right ventricle inferiorly. The aorta emerges from the cranial aspect and crosses to the left as the arch. The pulmonary artery extends cranially and bifurcates in the concavity of the aortic arch. The left pulmonary artery is attached to the concavity of the arch of the aorta, just distal to the origin of the left subclavian artery, by the ligamentum arteriosum. The pericardium is a strong fibrous sac that completely invests the heart and is attached to the diaphragm inferiorly. Pericardial tamponade can be created by less than 50 mL or up to more than 200 mL of blood.

8.4.3.4 THE AORTA AND GREAT VESSELS

The thoracic aorta is divided into three parts, the ascending aorta, arch, and descending aorta. The innominate artery is the first branch from the arch, passing upwards and to the right, posterior to the innominate vein. The left common carotid artery and left subclavian artery arise from the left side of the arch.

8.4.3.5 OESOPHAGUS

The oesophagus, approximately 25 cm long, extends from the pharynx to the stomach. It starts at the level of the sixth cervical vertebra and passes through the diaphragm about 2.5 cm to the left of the midline at the level of the 11th thoracic vertebra. The entire intrathoracic oesophagus is surrounded by loose areolar tissue, which allows for rapid spread of infection if the oesophagus is breached.

8.4.3.6 THORACIC DUCT

The duct arises from the *cysterna chyli* overlying the first and second lumbar vertebrae. It lies posteriorly and to the right of the aorta. It ascends through the oesophageal hiatus of the diaphragm between the aorta and the azygos vein, anterior to the right intercostal branches from the aorta. It overlies the right side of the vertebral bodies, and injury can result in a right-sided chylothorax. It drains into the venous system at the junction of the left subclavian and internal jugular veins.

8.5 DIAGNOSIS

Penetrating injuries to the chest may be clinically obvious. It is, however, important to log-roll the patient to make sure that the entire back has been examined. Log-rolling is just as important in patients with penetrating trauma as it is in blunt trauma, to rule out posterior injuries, and injury to the thoracic or lumbar spine.

The surgeon should auscultate each hemithorax, noting whether there are diminished or absent breath sounds.

Ultrasound has a role primarily in determining whether a patient has pericardial blood, assessing for the presence of pneumothoraces, with greater accuracy that with a supine plain chest x-ray (eFAST). It may also be superior to plain radiology in differentiating between fluid and lung contusion.[8]

Transoesophageal echocardiography is a useful adjunct in determining whether tamponade is present in the haemodynamically stable patient.

Computed tomography is not routinely used in patients with penetrating chest injury, except in *stable* patients with transmediastinal wounds. It may have some utility in determining the extent of pulmonary contusion caused by higher energy injuries or shotgun blasts but is not generally indicated in the initial resuscitation or treatment. CT angiography can be quite useful in the haemodynamically stable patient with penetrating injuries to the thoracic outlet or upper chest. This can detect arteriovenous fistulas and false aneurysms.

In the patient with penetrating injuries, a chest x-ray remains the 'gold standard' and should be obtained early. It is good practice to place metallic objects such as paper clips on the skin over any wounds on the chest wall. This is the key diagnostic study in penetrating injury, since not only will it reveal the presence of a pneumothorax and haemothorax, but also allow projection of a bullet track. Furthermore, missiles often leave metallic fragments outlining the path of the bullet, and areas of pulmonary contusion are additional indicators of the missile tract. It also can be useful for stab wounds. Tracking the missile helps the surgeon to determine which visceral organs may be injured and whether there is potential transgression of the diaphragm and/or mediastinum. Ultrasound will not show bullet tracks.

Non-operative management of mid-torso injuries is problematic until injury to the diaphragm or abdominal viscera has been excluded. Various modalities have been described to try to identify the trajectory of penetrating injuries in these regions, including triple contrast CT scan and recently, CT tractography with radiopaque contrast.[9] Thoracoscopy and laparoscopy have been successful in diagnosing diaphragm penetration. Laparoscopy may have a small advantage in that if the diaphragm has been penetrated, it also allows some assessment of the intraperitoneal viscera; however, in many ways, thoracoscopy is better for assessment of the diaphragm, particularly in the right hemithorax. The disadvantage is that once an injury has been detected, this does not rule out associated intraperitoneal injuries.

8.6 MANAGEMENT OF SPECIFIC INJURIES

Non-operative management can be used in most penetrating injuries. These patients should be observed in a monitored setting to ensure haemodynamic stability, monitoring of ventilatory status and output of blood from the pleural cavity.

Failures of non-operative management include patients who continue to bleed from the pleural cavity and those patients who go on to develop a clotted haemothorax. If there are retained clots, video-assisted thoracoscopy (VATS) is indicated, optimally within 72 hours of the injury to aid in the removal of these clots.[10]

8.6.1 Damage Control in the Chest

Damage control surgery can be applied to the chest, through packing and temporary vacuum closure.[11] Reconstruction can be carried out after physiological stabilisation. This often takes the form of myocutaneous flaps such as latissimus dorsi or pectoralis major particularly when cartilage or ribs must be debrided (see also Chapter 6).

8.6.2 Open Pneumothorax

The incidence of open pneumothorax or significant chest wall injuries following civilian trauma is low (less than 1% of all major thoracic injuries). Although all penetrating wounds are technically open pneumothoraces, the tissue of the chest wall serves as an effective seal. True open pneumothorax is most often associated with close-range shotgun blasts and high-energy missiles. There is usually a large gaping wound commonly associated with frothy blood at its entrance. Respiratory sounds can be heard, with to and from movement of air. The patient often has air hunger and may be in shock from associated visceral injuries.

The wound should be immediately sealed with an occlusive clean or sterile dressing such as petroleum-soaked gauze, thin plastic sheets, sealed on three sides to create a valve, or even aluminium foil as a temporary dressing. Once the chest wound has been sealed, it is important to realize that a tube thoracostomy may be immediately necessary because of the risk of converting the open pneumothorax into a tension pneumothorax, if there is associated parenchymal injury to the lung.

Large gaping wounds will invariably require debridement, including resection of devitalized tissue back to bleeding tissue, and removal of all foreign bodies including clothing, wadding from shotgun shells, or debris from the object that penetrated the chest. Most of these patients will require thoracotomy to treat visceral injuries and to control bleeding from the lung or chest wall.

After the wounds have been thoroughly debrided and irrigated, the size of the defect may necessitate reconstruction. The use of synthetic material to repair large defects in the chest wall has mostly been abandoned. Instead, myocutaneous flaps such as latissimus dorsi or pectoralis major have proven efficacy, particularly when cartilage or ribs must be debrided. The flap provides prompt healing and minimizes infection to the ribs or costal cartilages. If potential muscle flaps have been destroyed by the injury, a temporary dressing can be placed, and the patient stabilized in the intensive care unit and then returned to the operating room in 24–48 hours for a free myocutaneous graft or alternative reconstruction. Complications include wound infection and respiratory insufficiency, the latter usually due to associated parenchymal injury. Ventilatory embarrassment can persist secondary to the large defect. If the chest wall becomes infected, debridement, wound care and myocutaneous flaps should be considered.

8.6.3 Tension Pneumothorax (Haemo/Pneumothorax)

Tension pneumothorax is a threat to life. The importance of making the diagnosis is that it is the most easily treatable life-threatening surgical emergency in the emergency department. 'Simple' closed pneumothorax, which is not quite as dramatic, occurs in approximately 20% of all penetrating chest injuries. Haemothorax, in contrast, is present in about 30% of penetrating injuries, and haemopneumothorax is found in 40%–50% of penetrating injuries.

The diagnosis of tension pneumothorax can be difficult in a noisy ED. The classic signs are decreased breath sounds and percussion tympany on the ipsilateral side, and tracheal shift to the contralateral side. The diagnosis is clinical. In the patient who is dying, there should be no hesitation in performing a tube thoracostomy. Massive haemothorax is equally life-threatening.

8.6.4 **Massive Haemothorax**

Approximately 50% of patients with hilar, great vessel, or cardiac wounds expire immediately after injury. Another 25% live for periods of 5–6 minutes and, in urban centres, some of these patients may arrive alive in the ED after rapid transport. The remaining 25% live for periods of up to 30 minutes, and it is this group of patients who may arrive alive in the ED and require immediate diagnosis and treatment.

The diagnosis of massive haemothorax is invariably made by the presence of shock, ventilatory embarrassment, and a shift in the mediastinum.

Chest x-ray or eFAST will confirm the extent of blood loss, but most of the time tube thoracostomy is done immediately to relieve the threat of ventilatory embarrassment. If a gush of blood is obtained when the chest tube is placed, autotransfusion should be considered. There are simple devices for this that should be available in all major trauma resuscitation centres. The only contraindication to autotransfusion is a high suspicion of hollow viscus injury. Lesser forms of haemothorax are usually diagnosed by routine chest x-ray.

The treatment of massive haemothorax is to restore blood volume. In approximately 85% of patients with massive haemothorax, a systemic vessel has been injured such as the intercostal artery or internal mammary artery, and essentially, all such patients will require thoracotomy. In a few patients, there may be injury to the hilum of the lung or the myocardium. In about 15% of instances, the bleeding is from deep pulmonary lacerations. These injuries are treated by oversewing the lesion, making sure that bleeding is controlled to the depth of the lesion, or, in some instances, tractotomy or resection of a segment or lobe.

Complications of haemothorax or massive haemothorax are almost invariably related to the visceral injuries. Occasionally, there is a persistence of undrained blood that may lead to a cortical peel necessitating thoracoscopy or thoracotomy and removal of this peel. The aggressive use of two chest tubes should minimize the incidence of this complication. If that is not enough, early VATS evacuation of retained clots and fibrin is likely to be successful if performed within 72 hours.

8.6.5 **Tracheobronchial Injuries**[12]

Penetrating injuries to the tracheobronchial tree are uncommon and constitute less than 2% of all major thoracic injuries. Disruption of the tracheobronchial tree is suggested by massive haemoptysis, airway obstruction, progressive mediastinal air, subcutaneous emphysema, tension pneumothorax, and significant persistent air leak after placement of a chest tube. Fibreoptic bronchoscopy in the relatively stable patient, is a useful diagnostic adjunct in diagnosis, tube placement, post-operative tracheobronchial toilet and post-operative follow-up of tracheobronchial repairs.

Treatment for tracheobronchial injuries is straightforward. If it is a distal bronchus, there may be persistent air leak for a few days, but it will usually close with chest tube drainage alone. If, however, there is persistent air leak, or the patient has significant loss of minute volume through the chest tube, bronchoscopy is used to detect whether this is a proximal bronchus injury, and the involved area is explored usually through a posterolateral thoracotomy. If possible, the bronchus is repaired with monofilament suture. In some instances, a segmentectomy or lobectomy may be required.

8.6.6 **Oesophageal Injuries**

Penetrating injuries to the thoracic oesophagus are quite uncommon. Injuries to the cervical oesophagus are somewhat more frequent and are usually detected at the time of exploration of zone I and II injuries of the neck. In those centres where selective management of neck injuries is practised, the symptoms found are usually related to pain on swallowing and dysphagia. Occasionally, patients may present late with signs of posterior mediastinitis – a grave situation with a high mortality rate, even with aggressive and comprehensive treatment. Injuries to the thoracic oesophagus may present with pain, fever, pneumomediastinum, persistent pneumothorax despite tube thoracostomy, and pleural effusion with extravasation of contrast on a Gastrografin contrast swallow.

Treatment of cervical oesophageal injuries is relatively straightforward. As noted above, the injury is usually found during routine exploration of penetrating wounds beneath the platysma. Once found, a routine closure is performed. In more devitalizing injuries, it may be necessary to debride and close using drainage to protect the anastomosis. Injuries to the thoracic oesophagus should be repaired if the injury is less than 6 hours old and there is minimal inflammation and devitalized tissue present. A two-layer closure is all that is necessary. Post-operatively, the patient is kept on intravenous support and supplemental nutrition. Antibiotics may be indicated during the 24-hour perioperative period.

If the wound is between 6 and 24 hours old, a decision will be necessary to determine whether primary closure can be attempted or whether drainage and nutritional support is the optimal management. Almost all injuries older than 24 hours will not heal primarily when repaired. Open drainage, antibiotics, nutritional support and consideration of diversion is the optimal management. Complications following oesophageal injuries include wound infection, mediastinitis, and empyema.

The more recent technique of non-operative endoscopic expanding silicon-coated stent placement in selected cases is gaining acceptance in practice, although further experience is required to establish its correct application. Injuries of up to 30–40 mm in extent, with localized mural damage, and located in the middle and lower third of the oesophagus are suited to this technique. Cervical (upper third) and gastro-oesophageal junction injuries are not suitable, due to incomplete sealing by the stent. Some authorities advise a concomitant thoracotomy to place mediastinal drains when the stenting method is used. Accurate localization and assessment of the extent of the injury by contrast radiography and endoscopy is mandatory in selecting cases for stenting.

8.6.7 Diaphragmatic Injuries

See Section 9.3.2.

8.6.8 Pulmonary Contusion[13]

Pulmonary contusions represent bruising of the lung and are usually associated with direct chest trauma, high-velocity missiles, and shotgun blasts. The pathophysiology is the result of ventilation – perfusion defects and shunts. Its anatomical composition makes the extent of lung damage easily quantifiable on CT scanning.

The treatment of significant pulmonary contusion consists primarily of cardiovascular and tailored ventilatory support; adjunctive measures such as steroids and diuretics are used selectively as required to modulate the development of significant systemic inflammatory response (SIRS).

Antibiotics are not generally used, as this will simply select out nosocomial, opportunistic, and resistant organisms. It is preferable to obtain a daily Gram stain of the sputum and chest x-rays when necessary. If the Gram stain shows the presence of a predominant organism

with an associated increase in polymorphonuclear cells, antibiotics are indicated.

8.6.9 Flail Chest[13]

Traditionally, flail chest has been managed by internal splinting ('internal pneumatic stabilization') utilizing positive pressure ventilation. This modality remains the gold standard method of management, as it treats both the flail segment by splinting and the associated (often severe) pulmonary contusion.

While this is undoubtedly the method of choice in most instances, there has been increasing interest in the open reduction and fixation of multiple rib fractures. In uncontrolled trials, there have been considerable benefits shown, with a shortening of ventilation time and thus a reduction of risk for ventilator-associated pneumonia (VAP), and improved earlier mobilization resulting from reduced analgesic requirements (Table 8.1).

8.6.10 Fixation of Multiple Fractures of Ribs

A flail chest may be stabilized using pins, plates, wires, rods or, more recently, absorbable plates. Exposure for the insertion of these can be via a conventional posterolateral thoracotomy, or via incisions made over the ribs.

The Eastern Association Guidelines for the open reduction and internal fixation of rib fractures have guidelines in the PICO format[14] (see Tables 8.2 and 8.3).

8.6.11 Pulmonary Laceration

Lung preservation wherever possible is critically important, with conservative resections if required, using a combination of techniques such as tractotomy, wedge resection, and segmentectomy, reserving lobectomy or pneumonectomy for only the most critical patients. Currently available stapling devices are invaluable.

8.6.12 Air Embolism[15]

Air embolism is an infrequent event following penetrating trauma. It occurs in 4% of all major thoracic trauma. Sixty-five per cent of the cases are due to penetrating injuries. The key to diagnosis is to be aware of the possibility.

Table 8.1 Evidence Based Guidelines for Selective Non-Operative Management of Pulmonary Contusion-Flail Chest (PC-FC)

Level of Evidence	Recommendation
I	There are no recommendations for the management of PC-FC.
II	1. A pulmonary artery may be useful to avoid fluid overload during resuscitation. 2. Obligatory mechanical ventilation absence of respiratory failure solely the purpose of overcoming chest wall instability should be avoided. 3. Patients with PC-FC requiring mechanical ventilation should be supported in a manner based on institutional and physician preference and separated from the ventilator at the earliest possible time. Positive end expiratory pressure (PEEP) and continuous positive airway pressure (CPAP) should be included in the ventilatory regimen. 4. The use of optimal analgesia and aggressive chest physiotherapy should be applied to minimize the likelihood of respiratory failure and ensuing ventilatory support. Epidural catheter is the preferred mode of analgesia delivery in severe injury. 5. Steroids should not be used in therapy of pulmonary contusion.
III	1. A trial of mask CPAP should be considered in alert compliant patients with marginal respiratory status in combination with optimal regional anaesthesia. 2. There is insufficient evidence to prove the effectiveness of paravertebral analgesia in the trauma population. However, this modality may be equivalent to epidural analgesia and may be considered certain situations when epidural is contraindicated. 3. Independent lung ventilation be considered in severe unilateral PC when shunt cannot otherwise be corrected owing to maldistribution of ventilation, or when crossover bleeding is problematic. 4. High frequency oscillatory ventilation (HFOV) has not been shown to improve survival in blunt chest trauma patients with PC, but has been shown to improve oxygenation in certain cases where other modalities have failed. 5. Diuretics may be used in the setting of hydrostatic fluid overload, as evidenced by elevated pulmonary capillary wedge pressures in haemodynamically stable patients, or in the setting of known concurrent congestive cardiac failure. 6. Although improvement has not been definitively shown in any outcome parameters after surgical fixation of FC, this modality may be considered in cases of severe FC failing to wean from the ventilator, when thoracotomy is required for other reasons. Patient subgroups that would benefit of early fracture fixation has not been identified. 7. There is insufficient clinical evidence to recommend any type of proprietary implant for surgical fixation of rib fractures. However, in the trend studies indicate that replacing or wrapping devices are likely superior to intramedullary wires. 8. Self-activating multidisciplinary protocols for the treatment of chest wall injuries may improve outcome.

Source: Simon B et al. *J Trauma Acute Care Surg.* 2012 Nov;**73(5):**Suppl 4:S351–61.[13]

The pathophysiology is a fistula between a bronchus and the pulmonary vein. Those patients who are breathing spontaneously will have a pressure differential from the pulmonary vein to the bronchus that will cause approximately 22% of these patients to have haemoptysis on presentation. If, however, the patient has a Valsalva-type respiration or grunts, or is intubated with positive pressure in the bronchus, the pressure differential is from the bronchus to the pulmonary vein, causing systemic air embolism.

These patients present in one of three ways: focal or lateralizing neurological signs, sudden cardiovascular collapse, and froth when the initial arterial blood specimen is obtained. Any patient who has obvious chest injury, does not have obvious head injury and yet has focal or lateralizing neurological findings should be assumed

Table 8.2 The PICO Format

P	Patient, Population, or Problem	How would I describe the patient group?
I	Intervention, Prognostic Factor, or Exposure	Which main intervention, prognostic factor, or exposure is considered?
C	Comparison or Intervention (if appropriate)	What is the main alternative to compare with the intervention?
O	Outcome you would like to measure or achieve	What can be accomplished, measured, improved, or affected?

to have air embolism. Confirmation can occasionally be obtained by fundoscopic examination, which shows air in the retinal vessels. Patients who are intubated and have a sudden unexplained cardiovascular collapse with an absence of vital signs should be immediately assumed to have an air embolism to the coronary vessels. Finally, those patients who have a frothy blood sample drawn for initial blood gas determination will have air embolism.

When a patient comes in to the emergency department in extremis and an EDT is carried out, air should always be looked for in the coronary vessels. If air is found, the hilum of the offending lung should be clamped immediately to reduce the ingress of air into the vessels.

The treatment of air embolism is immediate thoracotomy, preferably in the operating room. In most patients, the left or right chest is opened depending on the side of penetration. If a resuscitative thoracotomy has been carried out, it may be necessary to extend this across the sternum into the opposite chest if there is no parenchymal injury to the lung on the left. Definitive treatment is to oversew the lacerations to the lung, in some instances perform a lobectomy, and only rarely a pneumonectomy.

Other resuscitative measures in patients who have asystolic arrest due to air embolism include internal cardiac massage and reaching up and holding the ascending aorta with the thumb and index finger for one or two beats – this will tend to push air out of the coronary vessels and thus establish perfusion. Adrenaline (epinephrine) 1:1000 can be injected intravenously or down the endotracheal tube to provide an alpha effect, driving air out of the systemic microcirculation. It is prudent to vent the left atrium and ventricle as well as the ascending aorta to remove all residual air once the lung hilum has been clamped. This prevents further air embolism when the patient is moved.

Using aggressive diagnosis and treatment, it is possible to achieve up to a 55% salvage rate in patients with air embolism secondary to penetrating trauma.

8.6.13 Cardiac Injuries

In urban trauma centres, cardiac injuries are most common after penetrating trauma, and constitute about 5%

Table 8.3 Eastern Association for the Surgery of Trauma Guidelines for Open Reduction and Internal Fixation of Rib Fractures

PICO	Recommendation
PICO Question 1: In adult patients with flail chest after blunt trauma, should rib ORIF be performed (versus non-operative management) to decrease mortality; DMV, ICU LOS, and hospital LOS; incidence of pneumonia and need for tracheostomy; and improve pain control?	In adult patients with flail chest after blunt trauma, we conditionally recommend rib ORIF to decrease mortality; shorten duration of mechanical ventilation (DMV); ICU LOS (intensive care unit length of stay), and hospital LOS; incidence of pneumonia and tracheostomy. We cannot offer a recommendation for pain control based on currently available evidence.
PICO Question 2: In adult patients with non-flail rib fractures after blunt trauma, should rib ORIF be performed (versus non-operative management) to decrease mortality and incidence of pneumonia; shorten DMV, hospital LOS; improve pain control; and decrease need for tracheostomy if applicable?	In adult patients with non-flail rib fractures after blunt trauma, we cannot offer a recommendation for any of the outcomes based on currently available evidence.

Abbreviations: ORIF, open reduction and internal fixation; DMV, duration of medical ventilation; ICU, intensive care unit; LOS, length of stay.

of all thoracic injuries. The diagnosis of cardiac injury is usually obvious. The patient presents with exsanguination, cardiac tamponade and, rarely, acute heart failure. In addition to the well described globular heart shape on x-rays, a straight left heart border has been associated with the presence of a haemopericardium. Patients with tamponade owing to penetrating injuries usually have a wound in proximity, decreased cardiac output, increased central venous pressure, decreased blood pressure, decreased heart sounds, narrow pulse pressure, and occasionally paradoxical pulse. Immediate clinician performed eFAST will usually demonstrate the presence of pericardial fluid, but in cases where the diagnosis of pericardial tamponade cannot be confirmed on clinical signs and on eFAST, formal echocardiogram is useful.

The treatment of all cardiac injuries is immediate thoracotomy, ideally in the operating room. In the patient who is in extremis, thoracotomy in the emergency department can be life-saving.

Complications from myocardial injuries include recurrent tamponade, mediastinitis and post-cardiotomy syndrome. The former can be avoided by placing a mediastinal chest tube or leaving the pericardium partially open following repair. Most cardiac injuries are treated through a left anterolateral thoracotomy, and only occasionally via a median sternotomy. If mediastinitis does develop, the wound should be opened (including the sternum), and debridement carried out with secondary closure in 4–5 days.

Another complication is herniation of the heart through the pericardium, which may occlude venous return and cause sudden death. This is avoided by loosely approximating the pericardium after the cardiac injury has been repaired.

8.6.14 Injuries to the Great Vessels

Injuries to the great vessels from penetrating forces are infrequently reported. The reason for this is that extensive injury to the great vessels results in immediate exsanguination into the chest, and most of these patients die at the scene of injury.

The diagnosis of penetrating great vessel injury is usually obvious. The patient is in shock, and there is an injury in proximity to the thoracic outlet or posterior mediastinum. If the patient stabilizes with resuscitation, angiography should be performed to localize the injury. Approximately 8% of patients with major vascular injuries

do not have clinical signs, stressing the need for angiography when there is a wound in proximity. These patients usually have a false aneurysm or arteriovenous fistula. Treatment of penetrating injuries to the great vessels can almost always be accomplished using lateral repair, since larger injuries that might necessitate grafts are usually incompatible with survival long enough to permit the patient to reach the emergency department alive.[16]

Complications of injuries to the great vessels include rebleeding, false aneurysm formation and thrombosis. A devastating complication is paraplegia, which usually occurs following blunt injuries but rarely after penetrating injuries, either because of associated injury to the spinal cord, or because at the time of surgery important intercostal arteries are ligated. The spinal cord has a segmental blood supply to the anterior spinal artery (artery of Adamkiewicz), and every effort should be made to preserve the intercostal vessels, particularly those that appear to be larger than normal, as these may constitute an important collateral feeder system.

8.7 CHEST DRAINAGE

8.7.1 Drain Insertion

Chest tubes are placed according to the technique described in the Advanced Trauma Life Support® programme (ATLS). The placement is in the triangle between the mid axillary line, anterior axillary line, via the fifth intercostal space – the triangle of safety. Care must be taken to avoid placement of the drain through breast tissue or the pectoralis major muscle. Drains should **not** be placed through pectoralis major muscle, and **never** through breast tissue. The optimal site is in the anterior axillary line.

In the conscious patient, a wheal of 1% lignocaine (Lidocaine) is placed in the skin, followed by a further 20 mL subcutaneously and down to the pleura.

Adequate local anaesthesia is critical. The aim is to block the relevant intercostal nerves.

Remember that local anaesthetic may take 5–10 minutes to work adequately. The chest is prepped and draped in the usual way, and after topical analgesia, an incision is made over about 2 cm in length, onto the underlying rib (Figure 8.5).

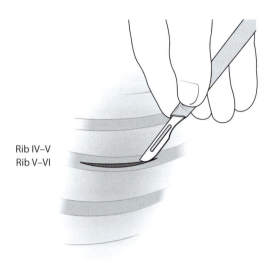

Rib IV–V
Rib V–VI

Figure 8.5 Anatomical placement of the incision for a chest drain.

Using blunt and forceps dissection, the tissue is lifted upwards off the rib, and penetration is made over the top of the rib towards the pleura (Figure 8.6). In this manner, damage to the intercostal neurovascular bundle is avoided.

Once the incision has been made, the wound is explored with the index finger for adults and the fifth finger for children. This ensures that the chest cavity has been entered and allows limited exploration of the pleural cavity (Figure 8.7). In patients with minor adhesions (e.g. following tuberculosis) it allows the lung tissue to be cleared from the path of the drain.

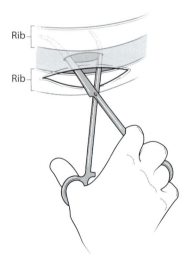

Rib
Rib

Figure 8.6 Blunt dissection over the top of the rib.

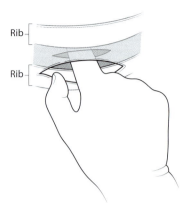

Rib
Rib

Figure 8.7 Use of a finger to clear adhesions.

Once the tract has been dilated with the finger, a large (34 or 36 FG) chest tube is inserted. The incision should be of sufficient size to allow the introduction of a finger *and* the tube together, allowing the tube to be directed cranially *behind* the lung towards the apex, via the posterior gutter (see Figure 8.8). This provides optimal drainage of both blood and air. When the chest tube is in place, it is secured to the chest wall with a size 0 monofilament suture as follows:

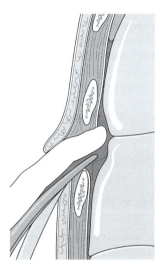

Figure 8.8 Finger and tube (held in forceps) inserted into chest cavity.

- A vertical mattress suture is inserted into the centre of the wound (Figure 8.9). A *single* throw is placed in the suture at skin level, and then the suture is *knotted* halfway up its length. After insertion of the tube, two simple sutures may be required as well to close the wound (Figure 8.10).

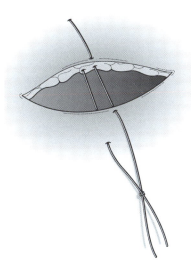

Figure 8.9 Insertion of a vertical mattress suture in the centre of the wound.

An additional simple suture may be required to close the wound in a linear fashion (Figure 8.10).

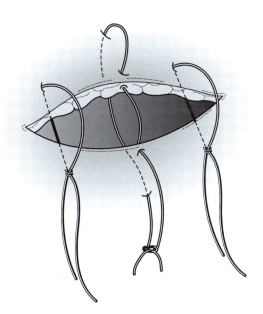

Figure 8.10 Additional simple sutures may be required for laterally for full closure.

- The suture is then wound around the chest tube until 1 cm before the 'halfway knot' mark is reached. The suture with knot is then threaded *under* the vertical mattress loop (Figure 8.11).

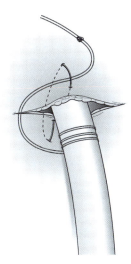

Figure 8.11 Securing the tube: first stage.

- The suture is then tied around the chest tube at the level of the knot, about 1 cm from the skin (Figure 8.12).

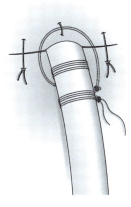

Figure 8.12 Securing the tube: second stage.

Pitfalls

- Do not use a 'purse-string' closure as this is both painful in the long term and less effective. Use a vertical mattress suture.
- Do **not** 'weave' the drain tie ('Roman Sandal technique') as if it becomes loose, the entire securing suture will be loose. The securing suture should be wound around the drain in one plane, as shown (Figure 8.10).

All connections are taped to prevent inadvertent disconnection or removal of the chest tube.

After the chest tube has been placed, it is prudent to obtain an immediate chest film or further ultrasound, to assess the adequate removal of air and blood, and the position of the tube. If, for any reason, blood accumulates and cannot be removed, another chest tube is inserted. Persistent air leak or bleeding should alert the surgeon that there is significant visceral injury that may require operative intervention.

Pitfall

- The surgeon should be aware that if blood continues to drain, the blood may be entering the chest via a hole in the diaphragm.

8.7.2 Drain Removal

The tube is removed once the lung has expanded. The suture is cut at the 'halfway knot'. The remaining suture is unwound, and the skin can then be pinched, or sealed with petroleum gauze, as the tube is withdrawn (Figure 8.13); the preplaced suture, now unwound, is then pulled tight and secured. The wound should thus be closed as a linear incision (Figure 8.14).

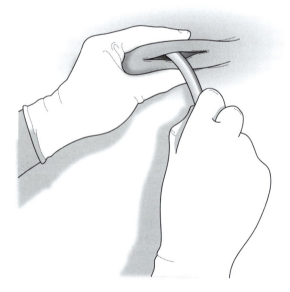

Figure 8.13 Removal of drain showing pinching of the skin.

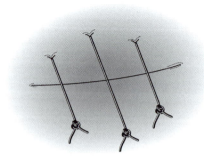

Figure 8.14 End result after drain removal.

Complications of tube thoracostomy include wound tract infection and empyema. With meticulous aseptic techniques, the incidence of both should be well under 1%.

There is enough (class I and II) data to recommend prophylactic antibiotic use in patients receiving tube thoracostomy following chest trauma. The data suggest there may be a reduction in the incidence of pneumonia but **not** empyema in trauma patients receiving prophylactic antibiotics when a tube thoracostomy is placed.[17]

Routine antibiotics are not a substitute for good surgical technique

On the frequently discussed issue of negative suction, a recent prospective study, concluded that negative suction confers **no** advantage in patients with uncomplicated traumatic pneumothorax, haemothorax, or haemopneumothorax.[18]

8.8 SURGICAL APPROACHES TO THE THORAX

The choice of approach to the injured thorax should be determined by three factors:

- The hemithorax and its contents.
- The stability of the patient.
- Whether the indication for surgery is acute or chronic (non-acute).

A useful distinction can be made with respect to indications (Table 8.4). It will be noted that the acute indications include all acutely life-threatening situations,

Table 8.4 Indications for Surgery in the Thorax	
Acute indications	**Chronic indications**
Cardiac tamponade	Unevacuated clotted haemothorax
Acute deterioration	Chronic traumatic diaphragmatic hernia
Vascular injury at the thoracic outlet	Traumatic atrioventricular fistula
Loss of chest wall substance	Traumatic cardiac septal or valvular lesions
Endoscopic or radiological evidence of tracheal, or oesophagus or great vessel injury	Missed tracheobronchial injury or tracheo-oesophageal fistula
Massive or continuing haemothorax	Infected intrapulmonary haematoma
Bullet embolism to the heart/pulmonary artery	
Penetrating mediastinal injury	

while the chronic or non-acute indications are essentially late presentations.

The surgical approaches in current use include:

- Anterolateral thoracotomy.
- Median sternotomy.
- Bilateral thoracotomy ('clamshell' incision).
- Posterolateral thoracotomy.
- The 'trapdoor' incision.

It is seldom necessary to resort to the remaining three approaches in the acute situation. Of these, the bilateral trans-sternal thoracotomy (the 'clamshell' incision) and the 'trapdoor' incision are complex and somewhat mutilating, with significant post-operative morbidity and difficulty in terms of access and closure.

In the *unstable* patient, the choice of approach usually will be an anterolateral thoracotomy or median sternotomy, depending upon the suspected injury. In the case of the *stable* patient, the choice of approach must be planned after proper evaluation and work-up has clearly identified the nature of the injury.

If time permits, intubation (or reintubation) with a double-lumen endotracheal tube, to allow selective deflation or ventilation of each lung, can be very helpful and occasionally life-saving, however advice should be sought from an experienced anaesthetist.

8.8.1 **Anterolateral Thoracotomy**

This is the approach of choice in most unstable patients and is utilized for EDT (Figure 8.15):

- This approach allows rapid access to the injured hemithorax and its contents.
- It is made with the patient in the supine position with no special positioning requirements or instruments.
- It has the advantages that it:
  - May be extended across the sternum into the contralateral hemithorax (the 'clamshell' incision or bilateral thoracotomy).
  - May be extended downwards to create a thoraco-abdominal incision.

This is the approach of choice in injury to any part of the left thorax or an injury above the nipple line in the right thorax. It should be noted that right lower thoracic injuries (i.e. below the nipple line) usually involve bleeding from the liver; the approach in these cases should initially be a midline laparotomy, the chest being entered only if no source of intra-abdominal bleeding is found.

8.8.1.1 TECHNIQUE

A slight tilt of the patient to the right is advisable; this is achieved by use of either a sandbag or other support, or by tilting the table.

The incision is made through the fourth or fifth intercostal space from the costochondral junction anteriorly to the mid-axillary line posteriorly, following the upper

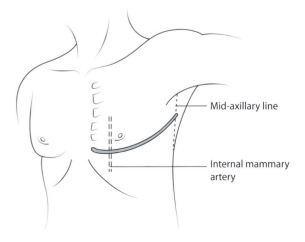

Figure 8.15 Anterolateral thoracotomy.

border of the lower rib in order to avoid damage to the intercostal neurovascular bundle.

The muscle groups are divided down to the periosteum of the lower rib. The muscle groups of the serratus anterior posteriorly and the intercostals medially and anteriorly are divided. The trapezius and the pectoralis major are avoided. Care should be taken at the anterior end of the incision, where the internal mammary artery runs and may be transected.

The periosteum is opened, leaving a cuff of approximately 5 mm for later closure. The parietal pleura is then opened, taking care to avoid the internal mammary artery adjacent to the sternal border. These vessels are ligated if necessary.

A Finochietto retractor is placed with the handle away from the sternum (i.e. laterally placed), the ribs are spread, and intrathoracic inspection for identification of injuries is carried out after suctioning. In cases of ongoing bleeding, an autotransfusion suction device is advisable.

Note that it is important to identify the phrenic nerve in its course across the pericardium if this structure is to be opened – the pericardiotomy is made 1 cm anterior and vertical to the nerve trunk in order to avoid damage and subsequent morbidity.

8.8.1.2 CLOSURE

Following definitive manoeuvres, the anterolateral thoracotomy is closed in layers over one or two large-bore intercostal tube drains and after careful haemostasis and copious lavage.

- The ribs and intercostal muscles should be closed with synthetic absorbable sutures.
- Closure of discrete muscle layers reduces both pain and long-term disability.
- The skin is routinely closed.

8.8.2 Median Sternotomy

This incision is the approach of choice in patients with a penetrating injury at the base of the neck (zone I) and the thoracic outlet, as well as to the heart itself. It allows access to the pericardium and heart, the arch of the aorta and the origins of the great vessels. It has the attraction of allowing upwards extension into the neck (as a Henry's incision), extension downwards into a midline laparotomy, or lateral extension into a supraclavicular approach (Figure 8.16). It has the relative disadvantage

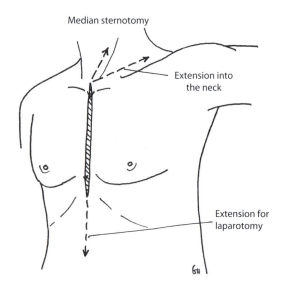

Figure 8.16 Median sternotomy.

of requiring a sternal saw or chisel (of the Lebsche type). In addition, the infrequent but significant complication of sternal sepsis may occur postoperatively, especially in the emergency setting.

8.8.2.1 TECHNIQUE

The incision is made with the patient fully supine, in the midline from the suprasternal notch to below the xiphoid cartilage. A finger-sweep is used to open spaces behind the sternum, above and below. Excision of the xiphoid cartilage may be necessary if this is large and intrusive and can be done with heavy scissors.

Split section (bisection) of the sternum is carried out with a saw (either oscillating or a braided-wire Gigli saw) or a Lebsche knife, commencing from above and moving downwards. This is an important point to avoid inadvertent damage to vascular structures in the mediastinum. In addition, be aware of the possible presence of the large transverse communicating vein, which may be found in the areolar tissue of the suprasternal space of Burns and must be controlled.

8.8.2.2 CLOSURE

- The pericardium is usually left open or only partially closed. It is advisable to close the pericardium with an absorbable suture to avoid adhesion formation.
- Two mediastinal tube drains are brought out through epigastric incisions.

- Closure of the sternotomy is made with horizontal sternal wires or encircling heavy non-absorbable suture (braided, non-absorbable).
- Closure of the linea alba should be by non-absorbable suture.

8.8.3 The 'Clamshell' Thoracotomy

This is the thoracic equivalent of the chevron or 'bucket handle' upper abdominal incision, providing wide exposure to both hemithoraces. It is usually necessary to use this incision only when it becomes necessary to gain access to both hemithoraces.

The 'clamshell' is essentially a bilateral fourth or fifth interspace thoracotomy, linked by division of the sternum, which allow the chest to be opened very widely anteriorly. The sternum is divided using a Gigli saw, chisel, or bone-cutting forceps (Figure 8.17).

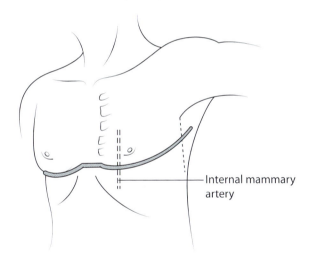

—Internal mammary artery

Figure 8.17 Bilateral trans-sternal thoracotomy ('clamshell') thoracotomy.

The incision is particularly effective in those situations where it is important to achieve rapid access to the *opposite* side of the chest, especially posteriorly, such as for:

- Transmediastinal injury.
- Lung injury.
- Injury on the right, where aortic control may be necessary.

As mentioned, earlier, it is the incision which allows access to the most thoracic structures. It has been recently demonstrated through cadaveric studies that the clamshell incision gives the access to most intrathoracic organs but it is inferior to median sternotomy in accessing upper mediastinal vascular structures.

Pitfall

It is essential to ligate the internal mammary arteries, and to ensure haemostasis prior to closure.

The clamshell incision carries a very high morbidity, a high risk of sternal non-union, and is very painful. It should only be considered if more limited exposure is impossible. Recovery is slower, with a high post-operative morbidity, and is often permanently incapacitating.

8.8.4 Posterolateral Thoracotomy

This approach requires appropriate positioning of the patient and is usually used in the elective setting for definitive lung and oesophageal surgery. It is not usually employed in the acute setting. It is more time-consuming in approach and closure, since the bulkier muscle groups of the posterolateral thorax are traversed, and scapular retraction is necessary.

8.8.5 'Trapdoor' Thoracotomy

The incision is considered *obsolete*.

8.9 EMERGENCY DEPARTMENT THORACOTOMY

8.9.1 History

Rapid emergency medical response times and advances in pre-hospital care have led to increasing numbers of patients arriving in resuscitation in extremis. Salvage of these patients often demands immediate control of haemorrhage and desperate measures to resuscitate them. This has often been attempted in hopeless situations, following both blunt and penetrating injury, and failure to understand the indications and sequelae will almost inevitably result in the death of the patient. With the increasing financial demands on medical care, and the increasing risk of transmission of communicable diseases, a differentiation must be made between the true EDT and futile care.

In 1874, Schiff described open cardiac massage, and in 1901, Rehn sutured a right ventricle in a patient presenting with cardiac tamponade. The limited success of EDT in most circumstances, however, prohibited the use of the technique for the next six or seven decades. A revival of interest occurred in the 1970s, when the procedure was initially revived by Ben Taub General Hospital in Houston for the treatment of cardiac injuries. It has subsequently been applied as a means of temporary aortic occlusion in exsanguinating abdominal trauma. More recently, there has been decreased enthusiasm, a more selective approach particularly with respect to blunt trauma, and consideration of other techniques such as resuscitative endovascular balloon occlusion of the aorta (REBOA) (see also Section 15.3). There is an extremely high mortality rate associated with all thoracotomies performed anywhere outside the operating theatre, especially when performed by non-surgeons.

It is important early on to differentiate between the definitions of thoracotomy:

- EDT for patients in extremis:
  - To control haemorrhage.
  - To control the aortic outflow (aortic 'cross-clamping').
  - To perform internal cardiac massage.
- *Planned* resuscitative thoracotomy, that is, in the operating room in acutely deteriorating patients for control of haemorrhage.

With EDT, it is also important to differentiate between:

- Patients with 'no signs of life'.
- Patients with 'no vital signs' in whom cardiac electrical activity, pupillary activity and/or respiratory effort is still evident. (This is where cardiac ultrasound can be very helpful.)

Obviously, the results of EDT in these two circumstances will differ.

8.9.2 **Objectives**

The primary objectives of EDT in this set of circumstances are to:

- Release cardiac tamponade.
- Control intrathoracic bleeding.

- Control air embolism or bronchopleural fistula.
- Permit open cardiac massage.
- Allow for temporary occlusion of the descending aorta to redistribute blood to the upper body and possibly limit subdiaphragmatic haemorrhage.

EDT has been shown to be most productive in life-threatening penetrating cardiac wounds, especially when cardiac tamponade is present. Patients requiring EDT for anything other than isolated penetrating cardiac injury rarely survive, even in established trauma centres. The outcome in the field is even worse. Indications for the procedure in military practice are essentially the same as in civilian practice.

EDT and the necessary rapid use of sharp surgical instruments, as well as exposure to the patient's blood, poses certain risks to the resuscitating surgeon. Contact rates of patient's blood to the surgeon's skin approximate to 20%. 'Invisible pathogens' such as human immunodeficiency virus (HIV), hepatitis C and others must be considered. The use of universal precautions and the selective use of EDT may minimize this risk.

8.9.3 **Indications and Contraindications**

There are instances where EDT has been shown to have clear benefit. These indications include:

- Those patients in whom there is a witnessed arrest and a high likelihood of isolated intrathoracic injury, especially penetrating cardiac injury ('salvageable' post-injury cardiac arrest).
- Those with severe post-injury hypotension (blood pressure <60 mm Hg) owing to cardiac tamponade, air embolism, or thoracic haemorrhage.

Less clear benefit occurs for:

- Patients presenting with moderate post-injury hypotension (blood pressure <80 mm Hg) potentially due to intra-abdominal aortic injury (e.g. an epigastric gunshot wound).
- Major pelvic fractures.
- Active intra-abdominal haemorrhage.

The first group of patients constitutes those in whom EDT is relatively indicated. One must consider the patient's age, pre-existing disease, signs of life, and injury mechanism, as well as the proximity of the ED to the operating theatre and the personnel available, when applying the principles related to EDT. Although optimal benefit from the procedure will be obtained with an experienced surgeon, in cases where a moribund patient presents with a penetrating chest wound, the emergency physician should not hesitate to perform the procedure.

EDT is *contraindicated*:

- When here has been cardiopulmonary resuscitation (CPR) in the absence of endotracheal tube intubation in excess of 5 minutes, or when there has been CPR for more than 10 minutes with or without endotracheal tube intubation.
- In cases of blunt trauma, when there have been no signs of life at the scene or only pulseless electrical activity is present in the ED.
- Consider the use of cardiac ultrasound to aid the diagnosis.

8.9.4 Results

The results of EDT vary according to the injury mechanism and location and to the presence of vital and life signs.

EDT has been shown to be beneficial in around 50% of patients presenting with signs of life after isolated penetrating cardiac injury, and only rarely in those patients presenting without signs of life (<2%). With non-cardiac penetrating wounds, 25% of patients benefit when signs of life and detectable vital signs are present, compared with 8% of those with signs of life only and 3% of those without signs of life.

Only 1%–2% of patients requiring EDT are salvaged after blunt trauma regardless of their clinical status on admission. A decision-making algorithm has been formulated based on these findings, and the four factors found to be most predictive of outcome following EDT are reported to be:

- Absence of signs of life at the scene.
- Absence of signs of life in the ED.
- Absence of cardiac activity at EDT.
- Systolic blood pressure less than 70 mm Hg after aortic occlusion.

At the scene, patients in extremis and without cardiac electrical activity are declared dead. Those with electrical activity are intubated, supported with CPR and transferred to the ED. If blunt injury is present, EDT is embarked only on if pulsatile electrical activity is present. (In penetrating trauma, all patients undergo EDT.) If no blood is present in the pericardial cavity and there is no cardiac activity, the patient is declared dead. All others are treated according to the type of injury, as above. Those with intra-abdominal injury who respond to aortic occlusion with a systolic blood pressure of more than 70 mm Hg and all other surviving patients are rapidly transported to the operating theatre for definitive treatment.

8.9.5 When to Stop EDT

EDT is a 'team event'. It should not be prolonged unduly but should have specific end points. If an injury is repaired and the patient responds, he or she should be moved to the operating room for definitive repair or closure.

EDT should be terminated if:

- Irreparable cardiac damage has occurred.
- The patient is identified as having massive head injuries.
- Pulseless electrical activity is established.
- Systolic blood pressure is less than 70 mm Hg after 20 minutes.
- Asystolic arrest has occurred.

8.9.6 Technique

8.9.6.1 INSTRUMENT REQUIREMENTS

The numbers of instruments and types of equipment necessary to perform EDT, and include only the following:

- A scalpel, with a #20 or #21 blade.
- Forceps.
- A suitable retractor such as Finochietto chest retractor or a Balfour abdominal retractor.
- A Lebsche knife and mallet or Gigli saw for the sternum.
- Large vascular clamps such as Satinsky vascular clamps (large and small).
- Mayo scissors.
- Metzenbaum scissors.
- Long needle-holders.
- Internal defibrillator paddles.
- Sutures, swabs, and Teflon pledgets.
- Sterile skin preparation and drapes.
- Good light.

8.9.6.2 APPROACH

Two basic incisions are used in EDT. These are applied according to the best incision for the injury suspected (based on the entrance and exit wounds, the trajectory and the most likely diagnosis from clinical examination), and may be extended in various ways according to need.

Routine immediate resuscitation protocols as per the ATLS® are instituted, and once indications for EDT have been fulfilled, EDT should follow without delay.

Pitfall

If the conditions are not fulfilled, you are embarking upon futile care.

The left anterolateral thoracotomy is the most common site for urgent access. The incision is placed in the fifth intercostal space through muscle, periosteum and parietal pleura from the costochondral junction anteriorly to the mid-axillary line laterally following the upper border of rib, and care is taken to avoid the internal mammary artery. This incision can be extended as a bilateral incision requiring horizontal division of the sternum and ligation of the internal mammary vessels bilaterally. It affords excellent access to both pleural cavities, pericardial cavity and even the abdominal cavity if required. The incision also may be extended cranially in the midline by dividing the sternum for penetrating wounds involving mediastinal structures. The same incision may be employed on the right side in hypotensive patients with penetrating right chest trauma in whom massive blood loss or air embolism is suspected. This, too, may be extended trans-sternally if a cardiac wound is discovered.

The median sternotomy affords the best exposure to the anterior and middle mediastinum, including the heart and great vessels, and is typically advocated for penetrating wounds, particularly of the upper chest between the nipples. This can be extended supraclavicularly for access to control subclavian and brachiocephalic vascular injuries.

8.10 SURGICAL PROCEDURES

8.10.1 Pericardial Tamponade

- Open the pericardium in a cranial to caudal direction, anterior to the phrenic nerve.

- The pericardial incision is initiated using either a knife or the sharp point of a pair of scissors, and blood and clots are evacuated.
- It is important to examine the whole heart to localize the source of bleeding.
- Deal with the source of bleeding.
- It is not essential to close the pericardium after the procedure.
- If the pericardium is closed, it should be drained to avoid a recurrent tamponade.

Pitfall

It is important to identify the phrenic nerve prior to opening the pericardium at least 1 cm anterior to this structure.

8.10.2 Cardiac Injury

Cardiac bleeding points on the ventricle are initially managed with digital pressure, and those on the atria and great vessels by partially occluding vascular clamps (e.g. Satinsky clamps).

If the heart is beating, repair should be delayed until initial resuscitation measures have been completed. If it is not beating, suturing precedes resuscitation.

- Wherever possible, initial control of a myocardial laceration should be digital, while the damage is assessed.
- Use 3-0 or 4-0 non-absorbable braided sutures tied gently to effect the repair. Pledgets may be helpful.
- Foley catheters may be used to temporarily control haemorrhage prior to definitive repair in the emergency department or operating theatre. A Foley catheter with a large balloon is preferable.

In inexperienced hands, and as a temporizing measure, a skin stapler will allow control of the bleeding, with minimal manipulation of the heart.

Pitfalls

- There is a real danger of extending the damage if the Foley balloon pulls through the laceration. Use a 30 mL balloon and avoid other than gentle traction.
- Care should be exercised near coronary arteries. Whereas a vertical mattress suture is normally

> - acceptable, it may be necessary to use a horizontal mattress suture under the vessel to avoid occluding it.
> - Staples often eventually tear out, so the repair should not be regarded as definitive.

Posterior wounds are more difficult as they necessitate elevation of the heart before their closure, which can lead to further haemodynamic compromise. With large wounds of the ventricle or inaccessible posterior wounds, temporary digital inflow occlusion might be necessary to facilitate repair.[19–21]

The great majority of low-pressure venous and atrial wounds can be closed with simple continuous sutures or horizontal mattress sutures of a 3/0 or 4/0 monofilament. Bolstering the suture with Teflon pledgets is NOT essential, but may occasionally be required, particularly if there is surrounding contusion, or there is proximity of the wound to a coronary artery.

If the stab wound or gunshot wound is in proximity to the coronary artery, care must be taken not to suture the vessels. This can be achieved by passing horizontal mattress sutures *underneath* the coronary vessels, avoiding ligation of the vessel.

If the coronary arteries have been transected, two options exist. Closure can be accomplished in the beating heart using a fine 6/0 or 7/0 polypropylene suture, under magnification if necessary. The second option is to temporarily initiate inflow occlusion and fibrillation. However, both measures have a high risk associated with them. Heparinization is optimally avoided in the trauma patient, and fibrillation in the presence of shock and acidosis may be difficult to reverse. Bypass is usually reserved for patients who have injury to the valves, chordae tendineae, or septum. In most instances, these injuries are not immediately life-threatening, but become evident over a few hours or days following the injury.

Most blunt injuries to the heart who survive the initial resuscitation and require operative intervention can likewise be treated with simple off pump methods although more complex injuries may require immediate cardiopulmonary bypass and advances techniques.

8.10.3 **Pulmonary Haemorrhage**

- Access is best achieved by anterolateral thoracotomy on the appropriate side.
- With localized bleeding sites, control can be achieved with a vascular clamp placed across the hilum, occluding the pulmonary artery, vein, and main-stem bronchus, or across the affected segment.
- The affected segment is then dealt with, preferably in controlled circumstances in the operating theatre by local oversewing, segmental resection, or pulmonary tractotomy.

Pulmonary tractotomy is a means of controlling tracts that pass through multiple lung segments where the extent of injury precludes pulmonary resection. It is a means of non-anatomical lung preservation in which linear staplers are passed along both sides of the tract formed, and the lung is divided to allow blood vessels and airways in the bases to be repaired; the divided edges are then oversewn.

With massive haemorrhage from multiple or indeterminate sites, or widespread destruction of lung parenchyma leaving large areas of non-viable tissue, hilar clamping with a large soft vascular clamp or a large doubled vessel loop, or a soft catheter across the hilar structures occluding the pulmonary artery, pulmonary vein and main-stem bronchus is employed until a definitive surgical procedure can be performed.

Air embolism is controlled by placing a clamp across the hilar structures, and air is evacuated by needle aspiration of the elevated left ventricular apex.

8.10.4 **Pulmonary Tractotomy**

- This is used where the injury crosses more than one segment, commonly caused by a penetrating injury. Anatomical resection may not be possible.
- Linear staplers can be introduced along both sides of the tract, the tract being divided and then oversewn.
- This procedure is also helpful in 'damage control' of the chest.

8.10.5 **Lobectomy or Pneumonectomy**[22]

- This is rarely performed, usually done to control massive haemorrhage from the pulmonary hilum.
- Lung preservation should be attempted wherever possible.
- A double-lumen endotracheal tube should be used whenever possible.
- For segmental pneumonectomy, use of the GIA stapler is helpful. The staple line can then be oversewn.

8.10.6 Thoracotomy with Aortic Cross-Clamping

This technique is employed to optimize oxygen transport to vital proximal structures (the heart and brain), maximize coronary perfusion, and possibly limit infra-diaphragmatic haemorrhage in both blunt and penetrating trauma.

The thoracic aorta is cross-clamped inferior to the left pulmonary hilum, and the area is exposed by elevating the left lung anteriorly and superiorly. The mediastinal pleura is dissected under direct vision, the aorta being separated by blunt dissection from the oesophagus anteriorly and the prevertebral fascia posteriorly. When properly exposed, the aorta is occluded using a large vascular clamp. It is important that the aortic cross-clamp time be kept to the absolute minimum, i.e. that the clamp is removed once effective cardiac function and systemic arterial pressure have been achieved, as the metabolic penalty rapidly becomes exponential once beyond 30 minutes.

8.10.7 Aortic Injury

- Most patients with these injuries do not survive to reach hospital.
- Cardiopulmonary bypass is preferable in order to avoid paraplegia.

8.10.8 Tracheobronchial Injury

- Flexible bronchoscopy is very helpful in assessment.
- Formal repair should be undertaken under ideal conditions, with removal of devitalized tissue.

8.10.9 Oesophageal Injury

- Surgical repair is mandatory.
- Two-layer repair (mucosal and muscular) is preferable.
- If possible, the repair should be wrapped in autogenous tissue.
- A feeding gastrostomy is preferable to a nasogastric tube through the area of repair, and the stomach should be drained.
- A cervical oesophagostomy may be required.

8.11 SUMMARY

The success in the management of thoracic injury in those cases requiring operation lies in the 'team approach', with good anaesthesia and rapid access to the thoracic cavity with good exposure. Thus, good lighting, appropriate instrumentation, functioning suction apparatus, and a 'controlled, aggressive but calm frame of mind' on the part of the team will result in acceptable, uncomplicated survival figures.

8.12 ANAESTHESIA FOR THORACIC TRAUMA

In all chest trauma, decision-making, assistance within the operation, and identifying and treating the injury, anaesthesia plays an important part. There are major differences in the presentation, treatment and prognosis of a penetrating or blunt thoracic injury. What they have in common is that if they arrive alive in hospital, with vigilant reception, on arrival, they stand a fighting chance.

8.12.1 Penetrating Thoracic Injury

Depending on the cause of the penetration the chances of the patient range from excellent (knife, low energy dispersing projectile) to very bad with structures (large vessels, heart) damaged beyond repair.

ATLS® 'ABC' principles should focus on signs of tamponade, pneumothorax, massive air leaks (emphysema), and should not miss hidden injuries such as penetration of the oesophagus in secondary survey. As a priority, remember to inspect the back of the patient immediately for an exit or entry wound and mark these with metal markers.

Penetrating thoracic injury is most often treated by chest tube insertion. A massive air leak will alert to large airway penetration, massive blood loss from cardiac and large vessel injury, and food from an oesophageal or stomach injury.

The massive air leak and a substantial airway bleeding should initially be treated by intubation, either with a normal endotracheal tube or a double lumen tube (DLT). This will allow a flexible bronchoscopy to identify the rupture site and isolate the rupture from the rest of the airway. The single lumen tube can be positioned past the rupture, the DLT can be used to identify the injured side. The single lumen tube will allow a type of bronchus blocker in a later stage to assist the operation.

Cardiac tamponade, massive cardiac or large vessel injury will all require an emergency thoracic intervention with anaesthesia prepared for very fast, large blood loss.

8.12.2 **Blunt Thoracic Injury**

Blunt thoracic injury commonly results from motor vehicle crashes (MVC), but may also be the result of a fall, being crushed under a large object, the result of a blast injury from an explosion, or a combination of the above. The injury usually works from the outside inwards: via the bony thoracic wall and spine, to the lungs, and the mediastinum. The severity of the damage will signify deep the damage is likely to be. The lungs provide some protection to the mediastinum. Sometimes, however, especially in case of a blast injury, the force can work from the inside out when the blast wave is swallowed or inhaled opening the deeper structures, lung, and oesophagus to the blast wave or rapid expanding shock wave.

Blunt trauma to the heart may lead to a cardiac contusion or chamber rupture. Myocardial contusion should be suspected based on the trauma mechanism and the additional trauma signs: rib fractures, lung contusion, dysrhythmias, sinus tachycardia, or ectopic beats. It can present as a progressive disease where an abnormal 12 lead ECG should lead to a cardiac ultrasound. Signs of left ventricle ischaemia ST-T changes and Q-waves may show. All types of atrio-ventricular blocks be a result of the oedema in the cardiac muscle. In the trans-thoracic (TTE) or trans-oesophageal (TOE) echo the valves should be inspected for ruptures and wall motion abnormalities should be excluded. Intra-aortic balloon counter-pulsation should be considered if there is cardiogenic shock.

Most deaths are from ventricular fibrillation. Management for valve damage may be operative, for the myocardial contusion just supportive.

For a free wall cardiac rupture, a rapid diagnosis needs to be made using eFAST, CT, TTE, and TOE. A sternotomy will be the most appropriate approach for an isolated cardiac injury. If cardiopulmonary bypass is available, this will facilitate the operation.

8.12.2.1 CONTAINED LARGE VESSEL RUPTURE/ANEURISM

A contained large vessel rupture can be dealt with by the cardiac surgeon or the interventional radiologist.

The thoracic aorta will most often tear at the *ligamentum arteriosum* where the vessel is restricted in its movement. Support for the intervention will be with a TOE and careful manipulation of the blood pressure to prevent shear stress on the tear. Open repair will follow the same techniques as an elective case with anaesthetic management consisting of a careful titration of vasodilation and inotropes on clamping and clamp release. A cardiopulmonary bypass may be necessary.

8.12.2.2 PULMONARY CONTUSION

The pulmonary contusion is an entity in development. The initial chest x-ray will not show the complete full-blown contusion in the stable patient; CT scan is the modality of choice. The contusion will very often be accompanied by a flail chest. The contusion is a complex of intra-parenchymal bleeding, oedema, and alveolar collapse owing to reduced surfactant production. This leads to ventilation–perfusion mismatch, shunting, and decreased compliance. Treatment consists of a ventilation strategy where one should realize that the ventilation stressors are primarily exerted on the healthier lung. Low volume, high PEEP, permissive hypercapnia, and maintaining a minimum oxygen saturation in order to avoid high oxygen concentrations, may be needed. If oxygenation to the required level is not achieved, extracorporeal membrane oxygenation (ECMO) can be considered, to bridge the time needed to reduce swelling and blood in the alveoli (see also Section 17.3).

8.12.2.3 LARGE AIRWAY DISRUPTION

The disruption of the trachea or a major bronchus can be potentially life threatening. The insertion of a chest tube may open the way for air following the path of least resistance away from the attached lung thus making ventilation impossible. With an avulsed lung (fallen lung sign on chest x-ray), spontaneous ventilation may be all that keeps the patient alive until the lungs are isolated.

A massive emphysema rising and falling with ventilation should instantly alert to a large airway leak. Lung separation can be achieved with advancing the endotracheal tube beyond the hole, or into the non-disrupted main bronchus. Flexible bronchoscopy may be supportive for identifying where the air leak is. Other options are a DLT or a bronchus blocker. For a large bronchial disruption, a rapid thoracotomy and clamping of the open bronchus can facilitate ventilation.

8.12.2.4 FLAIL CHEST

A flail chest can present itself on a scale ranging from an acceptable affliction to a near death experience where the pain makes breathing impossible. The pain can be treated with morphine, although this may complicate breathing as well, an epidural and/or ventilation assistance ranging from CPAP to intubation and assisted ventilation. This will depend on concomitant injury. Indications for operative fixation include flail chest, reduction of pain and disability, a chest wall deformity or defect, symptomatic non-union, thoracotomy for other indications, and open fractures. Minimal invasive techniques have been developed and are currently being used.

8.12.2.5 DIAPHRAGMATIC INJURY

Diaphragm rupture is easily missed especially on the right when covered by the liver. Anaesthetic management will depend on if a thoracic or abdominal approach is chosen. A gastric tube should be inserted to deflate the stomach, aspiration prevention measures should be utilised for intubation. Nitrous oxide should be avoided. If a thoracic approach is indicated lung separation is an option to facilitate the operation.

8.12.3 Anaesthetic Management of Thoracic Injury

When presented with a massive thoracic injury, preparation is essential. A guess needs to be made what surgery will be required, and the anaesthesia tailored to accommodate this. Will lung separation be helpful? A DLT makes a surgeon's life easy, but this is only a relative indication. Absolute indications include significant lung bleeding, contamination, overflow from lung abscess, and the inability to ventilate where isolation of the damaged lung is needed. Insert an arterial line for blood gases, and large bore cannulas.

8.13 ANAESTHETIC CONSIDERATIONS

- Penetrating trauma is most often treated by chest tubes.
- Wounds should be marked with metal markers before chest x-ray.
- Massive air leaks and a substantial airway bleeding should initially be treated by intubation with a normal endotracheal tube; preferably below the injury in the trachea, or in the healthy lung. A double lumen tube should only be used as a primary device if the anaesthesiologist is very experienced with this. Bronchus blocker might be considered at later stage.
- Several rib fractures or flail chest might indicate lung contusions with ventilation-perfusion mismatch, shunting, and decreased compliance. Treatment consists of analgesia, restriction of fluids, and ventilatory support – for example, early non-invasive ventilator support. ECMO might be considered in the extreme cases with persistent hypoxemia.
- Blunt trauma to the heart may lead to a cardiac contusion with arrythmias, ruptures, valvular defects, or intimal tear of the coronary vessels. Twelve lead ECG, troponins, and echocardiography are useful for diagnosis.
- Interventional radiology does not necessarily include general anaesthesia and endotracheal intubation.
- In diaphragmatic rupture a gastric tube should be inserted.
- Remember to use a cell salvage especially in thoracic injury. The blood loss may be significant, and it will be non-contaminated blood that can be rehung as full blood, or taken through the cell saver coming out as red cell concentrate.
- Autotransfusion should be considered in chest bleeding according to the institution's policy and experience.
- In the rare event of an emergency room thoracotomy close communication is necessary in order to evaluate the function and filling of the heart. During suturing on the penetrated heart low blood pressures are accepted and catecholamines are to be avoided.
- Do repeated blood gases to assist in steering lung protective ventilation.
- Do not forget associated head injuries and C-spine which are often also damaged and require a different approach to the ventilation strategies described above.
- A good pain management strategy may prevent a lot of co-morbidity in the casualty with massive thoracic injury.

REFERENCES AND RECOMMENDED READING

References

1. Mancini M, Smith LM, Nein A, Buechler KJ. Early evacuation of clotted blood and haemothorax using thoracoscopy: case reports. *J Trauma*. 1993 Jan;**34(1)**:144–7.

2. Kwan RO, Miraflor E, Yeung L, Strumwasser A, Victorino G. Bedside thoracic ultrasonography of the fourth intercostal space reliably determines safe removal of tube thoracostomy after traumatic injury. *J Trauma Acute Care Surg*. 2012 Dec;**73(6)**:1568–73. doi: 10.1097/TA.0b013e318265fc22.

3. Van As AB, Manganyi R, Brooks A. Treatment of thoracic trauma in children: literature review, Red Cross War Memorial Children's Hospital data analysis, and guidelines for management. *Eur J Pediatr Surg*. 2013 Dec;**23(6)**:434–43. doi: 10.1055/s-0033-1363160. Epub 2013 Dec 10. Review.

4. Kessel B, Dagan J, Swaid F, Ashkenazi I, Olsha O, Peleg K, Givon A. Rib fractures: comparison of associated injuries between pediatric and adult population. *Am J Surg*. 2014 Nov;**208(5)**:831–34. doi: 10.1016/j.amjsurg.2013.10.033. Epub 2014 Mar 26.

5. Lustenberger T, Talving P, Lam L, Inaba K, Mohseni S, Smith JA, et al. Penetrating cardiac trauma in adolescents: a rare injury with excessive mortality. *J Pediatr Surg*. 2013 Apr;**48(4)**:745–9. doi: 10.1016/j.jpedsurg.2012.08.020.

6. Lee LK, Rogers AJ, Ehrlich PF, Kwok M, Sokolove PE, Blumberg S, et al. Occult pneumothoraces in children with blunt torso trauma. *Acad Emerg Med*. 2014 Apr; **21(4)**:440–8. doi: 10.1111/acem.12344.

7. Bouhemad B, Zhang M, Lu Q, Rouby JJ. Clinical review: Bedside lung ultrasound in critical care practice. *Crit Care*. 2007;**11**:205. Review.

8. Advance Trauma Life Support Programme®. 10th Edn. Thoracic Skills. *American College of Surgeons*. 2018. Chicago, IL, USA. 346–7.

9. Bansal V, Reid CM, Fortlage D, Lee J, Kobayashi L, Doucet J, et al. Determining injuries from posterior and flank stab wounds using computed tomography tractography. *Am Surg*. 2014 April;**80(4)**:403–7.

10. Goodman M, Lewis J, Guitron J, Reed M, Pritts T, Starnes S. Video-assisted thoracoscopic surgery for acute thoracic trauma. *J Emerg Trauma Shock* 2013 Apr;**6(2)**:106–9. doi: 10.4103/0974-2700.110757.

11. O'Connor JV, DuBose JJ, Scalea TM. Damage-control thoracic surgery: Management and outcomes. *J Trauma Acute Care Surg*. 2014 Nov;**77**:660–65.

12. Welter S. Repair of tracheobronchial injuries. *Thorac Surg Clin*. 2014 Feb;**24(1)**:41–50. doi: 10.1016/j.thorsurg.2013.10.006. Review.

13. Simon B, Ebert J, Bokhari F, Capella J, Emhoff T, Hayward T, et al. Management of pulmonary contusion and flail chest: An Eastern Association for the Surgery of Trauma practice management guideline. *J Trauma Acute Care Surg*. 2012 Nov;**73(5)**:Suppl 4:S351–61. doi: 10.1097/TA.0b013e31827019fd.

14. Kasotakis G, Hasenboehler EA, Streib EW, Patel N, Patel MB, Mayur B, et al. Open reduction and Internal Fixation of rib fractures. An Eastern Association for the Surgery of Trauma Practice Management Guideline. *Journal of Trauma and Acute Care Surgery*. 2017 Mar;**82(3)**:618–26. doi: 10.1097/TA.0000000000001350.

15. Yee ES, Verrier ED, Thomas AN. Management of air embolism in blunt and penetrating thoracic trauma. *J Thorac Cardiovasc Surg*. 1983;**85**:661–7.

16. Mattox KL. Approaches to trauma involving the major vessels of the thorax. *Surg Clin N Am*. 1989;**69**:77–87.

17. Luchette FA, Barie PS, Oswanski MF, Spain DA, Mullins D, Palumbo F, et al. Practice Management Guidelines for Prophylactic Antibiotic Use in Tube Thoracostomy for Traumatic Hemopneumothorax: EAST Practice Management Guidelines Work Group. *J Trauma*. 2000 April;**48(4)**:753–7.

18. Morales CH, Mejía C, Roldan LA, Saldarriaga MF, Duque AF. Negative pleural suction in thoracic trauma patients: A randomized controlled trial. *J Trauma Acute Care Surg*. 2014 Aug;**77(2)**:251–5. doi: 10.1097/TA.0000000000000281.

19. Telich-Tarriba JE, Anaya-Ayala JE, Reardon MJ. Surgical repair of right atrial wall rupture after blunt chest trauma. *J Tex Heart Inst*. 2012;**39(4)**:579–81.

20. Lee CN, Leng SA, Sorokin V. Simple and quick repair of cardiac rupture due to blunt chest trauma. *Asian Cardiovasc Thorac Ann*. 2012;**20(1)**:64–5.

21. Nakajima H, Uwabe K, Asakura T, Yoshida Y, Iguchi A, Niinami H. Emergent surgical repair of left ventricular rupture after blunt chest trauma. *Ann Thorac Surg*. 2014 Aug;**98(2)**:e35–6. doi: 10.1016/j.athoracsur.2014.03.057.

22. Kamiyoshihara M. Igai H, Ibe T, Ohtaki Y, Atsumi J, Nakazawa S, et al. Pulmonary lobar root clamping and stapling technique: return of the "en masse lobectomy". *Gen Thorac Cardiovasc Surg*. 2013 May; **61(5)**:280–91. doi: 10.1007/s11748-012-0159-3. Epub 2012 Sep 28.

Recommended Reading

Burlew CC, Moore EE. Emergency Department Thoracotomy. In Moore EE, Mattox KL, Feliciano DV, eds. *Trauma*, 8th Edn. 2017;241–56.

DuBose JA, O'Connor JV. Lung, Trachea and Esophagus. In Moore EE, Mattox KL, Feliciano DV, eds. *Trauma*, 8th Edn. 2017;479–92.

Wall MJ, Tsai PI, Mattox KL. Heart and Thoracic Vascular Injuries. In Moore EE, Mattox KL, Feliciano DV, eds. *Trauma*, 8th Edn. 2017;492–522. McGraw-Hill Education New York, NY, USA.

The Abdomen 9

9.1 The Trauma Laparotomy

9.1.1 Overview

Delayed diagnosis and treatment of abdominal injuries are common causes of preventable death from blunt or penetrating trauma. Approximately 20% of abdominal injuries will require surgery. In the UK, Europe, and Australia, abdominal trauma is predominantly blunt in origin, while in the military context, as well as civilian trauma in South Africa, South America, and the larger US cities, it is predominantly penetrating.

The diagnosis of injury following blunt trauma can be difficult, and insight into the mechanism of injury can be helpful. Passenger restraints themselves may cause blunt trauma to the liver, duodenum or pancreas, and rib fractures are associated with hepatic or splenic injuries. Virtually all penetrating injury to the abdomen should be addressed promptly, especially in the presence of hypotension.

Pitfalls

- Blood is not initially a peritoneal irritant, and therefore it may be difficult to assess the presence or quantity of blood present in the abdomen.
- Bowel sounds may remain present for several hours after abdominal injury or may disappear soon after trivial trauma. This sign is therefore particularly unreliable.

Diagnostic modalities depend on the nature of the injury:

- Physical examination.
- Ultrasound – focused abdominal sonography for trauma (FAST).
- Computed tomography (CT) scanning (stable patients only).
- Diagnostic laparoscopy.
- Diagnostic peritoneal lavage.

It is important to appreciate the difference between abdominal surgery as part of the resuscitation process, and the definitive surgical treatment for abdominal trauma:

- Surgical resuscitation includes the technique of 'damage control resuscitation' and 'damage control surgery' and implies only that the surgical procedure is primarily life-saving by stopping bleeding and preventing further contamination, as the patient's physiological derangement preludes definitive repair (see also Sections 9.2 and 9.3).
- Definitive surgical treatment implies that the physiological state of the patient allows the definitive surgical repair to take place.

During resuscitation, standard Advanced Trauma Life Support® guidelines should be followed. These should include:

- Standard A-B-C-D-E priorities.
- Nasogastric or orogastric tube.
- Urinary catheter.

9.1.1.1 DIFFICULT ABDOMINAL INJURY COMPLEXES

There are at least four complex abdominal injury patterns:

- *Major liver injuries*: Management of actively bleeding hepatic injuries may be challenging. Improvement in

CT imaging has made it possible to treat more adult solid organ injury non-operatively. Unstable patients with major liver injury require urgent laparotomy, which is technically demanding for the general surgeon and the principle of appropriate mobilization and packing is the mainstay of treatment, followed by angio-embolization. The presence of a contrast blush on CT in a relatively stable patient may be handled with angio-embolization initially, if it is immediately available.

- *Pancreaticoduodenal injuries*: Difficulties in diagnosis and management are often encountered, as the extent of injury to the pancreas and bile ducts, as well as possible retropancreatic vascular injuries may not be immediately apparent. Missed injuries lead to significant morbidity and mortality.
- *Aortic and vena caval injuries*: Access to the retroperitoneal great vessels to obtain proximal and distal control is complicated in the presence of a large or enlarging retroperitoneal haematoma.
- *Complex pelvic fractures with associated open pelvic injury*: These are particularly difficult to treat and are associated with a high mortality.

Damage control approaches to these injuries may dramatically improve survival.

9.1.1.2 THE RETROPERITONEUM

The retroperitoneum is divided into:

- A central zone (zone I).
- Two lateral zones (zone II).
- A pelvic zone (zone III).

Injuries to retroperitoneal structures are associated with a high mortality and are often underestimated or missed. Exsanguinating vascular injuries need rapid and efficient access techniques. Large retroperitoneal haematomas often obscure the exact position and extent of the injury. The decision to explore a retroperitoneal haematoma is based on its location and the mechanism of injury, and whether the haematoma is pulsating or rapidly expanding.

Upper midline central retroperitoneal haematomas (zone I) as well as expanding lateral haematomas *must* be explored, as major abdominal vascular injury, or injury to the kidneys, ureters and renal vessels, pancreas, duodenum, and colon may be present. In the trauma patient, the retroperitoneum is always approached via a transperitoneal incision, because of the high incidence of intraperitoneal and retroperitoneal injuries occurring simultaneously.

Lateral retroperitoneal haematomas (zone II) need not be routinely explored unless expanding, unless perforation of the colon, or a ureteric injury is thought to have occurred. The source of bleeding is usually the kidney, and, the haematoma will probably not require surgery.

Non-expanding haematomas related to pelvic fractures (zone III) should not be explored. Ongoing bleeding from pelvic fractures is best managed with a combination of external fixation on the pelvis and angiographic embolization. Attempts at ligation of internal iliac vessels are usually unsuccessful. If angio-embolization is not available, expanding pelvic haematomas should be packed. Extraperitoneal packing is more effective than intraperitoneal pelvic packing and is advocated in unstable patients with pelvic fractures who require surgery for haemodynamic instability (see also Chapter 10).

9.1.1.3 NON-OPERATIVE MANAGEMENT OF PENETRATING ABDOMINAL INJURY

There is universal agreement that patients with generalized peritonism or haemodynamic instability should undergo urgent laparotomy after penetrating injury to the abdomen. In some institutions with a high volume of penetrating trauma to the abdomen, certain haemodynamically stable patients are managed non-operatively (see also Sections 9.4 and 9.5).

It is imperative that serial examination of these patients is undertaken in a meticulous fashion, and that a laparotomy is done if any concerns arise.

Most patients with penetrating abdominal trauma managed non-operatively may be discharged after 24 hours of observation in the presence of a reliable abdominal examination and minimal to no tenderness. In addition, diagnostic laparoscopy may be considered as a tool to evaluate diaphragmatic lacerations and peritoneal penetration to avoid unnecessary laparotomy (see also Section 15.1.7). If the laparoscopy is positive, one should convert to a full trauma laparotomy to explore the abdominal cavity fully for other injuries.

The Eastern Association for the Surgery of Trauma (EAST) Practice Management Guidelines provide the following evidence-based guidelines for the management of penetrating abdominal trauma (Table 9.1.1).[1]

Table 9.1.1 Evidence-Based Guidelines for the Management of Penetrating Injury of the Abdomen	
Level I	There are no level I evidence-based guidelines.
Level II	Patients who are haemodynamically unstable or who have diffuse abdominal tenderness after penetrating abdominal trauma should be taken for emergency laparotomy.
	Patients with an unreliable clinical examination (i.e. severe head injury, spinal cord injury, severe intoxication, or need for sedation or intubation) should be explored or further investigation done to determine if there is intraperitoneal injury.
	Others may be selected for initial observation. In these patients: 1. Triple-contrast (oral, intravenous, and rectal contrast) abdominopelvic computed tomography should be strongly considered as a diagnostic tool to facilitate initial management decisions, as this test can accurately predict the need for laparotomy. 2. Serial examinations should be performed, as physical examination is reliable in detecting significant injuries after penetrating trauma to the abdomen. Patients requiring delayed laparotomy will develop abdominal signs. 3. If signs of peritonitis develop, laparotomy should be performed. 4. If there is an unexplained drop in blood pressure or haematocrit, further investigation is warranted.
Level III	Most patients with penetrating abdominal trauma managed non-operatively may be discharged after 24 hours of observation in the presence of a reliable abdominal examination and minimal to no abdominal tenderness.
	Patients with penetrating injury to the right upper quadrant of the abdomen with injury to the right lung, right diaphragm, and liver may be safely observed in the presence of stable vital signs, reliable examination, and minimal to no abdominal tenderness.
	Angiography and investigation for and treatment of diaphragm injury may be necessary as adjuncts to the initial non-operative management of penetrating abdominal trauma.
	Mandatory exploration for all penetrating renal trauma is not necessary.

9.1.2 The Trauma Laparotomy

The trauma laparotomy is not for the faint-hearted, and whatever your opinion of the UK's Boy Scout movement, their motto of 'Be Prepared' is entirely germane to this topic. However, what the trauma surgeon has to 'be prepared' for, is the unexpected. Trauma does not follow guidelines, nor do penetrating injuries follow predictable patterns, so from the outset the surgeon is on a rollercoaster voyage of discovery and needs to be prepared for anything and everything.

Preparation of the OR and communication with the OR team prior to surgery is critical; it is necessary to explain what may be expected and what hazards are likely to be encountered. This sharing of information must include the anaesthetist and scrub nurse at the very least, but preferably the whole OR team. Further information on this can be found in Chapter 2 and in Appendix E.

The trauma laparotomy contains several essential steps:

- Rapid entry.
- Adequate (large) incision.
- Control of massive haemorrhage by:
  - Identification of all injuries.
  - Packing.
  - Direct control.
  - Proximal control (i.e. source control).
- Identification of injuries.
- Control of contamination.
- Reconstruction (if possible).

9.1.2.1 PRE-OPERATIVE ADJUNCTS

9.1.2.1.1 Antibiotics[2,3]

Routine single-dose pre-operative intravenous antibiotic prophylaxis should be employed. Subsequent antibiotic policy will depend on the intra-operative findings (Table 9.1.2).

Table 9.1.2 Practice Management Guidelines for Prophylactic Antibiotic Use in Penetrating Abdominal Trauma

Level I	There are sufficient class I and II data to recommend a single pre-operative dose of prophylactic antibiotics with broad-spectrum aerobic and anaerobic coverage as a standard of care for trauma patients sustaining penetrating abdominal wounds. Absence of a hollow viscus injury requires no further administration.
Level II	There are sufficient class I and class II data to recommend continuation of prophylactic antibiotics for only 24 hours in the presence of injury to any hollow viscus.
Level III	There are insufficient clinical data to provide meaningful guidelines for reducing infectious risks in trauma patients with hemorrhagic shock. Vasoconstriction alters the normal distribution of antibiotics, resulting in reduced tissue penetration. To circumvent this problem, the administered dose may be increased two- or threefold and repeated after every 10th unit of blood product transfusion until there is no further blood loss. Once haemodynamic stability has been achieved, antibiotics with excellent activity against obligate and facultative anaerobic bacteria should be continued for periods that depend on the degree of wound contamination. Aminoglycosides have been demonstrated to exhibit suboptimal activity in patients with serious injury, probably due to altered pharmacokinetics of drug distribution.

The antibiotics commonly recommended include a second-generation cephalosporin, plus metronidazole, or where available, amoxycillin/clavulanate. There is some evidence that aminoglycosides should not be used in acute trauma, partly because of the shift in fluids which requires substantially higher doses of aminoglycoside to reach the appropriate minimum inhibitory concentration (MIC), and partly because they work best in an alkaline environment (traumatized tissue is acidotic) (Table 9.1.3).

The administered dose should be increased twofold to threefold and repeated after every 10 units of blood transfusion until there is no further blood loss. If intra-abdominal bleeding is significant, it may be necessary to give a further dose of antibiotic therapy intraoperatively, owing to dilution of the preoperative dose.

9.1.2.1.2 Temperature Control[4]

Temperature control is fundamental in preventing complications in the injured patient. Minimizing patient hypothermia by raising the operating room temperature to a higher than normal level, and warming the patient with warm air blankets, warmed intravenous fluids, and warmed anaesthetic gases is very important.

Theatre preparations should, where possible, commence well before the arrival of the patient. These include warming of the operating theatre, warming of all intravenous fluids, warming of anaesthetic gases and activating external warming devices such as a Bair Hugger® (3M Corporation, St Paul, MN, USA).

9.1.2.1.3 Blood Collection and Autotransfusion

Preparations must be made for collection of blood in a saline and heparin primed drainage system, or a cell saving device, for autotransfusion if indicated.

9.1.2.2 **DRAPING**

During the trauma laparotomy, it may become necessary to extend the incision, if required. All patients should therefore be prepared and draped to allow access to the thorax, abdomen and groins if required (Figure 9.1.1).

Table 9.1.3 Antibiotic Prophylaxis and Empiric Therapy in Major Abdominal Injury after First Dose

No pathology found	No further antibiotics
Blood only	No further antibiotics
Small bowel or gastric contamination	Continuation for 24 hours only Copious peritoneal wash-out
Large bowel, minimal contamination	Continuation for 24 hours only
Large bowel, gross contamination	Copious peritoneal wash-out 24–72 hours of antibiotics

incision is that it may be extended easily upwards into a sternotomy or a right subcostal for difficult injuries of the right lobe of the liver, although in practice, this is rare. No time is wasted in chasing small bleeders from the wound edges with diathermy. These will stop on their own. Put gauze swabs over them and continue.

The next pass of the knife should be into the linea alba just superior (cranial) to the umbilicus – this being the quickest route to access the peritoneal cavity, as the parietal peritoneum is blended with the anterior abdominal wall at this point due to the umbilical cicatrix. This should obviate the need to pick up the peritoneum as a separate structure.

The peritoneum should be opened last, once the entire incision as indicated above has been performed. This is essentially for two reasons: firstly, a closed peritoneum maintains a tampon effect and keeps the incision visible, and secondly, this avoids losing time extending the incision in an abundantly bleeding situation. Usually, the peritoneum can be opened quickly with two fingers, or large Mayo's scissors without having to resort to any instrument (which may be dangerous).

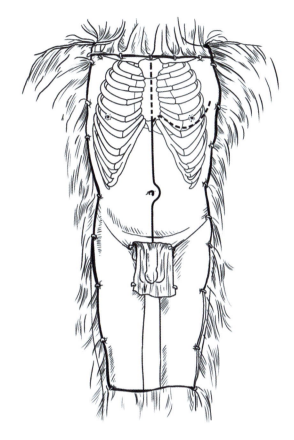

Figure 9.1.1 Exploration of the abdomen, showing extent of skin preparation and draping prior to surgery.

9.1.2.3 INCISION

Once the patient and staff are fully prepared, and the anaesthetist has indicated to the surgeon that they are ready for surgery to commence, the surgeon should waste no time entering the abdomen. A sharp knife, a profound knowledge of anatomy, and courage are all that are needed in the first 30–60 seconds!

All patients undergoing a laparotomy for abdominal trauma should be explored through a long midline incision, made with a scalpel. This incision is generally placed through, or to the left of, the umbilicus, to avoid the falciform ligament. The incision is made from the xiphisternum to the pubis, with one sweep of the blade, and if necessary, can be further extended into a sternotomy, or can be extended right or left as a thoracotomy for access to the liver, diaphragm, etc. (Figure 9.1.1).

A long, midline incision is made with a scalpel, from xiphisternum to pubis, in one sweep of the blade (preferably skirting the umbilicus, which should have been cleaned), down to the linea alba. The advantage of this

---

Pitfall

It may not easy to gain rapid entry to the abdominal cavity where previous surgery has been performed. This is termed a 'hostile abdomen' and may present the surgeon with extreme technical challenges to be able to safely enter the peritoneal space without injuring bowel or other structures adherent to the underlying abdominal scar(s). Identification of a hostile abdomen should forewarn the surgeon of difficult access and may be the occasion to resort to left anterior thoracotomy for aortic cross-clamping in the chest, or retrograde endovascular balloon occlusion of the aorta (REBOA) prior to laparotomy, in order to prevent exsanguination during difficult abdominal access.

In patients with gross haemodynamic instability, or who have had significant previous midline surgery, a bilateral subcostal ('clamshell' or 'chevron') incision extending from the anterior axillary line on each side transversely across the midline just superior to the umbilicus may be used.

9.1.2.4 INITIAL PROCEDURE

A quick exploratory 'trauma laparotomy' is performed to identify any other associated injuries:

1. As soon as the abdomen has been opened, large quantities of blood or other fluids may pour out,

and a Poole's sucker may be usefully introduced into the abdominal cavity whilst the incision is rapidly extended up and down using large Mayo's scissors to the full extent of the skin incision. Do NOT use fine dissection scissors, such as McIndoe's for this, as they will be badly blunted by the experience. Scoop out as much blood as possible into a receiver. Do not use a sucker at this time as it is too slow and will block with clots.

2. Eviscerate the small bowel. Perform a rapid exploration to any obvious site of large-volume (audible) bleeding. Assess the midline structures where packing is inefficient – the aorta, inferior vena cava (IVC), and mesentery, and if necessary, control with direct pressure or proximal control, for example, on the aorta. Active bleeding MUST be controlled before proceeding further with a laparotomy.

3. Once access has been achieved, blood and free abdominal contents should be scooped out using a small kidney dish or large gallipot, emptying it out into a large metal washbowl on a stand beside the surgeon. This allows the anaesthetist to view the contents and estimate blood loss; do not use suckers, as they are too slow, and will block with clots.

4. Having cleared most of the abdomen of blood and other contaminants into the large washbowl, dry, unfolded packs (for maximum absorption) should be inserted, starting from the places of suspected major bleeding, and working towards those areas which appear less involved. All areas of the abdominal cavity must be packed if injuries are not to be missed.

5. Perform packing using large dry abdominal swabs:
   - Under the left diaphragm.
   - In the left paracolic gutter.
   - In the pelvis.
   - In the right paracolic gutter.
   - Into the subhepatic pouch.
   - Above and lateral to the liver.
   - Directly on any other bleeding area.

Pitfalls

- **Use dry swabs throughout**: Dry swabs work better and will not cool the patient further. Pack them open, and loosely, into the above-mentioned anatomical areas. This type of packing is focused on identifying the origin of bleeding by removing the excess blood from the uninjured parts of the peritoneal cavity.

- **Never pass sharp instruments by hand**: The laparotomy is relatively uncontrolled. ALL sharps (scalpels, needles in needle holders, etc.) MUST be passed into and out of the operative field in a receiver (e.g. a kidney dish) to minimize the risk of a 'needle-stick'.

Packing does not control arterial bleeding.

6. Remove the abdominal packs, one at a time, starting in the area *least* likely to be the site of the bleeding. Then, apply pressure or compress the organ or area where active bleeding is identified.

7. Once the source of major haemorrhage has been identified – however approximately – the area has been firmly packed, and pressure applied to ensure no further significant bleeding occurs. Having established this, **STOP OPERATING!**

   This is the opportunity for the anaesthetist to catch up with adequate lines, fluid, and transfusion requirements, assess the blood gases, thromboelastogram (TEG), and core temperature, and discuss with the surgical team the likely injuries and options for repair, damage control, or 'bail-out' techniques.

Pitfall

Resources for possible options must be considered at this point, and if these are severely limited or non-existent, then the absolute minimum should be attempted to simply control bleeding and stop further contamination. Heroic surgery accompanied by frantic anaesthesia rarely results in a successful outcome. Decisions to transfer to a better equipped facility, if possible, or a higher care area to improve the patient's physiology must be made now – not after struggling for another hour or more with a coagulopathic, acidotic, cold patient, whose survival chances lessen by the minute, in the face of an absence of transfusion products, an intensive care unit – but for the obstinate ego of the surgeon.

9.1.2.5 PERFORM A TRAUMA LAPAROTOMY

Once access had been made into the peritoneal cavity, temporary control of haemorrhage made, and some time given to allow the anaesthetist to address the physiological needs of the patient, the compelling source of bleeding must now be addressed.

It is essential to treat first what kills first.

Methods of dealing with bleeding vary depending on whether the source is venous or arterial, and if a shunt or repair is required, or whether the vessel can be ligated without major deleterious effects. These techniques are described in the chapter on abdominal vascular injury (Section 9.2). Similarly, techniques for controlling contamination from the bowel (Section 9.3), biliary (Section 9.4), and urogenital tract (Section 9.8) are discussed in the relevant chapters.

When the major hazards have been dealt with, a full examination of the abdominal cavity must be made. Routines and patterns vary, but what matters is that the individual surgeon has a routine that they follow every time. One way is described here.

Starting from above and moving downwards, the integrity of the diaphragm is checked. It is often forgotten in complex and multi-cavity injuries. Both blunt and penetrating injuries may be responsible for diaphragmatic rupture.

Blunt chest or abdominal trauma may result in a rapid increase in thoracic or abdominal pressure, with traumatic rupture of the diaphragm. This is more common on the left, as the right lobe of the liver protects (to some extent) the right dome of the diaphragm. nevertheless, if blunt liver trauma of the right lobe is seen (segments VII and VIII especially) and the right triangular and coronary ligaments, along with the falciform ligament will need to be divided to inspect the dome of the right diaphragm properly.

Beware a large retrohepatic haematoma in blunt trauma; if it is not expanding, it is best left alone.

The left lobe of the liver is easy to see and mobilize if necessary, to check the diaphragm behind it. Small stab wounds that have entered the lower left chest may easily puncture the diaphragm, leaving the potential for either the stomach or a loop of bowel to be trapped in the defect, and leading to later necrosis of the bowel wall with spillage of gut content into the chest cavity. This may appear in the chest drain effluent and should give the clue to the diagnosis.

The epigastrium is crowded, and injuries are easy to miss. Specific organ injuries are dealt with in their relevant chapters, and only useful tips will be mentioned here.

Both sides of the stomach must be inspected; even so, it is easy to overlook a small penetrating injury that will store up trouble for the future. If the stomach is deflated, ask the anaesthetist to pass some air into the nasogastric tube, and squeeze the stomach gently, looking for bubbles appearing, or gastric contents, which may be bile-stained. An easy way to inspect the posterior surface of the stomach is by entering the gastrocolic omentum. Usually this is possible without needing to divide vessels.

The gall bladder, once decompressed by perforation, may be overlooked. The bile staining present may be assumed to come from the intestine, so care should be taken to carefully inspect the gall bladder for its integrity (see also Section 9.4).

Little time is spent on trying to preserve the spleen in trauma laparotomies, but there are some occasions when it matters, such as in children. For the most part, trauma to the spleen means splenectomy, which is a quick procedure and should take no more than 15 minutes. This topic is dealt with in Section 9.5.

This approach also gives a view of the superior surface of the pancreas and splenic vessels. It is sometimes possible to view the beginning of the portal vein at its formation from the joining of the splenic and superior mesenteric veins behind the neck of the pancreas. The head of the pancreas is examined by mobilizing the second part of the duodenum and rolling it gently to the left off the inferior vena cava, where the head of the pancreas will be seen in the 'C' of the duodenum. The inferior border of the pancreas is best seen by exposing it at the base of the mesentery, lifting the whole small bowel up and to the right. The tail of the pancreas is easily seen at the hilum of the spleen (see also Section 9.6).

Having mobilized the duodenal loop by Kocher's manoeuvre, the continuity of the whole small bowel should be assessed, placing Babcock or Duval tissue forceps on points of perforation or division, and rapidly stopping contamination by tying divided sections off with umbilical tapes or the long tags on abdominal swabs. If several holes are present within a relatively short segment of bowel, they may all be included in the tied-off loop, or it may be rapidly resected with a stapler.

It is helpful to have two pairs of eyes inspecting the bowel. However, the practice of passing it hand-to-hand, from surgeon to assistant, may result in missed injuries. Small perforations where the mesentery meets the bowel wall are difficult to find unless small haematomata there are carefully examined and/or explored.

Do not be side-tracked whilst making your examination – keep your focus.
One pair of hands, two pairs of eyes.

Once the caecum is reached, a decision may need to be made whether to explore any lateral haematoma in the right flank. If it is the result of blunt trauma and is neither expanding nor pulsatile, it may be left. If there has been penetrating trauma, the safe course of action is to explore it, even if it is neither expanding nor pulsatile. The reason for this is that it is not possible to rule out an injury to the retroperitoneal part of the ascending colon, nor an injury to the urinary tract. If both these injuries are present then the right kidney should be removed, as an infected urinoma and renal abscess will result. Both a colonic and urinary fistula are likely to occur.

The colon is systematically inspected, utilizing full right and left visceral rotations, and care being taken to minimize any faecal contamination. The gastrocolic omentum may need separating from the greater curve of the stomach to visualize the full circumference of the colon.

The rectum is partially retroperitoneal, and pelvic haematomata associated with penetrating trauma requires fine judgement in management if further major haemorrhage is to be avoided. Bullet or stab wounds in the buttocks or perineum may well have penetrated either or both bowel and bladder, and each needs full assessment. A urinary catheter should already have been placed so further drainage at damage control is unnecessary, but if blood has been found on the gloved finger on rectal examination, then a pararectal corrugated drain may be placed to exit the skin over the ischiorectal fossa.

At the initial laparotomy no stoma should be made in a damage control setting. The priority is to minimize time in the OR to the two essentials of stopping bleeding and further contamination – and leaving the reconstructive work to another time when the patient's physiology will withstand more surgery.

Gynaecological organs, unless the patient is pregnant, should not pose a problem, and are unlikely to be a major source of bleeding.

Injuries to the bladder may be difficult to diagnose, as blood in the catheter bag may have come from anywhere along the urinary tract. If the base of the bladder is thought to have been damaged, and no injury is found on initial examination, urethral and suprapubic catheters may be placed, and a bivalve of the bladder made at re-look laparotomy. If the site of injury is still not found, the ureter(s) may have been injured at the point of entry to the bladder and deep to the trigone. Which side – or both – may be identified by asking the anaesthetist to administer either a small injection of methylene blue or furosemide intravenously. Within less than a minute, whilst observing the bladder trigone from within, the ureteric orifices will squirt blue urine, or just a strong jet of normal coloured urine, demonstrating potency of the ureter on that or both sides.

Bladder, ureteric, and renal repairs can be found in Section 9.8.

9.1.2.5.1 Large Mesenteric Haematoma

The technique for separating the mesenteric root from the retroperitoneum is to mobilize the entire midgut loop, from transverse colon to the Ligament of Treitz. Start by 'Kocherizing' the duodenum and follow that plane around and behind the hepatic flexure of the colon, down the right paracolic gutter to the caecum. Then turn abruptly upwards (cephalad) again, behind the caecum and in front of the ureter and psoas, along the left-hand edge of the base of the mesenteric root. Continue this dissection, mobilizing the mesenteric root off the inferior vena cava and the aorta until the duodeno-jejunal flexure is seen, with the attachment of the Ligament of Treitz to its upper surface, passing behind the stomach to the right crus of the diaphragm.

At this point the entire midgut loop may be lifted clear of the abdominal cavity and placed into a sterile bag and left briefly on the chest of the patient. It is important to warn the anaesthetist about this procedure as the translocated bowel may rapidly become ischaemic if there is undue traction on the mesenteric base, which will result in a significant acidosis within a very short time, upsetting the smooth running of the anaesthetic and the patient's already disturbed physiology.

- Nevertheless, the manoeuvre quickly and clearly demonstrates whether the compelling source of bleeding is from mesenteric vessels or the retroperitoneum.
- Deal with lesions in order of their lethality:
  - Injuries to major blood vessels.
  - Major haemorrhage from solid abdominal viscera.
  - Haemorrhage from mesentery and hollow organs.
  - Retroperitoneal haemorrhage.
  - Contamination.

9.1.2.6 PERFORM DEFINITIVE PACKING

9.1.2.6.1 Definitive Packing

- *Use the folded dry packs 'flat' against the organ.*
- *Do not cover them in plastic – they will slip and will be too rigid.*

- *Preferably keep the dry swabs folded as it is easier to 'layer' them into a cavity.*
- *Place the packs flat against the organ.*
- *Packs must exert sufficient force on the organ to tamponade bleeding.*
- *Packs only work in venous injury (arteries must be controlled directly).*
- *Arterial perfusion should be preserved.*
- *Use the least number of packs that will achieve the desired result.*

9.1.2.6.1.1 *Liver (See also Section 9.4)*

When the initial packs are removed from the right upper quadrant, injury to the liver is assessed. It is prudent at this time to dissect the gastrohepatic ligament at the porta hepatis using blunt and sharp dissection so that a vessel loop (Rumel tourniquet) or vascular clamp can be placed across the portal triad.

The liver is mobilized only if necessary

Bleeding from the liver may require manual compression. If compression of the liver controls the bleeding, the bleeding is probably venous in nature, and can be arrested with definitive therapeutic liver packing. If not, Pringle's manoeuvre should be performed.

If a Pringle manoeuvre controls the bleeding, the surgeon should suspect hepatic artery or portal vein injury. Hepatorrhaphy is then performed to control intrahepatic vessels, alone or in combination with packing.

If a Pringle manoeuvre fails to control bleeding, the likely source is hepatic veins or IVC. Compression of the liver against the posterior abdominal wall and diaphragm can be useful, and packing should be performed.

9.1.2.6.1.2 *Spleen (See also Section 9.5)*

When the packs in the left upper quadrant are removed, and if there is associated bleeding from the spleen, a decision should be made on whether the spleen should be preserved or removed.

A vascular clamp placed across the hilum will allow temporary haemorrhage control.

9.1.2.6.1.3 *Pelvis (See also Chapter 10)*

If the pelvis seems to be a major source of bleeding, intraperitoneal packing should be converted to extra-peritoneal pelvic packing, once intra-abdominal haemorrhage has been achieved.

9.1.2.7 SPECIFIC ROUTES OF ACCESS

9.1.2.7.1 Lesser Sac

The stomach is grasped and pulled inferiorly, allowing the operator to identify the lesser curvature and the superior aspect of the pancreas visible through the lesser omentum. The coeliac artery and the body of the pancreas can also be accessed through this approach.

9.1.2.7.2 Greater Sac

The omentum is then grasped and drawn upwards. A window is made in the omentum (via the gastrocolic ligament) and provides access into the lesser sac posterior to the stomach. This allows excellent exposure of the entire body and tail of the pancreas, as well as the posterior aspect of the first part of the duodenum and the medial aspect of the second part. Any injuries to the pancreas can be easily identified. If there is a possibility of an injury to the head of the pancreas, a Kocher manoeuvre should be performed. Additional exposure can be achieved using the right medial visceral rotation.

9.1.2.7.3 Mobilization of the ascending colon (right hemicolon)

The hepatic flexure is retracted medially, dividing adhesions along its lateral border down to the caecum (Figure 9.1.2).

9.1.2.7.4 Kocher Manoeuvre

The Kocher manoeuvre is performed by initially dividing the lateral peritoneal attachment of the duodenum, allowing medial rotation of the duodenum (Figure 9.1.3).

The loose areolar tissue around the duodenum is bluntly dissected, and the entire second and third portions of the duodenum are identified and are mobilized medially with a combination of sharp and blunt dissection. This dissection is carried all the way medially to expose the IVC and a portion of the aorta.

The posterior wall of the duodenum can be inspected, together with the right kidney, porta hepatis, and IVC. By reflecting the duodenum and pancreas toward the anterior midline, the posterior surface of the head of the pancreas can be completely exposed (Figure 9.1.4). Better inspection of the third part and inspection of the fourth part of the duodenum can be achieved by mobilizing the ligament of Treitz and performing a right medial visceral rotation.

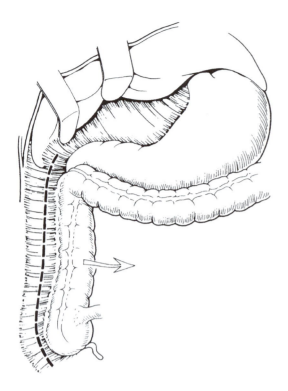

Figure 9.1.2 Mobilization of the right hemicolon.

9.1.2.7.5 Right Medial Visceral Rotation[5]

This was previously known as the Cattel and Braasch manoeuvre.

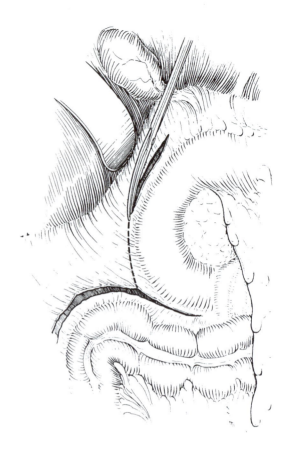

Figure 9.1.3 Kocher manoeuvre.

After mobilizing the right hemicolon from the hepatic flexure to the caecum, and performing a Kocher's manoeuvre, the small bowel mesentery is mobilized by sharply incising its retroperitoneal attachments from the right lower quadrant, to the ligament of Treitz, by progressively lifting up the caecum. The entire ascending colon and caecum are then reflected superiorly towards the left upper quadrant of the abdomen. A Kocher manoeuvre is performed as well. This will expose the right retroperitoneum (Figure 9.1.4). The small bowel mobilization is undertaken by sharply incising its retroperitoneal attachments from the right lower quadrant to the ligament of Treitz. The entire ascending colon and the caecum are then reflected superiorly towards the left upper quadrant of the abdomen.

As the dissection is carried further, the inferior border of the entire pancreas can then be identified and any injuries inspected. Severe oedema, crepitation, or bile staining of the periduodenal tissues implies a duodenal injury until proven otherwise. Mobilization of the whole duodenum is mandatory for exclusion of duodenal injury.

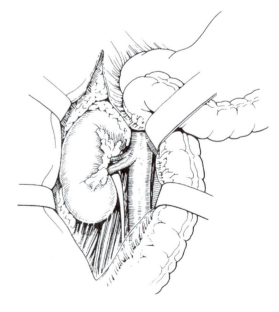

Figure 9.1.4 Reflection of the duodenum and right hemicolon to show the right kidney and IVC.

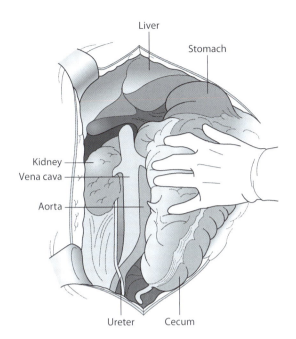

Figure 9.1.5 Right medial visceral rotation.

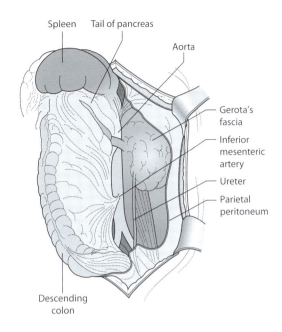

Figure 9.1.6 Left medial rotation.

These manoeuvres allow for complete exposure of the first, second, third, and fourth parts of the duodenum, along with the head, neck, and proximal body of the pancreas. Access to the vena cava and the renal vessels is also facilitated (Figure 9.1.5).

Exposure for repair of the aorta, and the distal body and tail of pancreas can be better obtained by performing a left medial visceral rotation.

9.1.2.7.6 Left Medial Visceral Rotation[6]

Medial rotation of the left side of the abdominal contents can be performed by mobilizing the spleen and descending colon, and then displacing the spleen, descending colon, and sigmoid colon to the right (left medial visceral rotation). This allows inspection of the left kidney, retroperitoneum, and tail of the pancreas.

Mobilize the splenorenal ligament and incise the peritoneal reflection in the left paracolic gutter, down to the level of the sigmoid colon. The left-sided viscera are then bluntly dissected free of the retroperitoneum and mobilized to the right. Care should be taken to remain in a plane anterior to Gerota's fascia, which covers the kidney. The entire anterior surface of the abdominal aorta and the origins of its branches are exposed by this technique. This includes the coeliac axis, the origin of the superior mesenteric artery, the iliac vessels, and the left renal pedicle (Figure 9.1.6). The dense and fibrous superior

mesenteric and coeliac nerve plexuses overlie the proximal aorta and need to be sharply dissected in order to identify the renal and superior mesenteric arteries.

If vascular access to the kidney is required, Gerota's fascia should be divided on the lateral aspect of the kidney, and the kidney rotated medially to allow access to the renal hilum, as well as the lateral side of the aorta, which can be controlled if necessary.

Pelvic haematomas should not be explored routinely. It is preferable to perform a combination of external pelvic fixation, pelvic packing, and angiographic embolization. Attempts at tying the internal iliac vessels are usually unsuccessful.

9.1.2.8 SPECIFIC ORGAN TECHNIQUES (SEE ALSO SPECIFIC ORGANS)

9.1.2.8.1 Hepatic Injury

In severe liver injury, after successful surgical treatment including the removal of devascularized necrotic tissue and resectional debridement in selected cases, the liver is packed, and the injured area compressed with warm pads. After complete exploration of the abdomen and treatment of other injuries and sources of bleeding, the liver packs are removed and any slight oozing on the surface of the liver can be arrested by sealing with fibrin and collagen fleece as described above. Fibrin glue cannot, however, compensate for inadequate surgical technique.

9.1.2.8.2 Splenic Injury

When possible, in the stable patient, the surgeon should try to achieve splenic repair that preserves as much of the damaged spleen as possible. For splenic preservation, the choice of procedure depends not only on the clinical findings, but also on the surgeon's experience of splenic surgery and the equipment available. In trauma cases, conservation of the spleen should not take significantly more time than would a splenectomy.

After using one of the surgical techniques described above, definitive treatment can be completed by the application of adhesives to secure the resected edge or the mesh-covered splenic tissue. Fibrin is sprayed on, and the collagen fleece is pressed on it for a few minutes. After removal of the compressing pad, a new layer of fibrin glue can help to ensure the prevention of rebleeding. In case of use of mesh, the collagen fleece and fibrin are placed directly on the injured splenic surface and then covered with the mesh. Additional fibrin spray may be then used.

9.1.2.8.3 Pancreatic Injury

When pancreatic injury is suspected, extended exploration of the whole organ is imperative. Parenchymal lacerations that do not involve the pancreatic duct can be sutured when the tissue is not too soft and vulnerable. With or without sutures, a worthwhile option in the treatment of such lacerations is fibrin sealing and collagen tamponade, for which adequate drainage is essential.

9.1.2.8.4 Retroperitoneal Haematoma

Injuries to the retroperitoneal vessels can cause haematomas of varying size, depending on the calibre of the vessels injured and the severity of the injury. Retroperitoneal haematomas can be treated by packing after surgical control of injured vessels and be followed by catheter embolization.

When the patient is stable, the packs may be removed after 24–48 hours. Rebleeding after removal of the packs can necessitate repacking. Slight bleeding can, however, be stopped effectively by spraying on adhesives.

9.1.3 **Closure of the Abdomen**

9.1.3.1 PRINCIPLES OF ABDOMINAL CLOSURE

On completion of the intra-abdominal procedures, it is important to adequately prepare for closure. This preparation includes:

- Careful evaluation of the adequacy of haemostasis and/or packing.
- Copious lavage and removal of debris within the peritoneum and wound.
- Placement of adequate and appropriate drains if indicated.
- Ensuring that the instrument and swab counts are completed and correct.

It is important to replace the small intestine in the abdominal cavity with great care at the conclusion of the operation.

9.1.3.2 CHOOSING THE OPTIMAL METHOD OF CLOSURE

Thal and O'Keefe[7] state that the optimal closure technique is chosen based on five principal considerations and list these as follows:

- The *stability* of the patient (and therefore the need for speed of closure).
- The amount of blood loss both prior to and during operation.
- The volume of intravenous fluid administered.
- The degree of intraperitoneal and wound contamination.
- The nutritional status of the patient and possible intercurrent disease.

These factors will also dictate the decision to plan for a relaparotomy, which will naturally influence the method chosen for closure. Other factors that should be taken into consideration are hypothermia, coagulopathy, and acidosis, which are indications to revert to damage control strategies.

Temporary abdominal closure is described in Chapter 6.

9.1.3.3 PRIMARY CLOSURE

Primary closure of the abdominal sheath (or fascia), the subcutaneous tissue and the skin is obviously the desirable goal and may be achieved when the conditions outlined above are optimal; that is, a stable patient with minimal blood loss and volume replacement, no or minimal contamination, no significant intercurrent problems, and a patient in whom surgical procedures are deemed to be completed with no anticipated subsequent operation. Should any doubt exist regarding these conditions at the conclusion of operation, it would be prudent to consider a technique of delayed closure.

The most commonly used technique at present is that of *mass closure* of the peritoneum and sheath using an monofilament suture with a continuous (preferable, since relatively quick) or an interrupted (discontinuous) application. Either absorbable material (e.g. 1 polydioxanone loop) or non-absorbable material (e.g. nylon, polypropylene) may be used. Chromic catgut is not a suitable material.

Whichever method is used, the most important technical point is that of avoiding excessive tension on the tissues of the closure. Remember the 'one centimetre-one centimetre' rule as described by Leaper et al.[8] (the so-called 'Guildford technique'; Figure 9.1.7). This uses 4 cm of material for every 1 cm advance. This spacing seems to minimize tension in the tissues, and thus also minimize compromise of the circulation in the area, as well as using the minimum acceptable amount of suture. The use of 0 or 1 looped polydioxanone as a continuous suture is recommended.

Retention sutures should be avoided at all costs. A wound that seems to require these is not suitable for primary closure.

Closure of such a wound may result in abdominal compartment syndrome; such a wound should be left open, with a vacuum dressing.

Skin closure as a primary manoeuvre may be done in a case with no or minimal contamination, using monofilament sutures or staples. These latter have the advantage of speed and, while being less haemostatic, nevertheless allow for a greater degree of drainage past the skin edges and less tissue reaction.

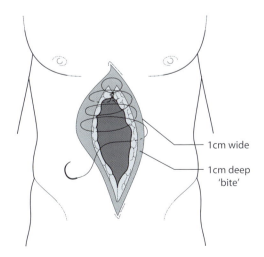

1cm wide

1cm deep 'bite'

Figure 9.1.7 The Guildford technique.

9.1.4 **Specific Tips and Tricks**

9.1.4.1 HEADLIGHT

Even in the most sophisticated of OR suites, clear, well-illuminated vision of the operating field is not optimal. For this reason, the use of a personal, battery-operated headlight of the LED variety is a good addition to the trauma surgeon's armamentarium. In military and austere environments, it is essential, as it may suddenly be the only light available; power cuts are common in the developing world, and generators fail at the most inappropriate moments. It is a good investment, along with plenty of spare batteries. Do not rely on rechargeable batteries.

9.1.4.2 STIRRUPS AND LITHOTOMY POSITION

In a complex patient, if the lithotomy position is used, then it is possible to position the scrub nurse (or an assistant) between the patients' legs – perhaps with a small Mayo table over the pubic area. This allows the scrub nurse to see the surgery, and anticipate the surgeon's needs, or allows an additional assistant without overcrowding the operative field.

Stirrups should always be in place for injuries that involve, or are suspected of involving, the perineum. In the female, gynaecological specula and retractors should also be available, and a good operating sigmoidoscope and light source for both sexes.

The OR scrub nurse should ensure that sterile legging drapes are immediately available should the patient need to be put up into the lithotomy position.

9.1.4.3 TABLE TILT

Easy operative access is the aim in all surgery; and just as the senior surgeon, when asked to assist his junior who is struggling, will frequently extend the incision to improve access, so too the use of a table tilt may make all the difference between an uncomfortable operative experience and one that is considerably easier.

A head-down tilt will move the small bowel up out of the pelvis and up under the diaphragm, where it can be held in place by a large roll of gauze. If a head-up tilt is combined with a table tilt to the left, then access to the right lobe of the liver and all the associated biliary anatomy is made easier. A head-up tilt and table tilt to the right will enable access to the spleen and the stomach, though a head-down tilt in this combination is better for repair to the diaphragm itself.

9.1.4.4 BE FLEXIBLE: MOVE!

Trauma surgery requires an open mind – although some knowledge is useful – with no preconceived ideas of exactly what is going to be found, and no rigid operative protocol on how to deal with the situation. This means that the surgeon and the operating team must be prepared to shift positions if unanticipated injury is found, or the procedure could be made technically easier by (for example) standing on the other side of the table or between the legs, raised in lithotomy poles.

The unscrubbed OR personnel should be ready to assist with such moves, along with repositioning of the operating lights. The latter move should not always be delegated to the anaesthetist, who is likely to be busy with resuscitative measures.

9.1.4.5 AORTIC COMPRESSION SPOON

This easily self-constructed adjunct to haemorrhage control was designed for use in control of the abdominal aorta in the subdiaphragmatic space, by direct downward pressure on the aorta upon the spine at the level of the diaphragmatic crura.

Its value lies in there being no need for difficult and time-wasting dissection of the aorta and division of the right crus. The oesophagus is pushed to the left, the left lobe of the liver is pushed caudally and to the right (the coronary ligament may need rapid division) and the spoon is then pushed vertically down against the spine, compressing the aorta.

The instrument is shaped so that the distal edge of the cup is removed with a coping saw, and the edge sanded down to a smooth, gently inverted 'U'. The spoon, being wooden, has the advantage of not slipping on the tissues, and has no moving parts – other than the assistant holding it. Clamps of all varieties frequently fail to enclose the whole of the aorta, as they slip off the vertebral body of the spine. Dissection around the aorta at this level, in order to place a Satinsky clamp, puts the phrenic and intercostal arteries in jeopardy and runs the risk of inadvertent damage to the posterior wall of the aorta, which is then difficult to repair.

9.1.4.6 PERICARDIAL WINDOW

Access to the pericardial sac can be made rapidly and easily from the abdomen by cutting directly backwards into the sac through the diaphragm from the xiphisternum. It is sometimes easier to do this by excising the xiphisternum in an inverted 'V', removing that cartilage in continuity with the backward incision.

Since the central tendon of the diaphragm and the pericardium share the same embryological origin from the septum transversum, there are no planes to dissect or get lost in. The entry should be immediately into the sac in front of the IVC and below the right atrium, from where it is easy to determine the presence or absence of pericardial tamponade.

9.1.4.7 WASHOUT

The solution to pollution is dilution.

Whether the peritoneal or thoracic cavity is to be washed out, it is a good rule of thumb to consider using at least six litres of warm saline – and then doubling it!

There is no advantage to using antiseptic solutions nor added antibiotics to the washouts.

If there has been contamination of the thoracic cavity through a small diaphragmatic hole, and bowel content has entered the thorax, it is wise to extend the diaphragmatic defect in a radial direction (to avoid the phrenic nerve and blood supply) allowing the passage of a hand into the thoracic cavity. This will allow a much more thorough lavage of the thorax, using the hand as a paddle, and less likelihood of retained bowel content and subsequent abscess formation. Always place a large bore intercostal basal drain, passed up *behind* the hilum of the lung in such cases, before closing the diaphragmatic defect.

Similarly, it is important to make sure that all peritoneal and retroperitoneal recesses are fully irrigated and washed out, though the bare area of the liver and the right suprahepatic space do not need to be disturbed if the right coronary ligament has not been transgressed.

If there have been through-and-through injuries to the liver, it is not a good idea to wash these out if they are not bleeding (see also Section 9.4).

Gross contamination with colonic contents within the peritoneum will require a second look and further washout in 24 hours, if the patient's physiology is robust enough.

9.1.4.8 DRAINS

There is no place for drains in the acute, damage-control laparotomy – with one exception; that is, to the pancreas and duodenum. Digestive enzymes free in the peritoneum are poor partners to a smooth recovery, and suction drains are recommended.

9.1.4.9 STOMAS

There is no place for stoma formation, either temporary or permanent, in an initial damage control laparotomy. At the first procedure, a temporary closure will have been used, and any divided bowel ends will have been sealed by one means or another 'clip/tie/staples and drop'. Even if the ends are ischaemic, they will not cause leakage for at least 48–72 hours, by which time a second look laparotomy should have been performed.

Temporary stomata may be formed if the patient's physiology is still precarious at second look, in preference to anastomosis, which is highly risky in the presence of persistent hypotension, or during the administration of inotropes. This may necessitate the formation of the 'split stoma', where both ends of what will become an anastomosis are brought out separately at different sites on the abdominal wall.

It is important to give thought to the main priority for their maintenance – that is, ease of nursing care. Thus, allowing enough space around the stoma for the application of adhesive bags, and the cleaning of the surgical wounds. Place stomas more laterally, higher (cranial direction) than normal.

Where a wound of the lower rectosigmoid has necessitated local excision, it is wise not to oversew the rectal stump as this creates a blind loop. Then, if the patient later exhibits signs of further sepsis in the ward or ICU, it will be very difficult to know whether an injury has been missed, the rectal stump has 'blown', or some other site of sepsis is responsible for the patient's decline. In the post-operative abdomen, it is virtually impossible to know – even on CT scanning – if the rectal stump is intact or not, as there will inevitably be murky fluid and post-operative exudate in the peritoneal cavity and pelvis.

It is therefore a good idea to bring up the rectal stump, open, into the lower extent of the laparotomy incision as a mucous fistula. This may require a little mobilization of the rectum to achieve, but it is a safer procedure than leaving a viable, peristaltic, blind-ended time-bomb in the pelvis of a critically ill patient. A tube or corrugated drain can be left coming out of the anus and sutured to the skin of the buttock for safety.

Another advantage of forming a rectal mucous fistula is that it makes the subsequent anastomosis of the colon to the rectum very easy, as the rectal stump is readily available to the surgeon, who does not then have to delve into matted pelvic adhesions to discover its whereabouts, risking further bowel perforation.

9.1.4.10 TEMPORARY CLOSURE

This is covered in detail elsewhere in this book. (See Section 6.3: Damage Control Surgery.)

9.1.4.11 TWO CATHETERS: BLADDER INJURY

Where there has been a bladder injury needing repair, it is a good idea to open the bladder by bivalving it in the sagittal plane (to avoid damaging its blood supply) so that the injury can be seen from both sides. This enables a sound repair to be performed that will include the bladder mucosa. (Like the oesophagus, the integrity of a bladder repair hinges mainly on good mucosal apposition.)

Once this has been achieved, in male patients, positioning both a suprapubic and a urethral catheter allows both greater safety in management, and more control.

The suprapubic catheter should not be brought out through the bivalve incision into the bladder as this will almost certainly create a urinary fistula, so it should be brought out of the bladder wall via a separate stab incision into the dome of the bladder and secured by an purse-string suture with absorbable material. It should then be brought out through another stab incision in the abdominal wall, away from the laparotomy incision, and again secured to the skin.

A urethral catheter in addition allows the surgeon to assess the patient's voiding ability – once withdrawn – without compromising the bladder repair's integrity. In this way, if the patient is unable to void, the suprapubic catheter acts as a safety valve, and can be released, having been clamped for 'trial-without-catheter' (TWoC). Usually, a few more days with suprapubic drainage is all that is required for the bladder to settle down, and the normal urethral mechanism to resume function.

Once the patient is again voiding good volumes and has a post-micturition sonar confirmation of an empty bladder, the suprapubic catheter may be removed with confidence.

9.1.4.12 EARLY TRACHEOSTOMY

In damage control situations it is important to anticipate physiological needs. Patients are in critical condition and do not tolerate multiple surgical insults easily. Surgery in trauma – albeit (hopefully) controlled – constitutes second, third, and even fourth 'hits' on the patient's physiology, so anticipation of future physiological need is necessary from the outset.

Within this remit, ventilatory support is a vital component, and the need for ongoing airway management via the formation of a tracheostomy in the future should be discussed at the first damage control laparotomy, or the second look at the latest: that is the case if the tracheostomy is to be performed in the OR by the surgical team. Newer, transcutaneous, Seldinger-type tracheostomies may now be performed quite easily in the ICU if required.

The point is that the procedure needs to be anticipated early on, and not postponed until the patient has gross retained bronchial secretions and is tipping into respiratory failure. This may then demand that regular bronchoscopy be performed until adequate bronchial toilet is achieved, and blood gases are returned to normal.

9.1.5 Briefing for Operating Room Scrub Nurses

A separate briefing for operating room scrub nurses forms Appendix E of this manual.

9.1.6 Summary

Think ahead.
This is the mantra for all on the trauma team, and means:
'Be ready for anything – because it will happen'.

The trauma laparotomy is a team event:
The anaesthesiologist and scrub staff
must be fully involved and informed of all
decision-making.

The laparotomy in trauma needs to be performed in a systematic fashion. The ease with which injuries can be missed, and the potentially catastrophic consequences of a missed injury, mandate that extreme care is taken to exclude injuries, based on the injury complexes, and the way in which the laparotomy is approached. Careful examination of each organ is essential.

Anaesthesia Considerations

- The trauma laparotomy may be performed for a myriad of reasons. Central, however, in the decision-making, is the evolution of physiological derangement. Vascular uncontained bleeding may dictate immediate transportation to the OR. Hollow viscus injury may allow for extensive time-consuming investigations. Solid organ injuries, in general, can go either way.
- In the physiological unstable patient, the team should realize that the investigations very often can be performed after the trauma laparotomy. This allows time to contain the bleeding, restore some measure of physiology, and proceed to more sophisticated injury focused investigations and procedures. The physiology also influences choices such as choosing for non-operative management, a laparoscopic intervention, or interventional radiology.
- Anaesthesia for the trauma laparotomy consists of essential procedures and secondary procedures. Essential procedures include two large bore IV cannulae, a gastric tube to guide surgery, and a urine catheter, followed by arterial and central lines and other monitors. These can be placed during the procedure and should be anticipated in the positioning of the patient and drapes. A rapid infuser is of course mandatory, with availability of large-bore lines. The fluid management should be a balance between the safety margin needed to maintain safe circulation parameters (the more blood that is lost and the faster it is lost the more margin you will need) and overfilling, resulting in abdominal compartment syndrome.
- The anaesthetist should monitor physiology and coagulation profiles and report the results to the team. Deep muscle relaxation must be maintained (the patient is not going to be extubated soon).
- Monitor safety in the surgical operation area: how much blood has been lost, haemostasis has been achieved, the timing of the damage control procedure, does the surgeon stick to damage control, and when time allows, organize the next steps in the treatment sequence.
- The trauma laparotomy influences anaesthesia. Opening the abdomen can release a torrential bleeding from the previously compressed vessel. Proximal and distal control of the aorta or the IVC or strangulation of the mesenteric blood flow can have profound effects on the circulation. Liver packing on to the diaphragm and the Pringle manoeuvre may obstruct venous return. A tear in the diaphragm with displacement of intra-abdominal organs into the chest cavity may prevent normal ventilation.

REFERENCES AND FURTHER READING

References

1. Como JJ, Bokhari F, Chiu WC, Duane T, Holevar MR, Tandoh MA, et al. Practice management guidelines for selective nonoperative management of penetrating abdominal trauma. *J Trauma*. 2010 Mar;**68(3)**:721–33. doi: 10.1097/TA.0b013e3181cf7d07.
2. Luchette FA, Borzotta AP, Croce MA, et al. Practice management guidelines for prophylactic antibiotics in penetrating abdominal trauma. Available from www.east.org (accessed online December 2018).
3. Goldberg SR, Anand RJ, Como JJ, Dechert T, Dente C, Luchette FA, et al. Prophylactic antibiotic use in penetrating abdominal trauma: An Eastern Association for the Surgery of Trauma practice management guideline. *J Trauma and Acute Care Surg*. 2012 Nov;Supplement **73(5)**:S321–25. doi: 10.1097/TA.0b013e3182701902.
4. Hardcastle TC, M Stander, N Kalafatis, E Hodgson, D Gopalan. External patient temperature control in emergency centres, trauma centres, intensive care units and operating theatres: A multi-society literature review. *S Afr Med J*. 2013;**103**:609–611.
5. Cattell RB, Braasch RW. A technique for the exposure of the third and fourth parts of the duodenum. *Surg Gynaecol Obstet*. 1960;**111**:379–85.
6. Mattox KL, McCollum WB, Jordan GL Jr, Beall AC Jr, DeBakey ME. Management of upper abdominal vascular trauma. *Am J Surg*. 1974 Dec;**128(6)**:823–8.
7. Thal ER, O'Keefe T. Operative exposure of abdominal injuries and closure of the abdomen. In *ACS Surgery: Principles and Practice*. New York: Web MD, 2007: Section 7 Chapter 9.
8. Leaper DJ, Pollock AV, Evans M. Abdominal wound closure: a trial of nylon, polyglycolic acid and steel sutures. *Br J Surg*. 1977 Aug;**64(8)**:603–6.

Recommended Reading

Hirshberg A. Mattox KL *Top Knife: The Art and Craft of Trauma Surgery*. Tfm Publishing Ltd 2005; Harley, United Kingdom.

Ogura T1, Lefor AT, Nakano M, Izawa Y, Morita H. Nonoperative management of hemodynamically unstable abdominal trauma patients with angioembolization and resuscitative endovascular balloon occlusion of the aorta. *J Trauma Acute Care Surg*. 2015;**78(1)**:132–5. doi: 10.1097/TA.00 00000000000473.

9.2 Abdominal Vascular Injury

9.2.1 **Overview**

Abdominal vascular injury presents a serious threat to life, where preparedness and anticipation are vital to a successful outcome. Consideration of both the possible injuries and the surgical approach to manage them is crucial. Adequate preparation is essential; an adequate incision will be required.

> *It is helpful to have available all the apparatus for massive transfusion, with activation of the massive transfusion protocol, ensuring rapid mobilization of packed cells, plasma and platelets to the ED and OR.*

Major vessel injuries within the abdominal cavity primarily present as haemorrhagic shock that does not respond to resuscitation; thus, immediate surgery becomes a part of the resuscitative effort. In penetrating injury, this may necessitate an emergency department thoracotomy (EDT) and aortic cross-clamp. Consideration should also be given to resuscitative endovascular balloon occlusion of the aorta (REBOA) (see also Section 15.3) which has a role in controlling abdominal and pelvic haemorrhage in a similar but less invasive manner to that of EDT[1] (see also Section 8.9).

> *However, the emergency department thoracotomy is not indicated in the severely shocked patient with blunt abdominal trauma, as the survival rate is close to zero.*

With an expanding haematoma, source control with direct or proximal control of the vessel is mandatory for success, where the surgeon should anticipate gaining control above the level of the injury. The steps in decision-making can be iterated thus:

1. **Is the patient's condition so parlous that immediate aortic cross-clamping must be undertaken via a thoracotomy?**

   Typically, this is the patient who has lost cardiac output (loss of palpable central pulse) immediately prior to reception in the resuscitation bay or is about to do so (drop in GCS, drop in end tidal CO_2, bradycardia). The cross-clamping will cut off the arterial bleeding distally, and preserve blood flow to the brain and coronary vesssels.

2. **Does the patient's condition permit expedited transfer to the OR for definitive haemorrhage control?**

   This is the patient in whom ongoing volume resuscitation is needed to maintain a coherent circulatory output and the threat of decompensation is ever-present.

3. **Does the patient's condition permit CT scan as a prelude to definitive operative repair (or transfer to the interventional radiology (IR) suite for embolization of amenable injury patterns)?**

   This patient will have responded to initial resuscitation such that they can withstand a 10–15 minute period of transfer to CT, loading on to the scanner, image acquisition, and then appraisal of images.

Pitfall

Step 3 must not be exploited as a means of deferring surgical control by those who are unfamiliar with, and therefore anxious about executing, the surgical interventions described in this chapter.

9.2.2 Retroperitoneal Haematoma

Haematomas are:

- Central (zone I).
- Lateral (zone II).
- Pelvic (zone III).

9.2.2.1 CENTRAL HAEMATOMA

Central haematomas can be further classified according to whether the apex lies in the *supracolic* or *infracolic*

portion of the abdomen, as judged by whether the apex is positioned with respect to the mesentery of the transverse colon. Haematomas that lie largely inferior (caudal) to this landmark involve the aortic bifurcation or the inferior mesenteric artery (IMA)-bearing portion and are exposed by transperitoneal or left-medial visceral rotation that may not need splenic, renal, or pancreatic mobilization. Haematomas that lie above (cranial) are due to the more challenging injuries of the juxtarenal and suprarenal aorta or injury to the superior mesenteric artery (SMA) or coeliac artery-bearing portions.

- If the apex of the central haematoma is to the right side of the midline, and observed bleeding is primarily venous in nature, the right colon should be mobilized to the midline, including the duodenum and head of the pancreas (right medial visceral rotation). This will expose the infrarenal cava and infrarenal aorta. It will also facilitate access to the portal vein.

- If the apex of the central haematoma is on the left side of the midline, and observed bleeding is primarily arterial in nature, it is best to approach the injury from the left. Left medial visceral rotation provides access to the aorta, the coeliac axis, the superior mesenteric artery, the splenic artery and vein, and the left renal artery and vein. In order to reach the posterior wall of the aorta, the kidney should be mobilized as well and rotated medially on its pedicle, taking great care not to cause further injury.

9.2.2.2 LATERAL HAEMATOMA

If these are not expanding or pulsatile, blunt injuries are best left alone, as the damage is usually renal. Renal injuries can generally be managed non-operatively including the use of selective embolization. However, with penetrating injury, because of the risk of damage to adjacent structures such as the ureter, it is safer to explore lateral haematomas. The surgeon must also be confident that there is no perforation of the posterior part of the colon in the paracolic gutters on either side.

9.2.2.3 PELVIC HAEMATOMA

If the patient is stable, contrast-enhanced CT in the emergency situation may demonstrate a large pelvic haematoma with a vascular 'blush' indicating ongoing arterial bleeding. In this case, it may be more appropriate to transfer the patient for immediate embolization.

- *Pelvic haematomas discovered at laparotomy should be considered in terms of patient stability.*
  - *Non-expanding haematoma in the context of a physiologically stable or improving patient are best left alone.*
  - *Expanding haematoma with patient instability must be dealt with.*

9.2.2.3.1 Extraperitoneal Pelvic Packing

In the context of blunt trauma (fractured pelvis) the first concern should be to ensure that a pelvic binder is correctly positioned to reduce pelvic volume. The next is to perform extra-peritoneal pelvic packing (EPP).[2] Haemostats are applied to the incised peritoneal edge located either side of the lower 25% of the laparotomy full-length incision. The pre-peritoneal plane is then developed laterally such that the haematoma is entered, and clot evacuated manually. It is important that the plane posterior to the rectum is fully developed before tightly packing this space with 2–3 large swabs. The manoeuvre should be repeated for the opposite side. If the packs remain dry, then no further adjunctive manoeuvres are required. If strike-through occurs then repack again. If strike-through occurs despite this then the relevant internal iliac artery should be ligated. Even if EPP controls the bleeding, the patient should be transferred to the interventional radiology (IR) suite for angiography, interrogation of vascular integrity and selective embolization at the completion of the damage-control laparotomy. Once haemostasis is fully secured in this manner, and the patient's haemodynamic state is more stable, consideration can be given to loosening of the pelvic binder in order to prevent pressure sores. Stabilization of the pelvis using external fixators or a C-clamp in the operating room can be considered, but this does not always provide adequate posterior fixation and is secondary to effective pelvic packing and embolization.

9.2.3 Surgical Approach to Major Abdominal Vessels

9.2.3.1 INCISION

The patient must be prepared 'from sternal notch to knee'. It is critical to gain proximal and distal control, and patient preparation should include the need to extend to a left lateral thoracotomy to gain access to the thoracic aorta, a median sternotomy to control the intracardiac IVC, and groin incisions to gain control of the iliac vessels.

9.2.3.2 MEDIAL VISCERAL ROTATION (SEE ALSO SECTION 9.1.2.7)

9.2.3.2.1 Aorta

Control of the aorta can be achieved at several different levels depending on the site of injury. The supracoeliac aorta can be exposed by the following steps:

a. Retracting the left lobe of liver toward patients right shoulder.
b. Retracting the body of the stomach toward left hip.
c. Making a window in the lesser omentum.
d. Visualizing the peritoneum covering the left crus of the diaphragm.
e. Sharply incising the peritoneum to expose the muscle fibres of the crus.
f. Splitting the fibres such that the pearly white adventitia of the aorta is seen.
g. Developing the plane either side of the aorta to admit the jaws of a straight vascular clamp (Figure 9.2.1).

Pitfall

Clamping the oesophagus rather than the aorta. Identification of the oesophagus, which lies to the left of the aorta, is aided by the prior placement of a nasogastric tube.

Exposure of the suprarenal aorta is difficult from the anterior approach, especially in the context of a supracolic haematoma overlying the coeliac and SMA regions. Exposure can be obtained by performing a left medial visceral rotation procedure. The entire abdominal aorta and the origins of its branches are exposed by this technique. This includes the coeliac axis, the origin of the superior mesenteric artery, the iliac vessels and the left renal pedicle. The dense and fibrous superior mesenteric and coeliac nerve plexuses, however, overlie the proximal aorta and need to be sharply dissected in order to identify the renal and superior mesenteric arteries.

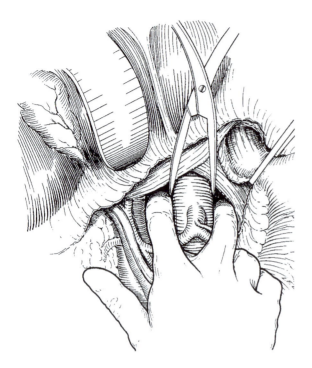

Figure 9.2.1 Control of the aorta by cross-clamping at the crura of the diaphragm.

Pitfall

Dissecting out the coeliac and superior mesenteric arteries is challenging owing to dense ganglionic tissues. It is strongly recommended that the supracoeliac aorta is controlled before entering the supracolic central haematoma. This can be done via two ways: either transperitoneal via the lesser omentum, or via the retroperitoneum. The latter route involves the fullest possible left medial visceral rotation (including kidney, spleen, and pancreas) with division of the left crus from the lateral aspect.

The distal aorta can be approached transperitoneally by retracting the small bowel to the right, the transverse colon superiorly, and the descending colon to the left. The aorta below the left renal vein can be accessed by incising the peritoneum over it and mobilizing the third and fourth parts part of the duodenum superiorly. Both iliac vessels can be exposed by distal continuation of the dissection. The ureters should be identified and carefully

preserved, especially in the region of the bifurcation of the iliac vessels.

Treatment of aortic or caval injuries is usually straightforward. Extensive lacerations are not compatible with survival, and it is uncommon to require graft material to repair the aorta. Caval injuries below the renal veins, if extensive, can be ligated, although lateral repair is preferred. Injuries above the renal veins in the cava should be repaired if at all possible (suture repair, patching, or inlay segmental grafting) as ligation at this level is usually not survivable.

9.2.3.3 COELIAC AXIS

The left colon is reflected to the right, together with the spleen and the tail of pancreas, to display the aorta and its branches. The coeliac trunk lies behind and inferior to the gastro-oesophageal junction. Injuries to this area are commonly missed, particularly in patients with stab wounds. Major vascular injury is particularly likely if there is a central retroperitoneal haematoma. In this situation, proximal vascular control prior to entering the haematoma is essential, either locally in the abdomen, or via a left lateral thoracotomy. Division of the left triangular ligament and mobilization of the lateral segment of the left lobe of the liver is also helpful.

It is difficult to 'repair' the coeliac axis as it is a short trunk-like vessel where access is by adherent ganglionic tissues and the branching origins of the left gastric, common hepatic and splenic vessels. Bleeding from this structure is more akin to haemorrhage from a direct injury to the front of the aorta and surgical control approximates to direct oversew of an identifiable haemorrhage point with 3-0 prolene with a secondary goal of maintenance of perfusion of its branches. End-organ ischaemia is not a likelihood assuming that the SMA and IMA remain intact.

The left gastric and splenic arteries can be ligated. The common hepatic artery can be safely tied provided that the injury is proximal to the gastroduodenal artery.

9.2.3.4 SUPERIOR MESENTERIC ARTERY[3]

The superior mesenteric artery is a vital artery for the viability of the small bowel, and should always be repaired, using conventional techniques. Proximally, the artery is accessible from the aorta at the level of the renal arteries

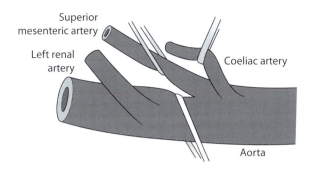

Figure 9.2.2 Anatomy of the superior mesenteric artery.

and is best approached with a left medial visceral rotation (Figure 9.2.2). More distally, the artery is accessed at the root of the small bowel mesentery.

If a period of ischaemia has elapsed, or the surgery is part of a damage control procedure, the artery should be shunted, using a plastic vascular shunt (e.g. Javid™ shunt – Bard Inc., Temple, AZ, USA), until repair can be effected.[4]

If repair is not possible, and replacement of the artery with a graft is required, it is best to place the graft on the infrarenal aorta, away from the pancreas and areas of potential leak.[5] Placement of the proximal end of the graft too high can result in kinking and subsequent occlusion of the graft when the bowel is returned to the abdominal cavity. The graft must be tailored so that there is no tension, and the aortic suture line must be covered to prevent an aortoenteric fistula.

The survival rate with penetrating injuries of the superior mesenteric artery is approximately 58%, falling to 22% if a complex repair is required.[5,6]

The superior mesenteric vein can be either shunted or simply ligated.[7]

9.2.3.5 INFERIOR MESENTERIC ARTERY

Injuries to the inferior mesenteric artery are uncommon, and the artery can generally be tied off. The viability of the colon should be checked before closure, with planned reoperation to evaluate viability of the colon.

9.2.3.6 RENAL ARTERIES

Preliminary vascular control is best obtained by accessing the renal arteries on the aorta using a standard infrarenal aortic approach. Access can also be obtained by mobilizing the viscera medially.

Repair is done using standard vascular techniques. However, the kidney tolerates warm ischaemia poorly, with 45 minutes of clamp time usually associated with permanent loss of function. Therefore, if there has been complete transection of the artery, and the kidney is of doubtful viability, preservation may not be in the best interest of the patient and an early nephrectomy considered.

9.2.3.7 ILIAC VESSELS

Proximal and distal control may be required, and distal control via a separate groin incision should be considered.

The iliac vessels are exposed by lifting the small bowel upwards, out of the pelvis. On the left, the sigmoid colon and its mesentery can be mobilized, and on the right, division of the peritoneal attachments over the caecum and mobilization of the caecum to the midline will aid exposure of the vessels.

The ureters must be formally identified as they cross the iliac bifurcation.

Pitfall

The common iliac veins are often strongly adherent to the back wall of the common iliac artery and attempts to 'sling' or encircle the arteries, or to mobilize the vein off the back of the artery, for purposes of control may result in torrential bleeding. A 'just enough' policy to dissection is advisable; with the operator gaining enough access to the front and sides of the common iliac artery/common iliac vein to allow room for a clamp above and below the injury zone; sometimes a side-biting clamp (e.g. a Satinsky clamp) is sufficient.

9.2.3.8 INFERIOR VENA CAVA[8]

9.2.3.8.1 Suprahepatic IVC (See also Section 9.4.8)

This is usually required for injuries affecting the retrohepatic IVC or hepatic veins. A frequently fatal injury complex heralded by profuse venous bleeding that emanates from the back of the liver not controlled by clamping of the portal triad and only controllable by direct downward pressure over the front of the liver such that the cava is firmly compressed.

Following exposure and clamping of the IVC above the renal vessels (see below) and whilst maintaining downward pressure on the liver, the coronary ligaments must be divided such that the liver can be displaced inferior-medially and the suprahepatic IVC seen. This manoeuvre is helped by splitting the central tendon of the diaphragm such that the portion of the IVC traversing the pericardium and diaphragm is revealed. The laparotomy incision can be extended across the costal margin in to the right chest as a further adjunct. Alternatively, access to the suprahepatic IVC can be obtained from within the chest by performing a median sternotomy and opening the pericardium. Alternatively, the surgeon must fully mobilize the liver by dividing the by incising the central tendon of the diaphragm, or by performing a median sternotomy and opening the pericardium.

9.2.3.8.2 Infrahepatic IVC

The infrahepatic vena cava can be exposed by means of a right medial visceral rotation procedure (Figure 9.2.3; see also Section 9.1.2.5).

The right colon is mobilized by taking down the hepatic flexure and incising the peritoneal reflection down the length of the right paracolic gutter. The colon is then reflected medially in a plane anterior to Gerota's fascia. If more exposure is required, the root of the mesentery can be mobilized by dividing the inferior mesenteric vein. Performance of a Kocher manoeuvre and medial mobilization of the duodenum and head of the pancreas will reveal the segment of vena cava immediately below the liver, and provide excellent exposure of the right renovascular pedicle.

Control is best achieved by direct pressure on the IVC above and below the injury, utilizing swabs (Figure 9.2.4).

If more definitive control is required, a combination of vascular clamps to the renal arteries and Rumel[9] tourniquets placed above the renal vessels (suprarenal), or above and below the injury, should be used (Figure 9.2.5).

Injuries to the posterior part of the IVC should always be expected with penetrating injury to the anterior part of the IVC. Not all bleeding posterior wounds need to be repaired.

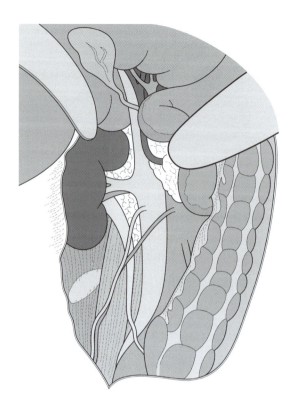

Figure 9.2.3 Right medial visceral rotation to expose the IVC.

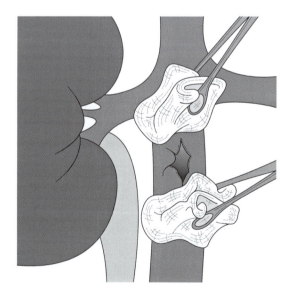

Figure 9.2.4 Control of the inferior vena cava using swab pressure.

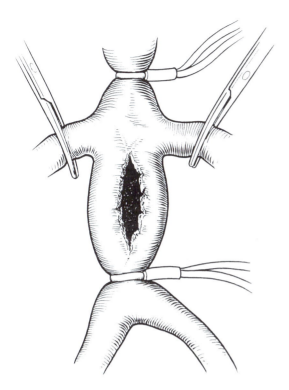

Figure 9.2.5 Control of the inferior vena cava with clamps and a two Rumel tourniquets.

It is very difficult to 'roll' the IVC to approach it posteriorly, owing to multiple lumbar veins, so all injuries should be approached transcavally. Not all non-bleeding posterior wounds require repair.

Provided it is infrarenal, ligation of the IVC is acceptable.

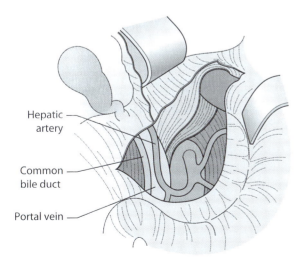

Hepatic artery

Common bile duct

Portal vein

Figure 9.2.6 Access to the portal vein.

9.2.3.9 PORTAL VEIN[10]

The portal vein lies in the free edge of lesser omentum, together with the common bile duct and the hepatic artery (Figure 9.2.6).

The portal vein, generally, can be controlled with a Pringle's manoeuvre. If the injury is more proximal, it may be necessary to reflect the duodenum medially, or divide the pancreas.

The portal vein should be shunted early to avoid venous hypertension of the bowel, which will make access to the area increasingly difficult. The stent can be left in place as part of a damage control procedure or repaired. Portocaval shunting is a possibility, and ligation as a last resort, which, however, carries a high mortality.

9.2.4 Shunting

If repair is not possible, or the procedure is being abbreviated, vascular shunting will restore circulation. It can be performed atraumatically, and rapidly (see also Section 6.1).

If a Javid™ or other proprietary shunts are available, these can be used. However, if they are not, a shunt can

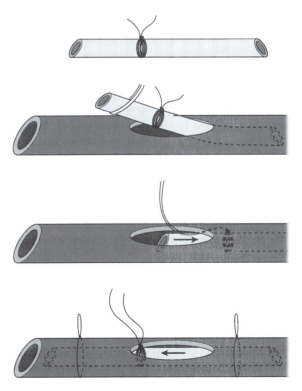

Figure 9.2.7 Diagrammatic representation of 'manufacture' and placement of a vascular shunt.

be fashioned from a suitable size of plastic tube, for example, a nasogastric tube, endotracheal tube, chest tube, etc.:

- The length required is three times the length of the defect.
- The diameter should be two-thirds of the diameter of the vessel to be shunted.

The shunt is fashioned as follows (Figure 9.2.7):

- Choose a plastic tube with the correct diameter.
- Cut the tube to length, as described above, bevelling the edges so that they can be passed into the vessel.
- Tie a length of silk around the tube, dividing it into a one third to two-thirds ratio.

Once the vessel has been controlled, using either clamps or Rumel tourniquets:

- Clamp one end of the shunt to prevent leakage.
- Pass the 'long' (two-thirds) end of the shunt up the vessel until the shunt is lying inside the vessel lumen or proximally, releasing the tourniquet to allow it to pass through.
- Using the silk as a 'handle', pull the shunt distally into the other end of the vessel.
- Secure it with ties.

There is no need for anticoagulation as the patients are often coagulopathic, and the rate of flow itself should prevent clot formation. The shunt can be left in place for 48–72 hours.

REFERENCES AND RECOMMENDED READING

References

1. Brenner ML, Moore LJ, DuBose JJ, Tyson GH, McNutt MK, Albarado RP, Holcomb JB, Scalea TM, Rasmussen TE. A clinical series of resuscitative endovascular balloon occlusion of the aorta for hemorrhage control and resuscitation. *J Trauma Acute Care Surg.* 2013 Sep;**75(3)**:506–11. doi: 10.1097/TA.0b013e31829e5416.2.

2. Smith WR, Moore EE, Osborn P, Agudelo JF, Morgan SJ, Parekh AA, et al. Retroperitoneal packing as a resuscitation technique for haemodynamically unstable patients with pelvic fractures: report of two representative cases and a description of technique. *J Trauma.* 2005 Dec;**59(6)**:1510–14.

3. Asensio JA, Berne JD, Chahwan S, Hanpeter D, Demetriades D, Marengo J, et al. Traumatic injury to the superior mesenteric artery. *Am J Surg.* 1999 Sep;**178(3)**:235–9.

4. Reilly PM, Rotondo MF, Carpenter JP, Sherr SA, Schwab CW. Temporary vascular continuity during damage control: intraluminal shunting for proximal superior mesenteric artery injury. *J Trauma.* 1995 Oct;**39(4)**:757–60.

5. Accola KD, Feliciano DV, Mattox KL, Burch JM, Beall AC Jr, Jordan GL Jr. Management of injuries to the superior mesenteric artery. *J Trauma.* 1986 Apr;**26(4)**:313–19.

6. Asensio JA, Britt LD, Borzotta A, Peitzman A, Miller FB, Mackersie RC, et al. Multi-institutional experience with the management of superior mesenteric artery injuries. *J Am Coll Surg.* 2001 Dec;**193(6)**:354–65; discussion 365–6.

7. Donahue TK, Strauch GO. Ligation as definitive management of injury to the superior mesenteric vein. *J Trauma.* 1988 Apr;**28(4)**:541–3.

8. Feliciano DV, Burch JM, Mattox K, Edelman M. Injuries of the inferior vena cava. *Am J Surg.* 1988 Dec;**156(6)**:548–52.

9. Welling DR, Rich NM, Burris DG, Boffard KD, Devries WC. Who was William Ray Rumel? *World J Surg.* 2008 Sep;**32(9)**:2122–5. doi: 10.1007/s00268-008-9599-4.

10. Stone HH, Fabian TC, Turkleson ML. Wounds of the portal venous system. *World J Surg.* 1982;**6**:335–41.

Selected Reading

At the time of publication the UK REBOA trial – randomising patients to Zone 1/Zone3 REBOA in addition to standard care versus standard care alone – is ongoing. (https://w3.abdn.ac.uk/hsru/REBOA/Public/Public/index.cshtml)

9.3 Bowel, Rectum, and Diaphragm

9.3.1 **Overview**

The surgeon must always bear in mind the three-dimensional nature of wound tracks in penetrating injury. An odd number of bowel enterotomies should prompt a second look for missed injury.

In all patients who are subjected to laparotomy after injury, the entire length of bowel, from the oesophagogastric junction, stomach, small bowel from the ligament of Treitz to the ileo-caecal valve, and large bowel from the caecum to the rectum, and their mesenteries should be inspected (see also Section 9.1).

Pitfall

- Failure to inspect the diaphragm, particularly in the presence of penetrating injury, especially if below the 5th intercostal space.
- Both the surgeon and the assistant independently inspect the same segment of bowel at the same time. Ideally, only one operator handles the bowel at any time, as otherwise each operator thinks that the other is doing the inspection.

Two hands, but four eyes.

The commonest sites of missed organ injury in the abdomen are:

- Diaphragm.
- Oesophagogastric junction.
- Along the lesser or greater curvature of the stomach (a penetrating injury can be obscured by the fatty envelope of the vessels in these locations).
- The posterior aspect of stomach and adjacent pancreas (in the lesser sac; a missed injury here led to the death of President McKinley in 1902[1]).
- Small bowel (a small penetrating injury to small bowel can be easy to miss).
- Retroperitoneal colon and rectum.

9.3.2 **Diaphragm**

The diaphragm divides the torso into thoracic and abdominal components. Particularly with penetrating injury, the penetration may go through the diaphragm, and give misleading signs. For example, a stab wound of the lower chest with a haemothorax may reflect an intra-abdominal injury to the liver, spleen, or kidney, with blood draining through the diaphragm into the chest. All diaphragmatic injuries benefit from early diagnosis and repair. The presence of a defect poses significant risk of herniation of abdominal contents (most commonly stomach or colon) into the chest, because the thoracic cavity is at negative pressure compared to the abdominal cavity. Herniation may occur during the acute trauma phase or may be delayed by months to years and may be acutely life-threatening due to strangulation and/or tension gastrothorax or colothorax.

Diagnosis of a diaphragmatic defect is not possible with imaging, *unless herniation has occurred*. In the case of herniation, chest x-ray may demonstrate the appearance of a raised hemidiaphragm or the presence of a hollow viscus in the chest. Passage of a nasogastric tube prior to performing a chest x-ray will show the presence of a herniated stomach in the left thoracic cavity. CT is helpful to demonstrate hollow, as well as solid viscera in the chest. In the event of blunt trauma with acute herniation through the left hemidiaphragm, it is important to rule out an oesophageal blow-out injury (i.e. look for gas in the posterior mediastinum in the vicinity of the thoracic oesophagus). Although rare, missing this injury is potentially life-threatening.

When herniation has not occurred through a diaphragmatic injury, the only way to diagnose it is by *direct inspection*. Penetrating trauma to the *left* thoracoabdominal region (the ribcage below the fifth intercostal space) may be associated with as high as 40% likelihood of a diaphragmatic defect.[1] If such a patient is stable and has no indication for laparotomy, laparoscopy or video-assisted thoracoscopy (VATS) is helpful for inspection of the diaphragm. VATS is useful in patients who may benefit from the simultaneous management of a pleural collection, otherwise many surgeons prefer laparoscopy. However, if an indication for laparotomy exists, it remains preferable to laparoscopy (see also Chapter 15). Laparoscopic or thoracoscopic repair of the diaphragm is indicated if a defect is found, regardless of the size of the defect.

The EAST PICO Guidelines may be helpful (Tables 9.3.1 and 9.3.2).[2]

Table 9.3.1 PICO Format for Recommendations

P	Patient, Population, or Problem	How would I describe the patient group?
I	Intervention, Prognostic Factor, or Exposure	Which main intervention, prognostic factor, or exposure is considered?
C	Comparison or Intervention (if appropriate)	What is the main alternative to compare with the intervention?
O	Outcome you would like to measure or achieve	What can be accomplished, measured, improved, or affected?

Table 9.3.2 PICO Recommendation for Diaphragmatic Injury

	Question	Guidelines
1	In left-sided thoraco-abdominal stab wound patients who are haemodynamically stable and without peritonitis (P), should laparoscopy (I) or computed tomography (C) be performed to decrease the incidence missed diaphragmatic injury (O)?	In left thoraco-abdominal stab wound patients who are haemodynamically stable and without peritonitis (P), we conditionally recommend laparoscopy (I) rather that computed tomography (C) to decrease the incidence missed diaphragmatic injury (O).
2	In penetrating thoraco-abdominal trauma patients who are haemodynamically stable without peritonitis and in whom a right diaphragm injury is confirmed or suspected (P), should operative (I) or non-operative (C) management be undertaken to minimize both the need for delayed operation for diaphragmatic hernia and risk of surgical morbidity (procedural complications, LOS, surgical site infection, and empyema) (O)?	In haemodynamically stable trauma patients with acute diaphragm injuries, we conditionally recommend (P) the abdominal (I) rather than the thoracic (C) approach to repair the diaphragm to decrease mortality, delayed herniation, missed thoraco-abdominal organ injury, and surgical approach-associated morbidity (procedural complications, LOS, surgical site infection, and empyema) (O).
3	In haemodynamically stable trauma patients with acute diaphragm injuries (P) should the abdominal (I) or thoracic (C) approach be used to repair the diaphragm to decrease mortality, delayed herniation, missed thoraco-abdominal organ injury, and surgical approach-associated morbidity (procedural complications, LOS, surgical site infection, and empyema) (O)?	In haemodynamically stable trauma patients with acute diaphragm injuries, we conditionally recommend (P) the abdominal (I) rather than the thoracic (C) approach to repair the diaphragm to decrease mortality, delayed herniation, missed thoraco-abdominal organ injury, and surgical approach-associated morbidity (procedural complications, LOS, surgical site infection, and empyema) (O).
4	PICO 4: In patients who present with delayed visceral herniation through a traumatic diaphragmatic injury (P), should the abdominal (I) or thoracic (C) approach be used to decrease mortality and surgical approach-related morbidity (procedural complications, surgical site infection, LOS, empyema) (O)?	In patients who present with delayed visceral herniation through a traumatic diaphragmatic injury (P), we make no recommendation in regard to the routine surgical approach, abdominal (I) or thoracic (O) to decrease mortality and surgical approach-related morbidity (procedural complications, surgical site infection, LOS, empyema) (O).
5	PICO 5: In patients with acute penetrating diaphragmatic injuries without concern for other intra-abdominal injuries (P), should laparoscopic (I) or open (C) repair be performed to decrease mortality, delayed herniation, missed thoraco-abdominal organ injury, and surgical approach-associated morbidity (procedural complications, LOS, surgical site infection, and empyema) (O)?	In patients with acute penetrating diaphragmatic injuries without concern for other intra-abdominal injuries (P), we conditionally recommend laparoscopic (I) over open (C) repair in weighing the risks of mortality, delayed herniation, missed thoraco-abdominal organ, and surgical approach-associated morbidity (procedural complications, LOS, surgical site infection, and empyema) (O).

Note: As it is generally accepted that penetrating injuries to the left diaphragm require repair, no PICO question was formulated to study this topic.

Note that penetrating injury to the *right* thoraco-abdominal region does not routinely require the above-mentioned approach, since the liver tends to act as a barrier and herniation on this side is uncommon.

Herniation through the diaphragm mandates exploratory laparotomy in most cases, to exclude subdiaphragmatic visceral injuries.

Repair of the diaphragm at laparotomy is relatively straightforward. It is crucial to hold the laceration at its apices with two Littlewoods or Allis tissue forceps and to *pull the diaphragm out toward oneself*. This greatly facilitates repair, as opposed to struggling in the depths of the abdomen. The laceration can be sutured in a continuous fashion using a non-absorbable suture. There is *no* evidence that a braided suture or interrupted sutures make much difference; however, interrupted sutures may be helpful when dealing with a jagged laceration or a blown-out laceration which stretches in two or three directions. The use of synthetic material to close large defects from high velocity missile or shotgun injuries is only rarely indicated. If the defect is so large that the edges cannot be opposed, it can be closed with a patch, such as polytetrafluoroethylene (PTFE). Ideally this is done using a trans-thoracic approach.

If the laceration is close to the pericardium, extra care must be taken not to inadvertently include the pericardium in the suture.

If there is major contamination of the abdominal cavity, then the thoracic cavity must be thoroughly washed out as well, using copious amounts of normal saline, and a chest drain placed. It may be necessary to enlarge the diaphragmatic defect in order to facilitate adequate chest washout. The laceration can be enlarged radially towards the chest wall (cutting the diaphragm transversely may divide branches of the phrenic nerve), or if the injury is peripheral, the defect may be enlarged transversely along the chest wall. The diaphragmatic defect should be closed prior to washing out the abdominal cavity to avoid further contamination.

The complications of injuries to the diaphragm are primarily related to late diagnosis with hernia formation and incarceration. Phrenic nerve palsy is another complication, but this is uncommon after penetrating trauma.

9.3.3 **Stomach**

The stomach is lifted and pulled caudally, using two Babcock forceps, and the anterior surface inspected. It is helpful if there is a nasogastric tube in place; place the forceps around the tube, forming a useful gastric retractor. The lesser sac should be entered through the greater omentum, and the stomach can then be lifted to allow inspection of its posterior surface (as well as the body and tail of the pancreas).

The stomach is highly vascular, and in all injuries, life-threatening bleeding can result. All holes should be repaired using a continuous, full-thickness 2/0 or 3/0 non-absorbable suture. Simple gastric injuries can be minimally debrided and closed; more complex gastric injuries should be controlled by non-anatomic resection, with reconstruction deferred to the re-look laparotomy.

Pitfall

In all penetrating injuries in which a hole is found on the anterior surface of the stomach, it is important to seek the corresponding hole on the posterior wall of the stomach. If this cannot be found, enlarge the anterior hole and inspect the stomach from within: 'penetrating holes generally go in pairs – one in, one out'. Carefully inspect the lesser and greater curvatures where a small defect may be obscured by the fatty envelopes of the gastric vasculature.

9.3.4 **The Duodenum**

The duodenum must be carefully inspected from the pylorus to the ligament of Treitz. If there is a haematoma on the duodenum, it is mandatory to perform a Kocher manoeuvre, and inspect the posterior surface of the duodenum. A Duval forceps is useful in providing the gentle retraction needed when working with the duodenum (see also Section 9.6).

9.3.5 **Small Bowel**

The fundamental decision to be made on every patient is: damage control or definitive surgery.

The decision will depend on the context; that is, the injury pattern, the physiological status of the patient, and the nature and volume of other patients waiting. If a decision is made to 'damage control' the patient, then management of visceral injury is usually simple. The stomach will require haemostatic sutured closure; the rest of the bowel will usually be dealt with by resecting damaged gut and leaving it stapled or tied off in discontinuity ('clip-and-drop'). Definitive intestinal surgery can be undertaken at re-look surgery, when the patient should be in a better physiological state.

Starting at the ligament of Treitz, each segment of small bowel is inspected and then flipped over to examine the opposite side. The mesentery is carefully inspected as well. If the bowel is accidentally dropped, start again at the ligament of Treitz.

9.3.5.1 THE STABLE PATIENT

Small bowel injuries should be closed, with primary repair or resection and primary anastomosis as appropriate. Consider one resection and anastomosis when several wounds are localized close to each other. Be mindful, however, that bowel should be preserved wherever possible.

Where multiple small wounds are present (e.g. following a shotgun injury), a skin stapler (35W) can be used to close individual holes safely.

9.3.5.2 THE UNSTABLE PATIENT

If the patient is haemodynamically unstable, damage control is likely, and bowel injuries should be treated using damage control procedures. The priority is to treat the haemorrhage, and then to control contamination.

Small wounds can be closed rapidly, using a 35W skin stapler or with mass closure. In patients with more extensive injuries requiring damage control, simple proximal and distal closure of the injured bowel using a GastroIntestinal Anastomosis (GIA)-type stapler or umbilical tape (with rapid resection of the injured segment) is the best way to prevent ongoing soiling.

Neither any anastomosis nor any stoma should be performed at this stage, as these can be time-consuming, the tissue viability is uncertain, and the leak rate is much higher, especially in the presence of concomitant contamination. At the time of re-look laparotomy, the feasibility of anastomosis versus the need for ileostomy or colostomy is assessed.

Pitfall

In wounds caused by small penetrating missiles, for example with a shotgun, it is easy to miss multiple holes, which

are often less than 2 mm in diameter. It is recommended that in these cases, the bowel be passed through a bowl of water, so that any air leak will show itself as bubbles. All such injuries should be re-inspected at 36–48 hours, and the procedure repeated.

9.3.6 **Large Bowel**[3,4]

World War II experience of poor outcomes following complications of repair or anastomosis after colonic injury led to a policy of mandatory colostomy for colon injury that continued into civilian practice in the post-war years. In 1979, a randomized trial found that primary repair was associated with fewer complications than diversion; however, throughout the trial, approximately half of the total patients with colonic injury were excluded from randomization and had a mandatory colostomy due to the presence of factors assumed to increase risk of complications (shock, extensive faecal contamination, prolonged delay from injury to operation, destructive colonic injury, or multiple associated injuries). Subsequent trials and a meta-analysis confirmed mortality was not significantly different between diversion and repair; however, morbidity was significantly less with primary repair. A further important consideration when considering optimal primary surgery is the morbidity inherent in colostomy reversal; complications following closure after colon injury have been reported to occur in up to half of patients.

In a civilian major trauma centre, primary repair appears safe even when the colonic injury is severe; however, a multicentre prospective study on destructive colon wounds confirmed that abdominal complications are more likely if the patient was critically injured and the transfusion requirement was ≥4 units of blood or there was severe faecal contamination associated with the bowel injury. Importantly, the actual surgical method of colon wound management (colostomy or repair/anastomosis) made no difference.

Pragmatic recommendations for the management of patients with colonic injury were produced in the early years of this century; patients with non-destructive injuries should undergo minimal debridement of the colonic injury and primary repair, patients with destructive wounds of the colon but without co-existent serious injury, comorbidities or large transfusion requirement should undergo resection and anastomosis, while patients with destructive wounds, co-existing critical injury, significant medical illness, or transfusion requirements of

>6 units should undergo faecal diversion. Utilizing these guidelines led to colostomy being undertaken for <10% of all colon wounds with acceptable morbidity.

9.3.6.1 THE STABLE PATIENT

For colonic injuries, indications for colostomy are still debated. Time from injury, haemodynamic status, co-morbid conditions and degree of contamination will influence the decision. More primary repairs/primary anastomoses are being performed, with fewer colostomies. Simple colonic injuries can be treated in much the same way as a simple small bowel injury, with local debridement and primary repair. When there are multiple small and large bowel lacerations, a protective ileostomy can be helpful.

9.3.6.2 THE UNSTABLE PATIENT

In the unstable patient undergoing a damage control procedure, small wounds can simply be sutured using a 2/0 or 3/0 nonabsorbable suture. The wounds can be re-inspected at the re-look procedure.

Larger wounds should be excluded in the same manner as small bowel. All macroscopic contamination should be washed out using copious amounts of warmed saline before (temporary) closure. This washout may serve the added purpose of core rewarming if necessary.

Destructive colonic injuries should be treated with resection and stapling or tying off in discontinuity. The decision to restore continuity by anastomosis or divert is made at re-look laparotomy. In a recent series, up to 75% of patients with colon injury undergoing damage control laparotomy (DCL) had anastomosis at subsequent laparotomy with acceptable rates of complications. If a damage control patient remains critically unwell at time of first re-look (typically at 48 hours) with inotropes still required, if they have a large burden of injury, or if they have had a massive transfusion, it is advisable to avoid a colonic anastomosis and opt for colostomy at the final procedure when definitive closure was intended. if a stoma is considered the most appropriate management for the patient, surgeons should be aware that early colostomy closure can be achieved safely.

Pitfalls

- No stomas should be performed in the unstable patient as this prolongs the surgical time and may make things more complex in the presence of competing injury.
- Stomas should be performed only at the last damage control procedure.
- Stomas should be placed more laterally (away from the skin edge), and at the level of the umbilicus.

9.3.7 **Rectum**[5]

Surgeons consider the rectum in distinct parts: the intra-peritoneal upper third and the extraperitoneal lower two thirds. Diagnosis of rectal injury can be difficult and, as low rectal injuries are, by definition, not within the peritoneal cavity, they can easily be missed. Any penetrating injury at the level of the lower abdomen, hips, or thighs (such as penetrating injury to the buttocks) may be associated with a rectal injury. Major pelvic fracture can also cause injury to the rectal muscle tube.

Suspicion of rectal injury mandates specific investigation; luminal examination with a flexible sigmoidoscope is much more likely to identify a rectal injury than rigid sigmoidoscopy, which can have a high false negative rate. Pre-operative CT (in a stable patient) may be helpful in delineating a bullet track and/or suggesting the likelihood of rectal injury in the form of perirectal gas and/or extravasation of rectal contrast. In this setting, CT has the added benefit of demonstrating injuries to other pelvic structures such as the ureters, bladder, blood vessels, and internal female structures – invaluable for pre-operative planning.

An intraperitoneal rectal injury should be debrided and repaired and should best be covered by proximal diversion (loop sigmoid colostomy).

An extraperitoneal rectal injury is usually inaccessible and is treated by proximal diversion only.

Pitfall

Do not use routine presacral drainage or distal rectal washout. This will increase the risk of contamination, or secondary infection (Table 9.3.3).

9.3.8 **Mesentery**

Arterial bleeders should be tied off. Do not extend mesenteric lacerations, and if necessary oversew bleeding wounds. Watch for bowel ischaemia once the mesentery has been dealt with in this manner.

Table 9.3.3 Management of Penetrating Extraperitoneal Rectal Injuries: An Eastern Association for the Surgery of Trauma Practice Management Guidelines

	Question	Guidelines
1	In patients with non-destructive penetrating extraperitoneal rectal injuries (P), should proximal diversion (I) be performed versus no proximal diversion with primary repair (if feasible) (C) to decrease the incidence of complications (O)?	Despite the overall quality of evidence being very low, the panel considered that most patients would place a high value on avoidance of mortality and infectious complications. All of these factors resulted in the formulation of a conditional recommendation by the committee. The committee concludes that the desirable effects of adherence to a recommendation probably outweigh the undesirable effects. Thus, in patients with non-destructive penetrating extraperitoneal rectal injuries, we conditionally recommend proximal diversion (versus non-diversion).
2	In patients with non-destructive penetrating extraperitoneal rectal injuries (P), should presacral drainage (I) versus no presacral drainage (C) be performed to decrease the incidence of complications (O)?	In patients with non-destructive extraperitoneal rectal injuries, we conditionally recommend against the routine use of presacral drains.
3	In patients with non-destructive penetrating extraperitoneal rectal injuries (P), should distal rectal washout be performed (I) versus no distal rectal washout (C) to decrease the incidence of complications (O)?	In patients with non-destructive extraperitoneal rectal injuries, we conditionally recommend against the routine use of presacral drains.

9.3.9 Adjuncts

9.3.9.1 ANTIBIOTICS

Practice management guidelines for prophylactic antibiotic use in penetrating abdominal trauma are given in Chapter 9.2.

REFERENCES AND SELECTED READINGS

References

1. Mjoli M, Oosthuizen G, Clarke D, Madiba T. Laparoscopy in the diagnosis and repair of diaphragmatic injuries in left-sided penetrating thoracoabdominal trauma: laparoscopy in trauma. *Surg Endosc.* 2015; **29(3)**:747–52. doi: 10.1007/s00464-014-3710-8.

2. McDonald, AA, Robinson Bryce RH, Alarcon L, Bosarge PL, Dorion, H. Valuation and management of traumatic diaphragmatic injuries: A Practice Management Guideline from the Eastern Association for the Surgery of Trauma. *J Trauma Acute Care Surg.* 2018 Jul;**85(1)**:198–207. doi: 10.1097/TA.0000000000001924.

3. Sharpe JP, Magnotti LJ, Fabian TC. Evolution of the operative management of colon trauma. *Trauma Surg & Acute Care Open.* 2017;**2**:e000092. doi: 10.1136/tsaco-2017-000092.

4. Berne JD, Velmahos GC, Chan LS, Asensio JA, Demetriades D. The high morbidity of colostomy closure after trauma: further support for the primary repair of colon injuries. *Surgery.* 1998 Feb;**123(2)**:157–64.

5. Bosarge PL, Como JJ, Fox N, Falck-Ytter Y, Haut ER, Dorion HA, et al. Management of penetrating extraperitoneal rectal injuries: An Eastern Association for the Surgery of Trauma practice management guideline. *J Trauma Acute Care Surg.* 2016 Mar;**80(3)**:546–51. doi:10.1097/TA.0000000000000953.

Selected Readings

Weinberg JA, Croce MA. Penetrating Injuries to the Stomach, Duodenum, and Small Bowel. *Curr Trauma Rep.* 2015; **1(2)**:107–112. https://doi.org/10.1007/s40719-015-0010-2.

Trust MD, Brown CVR. Penetrating Injuries to the Colon and Rectum. *Curr Trauma Rep.* 2015; **1(2)**:113–118. https://doi.org/10.1007/s40719-015-0013-z.

9.4 The Liver and Biliary System

9.4.1 Overview

Most liver injuries are diagnosed on the trauma CT, are relatively asymptomatic, low grade, and do not require surgical intervention. Operative management of high-grade hepatic lesions is technically very challenging and can be a devastating experience. Exquisite decision-making, thorough understanding of hepatic anatomy including the arterial supply, portal venous supply, and the hepatic venous drainage, and advanced operative techniques are essential. The evolution in management of hepatic injury has evolved since packing was first described over 100 years ago, through aggressive surgery, to refinement of techniques, and the increasing role of non-operative management of most injuries.[1]

Richardson and co-workers managed approximately 1200 blunt hepatic injuries over a 25-year period. Non-operative management was used in up to 80% of cases. Deaths secondary to injury dropped from 8% to 2%.[2] They proposed four reasons for the decrease in mortality from liver injury:

- Improved results with packing and re-operation (damage control).
- Use of angiography and embolization.
- Advances in operative techniques for major hepatic injury.
- Decrease in the number of patients undergoing exploration for hepatic venous injury (surgeons were not exacerbating the injury).[1]

The key to success is the appreciation of the patient's physiology as this is the fundamental deciding factor between operative and non-operative approaches, rather than anatomical injury grading.

The liver is comprised of a right and a left half, defined by Cantlie's line separating the two. Cantlie's line runs from the gallbladder fossa to the IVC. The liver is divided into eight Couinaud's segments. Segment 1 is the caudate lobe, segments II–IV make up the left hemi-liver, and the right hemi-liver includes segments V–VIII (Figure 9.4.1).

The structures within the porta hepatis include the hepatic artery, portal vein, and bile duct. The portal triad is encased in an extension of Glisson's capsule, and thus relatively resistant to injury. The portal triad runs *within* the segments of the liver. The major hepatic veins (right, left and middle) have no valves, are not protected by an extension of Glisson's capsule and run *between* the segments of the liver. Difficult to control, life-threatening haemorrhage in the operating room is generally related

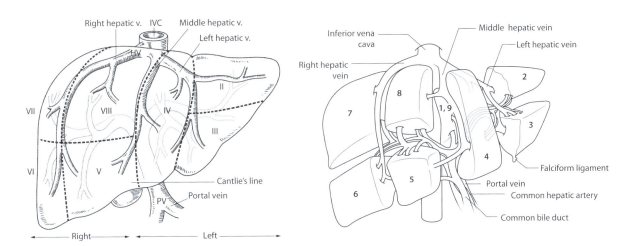

Figure 9.4.1 Hepatic anatomy. Segments of the liver are numbered.

to hepatic vein or retrohepatic IVC injury. The liver generally encases a portion of the retrohepatic cava, at times circumferentially. Full mobilization of the liver to expose the retrohepatic IVC requires division of this attachment. The major hepatic veins are 8–12 cm in length, the majority of which is intrahepatic. Injury to the major hepatic veins is generally to this portion of the veins and can be controlled by compression or suture ligation. The extrahepatic segments of the major hepatic veins are <2 cm in length and are less commonly injured. Injury to the extrahepatic portion of the major hepatic veins generally presents as exsanguinating haemorrhage and carries a high mortality.[2] In addition, 3 to 11 short hepatic veins run directly from the liver to the IVC, can also be a source of haemorrhage, and must be identified and controlled if liver resection is necessary. The short hepatic veins can be large, especially if the right hepatic vein is found to be diminutive Finally, the liver parenchyma will tolerate ligation or embolization of hepatic artery branches, but the bile ducts will not. The bile ducts depend on the hepatic artery for their blood supply (Figure 9.4.2).[3]

Knowledge of this hepatic anatomy is important, as it explains some of the patterns of injury that follow blunt trauma. In addition, there are differences in tissue elasticity that also determine injury patterns. Segmental anatomical resection has been well documented but is usually not applicable to trauma.

The forces from blunt injury are usually direct compressive forces or shear forces. The elastic tissue within arterial blood vessels makes them less susceptible to tearing than other structures within the liver. Venous and biliary ductal tissue are moderately resistant to shear forces, whereas the liver parenchyma is not. Thus, fractures within the liver parenchyma tend to occur along segmental fissures (remember this is where the major hepatic veins course) or directly in the parenchyma. This causes shearing of branches emanating from the major hepatic and portal veins. With severe deceleration injury and traction injury, the origin of the short retro-hepatic veins may be ripped from the cava causing devastating haemorrhage (these veins may be as large as 1 cm in diameter). Similarly, the small branches from the caudate lobe entering directly into the cava are at high risk for shearing with linear tears on the caval surface. Direct compressive forces usually cause tearing between segmental fissures in an anterior-posterior vector. Horizontal fracture lines into the parenchyma give the characteristic burst pattern to such liver injuries. If the fracture lines are parallel, these have been dubbed 'bear claw' type injuries and probably represent where the ribs have been compressed directly into the parenchyma. This can cause massive haemorrhage if there is direct extension or continuity with the peritoneal cavity.

Appropriate decision-making is critical to a good outcome:

- The patient's physiology drives decision-making – unstable physiology requires surgery whereas stable physiology does not regardless of grade of liver injury.
- Patients actively bleeding from major liver injury must be taken to the operating room promptly, with rapid haemorrhage control. Any delay in doing so increases risk of coagulopathy and mortality.
- If operation is indicated, the simplest, quickest technique that can restore haemostasis is the most appropriate.

**Be a minimalist – if you have controlled the liver bleeding in an unstable patient:
STOP – PACK – LEAVE THE OR**

- Do NOT abort the operation and leave the OR if surgical bleeding is not controlled. Damage control and truncating the operation is indicated for medical bleeding (coagulopathy).
- If simple manoeuvres fail to control haemorrhage, the decision to proceed with hepatorrhaphy or resectional debridement must be made quickly, and surgeons must equip themselves with the appropriate skills to undertake this.

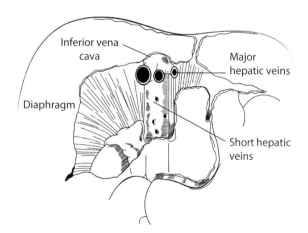

Figure 9.4.2 Retrohepatic anatomy of the liver. The major hepatic veins and short hepatic veins are shown.

9.4.2 **Resuscitation**

The haemodynamically *stable* patient without signs of peritonitis or other indication for operation is generally managed non-operatively (>80% of blunt liver injuries). The haemodynamically *unstable* patient with liver injuries requires immediate surgical exploration to achieve haemostasis and exclude other sources of bleeding. The patient in whom a surgical approach is decided upon or is mandated by haemodynamic instability should be transferred to the operating room as rapidly as possible after the following are completed.

Consider early damage control and packing before the coagulopathy is established.
Once the patient is cold, coagulopathic, and in irreversible shock, the battle usually is lost.
Call for senior help early in the operation.

Pitfall

REBOA should be considered with huge caution in severe liver injury as Zone I REBOA may simply increase the risk of hepatic venous bleeding whilst delaying transfer to the operating room.

9.4.3 **Diagnosis**

Control of bleeding takes priority over any diagnostic procedure (including CT).

Any delay to control of bleeding will increase mortality. Surgery should not be delayed by multiple emergency department procedures such as limb x-rays, unnecessary ultrasonography, and vascular access procedures. CT of the brain should be delayed until the patient is stable. Hypotension significantly increases mortality for traumatic brain injury. The anaesthesiologist can continue resuscitation in the operating room.

In the patient with blunt injury, there may be an absence of clear clinical signs such as rigidity, distension, or unstable vital signs may be absent. Up to 40% of patients with significant haemoperitoneum have no obvious signs. FAST may be particularly useful in the setting of blunt injury and haemodynamic instability, since the presence of free fluid in the abdominal cavity will direct you quickly to the operating room in a hypotensive patient. With a haemodynamically *stable* patient,

CT is an invaluable diagnostic aid and allows the surgeon to make decisions on the need for embolization or operative management. Diagnostic peritoneal lavage is rarely required these days owing to availability of FAST, but if available in the blunt trauma setting may be useful, particularly when CT support services are inadequate or unavailable.

The purpose of diagnostic investigation in the stable patient is to help identify those patients who can be safely managed non-operatively, to assist decision-making in non-operative management, and to act as a baseline for comparison in future imaging studies. Accurate, good quality contrast enhanced CT has enhanced our ability to make an accurate diagnosis of liver injuries.

Penetrating wounds of the liver usually do not present a diagnostic problem, as most surgeons would advocate laparotomy. CT scan using contrast for penetrating liver injury can be useful in very select circumstances – in the haemodynamically stable patient who is suspected to have an injury of the right upper quadrant, isolated to the liver only. In this setting trajectory of the injury can be confirmed, delineation of vascular viability, and assistance with the decision of whether to treat the injury non-operatively versus operatively, with or without embolization.

9.4.4 **Liver Injury Scale[4]**

The American Association for the Surgery of Trauma's Committee on Organ Injury Scaling has developed a grading system for classifying injuries to the liver (Table 9.4.1).

Hepatic injuries are graded on a scale of I to VI, with I representing superficial lacerations and small subcapsular haematomas and VI representing avulsion of the liver from the vena cava. Isolated injuries that are not extensive (grades I–III) are usually managed non-operatively; however, extensive parenchymal injuries and those involving the juxtahepatic veins (grades IV and V) may require complex manoeuvres for successful treatment. Hepatic avulsion (grade VI) is generally lethal.

Eighty per cent of blunt liver injuries are grades I–III. Grades IV and V comprise 15%–20% of blunt liver injuries and these are the patients who are unstable and require laparotomy for control of haemorrhage. In general, if the patient with blunt liver injury is stable enough for CT, the patient can be managed non-operatively. In the patient who is truly stable, without active bleeding, this generally applies irrespective of the grade of liver injury or amount of haemoperitoneum.

Table 9.4.1 Liver Injury Scale 2018 Revision

AAST Grade	AIS Severity	Imaging Criteria (CT Findings)	Operative Goals	Pathologic Criteria
I	2	**Haematoma** Subcapsular haematoma <10% surface area **Laceration** Parenchymal laceration <1 cm in depth	**Haematoma** Subcapsular haematoma <10% surface area **Laceration** Parenchymal laceration <1 cm in depth Capsular tear	**Haematoma** Subcapsular haematoma <10% surface area **Laceration** Parenchymal laceration <1 cm Capsular tear
II	2	**Haematoma** Subcapsular haematoma 10%–50% surface area Intraparenchymal haematoma <10 cm in diameter **Laceration** Laceration 1–3 cm in depth and <10 cm length	**Haematoma** Subcapsular haematoma 10%–50% surface area Intraparenchymal haematoma <10 cm in diameter **Laceration** 1–3 cm in depth and >10 cm length	**Haematoma** Subcapsular haematoma 10%–50% surface area Intraparenchymal haematoma <10 cm in diameter **Laceration** Laceration 1–3 cm depth and >10 cm length
III	3	**Haematoma** Subcapsular haematoma >50%, surface area Ruptured subcapsular or parenchymal haematoma Intraparenchymal haematoma >10 cm **Laceration** Laceration >3 cm depth Any injury in the presence of a liver vascular injury or active bleeding contained within liver parenchyma	**Haematoma** Subcapsular haematoma >50%, surface area or expanding; ruptured subcapsular or parenchymal haematoma Intraparenchymal haematoma >10 cm **Laceration** Laceration >3 cm in depth	**Disruption** Parenchymal disruption involving 25%–75% of a hepatic lobe
IV	4	**Disruption** Parenchymal disruption involving 25%–75% of a hepatic lobe **Vascular injury** Active bleeding extending beyond the liver parenchyma into the peritoneum	**Disruption** Parenchymal disruption involving 25%–75% of a hepatic lobe	**Disruption** Parenchymal disruption >75% of hepatic lobe
V	5	**Disruption** Parenchymal disruption >75% of hepatic lobe **Vascular injury** Juxtahepatic venous injury to include retrohepatic vena cava and central major hepatic veins	**Disruption** Parenchymal disruption >75% of hepatic lobe **Vascular injury** Juxtahepatic venous injury to include retrohepatic vena cava and central major hepatic veins	**Vascular injury** Juxtahepatic venous injury to include retrohepatic vena cava and central major hepatic veins

Note: Vascular injury is defined as a pseudoaneurysm or arteriovenous fistula and appears as a focal collection of vascular contrast that decreases in attenuation with delayed imaging, Active bleeding from a vascular injury presents as vascular contrast, focal or diffuse, that increases in size or attenuation in delayed phase. Vascular thrombosis can lead to organ infarction.
Grade based on highest grade assessment made on imaging, at operation or on pathologic specimen.
More than one grade of liver injury may be present and should be classified by the higher grade of injury.
Advance one grade for multiple injuries up to a grade III.

9.4.5 **Management**

Traditionally, discussion of liver injuries differentiates between those arising from blunt and those arising from penetrating trauma. In general, blunt hepatic injury carries higher mortality than penetrating liver injury owing to the magnitude of parenchymal injury. Most stab wounds cause relatively minor liver injury unless a critical structure such as the hepatic vein, the intrahepatic cava, or the portal structures is injured. In contrast, gunshot wounds, particularly high energy injuries, and shotgun blasts can be devastating. High grade parenchymal liver injury (grades IV and V) or juxtahepatic caval injury from severe blunt trauma carry high mortality and continue to be the most challenging for the surgeon.

9.4.5.1 SUBCAPSULAR HAEMATOMA

An uncommon but troublesome hepatic injury is subcapsular haematoma, which arises when the parenchyma of the liver is disrupted by blunt trauma, but Glisson's capsule remains intact. Subcapsular haematomas range in severity from minor blisters on the surface of the liver to ruptured central haematomas accompanied by severe haemorrhage. They may be recognized either at the time of the operation or in the course of CT scanning. If a grade I or II subcapsular haematoma (i.e. a haematoma involving less than 50% of the surface of the liver that is not expanding and is not ruptured) is discovered during an exploratory laparotomy, it should be left alone. If the haematoma is explored, meatotomy with selective ligation may be required to control bleeding vessels. Even if effective, one must still contend with diffuse haemorrhage from the large denuded surface, and packing may also be required. A haematoma that is expanding during operation (grade III) may have to be explored. Such lesions are often the result of uncontrolled arterial haemorrhage and packing alone may not be successful. An alternative strategy is to pack the liver to control venous haemorrhage, close the abdomen, and perform hepatic arteriography and embolization of the bleeding vessels. Ruptured grades III and IV haematomas are treated with exploration and selective ligation, with or without packing (Figure 9.4.3).

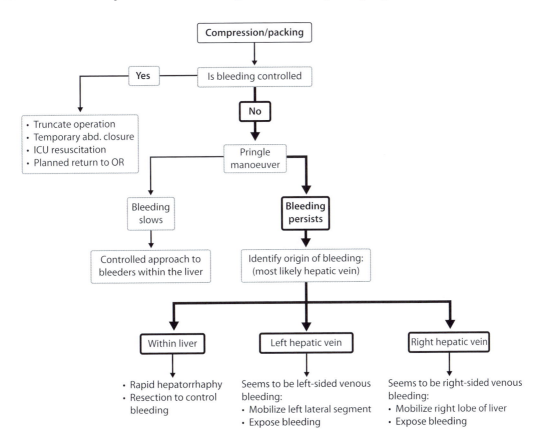

Figure 9.4.3 Surgical decision-making algorithm in major hepatic trauma.

9.4.5.2 NON-OPERATIVE MANAGEMENT (NOM)[5,6]

Nearly all children and 50% to 80% of adults with blunt hepatic injuries can be treated without laparotomy. This change in approach has been occasioned by the increasing availability of rapid ultrasound, helical CT, and interventional radiology (Table 9.4.2).

The primary requirement for non-operative therapy is haemodynamic stability. To confirm stability, frequent assessment of vital signs and monitoring of the haematocrit and lactate or base deficit are necessary, in conjunction with CT as required. Continued haemorrhage occurs in 1%–4% of patients. Hypotension may develop, usually within the first 24 hours after hepatic injury, but sometimes several days later. Failure rates from non-operative management in well selected patients are extremely low (1%).

The presence of extravasation of contrast on CT denotes active bleeding depending on the phase of the scan. The hepatic arteries are relatively protected by Glisson's capsule and although can be injured in isolation in penetrating trauma, in blunt injury there is likely to be associated hepatic venous and portal venous bleeding. In isolated arterial haemorrhage; therapeutic angiography with embolization should be applied early, otherwise, operative intervention will become necessary. Angiography/embolization may also be used postoperatively as a component of damage control for major liver injury.

Table 9.4.2 Evidence-Based Guidelines for Selective Non-Operative Management of Hepatic Injury

Level of Evidence	Recommendation
I	Patients who have diffuse peritonitis or who are haemodynamically unstable after blunt abdominal trauma should be taken urgently for laparotomy.
II	1. A routine laparotomy is not indicated in the haemodynamically stable patient without peritonitis presenting with an isolated blunt hepatic injury. 2. In the haemodynamically stable blunt abdominal trauma patient without peritonitis, an abdominal CT with intravenous contrast should be performed to identify and assess the severity of injury to the liver. 3. The severity of hepatic injury (as suggested by CT grade or degree of haemoperitoneum), neurologic status, age >55 and/or the presence of associated injuries are not contraindications to a trial of non-operative management in a haemodynamically stable patient. 4. Angiography with embolization should be considered in a haemodynamically stable patient with evidence of active extravasation (a contrast blush) on abdominal CT. 5. Non-operative management of hepatic injuries should only be considered in an environment that provides capabilities for monitoring, serial clinical evaluations, and an operating room available for urgent laparotomy.
III	1. After blunt hepatic injury, clinical factors such as a persistent systemic inflammatory response, increasing/persistent abdominal pain, or an otherwise unexplained drop in haemoglobin should prompt re-evaluation by CT. 2. Interventional modalities such as endoscopic retrograde cholangiopancreatography (ERCP) angiography, laparoscopy, or percutaneous drainage, may be required to manage complications (bile leak, biloma, bile peritonitis, hepatic abscess, bilious ascites, and haemobilia), that arise as a result of non-operative management of blunt hepatic injury. This is most likely to be necessary in grade IV and V hepatic injuries. 3. Pharmacologic prophylaxis to prevent venous thromboembolism can be used for patients with isolated blunt hepatic injuries without increasing the failure rate of non-operative management, although the optimal timing of safe initiation has not been determined.
Unanswered Questions	1. Frequency of haemoglobin measurements. 2. Intensity and duration of monitoring. 3. Duration and intensity of restricted activity (both in hospital and after discharge). 4. Optimum length of stay both for the intensive care unit and the hospital.

Source: Buckman RF Jr. et al. *J Trauma.* 2000 May;48(5):978–84.

A persistently falling haematocrit should be treated with packed red blood cell (pRBC) transfusions. If the haematocrit continues to fall after two or three units of pRBCs within 24 hours, embolization in the interventional radiology suite or laparotomy should be considered.

9.4.5.3 SUBCAPSULAR HAEMATOMA

An uncommon but troublesome hepatic injury is subcapsular haematoma, which arises when the parenchyma of the liver is disrupted by blunt trauma, but Glisson's capsule remains intact. Subcapsular haematomas range in severity from minor blisters on the surface of the liver to ruptured central haematomas accompanied by severe haemorrhage. They may be recognized either at the time of the operation or in the course of CT scanning. If a grade I or II subcapsular haematoma (i.e. a haematoma involving less than 50% of the surface of the liver that is not expanding and is not ruptured) is discovered during an exploratory laparotomy, it should be left alone. If the haematoma is explored, meatotomy with selective ligation may be required to control bleeding vessels. Even if effective, one must still contend with diffuse haemorrhage from the large denuded surface, and packing may also be required. A haematoma that is expanding during operation (grade III) may have to be explored. Such lesions are often the result of uncontrolled arterial haemorrhage and packing alone may not be successful. An alternative strategy is to pack the liver to control venous haemorrhage, close the abdomen, and perform hepatic arteriography and embolization of the bleeding vessels. Ruptured grades III and IV haematomas are treated with exploration and selective ligation, with or without packing.

9.4.5.4 OPERATIVE (SURGICAL) MANAGEMENT

Most injuries requiring surgical intervention are managed simply by evacuating the free intraperitoneal blood and washing out the peritoneal cavity; some will require drainage of the injury because of a possible bile leak. However, 25% of liver injuries requiring surgical intervention require direct control of more major hepatic bleeding. Most bleeding from hepatic injury is venous in nature and therefore can be controlled by direct compression and liver packs. Tissue sealants may be a useful adjunct.[7] Caution must be exercised since bile within the peritoneal cavity is not always well tolerated, and closed suction drainage should be routine in these patients.

9.4.6 **Surgical Approach**[8–10]

During treatment of a major hepatic injury, ongoing haemorrhage may pose an immediate threat to the patient's life, and temporary control will give the anaesthesiologist time to restore the circulating volume before further blood loss occurs. This is best achieved immediately upon entry into the abdomen by direct manual compression of the liver. The goal is to restore the normal anatomy by manual compression and then maintain it with packing. Compress right and liver halves of the liver back to normal anatomy and simultaneously push the liver posteriorly to tamponade potential retrohepatic venous bleeding.

Additionally, multiple bleeding sites beyond the liver are common with both blunt and penetrating trauma. Even if the liver is not the highest priority, temporary control of hepatic bleeding allows repair of other injuries without unnecessary blood loss. As always, the most active/life-threatening bleeding must be controlled first.

- Perihepatic packing.
- Pringle manoeuvre.
- Tourniquet or liver clamp application.
- Electrocautery, Aquamantys® bipolar sealer (Medtronic, Minneapolis, MN), or Argon beam coagulator.
- Haemostatic agents and glues.
- Hepatic suture.
- Hepatorrhaphy and non-anatomic resection (resectional debridement).

9.4.6.1 INCISION

The patient is placed in the supine position.

- Warming devices are placed around the upper body and lower limbs.
- The chest and abdomen are surgically prepared and draped – prepare the patient from chin to mid thighs and table-to-table laterally.
- The instruments necessary to extend the incision into a sternotomy or thoracotomy must be available.
- A generous midline incision from pubis to xiphisternum is the minimum incision required. On rare occasion, for the patient 'in extremis', a combined sternotomy and midline laparotomy approach is recommended from the outset to allow access for internal cardiac massage and vena caval vascular control. Supradiaphragmatic intrapericardial inferior vena caval control is often easier than abdominal control

adjacent to a severe injury. However, this opens another body cavity and is uncommonly necessary.

- Do not hesitate to extend the midline incision with a right subcostal incision if there is difficulty exposing the IVC, hepatic veins or right lobe of the liver.
- A table-mounted retractor, such as the 'Omnitract' or Bookwalter type automatic retractor greatly facilitates access. Apply the retractor to pull the ribcage cephalad and anteriorly to optimize exposure.

9.4.6.2 INITIAL ACTIONS

Once the abdomen has been opened, intraperitoneal blood is evacuated, bleeding controlled, and if there is evidence of hepatic bleeding, the liver should be initially packed, and the abdomen rapidly examined to exclude extrahepatic sites of blood loss. Autotransfusion should be considered. Once the anaesthetist has had an opportunity to restore intravascular volume and haemostasis has been achieved for any extrahepatic injury, the liver injury then can be approached.

In dealing with liver injury, be a minimalist – if the lesion has ceased bleeding, nothing more needs to be done in most cases and above all, the non-bleeding lesion should **not** be explored further. If further surgery is required, adequate exposure and mobilization of the liver are necessary. Most injuries do not require formal mobilization of the injured lobe to permit repair or packing.

> **Perfection is the enemy of good!**
> **The non-bleeding liver should not be explored further.**
> **Call early for senior help for complex liver injuries that continue to bleed**

9.4.6.3 TECHNIQUES FOR TEMPORARY CONTROL OF HAEMORRHAGE

- Perihepatic packing.
- Hepatic 'tourniquet'.
- Tract tamponade balloons.
- Pringle manoeuvre.
- Tractotomy, direct suture ligation, or hepatic resection.
- Hepatic artery ligation.
- Hepatic vascular isolation.
- Techniques to control retrohepatic caval bleeding:
  - Moore-Pilcher balloon.
  - Veno-venous bypass (uncommonly needed).

9.4.6.3.1 Perihepatic Packing

The philosophy of packing has altered, and packs are used to restore the anatomical relationship of the components, and secondarily to act as compressive agent. Packs for a liver wound should *not* be pushed into the wound itself as this worsens the injury and causes further bleeding.

Liver packing can also be definitive treatment, particularly with bilobar injury, or to buy time if the patient develops coagulopathy, hypothermia, or there are no blood resources. Liver packing is the method of choice where expertise in more sophisticated techniques is not available. If packing is successful, and the bleeding is controlled, no further action may be required – this decision must be made early in the operation before the patient has received large numbers of red blood cells (RBCs) in transfusion. If simple actions fail to control bleeding, then a more complex operation will be necessary. Furthermore, surgical expertise and speed are essential to rapidly control the bleeding. Remember that mortality in trauma patients is 25% after 10 units of RBCs and 50% after 20 units of RBCs. Thus, bleeding should ideally be controlled prior to 10 units and certainly by 20 units of transfusion

> *Blood loss not time is your 'clock' when dealing with major hepatic injury.*

Packing is initially performed using large *dry* flat abdominal packs, placed laterally, inferiorly, medially, and around the liver. Ideally it is not necessary to unfold these. Careful placement of packs is capable of controlling haemorrhage from most hepatic venous injuries.

Restore the anatomy of the liver by direct manual compression (Figure 9.4.4a):

- Place the first pack(s) across the injury to stabilize the damaged tissue.
- Additional packs may be placed between the liver and the diaphragm, posteriorly and laterally, and between the liver and the anterior chest wall.
- There is no benefit in placing multiple packs between the dome of the liver and the diaphragm, which will only have the effect of raising the diaphragm.
- Pack the inferior surface of the liver from the porta hepatis laterally. This moves the right lobe of the liver laterally (Figure 9.4.4b).
- Then pack the liver 'backwards' between the subcostal margin and the anterior surface of the right lobe. The liver should not be packed so tightly as to cause compression of the vena cava which will reduce venous return.

(a)

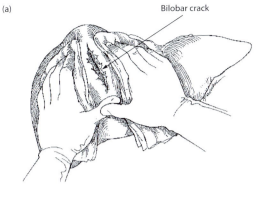

Bilobar crack

(b)

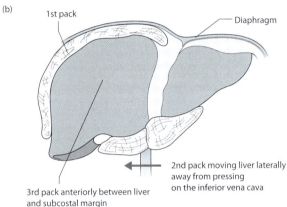

1st pack

Diaphragm

2nd pack moving liver laterally away from pressing on the inferior vena cava

3rd pack anteriorly between liver and subcostal margin

Figure 9.4.4 (a) Manual use of swabs for the restoration of anatomy of the liver. (b) Final packing for liver.

If necessary, the liver can be mobilized by division of the hepatic ligaments (see Section 9.4.6.4) until the bleeding has been controlled. Several packs may be required to control the haemorrhage from an extensive right lobar injury. The minimum number of packs to achieve haemostasis should be used.

Pitfall

Packing is not as effective for injuries of the left lobe, because with the abdomen open, there is insufficient abdominal and thoracic wall anterior to the left lobe to provide adequate counter-compression. Fortunately, haemorrhage from the left lobe can be controlled by dividing the left triangular and coronary ligaments and compressing the lobe between the hands – segments 2 and 3 can be resected rapidly if needed.

Key factors for success in packing the liver are:

- Use dry abdominal swabs. Wet swabs are less absorbent and exacerbate hypothermia.
- Use them 'folded' as it is easier to layer them for even pressure.
- Ensure that they have radio-opaque markers included in their manufacture.
- Do *not* cover them with plastic as they will not hold position.
- Ongoing bleeding despite initial packing, mandates repacking or other haemostatic procedure and consideration of embolization.

During the period that the packs are placed, it is important to establish more intravenous access lines and other monitoring devices as needed. Hypothermia should be anticipated, and corrective measures taken. After haemodynamic stability has been achieved, the packs are removed, and the injury to the liver rapidly assessed. The control of haemorrhage is the first consideration, followed by control of contamination. If the bleeding has stopped, nothing further may be required.

If in doubt, apply damage control techniques, with definitive packing of the liver.

- Consider angiography and embolization following damage control surgery.
- Packs should preferably be removed within 24–72 hours. If removed too early, bleeding may recur. A higher risk of perihepatic infection results from packs remaining longer than 72 hours.
- The packs should be carefully removed to avoid precipitating further bleeding.
- If there is no bleeding, the packs can be left out, and closed suction drains placed.
- Necrotic tissue should be resected.

Two complications may be encountered with the packing of hepatic injuries. First, tight packing compresses the inferior vena cava, decreases venous return, and reduces right ventricular filling; hypovolaemic patients may not tolerate the resultant decrease in cardiac output. Second, perihepatic packing forces the right diaphragm to move superiorly and impairs its motion; this may lead to increased airway pressures and decreased tidal volume.

If compression and packing is unsuccessful, then it will be necessary to achieve direct access to the bleeding vessel and direct suture ligation. This will often necessitate extension of the wound to gain access and view the bleeding point. During this direct access, bleeding can be temporarily controlled by direct compression, which requires a capable assistant. Temporary clamping of the porta hepatis (Pringle's manoeuvre) is also a useful adjunctive measure. Other adjunctive measures include interruption of the venous or arterial inflow to a segment or lobe (less than 1% of all liver injuries), haemostatic agents such as crystallized bovine collagen, fibrin adhesives, gel foam, and use of the argon laser or harmonic scalpel.

9.4.6.3.2 Hepatic Tourniquet

When faced with bleeding from the left lobe of the liver, it is easier to rather suture the actively bleeding liver. If this is not possible, once the bleeding lobe has been mobilized, Penrose tubing can be wrapped around the liver near the anatomic division between the left lobe and the right. The tubing is stretched until haemorrhage ceases, and tension is maintained by clamping the drain. Unfortunately, tourniquets are difficult to use, and they tend to slip off or tear through the parenchyma if placed over an injured area. An alternative is the use of a liver clamp; however, the application of such devices is hindered by the variability in the size and shape of the liver. Bleeding from the left lateral segment can be definitively and rapidly controlled with resection using the stapling devices.

9.4.6.3.3 Tract Tamponade Balloons[11]

These can be useful in haemostasis of a tract, from stab or gunshot wounds. The balloon is threaded down the tract and inflated, to tamponade the bleeding from inside out. The balloon can be either manufactured by the surgeon using Penrose rubber tubing, or even a condom and a nasogastric tube. A Sengstaken-Blakemore tube for tamponade of oesophageal varices is ideal.

9.4.6.3.4 Pringle's Manoeuvre

Pringle's manoeuvre is often used as an adjunct to packing, for the temporary control of haemorrhage. When encountering life-threatening haemorrhage from the liver, the hepatic pedicle should be compressed manually. The compression of the hepatic pedicle via the Foramen of Winslow is known as Pringle's manoeuvre. The liver then should packed as above. The hepatic pedicle is best clamped from the left side of the patient, by digitally dissecting a small hole in the lesser omentum, near the pedicle, and then placing a soft clamp over the pedicle from

the left-hand side, through the Foramen of Winslow. The advantage of this approach is the avoidance of injury to the structures within the hepatic pedicle, and the assurance that the clamp will be properly placed the first time. The pedicle can be left clamped for up to an hour. However, this is probably true only in the haemodynamically stable patient. In the hypotensive patient, intermittent clamping produces less ischaemia than continuous clamping; leave the clamp on for 10 minutes at a time, with 5 minutes of reperfusion between clamp placement. The clamp should be replaced as soon as possible with a Rumel vascular sling.

The Pringle's manoeuvre is both therapeutic and diagnostic. If bleeding within the liver stops with the Pringle's manoeuvre, haemorrhage is from branches of the hepatic artery or the portal vein – these bleeding sites should be controlled. If haemorrhage persists with the clamp on the porta hepatis, the source of bleeding is generally from the hepatic veins or the retrohepatic vena cava, or less commonly aberrant extrapedicular arterial supply to the left or right lobes.

9.4.6.3.4.1 *Getting Access to Deeper Bleeding within the Liver*

At times, extension of the liver injury may be needed to gain access to deeper bleeding, preferably using the 'finger fracture' technique. Remember as you proceed more deeply within the liver, the vessels become larger.

9.4.6.3.4.2 *Finger Fracture*

To provide the above access, 'finger fracture' through normal liver tissue, to get to the injured vessels deep in the parenchyma. The normal capsule is 'scored' using diathermy or scalpel. Then the normal liver tissue is gently compressed between thumb and forefinger, rubbing the normal parenchymal tissue away, leaving just the intact vessels for ligation or clipping. Avoid forceful pinching or crushing of the liver tissue, as this may disrupt the hepatic vasculature, increasing the haemorrhage.

9.4.6.3.4.3 *Stapling Devices*

Stapling devices provide an even more rapid method to resect/divide liver parenchyma. Crushing staples with a vascular load are best. The Ligasure® (Johnson and Johnson, Brunswick, NJ, USA) or equivalent may also be used to quickly divide liver parenchyma.

As with any liver surgery, be certain to protect normal/non-insured vasculature and bile ducts as you perform these manoeuvres. Knowledge of hepatic anatomy is critical.

Do not cross Cantlie's line as you resect a lobe or segment.

9.4.6.3.5 Hepatic Suture

Suturing of the hepatic parenchyma is not routinely recommended to control more superficial lacerations which continue to bleed but may be used if other methods are ineffective. If, however, the capsule of the liver has been stripped away by the injury, sutures which are tied over the capsule are far less effective.

The liver is usually sutured using a large curved needle blunt nosed needle with 0 or 2/0 resorbable sutures. The large diameter prevents the suture from pulling through Glisson's capsule. At times, this may be life-saving. On the other hand, deeper injury may be present with resultant haemorrhage, abscess, or biloma. For shallow lacerations, a simple continuous suture may be used to approximate the edges of the laceration. For deeper lacerations, interrupted horizontal mattress sutures may be placed parallel to the edges, and tied over the capsule. The danger of suturing, is that sutures tied too tight may cut off the blood supply to viable liver parenchyma, resulting in necrosis.

Most sources of venous haemorrhage can be managed with intraparenchymal sutures.

Pitfall

The best way of ensuring haemostasis is to ensure that the damaged liver anatomy is 'reconstituted', and that the injured surfaced are in contact with one another. This is best treated by meticulous packing.

9.4.6.3.6 Hepatic Resection[8,12]

In elective circumstances anatomic resection produces good results, but in the uncontrolled circumstances of trauma, mortality has been recorded in excess of 50%. Anatomic lobectomy should be reserved for patients with:

- Extensive injuries of the lateral segments of the left lobe where bimanual compression is not possible.
- Delayed lobectomy in patients where packing initially controls the haemorrhage, but where there is a segment of the liver that is non-viable.
- Almost free segments of liver.
- Devitalized liver at the time of pack removal.

9.4.6.3.7 Hepatic Shunts

The atriocaval shunt was designed to achieve hepatic vascular isolation while still permitting some venous blood

from below the diaphragm to flow through the shunt into the right atrium. A shunt can be introduced from above via the left atrial appendage, or from below via the sapheno-femoral junction.

The mortality remains high with this approach, and it is no longer in general use.

9.4.6.4 MOBILIZATION OF THE LIVER

In general, and for most injuries, it is *not* necessary to mobilize the liver; injuries can be managed without resorting to full mobilization. However, in some situations, particularly with injury to the superior or posterior aspects, mobilization is necessary.

Ensure that the table-mounted self-retaining retractor (Omnitract®, Bookwalter®, Rochard®, etc.) is lifting the costal margin in both a cephalad and anterior direction. Lifting the ribcage anteriorly (away from the table) is critical for adequate exposure. Access to the right lobe of the liver is restricted due to the right subcostal margin and the posterior attachments. If a self-retaining retractor is not immediately available, the costal margin can be elevated, initially with a Morris retractor, and then with a Kelly or Deaver retractor. The right triangular and coronary ligaments are divided with scissors or cautery. Avoid entering the diaphragm or liver parenchyma as you do so. This usually can be done under vision but in the larger subject it can be accomplished blindly from the patient's left side. The superior coronary ligament is divided, avoiding the lateral wall of the right hepatic vein. The inferior coronary ligament is divided, taking care not to injure the right adrenal gland (which is vulnerable because it lies directly beneath the peritoneal reflection) or the retrohepatic vena cava. When the ligaments have been divided, the right lobe of the liver can be rotated medially into the surgical field. Sudden onset or aggravation of bleeding during mobilization of the right liver attests to hepatic vein or retrohepatic caval injury and mandates immediate replacement of the mobilized liver and damage control packing.

The left lobe can be easily mobilized by dividing the left triangular ligament under vision, avoiding injury to the left inferior phrenic vein and the left hepatic vein.

Pitfall

In the event of a retrohepatic haematoma being evident, rotation of the right lobe of the liver should be avoided unless strong indications are present, and adequate expertise is available. Packing and transport to a higher-level centre may be a safer option.

If exposure of the junction of the hepatic veins and the retrohepatic vena cava is necessary, the midline abdominal incision can be extended by means of a median sternotomy, or a lateral subcostal extension. The pericardium and the diaphragm then can be divided in the direction of the IVC. In an unstable patient, a more rapid means to access the suprahepatic IVC is via the abdomen through the central diaphragm/pericardium, and approach via the intracardiac route.

9.4.6.5 HEPATIC ISOLATION

Hepatic vascular isolation is accomplished by occlusion of the blood vessel access to the liver:

- Clamping the aorta at the diaphragm.
- Executing a Pringle manoeuvre.
- Clamping the IVC above the right kidney (infrahepatic/suprarenal).
- Clamping the IVC above the liver (suprahepatic).

The time limit for isolation is about 30 minutes. The technique is not straightforward and is best achieved by those experienced in its use. In patients scheduled for elective procedures, this technique has enjoyed nearly uniform success, but in trauma patients, the results have been disappointing.

Access to the suprarenal, infrahepatic IVC is through a Kocher rotation of the duodenum, and then clamping the IVC under direct vision.

Access to the suprahepatic infradiaphragmatic IVC is obtained mobilization of the suspensory ligaments, gently pulling the right lobe of the liver caudally and antero-medially, then applying a curved vascular clamp over the dome of the liver on the right and clamping the IVC at the diaphragmatic hiatus. A headlight may be useful.

In certain circumstances, it is easier to control the suprahepatic IVC *above* the diaphragm:

9.4.6.5.1 Intrapericardial control of the inferior vena cava

A small hole is made in the diaphragmatic pericardium as superiorly as possible. Be careful to avoid injury to the heart with this manoeuvre (Figure 9.4.5a). The

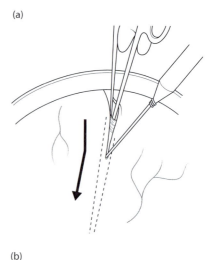

(a)

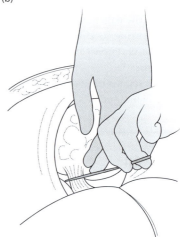

(b)

Figure 9.4.5 (a) Splitting of the diaphragm; (b) clamping of the suprahepatic IVC above the diaphragm.

pericardium is bluntly dissected from the posterior aspect of the sternum. With a clamp or finger protecting the heart, electrocautery or scissors is used the split the central diaphragm posteriorly. Curve toward the patient's right as you approach entry of the IVC into the pericardium. The heart is lifted cephalad and anteriorly with your left hand; a vascular clamp is placed on the IVC[8] (Figure 9.4.5b).

9.4.7 Perihepatic Drainage

Several prospective and retrospective studies have demonstrated that the use of either Penrose or sump drains carries a higher risk of intra-abdominal infection than the use of either closed suction drains or no drains at all. If drains are to be used, closed suction devices are preferred.

Pitfall

Patients who are initially treated with perihepatic packing may also require drainage; however, drainage is *not* indicated at the initial damage control procedure, given that the patient will be returned to the OR within the next 36–48 hours. The primary function is to drain bile, not blood.

The best treatment for a post-operative bile leak is prevention. This is usually not done. Ideally, as a routine part of the definitive operation for major hepatic injury (generally the re-look operation after damage control), a cholangiogram should be obtained. This defines the biliary anatomy and will identify major ductal injury while in the OR. Inject saline intermittently through a catheter in the cystic duct remnant (cholecystectomy performed) to identify and oversew leaking bile ducts.

9.4.8 Complications

Overall mortality for patients with hepatic injuries is approximately 10%. The most common cause of death is exsanguination, followed by multiple organ dysfunction syndrome (MODS) and intracranial injury.

- Morbidity and mortality increase in proportion to the injury grade and to the complexity of repair.
- Hepatic injuries caused by blunt trauma carry a higher mortality than those caused by penetrating trauma.
- Infectious complications occur more often with penetrating trauma.

Post-operative haemorrhage occurs in a small percentage of patients with hepatic injury. The source may be either a coagulopathy or a missed vascular injury (usually to an artery). In most instances of persistent post-operative haemorrhage, the patient is best served by return to the OR. Arteriography with embolization may be considered in selected patients. If coagulation studies indicate that a coagulopathy is the likely cause of post-operative haemorrhage, then correction of the coagulopathy must be a critical part of the strategy.

Perihepatic infections occur in fewer than 5% of patients with significant hepatic injury. They develop more often in patients with penetrating injuries than in patients with blunt injuries, presumably because of the greater frequency of enteric contamination. An elevated temperature and a rising white blood cell count should prompt a search for intra-abdominal infection. In the absence of pneumonia, an infected line, or urinary tract infection, an abdominal CT with intravenous and upper gastrointestinal contrast should be obtained.

Many perihepatic infections (but not necrotic liver) can be treated with CT or ultrasound-guided drainage. In refractory cases, especially for posterior infections, right 12th rib resection remains an excellent approach.

Bilomas are loculated collections of bile that may become infected. They are best drained percutaneously under radiological guidance. If a biloma is infected, it should be treated as an abscess and drained; if it is sterile, it will eventually be resorbed.

Biliary ascites is caused by disruption of a major bile duct and requires reoperation and the establishment of appropriate drainage. Even if the source of the leaking bile can be identified, primary repair of the injured duct can be difficult to achieve. It is best to wait until a firm fistulous communication is established with adequate drainage. Adjunctive, transduodenal drainage by endoscopic retrograde cholangiopancreatography (ERCP) and papillotomy (ductotomy), or stent placement may be of benefit in selected cases. Secondary infection of biliary ascites may lead to biliary peritonitis which may require urgent drainage by laparotomy or laparoscopy with appropriate use on antibiotics.

Biliary fistulae occur in up to 15% of patients with major hepatic injury. They are usually of little consequence and generally close without specific treatment. In rare instances, a fistulous communication with intra-thoracic structures forms in patients with associated diaphragmatic injuries, resulting in a bronchobiliary or pleurobiliary fistula. Because of the pressure differential between the biliary tract and the thoracic cavity, most of these fistulae must be closed operatively.

Haemorrhage from hepatic injuries is often treated without identifying and controlling each bleeding vessel individually, and arterial pseudoaneurysms may develop. As the pseudoaneurysm enlarges, it may rupture into the parenchyma of the liver, into a bile duct, or into an adjacent branch of the portal vein. Rupture into a bile duct results in haemobilia, which is characterized by intermittent episodes of right upper quadrant pain, upper gastrointestinal haemorrhage, and jaundice;

rupture into a portal vein may result in portal vein hypertension with bleeding varices. Both complications are rare and are best managed with hepatic arteriography and embolization.

9.4.9 Injury to the Retrohepatic Vena Cava

Approximately 2% of all liver injuries are complex and represent injuries to major hepatic venous structures, portal triad, the intrahepatic cava, the injuries are bilobar, or are difficult to control because of hypothermia and coagulopathy. Injuries to the hepatic vein or retrohepatic cava can be approached in the following ways:

- Direct compression (may require extension of the laceration).
- Atriocaval shunt.
- Temporary clamping of the porta hepatis, suprarenal cava, and suprahepatic cava (see also Section 9.4.6.5).
- Veno-venous bypass (Heaney technique).
- Packing.

Direct compression and control of hepatic venous injuries can be accomplished in some patients. Major liver injury requires manual compression and simultaneous medial rotation and retraction – a difficult manoeuvre. Ideally, two experienced surgeons are now in the operating room. In such a situation the most senior surgeon should be the one doing the direct compression and the assistant should do the actual suturing of the hepatic vein or cava.

Adequate exposure, experienced surgeons, good anaesthesia help and a deep blood bank are essential in salvaging these patients.

However, in many cases, especially with blunt injury, packing the liver against the cava secures haemostasis as part of damage control, and the definitive care can take place later.

Hepatic vascular isolation, by clamping of the porta hepatis, suprarenal cava and suprahepatic cava can be done on a temporary basis (see also Section 9.4.6.5). This requires considerable experience by the anaesthesiologist and a surgeon capable of dealing with the problems rapidly.

Veno-venous bypass has been used successfully in liver transplant surgery and with new heparin free pumps and tubing, may have a place in the trauma patient.

Is bilobar injury, or it can simply buy time if the patient develops a coagulopathy, hypothermia, or there are no blood resources. Liver packing is the method of choice where expertise in more sophisticated techniques is not available, or when it is therapeutic in controlling the bleeding.

9.4.10 Injury to the Porta Hepatis[13]

If there is a haematoma in the porta hepatis, there is a high probability of injury to the vessels of the portal triad, often in association with injury to the common bile duct.

The key is to obtain source control.

- Before entering the haematoma, perform a Pringle's manoeuvre, preferably with a Rumel tourniquet.
- Control bleeding vessels in the porta, initially with finger compression, and subsequently with vascular clamps. *Do not clamp blindly!*
- Do NOT place sutures or ties until the common bile duct has been identified.
- When in doubt, *shunt* the portal vein.
- The hepatic artery can by ligated if necessary.

Injuries to the porta hepatis also can be exsanguinating. Common hepatic, right and left hepatic arteries usually can be managed by simple ligation. Remember that hepatic artery ligation or embolization is well tolerated by the liver parenchyma (via portal vein flow) but not by the bile ducts (depend on arterial flow).

Injury to the left or right portal vein can be ligated. Ligation of the main portal vein has been reported to be successful, however, shunting as part of damage control, and subsequent repair is recommended whenever possible.

Packing should be removed in the standard damage control sequence (when the patient is warm, appropriately transfused and haemodynamic and respiratory parameters have been normalized); It is recommended that lateral and medial suction drains be placed after packs have been removed, as biliary leak is relatively common.

9.4.11 Injury to the Bile Ducts and Gallbladder[14,15]

Injuries to the extrahepatic bile ducts, although rare, can be caused by either penetrating or blunt trauma. The diagnosis is usually made by noting the accumulation of bile in the upper quadrant during laparotomy for treatment of associated injuries.

9.4.12 **Anaesthetic Considerations**

- Establishment of adequate upper limb large bore vascular access and initiation of resuscitation fluids. Infuse blood products early and preferentially if the patient is profoundly hypotensive. Avoid excessive crystalloid infusion.
- Avoid IV access below the diaphragm as this may exacerbate bleeding from the liver or IVC.
- Initiation of the massive haemorrhage (massive transfusion) protocol.
- REBOA should be considered with *huge caution* in severe liver injury as zone I REBOA may simply increase the risk of hepatic venous bleeding whilst delaying transfer to the operating room.
- The patient's physiology drives decision-making – unstable physiology requires surgery whereas stable physiology does not regardless of grade of liver injury.
- Patients actively bleeding from major liver injury must be taken to the operating room promptly, with rapid haemorrhage control. Any delay in doing so increases risk of coagulopathy and mortality.
- Resuscitation of patients with liver injury is best done simultaneously with the surgery.
- When the surgeon is packing the liver, monitor venous return to avoid occlusion of the IVC by the packing.

Bile duct injuries can be divided into those below the confluence of the cystic duct and common duct and those above the cystic duct. Treatment of common bile duct (CBD) injuries after external trauma is complicated by the small size and thin wall of the normal duct.

For the lower ductal injuries (those injuries below the cystic duct), when the tissue loss is minimal, the lesion can be closed over a T-Tube (as with exploration of the CBD for stones). A choledochoduodenostomy can be performed if the duodenum has not been injured. If the duodenum has been injured, or there is tissue loss, since the common duct is invariably small, a modification of the Carrel patch can be utilized. From blunt trauma, the common bile duct can be transected at the superior border of the pancreas. This is best treated with Roux-en-Y hepatojejunostomy.

In higher ductal injuries between the confluence of the cystic duct and the common duct and the hepatic parenchyma, a hepatojejunostomy with an internal splint is recommended. An adjunctive measure is to bring the Roux-en-Y end to the subcutaneous tissue so that access can be gained later if a stricture develops. Percutaneous intubation of the Roux-en-Y limb is then possible with dilatation of the anastomosis.

Treatment of injury to the left or right hepatic duct is even more difficult. If only one hepatic duct is injured, a reasonable approach is to ligate it and deal with any infections or atrophy of the lobe rather than to attempt repair. If both ducts are injured, each should be intubated with a small catheter brought through the abdominal wall. Once the patient has recovered sufficiently, delayed repair is performed under elective conditions with a Roux-en-Y hepatojejunostomy.

REFERENCES

1. Pachter HL. Prometheus bound: evolution in the management of hepatic trauma-from myth to reality. 2011 Fitts Oration. *J Trauma*. 2012 Feb;**72(2)**:321–9. doi: 10.1097/TA.0b013e31824b15a7.

2. Richardson JD, Franklin GA, Lukan JK, Carrillo EH, Spain DA, Miller FB, et al. Evolution in the management of hepatic trauma: a 25-year perspective. *Ann Surg*. 2000 Sep;**232(3)**:324–30.

3. Buckman RF Jr, Miraliakbari R, Badellino MM. Juxtahepatic venous injuries: a critical review of reported management strategies. *J Trauma*. 2000 May;**48(5)**:978–84.

4. Kozar RA, Crandall M, Shanmuganathan K, Zarzaur B, Coburn M, Cribari C, et al. Organ injury scaling 2018 update: Spleen, liver and kidney. *J Trauma Acute Care Surgery*. 2018 Dec;**85(6)**:1119–22. doi: 10.1097/TA.0000000000002058.

5. Stassen NA, Bhullar I, Cheng JD, Crandall M, Friese R, Guillamondegui O, et al. A Non-operative management of blunt hepatic injury: An Eastern Association for the Surgery of Trauma Practice Management Guideline. *J Trauma Acute Care Surg*. 2012;**73:5 Supplement 4**: S289–300. In: Trauma Practice Management Guidelines. Eastern Association for the Surgery of Trauma. http://www.east.org. doi: 10.1097/TA.0b013e318270160d (accessed online January 2015).

6. Polanco PM, Brown JB, Puyana JC, Billiar TR, Peitzman AB, Sperry JL. The swinging pendulum: A national perspective of nonoperative management in severe blunt liver injury. *J Trauma Acute Care Surgery*. 2013 Oct;**75(4)**:590–5. doi: 10.1097/TA.0b013e3182a53a3e.

7. Ochsner MG, Maniscalco-Theberge ME, Champion HR. Fibrin glue as a haemostatic agent in hepatic, splenic trauma. *J Trauma*. 1990 July;**30(7)**:884–7.

8. Peitzman AB, Marsh JW. Advanced operative techniques in the management of complex liver injury. *J Trauma and Acute Care Surgery*. 2012 Sep;**73(3)**:765–70. doi: 10.1097/TA.0b013e318265cef5.

9. Kozar RA, Feliciano DV, Moore EE, Moore FA, Cocanour CS, West MA, et al. Western Trauma Association / Critical decision in trauma: operative management of blunt hepatic injury. *J Trauma*. 2011 Jul;**71(1)**:1–5. doi: 10.1097/TA.0b013e318220b192.

10. American College of Surgeons. Operative Exposure in abdominal trauma: exposure of liver injuries. ASSET: Advanced Operative Skills for Exposure in Trauma, Chicago, 2019.

11. Poggetti RS, Moore EE, Moore FA, Mitchell MB, Read RA. Balloon tamponade for bilobar transfixing hepatic gunshot wounds. *J Trauma*. 1992 Nov;**33(5)**:694–7. Review.

12. Polanco P, Leon S, Pineda J, Puyana JC, Ochoa JB, Alarcon L, et al. Hepatic resection in the management of complex injury to the liver. *J Trauma*. 2008 Dec;**65(6)**:1264–9; discussion 1269-70. doi: 10.1097/TA.0b013e3181904749.

13. Sheldon GF, Lim RC, Yee ES, Petersen SR. Management of injuries to the porta hepatis. *Ann Surg*. 1985 Nov; **202(5)**:539–45.

14. Bade PG, Thomson SR, Hirshberg A, Robbs JR. Surgical options in traumatic injury to the extrahepatic biliary tract. *Br J Surg*. 1989 Mar;**76(3)**:256–8.

15. Feliciano DV, Bitondo CG, Burch JM, Mattox KL, Beall AC Jr, Jordan GL Jr. Management of traumatic injuries to the extrahepatic biliary ducts. *Am J Surg*. 1985 Dec; **150(6)**:705–9.

Recommended Reading

Coccolini F, Catena F, Moore EE, Ivatury R, Biffl W, Peitzman A, et al. WSES classification and guidelines for liver trauma. *World J Emerg Surg*. 2016 Oct;10;**11**:50. eCollection.

Ivatury RR (ed). *Operative techniques for severe liver injury*. Springer, 2015, New York.

Piper GL, Peitzman AB. Current management of hepatic trauma. *Surg Clin North America*. 2010;**90**:775–785.

Posner MC, Moore EE. Extrahepatic biliary tract injury: operative management plan. *J Trauma*. 1985;**25**:833–7.

9.5 Spleen

9.5.1 Overview

The conventional management of splenic injury used to be splenectomy. However, stimulated by the success of non-operative management (NOM) in children and the recognition of the importance of splenic function, there has been a shift in strategy. Today, the management of splenic injury should rely primarily on the haemodynamic status of the patient on presentation, although splenic injury grade, patient age, associated injuries, and institutional specific resources must be taken in consideration.

9.5.2 Anatomy

The splenic artery, a branch of the coeliac axis, provides the principal blood supply to the spleen. The artery gives rise to a superior polar artery, from which the short gastric arteries arise. The splenic artery also gives rise to superior and inferior terminal branches that enter the splenic hilum. The artery and the splenic vein are embedded in the superior border of the pancreas.

Three splenic suspensory ligaments maintain the intimate association between the spleen and the diaphragm (lienophrenic ligament), left kidney (lienorenal ligament) and splenic flexure of the colon (lienoocolic ligament). The gastrosplenic ligament contains the short gastric arteries. These attachments place the spleen at risk of avulsion during rapid deceleration. The spleen is also relatively delicate and can be damaged by impact from the overlying ribs.

9.5.3 Diagnosis

9.5.3.1 CLINICAL

The patient may complain of left upper quadrant pain or referred pain to the left shoulder, and there may be local tenderness. Signs of hypovolaemia (tachycardia or hypotension) might be present.

9.5.3.2 ULTRASOUND

Ultrasonic diagnosis has the great advantage that it can be performed in the emergency room during resuscitation. Focused abdominal sonography for trauma (FAST) ultrasound can detect free fluid around the spleen and in the paracolic gutter, indicating splenic injury. It will not show whether active arterial bleeding is taking place.

9.5.3.3 COMPUTED TOMOGRAPHY (CT) SCAN

In the haemodynamically stable patient with blunt abdominal trauma, CT scan is the preferred diagnostic modality to identify and grade splenic injury. CT will show the parenchymal lesions and any blood collection, and a contrast blush will indicate whether there is still active bleeding. If so, angiography with embolization (AE) should be considered if available.

9.5.4 Splenic Injury Scale[1]

The Organ Injury Scale of the American Association for the Surgery of Trauma is based on the most accurate assessment of injury, whether it is by radiological study, laparotomy, laparoscopy, or autopsy evaluation (Table 9.5.1).

9.5.5 Management

9.5.5.1 NON-OPERATIVE MANAGEMENT[2]

The approach of NOM for blunt splenic injuries in the paediatric population is well described, with a splenic preservation rate of more than 90%. Stimulated by the success of NOM in children, there has been a similar trend in haemodynamically stable adults with splenic injury. The advantages of NOM include the avoidance of non-therapeutic laparotomies with their associated cost and morbidity, a lower rate of intra-abdominal complications and reduced transfusion risk.

After resuscitation and completion of the trauma work-up, haemodynamically stable patients will undergo CT scan. Patients with grade I, II, or III splenic injuries, who have no associated intra-abdominal injuries requiring surgical intervention, and no co-morbidities to preclude close observation, are obvious candidates for NOM. However, the failure rate of NOM for splenic

injuries in adults increases with the grade of splenic injury. Associated injuries must be excluded on admission.[3]

Angiographic embolization, if available, is a useful adjunct to NOM.[4,5] The indications include evidence of ongoing bleeding with a significant drop in haemoglobin level and tachycardia, or contrast extravasation outside or within the spleen on CT as well as formation of a pseudoaneurysm.

Patients with high grade splenic injuries treated non-operatively should be monitored closely to detect any signs that indicate the need for intervention. There is, however, no evidence that bed rest or restricted activity is beneficial. Moreover, there is little evidence to support the use of serial CT scans, without clinical indications, to monitor progress.[6]

The advantages of NOM include the avoidance of non-therapeutic laparotomies (with associated cost and morbidity), fewer intra-abdominal complications, and reduced transfusion risk. The risk of delayed re-bleeding of the spleen after non-operative management is acceptably low, reportedly in the range of 1%–8%. Rebleed is considered more likely if a higher-grade injury (grade IV/V) has been managed non-operatively. However, prophylactic AE of the splenic artery in adults with grade IV and V injuries has been reported to result in a NOM success rate of 96% (Table 9.5.2).[3]

9.5.5.2 OPERATIVE MANAGEMENT

If a patient with splenic injury is haemodynamically unstable, operative treatment is necessary. Although splenic preservation is desirable, most patients who require an operation due to splenic bleeding will have a splenectomy performed.

Non-operative management is contraindicated and urgent open surgical intervention is indicated[7] when there is:

- Haemodynamic instability.
- Risk of concurrent abdominal hollow organ injury, or associated intra-abdominal injury requiring surgery.
- Evidence of continued splenic haemorrhage.
- Replacement of greater than 50% of the patient's blood volume.

9.5.6 Surgical Approach

Access to the spleen in trauma is best performed via a long midline incision. When indicated, the spleen is

Table 9.5.1 Splenic Injury Scale 2018 Revision

AAST Grade	AIS Severity	Imaging Criteria (CT Findings)	Operative Goals	Pathologic Criteria
I	2	**Haematoma** Subcapsular haematoma <10% surface area **Laceration** Parenchymal laceration <1 cm depth	**Haematoma** Subcapsular haematoma <10% surface area **Laceration** Parenchymal laceration <1 cm depth Capsular tear	**Haematoma** Subcapsular haematoma <10% surface area **Laceration** Parenchymal laceration <1 cm depth Capsular tear
II	2	**Haematoma** Subcapsular haematoma 10%–50% surface area; Intraparenchymal haematoma <5 cm in **Laceration** Laceration 1–3 cm	**Haematoma** Subcapsular haematoma 10%–50% surface area Intraparenchymal haematoma <5 cm in diameter **Laceration** 1–3 cm	**Haematoma** Subcapsular haematoma 10%–50% surface area Intraparenchymal haematoma <5 cm in diameter **Laceration** Laceration 1–3 cm depth
III	3	**Haematoma** Subcapsular haematoma >50%, surface area; Ruptured subcapsular or intraparenchymal haematoma ≥5 cm **Laceration** Parenchymal laceration >3 cm depth Any injury in the presence of a liver vascular injury or active bleeding contained within liver parenchyma	**Haematoma** Subcapsular haematoma >50%, surface area; Ruptured subcapsular or intraparenchymal haematoma ≥5 cm **Laceration** Laceration >3 cm in depth	**Haematoma** Subcapsular haematoma >50%, surface area; Ruptured subcapsular or intraparenchymal haematoma ≥5 cm **Laceration** Parenchymal laceration >3 cm depth
IV	4	**Laceration** Parenchymal laceration involving segmental or hilar vessels producing >25% devascularisation **Disruption** Any injury in the presence of a splenic vascular injury, or active bleeding confined within the splenic capsule	**Laceration** Parenchymal laceration involving segmental or hilar vessels producing >25% devascularisation	**Laceration** Parenchymal laceration involving segmental or hilar vessels producing >25% devascularisation
V	5	**Vascular injury** Any injury in the presence of splenic vascular injury with active bleeding extending beyond the spleen into the peritoneum **Disruption** Shattered spleen	**Vascular injury** Hilar vascular injury which devascularises the spleen **Disruption** Shattered spleen	**Vascular injury** Hilar vascular injury which devascularises the spleen **Disruption** Shattered spleen

Note: Vascular injury is defined as a pseudoaneurysm or arteriovenous fistula and appears as a focal collection of vascular contrast that decreases in attenuation with delayed imaging. Active bleeding from a vascular injury presents as vascular contrast, focal or diffuse, that increases in size or attenuation in delayed phase. Vascular thrombosis can lead to organ infarction.

Grade based on highest grade assessment made on imaging, at operation, or on pathologic specimen.

More than one grade of splenic injury may be present and should be classified by the higher grade of injury.

Advance one grade for multiple injuries up to a grade III.

Table 9.5.2 Evidence-Based Guidelines for Selective Non-Operative Management of Splenic Injury

Level of Evidence	Recommendation
I	Patients who have diffuse peritonitis or who are haemodynamically unstable after blunt abdominal trauma should be taken urgently for laparotomy.
II	1. A routine laparotomy is not indicated in the haemodynamically stable patient without peritonitis presenting with an isolated splenic injury. 2. The severity of splenic injury (as suggested by CT grade or degree of haemoperitoneum), neurologic status, age >55 and/or the presence of associated injuries are not contraindications to a trial of non-operative management in a haemodynamically stable patient. 3. In the haemodynamically normal blunt abdominal trauma patient without peritonitis, an abdominal CT scan with intravenous contrast should be performed to identify and assess the severity of injury to the spleen. 4. Angiography should be considered for patients with American Association for the Surgery of Trauma (AAST) grade of greater than III injuries, presence of a contrast blush, moderate haemoperitoneum, or evidence of ongoing splenic bleeding. 5. Non-operative management of splenic injuries should only be considered in an environment that provides capabilities for monitoring, serial clinical evaluations, and an operating room available for urgent laparotomy.
III	1. After blunt splenic injury, clinical factors such as a persistent systemic inflammatory response, increasing/persistent abdominal pain, or an otherwise unexplained drop in haemoglobin should dictate the frequency of and need for follow-up imaging for a patient with blunt splenic injury. 2. Contrast blush on CT scan alone is not an absolute indication for an operation or angiographic intervention. Factors such as patient age, grade of injury, and presence of hypotension need to be considered in the clinical management of these patients. 3. Angiography may be used either as an adjunct to non-operative management for patients who are thought to be at high risk for delayed bleeding or as an investigative tool to identify vascular abnormalities such as pseudoaneurysms that pose a risk for delayed haemorrhage. 4. Pharmacologic prophylaxis to prevent venous thromboembolism can be used for patients with isolated blunt splenic injuries without increasing the failure rate of non-operative management, although the optimal timing of safe initiation has not been determined.
Unanswered Questions	1. Frequency of haemoglobin measurements. 2. Frequency of abdominal examinations. 3. Intensity and duration of monitoring. 4. Is there a transfusion trigger after which operative or angiographic intervention should be considered? 5. Time to reinitiating oral intake. 6. The duration and intensity of restricted activity (both in-hospital and after discharge). 7. Optimum length of stay for both the intensive care unit (ICU) and hospital. 8. Necessity of repeated imaging. 9. Timing of initiating chemical deep venous thrombosis (DVT) prophylaxis after a splenic injury. 10. Should patients with severe injuries/or embolized injuries receive post-splenectomy vaccines? 11. Is there an immunologic deficiency after splenic embolization?

Source: Stassen NA et al. *J Trauma.* 2012;73(5):S294–300. Available from: www.east.org (accessed online January 2015).

mobilized under direct vision. In paediatric patients, a midline incision should also be used, rather than a subcostal incision, since there is better access to the entire abdominal cavity if there is injury to other intra-abdominal structures.

The spleen is best approached by a surgeon standing on patient's right-hand side. The table can be rotated slightly to the right. The spleen is mobilized under direct vision. Great care and gentle handling are necessary to avoid pulling on the spleen, avulsing the capsule, making a minor injury worse by stripping the capsule off the lower pole.

Medial traction by the operator's non-dominant hand will give access to the lienophrenic, lienorenal, and lienocolic ligaments.

- The spleen is gently pulled upwards and medially, and the lienorenal and lienocolic ligaments are divided.
- The spleen is then gently pulled downwards, and the lienophrenic ligaments are divided with scissors, close to the spleen, between the spleen and the diaphragm.
- The short gastric vessels between the greater curvature of the stomach and the spleen must be divided between ligatures. These vessels must be divided *away* from the greater curvature, as there is a danger of avascular necrosis of the stomach if they are divided too close to the stomach itself.
- The spleen is pulled forward, and several packs can be placed in the splenic bed to hold it forward so that it can be inspected.

In the presence of other competing other major injuries, haemodynamic instability or if the spleen has sustained damage at the hilum, a routine splenectomy should be performed. In the stable patient and in the absence of other life-threatening injuries, splenic preservation should be considered.

9.5.6.1 SPLEEN NOT ACTIVELY BLEEDING

If not actively bleeding, the spleen can be left alone.

9.5.6.2 SPLENIC SURFACE BLEED ONLY

These bleeds will usually stop with a combination of manual compression, packing, diathermy, argon beam, or fibrin adhesives in combination with collagen fleece.

9.5.6.3 MINOR LACERATIONS

These may be sutured using absorbable sutures, with or without Teflon pledgets. Suturing is time-consuming and mostly not helpful in trauma patients. The superficial lacerations are best treated with fibrin adhesive and collagen tamponade. These measures are best taken at the beginning of the operation and the spleen packed; upon completion of the operation, the pack can be removed without displacing the collagen fleece.

9.5.6.4 SPLENIC TEARS

If the lacerations are deep and involve both the concave and convex surfaces, the spleen is best and most effectively preserved with a mesh splenorrhaphy. If the lacerations involve only one pole or one half of the organ, the respective vessels should be ligated, and a partial splenectomy performed. Owing to the technical problems, these are rarely used.

9.5.6.5 PARTIAL SPLENECTOMY

This is *rarely* used in the trauma patient. Injuries involving only one pole of the spleen can be treated with partial resection. Prior to resection, the spleen should be mobilized. Stapler resection makes organ conservation possible in many cases, and it represents a valuable alternative to sutured partial splenectomy or splenorrhaphy. Its greatest advantages are simplicity of use, the practicality of the instrument itself and the reduction in time and blood transfusion.

9.5.6.6 MESH WRAP

If the spleen is viable, it can be wrapped in an absorbable mesh to tamponade the bleeding.

The prerequisite for mesh splenorrhaphy is complete mobilization and elevation of the spleen. An absorbable mesh should be chosen (e.g. Vicryl®).

9.5.6.7 SPLENECTOMY

In the presence of other major injuries, with haemodynamic instability or if the spleen has sustained damage at the hilum, a routine splenectomy should be carried out following careful mobilization of the spleen.

Access to the splenic pedicle can be anterior or posterior. Care must be taken to avoid injuring the tail of the pancreas, which lies very close to the hilum of the spleen.

Table 9.5.3 Post-Splenectomy Vaccination Guidelines	
Evidence	**Recommendation**
Level 1	• None
Level 2	• Non-elective splenectomy patients should be vaccinated at least 14 days post-splenectomy or at time of discharge from the hospital. • Asplenic patients should be re-vaccinated at the appropriate time interval for each vaccine.

Level 3	• Asplenic or immunocompromised patients (with an intact but non-functional spleen) should be vaccinated as soon as the diagnosis is made.
	• When adult vaccination is indicated, the following FIVE vaccinations should be administered:
	  ○ Pneumococcal vaccine naïve: Conjugate pneumococcal vaccine (PCV13) followed by polyvalent pneumococcal vaccine (PPSV23) ≥8 weeks later.
	  ○ Previous PPSV23 vaccination: PCV13 ≥1 year after PPSV23.
	  ○ MenACWY (Menactra®), two doses, given at least two months apart.
	  ○ MenB-FHbp (three-dose series) at 0, 2, and 6 months OR MenB-04C (two dose series) at least one month apart.
	  ○ *Haemophius influenzae b vaccine* (HibTITER).
	• Paediatric vaccination should be performed according to the recommended paediatric dosage and vaccine types with special consideration made for children less than 2 years of age.

Vaccine	Dose (mL)	Route	Re-vaccination
13-valent pneumococcal (PCV13, Prevnar 13)	0.5	IM	None
23 valent pneumococcal (PPSV23, Pneumovax®)	0.5	IM or SC	Once at 5 years
Meningococcal/diphtheria conjugate (MENACWY)	0.5	IM	At 2 months and every 5 years
Serogroup B Meningococcal (MENB-FHbp)	0.5	IM	At 2 months and 6 months
Serogroup B Meningococcal (MENB-4C)	0.5	IM	Once at ≥1 month
Haemophilus b conjugate	0.5	IM	None

9.5.6.8 DRAINAGE

The splenic bed is *not* routinely drained after splenectomy. If the tail of the pancreas has been damaged, a closed suction drain should be placed in the area affected.

9.5.7 Outcome

• Many publications support NOM in the haemodynamically stable patient, with a high success rate. The risk of delayed rebleeding of the spleen after NOM is acceptably low, reportedly in the range 1%–8%.
• Subphrenic abscess can be seen in patients treated operatively, but may be treated by percutaneous drainage.
• Pleural effusion, pulmonary atelectasis, and pneumonia are not uncommon in patients treated either non-operatively or operatively.
• Pseudoaneurysm development can be successfully treated with embolization.

• After splenectomy, there is a small but lifelong risk of overwhelming post-splenectomy sepsis. Patients should be informed of the defect in their immune system and be encouraged to keep their pneumococcus and influenza immunizations current. These patients are more susceptible to malaria than the rest of the population.[8,9]

See Table 9.5.3: Post-Splenectomy Vaccination Guidelines.

9.5.8 Opportunistic Post-Splenectomy Infection

If the spleen is removed, or devascularized, resulting in functional asplenia, the loss of function places the individual at high risk of infection with the risk of opportunistic post-splenectomy infection (OPSI) by organisms such as *Streptococcus pneumoniae*, *Haemophylus influenzae* type B, and *Neisseria meningitidis*. The incidence is estimated at 0.05%–2% of such patients, with a mortality reportedly as high as 50%.

REFERENCES AND RECOMMENDED READING

References

1. Kozar RA, Crandall M, Shanmuganathan K, Zarzaur B, Coburn M, Cribari C, et al. Organ injury scaling 2018 update: Spleen, liver and kidney. *J Trauma Acute Care Surgery.* 2018 Dec;**85(6)**:1119–1122. doi: 10.1097/TA.000 0000000002058.

2. Stassen NA; Bhullar I, Cheng JD, et al. Practice Management Guidelines for the selective nonoperative management of blunt splenic injury. *J Trauma.* 2012;**73(5)**:S294–S300, Available from www.east.org (accessed January 2015).

3. Skattum J, Naess PA, Eken T, Gaarder C. Refining the role of splenic angiographic embolization in high-grade splenic injuries. *J Trauma Acute Care Surg.* 2013;**74(1)**:100–3; discussion 103-4.

4. Haan JM, Biffl W, Knudson MM, et al. Splenic Embolization Revisited: A Multicenter Review. *J Trauma.* 2004;**56**:542–547.

5. Raikhlin A, Baerlocher MO, Asch O, Myers A. Imaging and transcatheter arterial embolization for traumatic splenic injuries: review of the literature. *Can J Surg.* 2008;**51**:464–472.

6. Haan JM. Follow-up abdominal CT is not necessary in low-grade splenic injury. *Am Surg.* 2007;**73**:13–18.

7. Peizman AB, Harbrecht BG, Rivera L, Heil B. Failure of observation of blunt splenic injury in adults: variability in practice and adverse consequences. *J Am Coll Surg.* 2005;**201**:179–87.

8. Shatz DV. Vaccination practices among North American trauma surgeons in splenectomy for trauma. *J Trauma.* 2002;**53**:950–56.

9. Post-Splenectomy Vaccine Prophylaxis. A surgicalcritical-care.net guideline. 2015 Jul; Available from: http://www.surgicalcriticalcare.net/Guidelines/post%20splenectomy%20vaccines%202015.pdf (accessed online Dec 2018).

Recommended Reading

Peitzman AB, Heil B, Rivera L, et al. Blunt splenic injury in adults: multi-institutional study of the Eastern Association for the Surgery of Trauma. *J Trauma.* 2000;**49**:177–87.

Savage SA, Zarzaur BL, Magnotti LJ, et al. The evolution of blunt splenic injury: resolution and progression. *J Trauma.* 2008;**64**:1085–92.

Smith J, Armen S, Cook CH, Martin LC. Blunt splenic injuries: have we watched long enough? *J Trauma.* 2008;**64**:656–65.

9.6 Pancreas

9.6.1 **Overview**

Pancreatic and combined pancreaticoduodenal injuries remain a dilemma for most surgeons and, despite advances and complex technical solutions, they still carry a high morbidity and mortality. The increase in penetrating injuries throughout the world, and the increase in wounding energy from gunshots, has made the incidence of pancreatic injury more common. Pancreatic injury must be suspected in all patients with abdominal injuries, even those who initially have few signs. Since the pancreas is retroperitoneal, it usually does not present with peritonitis. It requires a high level of suspicion and significant clinical acumen, as well as aggressive radiographic imaging to identify an injury early.

The pancreas and duodenum are difficult areas for surgical exposure and represent a major challenge for the operating surgeon when these organs are substantially injured. Although the retroperitoneal location of the pancreas means that it is commonly injured, its position also contributes to the difficulty in diagnosis as the organ is concealed, resulting in delay in diagnosis, with an attendant increase in morbidity.

Management varies from simple drainage to highly challenging procedures depending on the severity, the site of the injury, and the integrity of the duct. Accurate intra-operative investigation of the pancreatic duct is particularly challenging. To compound this, pancreatic trauma is associated with a high incidence of injury to adjoining organs (duodenum, kidney, liver) and major vascular structures, which adds to the high morbidity and mortality.[1]

The surgeon must always be critically aware of the patient's changing physiological state and be prepared to forsake the technical challenge of definitive repair for life-saving damage control.

9.6.2 **Anatomy**

The pancreas lies at the level of the pylorus and crosses the first and second lumbar vertebrae. It is about 15 cm long from the duodenum to the hilum of the spleen, 3 cm wide and up to 1.5 cm thick. The head lies within the concavity formed by the duodenum, with which it shares its blood supply through the pancreaticoduodenal arcades.

The pancreas has an intimate anatomical relationship with the upper abdominal vessels. It overlies the inferior vena cava, the right renal vessels, and the left renal vein. The uncinate process encircles the superior mesenteric artery and vein, while the body covers the suprarenal aorta and left renal vessels. The tail is closely related to the splenic hilum and left kidney, and overlies the splenic artery and vein, with the artery marking a tortuous path at the superior border of the pancreas.

There are several named arterial branches to the head, body and tail that must be ligated in spleen-sparing procedures. Studies have shown that between seven and 10 branches of the splenic artery, and 13–22 branches of the splenic vein run into the pancreas.

9.6.3 **Mechanisms of Injury**

9.6.3.1 BLUNT TRAUMA

The relatively protected location of the pancreas means that a high-energy force is required to damage it. Most injuries result from motor vehicle accidents in which the energy of the impact is directed to the upper abdomen – epigastrium or hypochondrium – commonly through the steering wheel of an automobile. This force results in crushing of the retroperitoneal structures against the vertebral column, which can lead to a spectrum of injury from contusion to complete transection of the body of the pancreas.

9.6.3.2 PENETRATING TRAUMA

The rising incidence of penetrating trauma has increased the incidence of injury to the pancreas. A stab wound damages tissue only along the track of the knife, but in gunshot wounds the passage of the missile and its pressure wave will result in injury to a wider region. Consequently, the pancreas and its duct must be fully assessed for damage in any penetrating wound that approaches the substance of the gland. Injuries to the pancreatic duct occur in 15% of cases of pancreatic trauma and are usually a consequence of penetrating trauma.

9.6.4 **Diagnosis**

The central retroperitoneal location of the pancreas makes the investigation of pancreatic trauma a diagnostic challenge: the specific diagnosis is often unsuspected, until laparotomy, especially if there are competing life-threatening vascular and other intra-abdominal organ injuries. In recent years, there has been debate about the need for accurate assessment of the integrity of the main pancreatic duct. Bradley[2] showed that mortality and morbidity were increased when there was failure or delay in recognising ductal injury. When these results are reviewed in conjunction with earlier work, that showed an increase in late complications if ductal injuries were missed,[3] the importance of evaluating the duct is evident.

9.6.4.1 CLINICAL EVALUATION

In a patient with an isolated pancreatic injury, even ductal transection may be initially asymptomatic or have only minor signs, and the possibility must be kept in mind. Clinical examination is notoriously *unreliable*.

9.6.4.2 SERUM AMYLASE AND SERUM LIPASE

The level of the serum amylase and serum lipase is not related to pancreatic injury in either blunt or penetrating trauma. A summary on serum amylase in blunt abdominal trauma by Biffl[4] showed a positive predictive value of 10% and a negative predictive value of 95% for pancreatic injury, although more recent work has suggested that accuracy may be improved when the activity is measured more than 3 hours after injury.[5] At present, serum amylase has little value in the initial evaluation of pancreatic injury. There is increasing interest in the value of lipase in trauma but to date there remains little data to support this and neither should be relied upon to rule out pancreatic injury.

9.6.4.3 ULTRASOUND

The posterior position of the pancreas almost completely masks it from diagnostic ultrasound.

9.6.4.4 DIAGNOSTIC PERITONEAL LAVAGE (DPL)

DPL has been largely superseded. The retroperitoneal location of the pancreas renders diagnostic peritoneal lavage inaccurate in the prediction of isolated pancreatic injury. However, the numerous associated injuries that may occur with pancreatic injury may make the lavage diagnostic if the level of the amylase in the lavage fluid is checked.

9.6.4.5 COMPUTED TOMOGRAPHY

CT scan has been advocated as the best investigation for evaluation of the retroperitoneum. In a haemodynamically stable patient, CT scanning with contrast enhancement has a sensitivity and specificity as high as 80%. However, particularly in the initial phase, CT scanning may miss or underestimate the severity of a pancreatic injury,[6] so normal findings on the initial scan do not exclude appreciable pancreatic injury, and a repeat scan in the light of continuing symptoms may improve its diagnostic ability.

9.6.4.6 ENDOSCOPIC RETROGRADE CHOLANGIOPANCREATOGRAPHY

There are two phases in the investigation of pancreatic injury in which endoscopic retrograde cholangiopancreatography (ERCP) may have a role.[7]

9.6.4.6.1 Acute Presentation

A very small number of patients with isolated pancreatic trauma occasionally have initially benign clinical findings. ERCP has no practical role in the investigation of pancreatic duct injury in the acute phase as most patients will not be stable enough and their injuries will not allow positioning for ERCP. In those patients who do not settle with conservative management and there is suspicion of ductal injury, ERCP will give detailed information about the ductal system although cannulation of the pancreatic duct can itself cause pancreatitis. There is increasing discussion of the role of ERCP placed pancreatic duct stents for ductal injury; however, there is limited literature to support this.

9.6.4.6.2 Delayed Presentation

A small number of patients present with symptoms months to years after the initial injury potentially with a retroperitoneal collection or pancreatic fistula. Magnetic resonance cholangiopancreatography (MRCP) is likely to be the initial investigation however ERCP can be used to assess the integrity of the duct and consider pancreatic duct stenting.

9.6.4.7 MAGNETIC RESONANCE CHOLANGIOPANCREATOGRAPHY

MRCP is the mainstay of evaluation of the pancreaticobiliary tree in the non-acute setting. There is no role in the initial evaluation of the injured patient, but there is value in the assessment for ductal injury in those patients who have developed a complication such as a pseudocyst or pancreatic fistula.[8] MRCP can allow better selection of patients with suspected injuries than can ERCP, because patients with an intact pancreatic duct or minor injury can be successfully treated conservatively. Some authors believe that it will have an increasing role in identifying patients who are unlikely to benefit from endoscopic intervention, those with an intact pancreatic duct (or very minor injury) and those with severe duct strictures or obstruction).

9.6.4.8 INTRA-OPERATIVE PANCREATOGRAPHY

Intra-operative visualization of the pancreatic duct has been advocated in the investigation of the duct, particularly when it is not possible to assess its integrity by examination. Nevertheless, in the opinion of Subramanian et al., simple examination of the area of injury for several minutes with loupe magnification reveals clear pancreatic fluid leakage in most injuries that involve the pancreatic duct.[9] An accurate assessment of the degree of injury to the duct will reduce the complication rate indicate the most appropriate operation and, when no involvement is found, allow a less aggressive procedure to be undertaken. However, the ductal system frequently cannot be found due to its small size in previously normal patients. Therefore, the invasive nature of intra-operative investigation by transduodenal pancreatic duct catheterization, distal cannulation of the duct in the tail, or needle cholecystocholangiogram makes this unattractive and rarely indicated.

Intra-operative ultrasound can be used to help diagnose a parenchymal or ductal laceration.[10]

9.6.4.9 OPERATIVE EVALUATION

Operative evaluation of the pancreas necessitates complete exposure of the organ. A central retroperitoneal haematoma must be thoroughly investigated, and intra-abdominal bile staining makes a complete evaluation essential to find the pancreatic or duodenal injury. In this case, a ductal injury must be assumed until excluded.

If the sphincter of Oddi and the distal biliary tract are intact, it is wise to attempt to preserve the head and neck of the pancreas. Major injuries to the body of the pancreas are usually treated by a distal pancreatectomy with splenectomy. If the injury is to the head of the pancreas, involving the duct and sphincter, a Whipple procedure must be contemplated. Increasingly, there is a move toward lesser procedures since the mortality of a Whipple procedure continues to be significant in the severely injured trauma patient. These injuries continue to be a major challenge for the trauma surgeon. It is essential to understand the manoeuvres necessary for gaining complete control of the duodenum and pancreas in order to completely explore and identify any injuries.

9.6.5 Pancreas Injury Scale

The organ injury scale developed by the American Association for the Surgery of Trauma (AAST)[11] has been accepted by most institutions that regularly deal with pancreatic trauma (Table 9.6.1).

9.6.6 Management

9.6.6.1 NON-OPERATIVE MANAGEMENT

In isolated blunt pancreatic injuries, exclusion of a major pancreatic duct injury with ERCP followed by expectant non-operative management is gaining popularity. Recent reports utilizing early ERCP to identify and sometimes treat blunt pancreatic injuries by transpapillary stent insertion are showing promising results,[12,13] and can decrease the incidence of pancreatic-related complications and failure rate of non-operative management. A pancreatic duct stent appears useful for a proximal pancreatic fistula, but may be complicated by a long-term stricture, whereas ductal stenting in the acute phase is potentially dangerous in that it may lead to a delay in necessary laparotomy and definitive repair of the pancreatic injury.[14] Because of the small size of the pancreatic duct distal to the ampulla, stenting is ordinarily not used in this location.[15] Recent evidence suggests that endoscopic interventions are more successful in managing pancreatic fistulae and pseudocysts than in managing patients with main pancreatic duct stricture.[9,15]

NOM of low-grade (grades I and II) blunt pancreaticoduodenal injuries is safe despite occasional failures. Missed diagnosis continues to occur despite advances in CT scanning, but does not seem to cause an adverse outcome in most patients.[16] The vogue for conservative management of body and tail pancreatic duct injury has more recently been challenged with distal pancreatectomy shown to have relatively low morbidity and mortality.

Grade[a]	Type of Injury	Description of Injury
Table 9.6.1 Pancreas Injury Scale		
I	Haematoma	Minor contusion without duct injury
	Laceration	Superficial laceration without duct injury
II	Haematoma	Major contusion without duct injury or tissue loss
	Laceration	Major laceration without duct injury or tissue loss
III	Laceration	Distal transection or parenchymal injury with duct injury
IV	Laceration	Proximal[b] transection or parenchymal injury involving the ampulla
V	Laceration	Massive disruption of the pancreatic head

Note: See also Appendix B.
[a] Advance one grade for multiple injuries up to grade III.
[b] The proximal pancreas is deemed to be that part of the pancreas to the *right* of the superior mesenteric artery and vein.

9.6.6.2 OPERATIVE MANAGEMENT

Many pancreatic injuries will only be confirmed following a CT scan, or at the time of surgery. The surgical approach is often for that of the presenting sign (e.g. peritonitis), and the pancreatic injury will be found at laparotomy. Commonly, there are associated injuries of the duodenum, bowel mesentery, etc.

9.6.7 Surgical Approach

9.6.7.1 INCISION AND EXPLORATION (SEE ALSO SECTION 9.1)

Access to the pancreas in trauma is gained via a long midline incision.

Penetrating pancreatic trauma should be obvious. Once the retroperitoneum has been violated in penetrating trauma, it is imperative for the surgeon to do a thorough exploration of the central region.

Diagnosis of blunt pancreatic trauma is much more problematic. As the pancreas is a retroperitoneal organ, there may be no anterior peritoneal signs. The history can be helpful if information from the paramedics indicates that the vehicle's steering column was bent, or if the patient can give a history of epigastric trauma.

For complete evaluation of the gland, it is essential to see the pancreas from both the anterior and posterior aspects. To examine the anterior surface of the gland, it is necessary to divide the gastrocolic ligament and open the lesser sac. An extended Kocher manoeuvre is required so that the duodenum can be mobilized and an adequate view gained of the pancreatic head, uncinate process, and posterior aspect. Injury to the tail requires mobilization of the spleen and left colon to allow medial reflection of the pancreas and access to the splenic vessels. Division of the ligament of Treitz and reflection of the fourth part of the duodenum and duodenojejunal flexure gives access to the inferior aspect of the pancreas. Any parenchymal haematoma of the pancreas should be thoroughly explored, including irrigation of the haematoma, to exclude possible injury of the duct.

9.6.7.1.1 Access via the Lesser Sac

The stomach is then grasped and pulled inferiorly, allowing the operator to identify the lesser curvature and the pancreas through the lesser sac. Frequently, the coeliac artery and the body of the pancreas can be identified through this approach. The omentum is then grasped and drawn upwards. An otomy is made in the omentum, and the operator's hand is passed into the lesser sac posterior to the stomach. This allows excellent exposure of the entire body and tail of the pancreas. Any injuries to the pancreas can be easily identified.

9.6.7.1.2 Duodenal Rotation (Kocher's Manoeuvre)

If there is the possibility of an injury to the head of the pancreas, a Kocher manoeuvre is performed. The loose areolar of tissue around the duodenum is bluntly dissected, and the entire second and third portions of the duodenum re-identified and mobilized medially. This dissection is carried all the way medially to expose the inferior vena cava and a portion of the aorta. By reflecting the duodenum and pancreas toward the anterior midline, the posterior surface of the head of the pancreas can be completely inspected.

9.6.7.1.3 Right Medial Visceral Rotation

The inferior border of the proximal portion of the pancreas can be identified by performing a right medial visceral rotation. This is performed by taking down the ascending colon and then mobilizing the caecum, the terminal ileum, and the mesentery toward the midline. The entire ascending colon and caecum are then reflected superiorly towards the left upper quadrant of the abdomen. This gives excellent exposure of the entire vena cava, the aorta, and the third and fourth portions of the duodenum.

9.6.7.1.4 Left Medial Visceral Rotation

The descending colon on the left is mobilized, together with the spleen and the tail of the pancreas. These are rotated medially, allowing inspection of the tail and posterior and inferior aspects of the pancreas.

These manoeuvres allow for complete exposure of the first, second, third, and fourth portions of the duodenum along with the head, neck, body, and tail of the pancreas.

When pancreatic injury is suspected, extended exploration of the whole organ is imperative. Parenchymal lacerations that do not involve the pancreatic duct can be sutured when the tissue is not too soft and vulnerable. With or without the use of sutures, a worthwhile option in the treatment of such lacerations is fibrin sealing and collagen tamponade, and adequate drainage is essential.

9.6.7.2 PANCREATIC INJURY: SURGICAL DECISION-MAKING

9.6.7.2.1 Contusion and Parenchymal Injuries

Relatively minor pancreatic lacerations and contusions (AAST grades I and II) comprise most injuries to the pancreas. If there is obvious disruption to the pancreatic duct, it should be ligated with distal pancreatic resection and in the unstable trauma patient with splenectomy.

> **Pitfall**
>
> Suturing of parenchymal lesions (AAST grades I and II) to gain haemostasis simply leads to necrosis of the pancreatic tissue.

9.6.7.2.2 Drainage Alone

Injuries to the tail and body of the pancreas that do not involve the duct can be drained, and with haemostasis this has become standard practice. Suction drainage should be used, as fewer intra-abdominal abscesses develop and there is less skin excoriation with a closed suction system.[18]

9.6.7.2.3 Distal Pancreatectomy

In most cases in which there is a major parenchymal injury of the pancreas to the left of the superior mesenteric vessels (AAST grades II or III), a distal pancreatectomy is the procedure of choice, independent of the degree of ductal involvement. After mobilization of the pancreas and ligation of the vessels, the pancreatic stump can be closed with sutures and the duct ligated separately, or it can be closed with a stapling device. A drain should be placed at the site of transection as there is a postoperative fistula rate of 14%. Suction drains are again preferable.

> **Pitfall**
>
> Avoid the use of a linear guillotine stapler (GIA type), as the margin between the cutr edge and the very small staples is unsafe. Rather, use a transverse anastomosis (TA type) staple, and all 5 mm of tissue at the cut edge, outside of the staples.

Most authors agree that a pancreatectomy to the *left* of the superior mesenteric vessels usually leaves enough pancreatic tissue resulting in an acceptably low rate of insulin-dependent diabetes. Procedures associated with resection of greater than 80% of the pancreatic tissue are associated with a risk of adult-onset diabetes mellitus.

9.6.6.2.4 Splenic Salvage in Distal Pancreatectomy

Splenic salvage has been advocated where possible, in *elective* distal pancreatectomy. However, this should be saved for the rare occasions when the patient is haemodynamically stable, and the injury is limited to the pancreas.

> **Pitfall**
>
> The technical problems of dissecting the pancreas free from the splenic vessels and ligating the numerous tributaries make the procedure contraindicated in an unstable patient with multiple associated injuries. When this operation is considered, the surgeon must clearly balance the extra time that it takes and the problems associated with lengthy operations in injured patients against the small risk of the development of OPSI post-operatively.

9.6.7.2.5 Ductal Injuries: Combined Injuries of the Head of the Pancreas and Duodenum

The injuries that vex the surgeon most, however, are those to the head of the gland, particularly those juxtaposed with, or also involving the duodenum. Resection (Whipple procedure) is usually reserved for those patients who have destructive injuries or those in whom the blood supply to the duodenum and pancreatic head has been compromised. As assessment of the damage is often difficult, damage control surgery is usually required, with preservation of all potentially viable tissue.

Severe combined pancreaticoduodenal injuries account for less than 10% of injuries to these organs, and are commonly associated with multiple intra-abdominal injuries, particularly of the vena cava.[19] They are usually the result of penetrating trauma. The integrity of the distal common bile duct and ampulla on cholangiography, and the severity of the duodenal injury, will dictate the operative procedure. If the duct and ampulla are intact, simple repair with variations of drainage and pyloric exclusion. This includes extensive closed (suction) drainage around the injury site. Common duct drainage is not indicated.

9.6.7.2.6 Damage Control

Patients with severe pancreatic or pancreaticoduodenal injury (AAST grades IV and V) are not stable enough to undergo complex reconstruction at the time of initial laparotomy. Damage control with the rapid arrest of

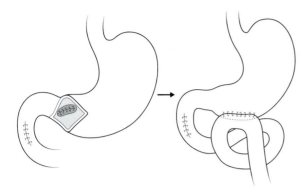

Figure 9.6.1 Pyloric exclusion and gastric bypass.

haemorrhage and bacterial contamination, and placement of drains and packing, is preferable. It may be helpful to place a tube drain directly into the duct, both for drainage and to allow easier isolation of the duct at the subsequent operation. The damage control laparotomy is followed by a period of intensive care and continued aggressive resuscitation to correct physiological abnormalities and restore reserve before the definitive procedure.

9.6.7.2.7 Pyloric Exclusion[17]

Pyloric exclusion has been widely reported for the management of severe combined pancreaticoduodenal injuries without major damage to the ampulla or the common bile duct. The rationale is to minimize exocrine pancreatic stimulation caused by gastric acid, and filling of the duodenum. The technique involves the temporary diversion of enteric flow away from the injured duodenum by closure of the pylorus. This is best achieved with access from the stomach through a gastrotomy and the use of a slowly absorbable suture. The alternative is a TA stapler across the pylorus. (NB: The GIA type of staple cannot be used owing to its integral guillotine) (Figure 9.6.1).

Contrast studies have shown that the pylorus re-opens within 2–3 weeks in 90%–95% of patients, allowing flow through the anatomical channel. The stomach is decompressed with a gastrojejunostomy.[21] Once the pylorus is open, the gastrojejunostomy usually closes spontaneously. There has been recent debate as to the need the procedure, since even a nasogastric tube and use of proton pump inhibitors will be as effective.[20] Although the technique remains controversial, pyloric exclusion may be a useful option for grade III and IV combined pancreaticoduodenal injuries.

9.6.7.2.8 T-Tube Drainage

Some surgeons advocate closing the injury over a T-tube in combined injuries where the second part of the duodenum is involved. This ensures adequate drainage and allows the formation of a controlled fistula once the track has matured.

9.6.7.2.9 Pancreaticoduodenectomy (Whipple's Procedure)

This is a major procedure to be practised in trauma only if no alternative is available[22] and will be required in less than 10% of combined injuries. Damage control with control of bleeding and of bowel contamination, and ligation of the common bile and pancreatic ducts should be the rule. Indications for considering a pancreaticoduodenectomy are massive disruption of the pancreaticoduodenal complex, devascularization of the duodenum, and sometimes extensive duodenal injuries of the second part of the duodenum involving the ampulla or distal common bile duct.

The Whipple procedure (as first described for carcinoma of the ampulla[23]), is indicated only in the rare stable patient with this type of injury. The nature and severity of the injury and the co-existing damage to vessels is often accompanied by haemodynamic instability, and the surgeon must therefore control the initial damage and delay formal reconstruction until the patient has been stabilized. The results of this operation vary, and when patients with major retroperitoneal vascular injuries are included. mortality can approach 50%. More recently in the largest series to date, patients who underwent a DCS or staged Whipple procedure for complex pancreaticoduodenal trauma and the largest series with blunt trauma, in-hospital mortality was 13%.[24]

Damage control is an integral part of the approach to these devastating injuries. Krige et al. have reported their use of DCS in pancreatic trauma, in a series of predominately penetrating trauma and associated vascular injury they reported a salvage rate of 45% using DCS.[25,26]

The role of pancreaticoduodenectomy in trauma is best summarized by Walt[27] in 1996:

Finally, to Whipple or not to Whipple, that is the question. In the massively destructive lesions involving the pancreas, duodenum and common bile duct, the decision to do a pancreaticoduodenectomy is unavoidable; and, in fact, much of the dissection may have been done by the wounding force. In a few patients, when the call is of necessity close, the overall physiologic status of the patient and the extent of damage become the determining factors in the decision. Though few in gross numbers, more patients are eventually salvaged by drainage, TPN [total parenteral nutrition] and meticulous overall care than by a desperate pancreaticoduodenectomy in a marginal patient.

9.6.8 Adjuncts

9.6.8.1 SOMATOSTATIN AND ITS ANALOGUES

Somatostatin and its analogue octreotide have been used to reduce pancreatic exocrine secretion in patients with acute pancreatitis. Despite meta-analysis, its role has not been clearly defined. Buchler et al.[28] reported a slight but not significant reduction in the complication rate in patients with moderate-to-severe pancreatitis, but this was not verified by Imrie's group in Glasgow,[29] who found that somatostatin gave no benefit.

Retrospective work on the role of octreotide in pancreatic trauma, however, differs. Somatostatin cannot be recommended in trauma on the current evidence, and a level 1 study is required.

9.6.8.2 NUTRITIONAL SUPPORT

Whether nutritional support is required should be considered at the definitive operation. Major injuries that precipitate prolonged gastric ileus and pancreatic complications may preclude gastric feeding. A feeding jejunostomy can be used but can lead to technical complications. Sometimes a long nasojejunal feeding catheter can be negotiated past the duodenojejunal flexure, providing a non-invasive alternative. The creation of a percutaneous feeding jejunostomy via the abdominal wall, with the tip sited 15–30 cm distal to the duodenojejunal flexure, will allow early enteral feeding. We prefer elemental diets that are less stimulating to the pancreas and have no greater fistula output than total parenteral nutrition. Total parenteral nutrition is far more expensive but may be used if enteral access distal to the duodenojejunal flexure is impossible.

9.6.9 Pancreatic Injury in Children

The pancreas is injured in up to 10% of cases of blunt abdominal trauma in children, usually as a result of a handlebar injury. Whether these children with high grade pancreatic injury should be operated upon or managed conservatively (the current vogue for the management of solid organ injuries in children) has been controversial. In most cases, a NOM approach is used,

although considerable variability exists regarding NOM strategies.[30] However, there are increasing advocates of distal pancreatectomy in children with body/tail transection providing an overall improved outcome.

9.6.10 Complications

Pancreatic trauma is associated with up to 19% mortality. Early deaths result from the associated intra-abdominal vascular and other organ injuries, and later deaths from sepsis and the systemic inflammatory response syndrome. Pancreatic injuries have post-operative complication rates of up to 42%, and the number rises with increasing severity of injury; with combined injuries and associated injuries, the complication rate approaches 62%.

Most complications are treatable or self-limiting, however, and could be avoided by an accurate assessment of whether the pancreatic duct was damaged pancreatic complications can be divided into those occurring early and those occurring late in the post-operative period.

9.6.10.1 EARLY COMPLICATIONS

9.6.10.1.1 Pancreatitis

Post-operative pancreatitis may develop in about 7% of patients. It may vary from a transient biochemical leak of amylase to a fulminant haemorrhagic pancreatitis. Fortunately, most cases run a benign course and respond to bowel rest and nutritional support.

9.6.10.1.2 Fistula

The development of a postoperative pancreatic fistula is the most common complication, increasing when the duct is involved, and the rate may be as high as 37% in combined injuries. Most fistulae are minor (less than 200 mL of fluid per day), and self-limiting when there is adequate external drainage. However, high-output fistulae (>7000 mL per day) may require surgical intervention for closure or prolonged periods of drainage with nutritional support. Management is directed locally at early adequate nutrition (preferably with distal enteral feeds through a feeding jejunostomy), adequate drainage, and transpapillary pancreatic stenting of confirmed ductal injuries.

9.6.10.1.3 Abscess Formation

Most abscesses are peripancreatic and associated with injuries to other organs, specifically the liver and intestine. A true pancreatic abscess is uncommon and usually results from inadequate debridement of necrotic tissue. For this reason, simple percutaneous drainage is generally not enough, and further debridement is required.

9.6.10.2 LATE COMPLICATIONS

9.6.10.2.1 Pseudocyst

Accurate diagnosis and surgical treatment of pancreatic injuries should result in a rate of pseudocyst formation of about 2%–3%. Accurate evaluation of the state of the duct will dictate management, and if the duct is intact, percutaneous drainage is likely to be successful. However, a pseudocyst together with a major ductal disruption will not be cured by percutaneous drainage, which will convert the pseudocyst into a chronic fistula. Current

options include cystogastrostomy (open or endoscopic), endoscopic stenting of the duct, or resection.

9.6.10.2.2 Exocrine and Endocrine Deficiency

Pancreatic resection distal to the mesenteric vessels will usually leave enough tissue for adequate exocrine and endocrine function, as work has shown that a residual 10%–20% of pancreatic tissue is usually enough. Patients who have procedures that leave less functioning tissue will require exogenous endocrine and exocrine enzyme replacement.

9.6.11 **Summary of Evidence Based Guidelines**[31,32]

Table 9.6.2 gives a summary of the evidence-based guidelines for pancreatic trauma.

Table 9.6.2 Summary of EAST Evidence-Based Guidelines for Pancreatic Trauma

PICO Format	
P	Patient, Population, or Problem
I	Intervention, Prognostic Factor, or Exposure
C	Comparison or Intervention (if appropriate)
O	Outcome you would like to measure or achieve
PICO	**Recommendation**
PICO Question 1: For adults with grade I/II injury to the pancreas identified by CT scan (P), should operative intervention (I) or non-operative management (C) be performed?	We conditionally recommend non-operative management for grade I/II pancreatic injuries diagnosed by CT scan. Non-operative management appears to have low morbidity. If the pancreatic duct is not definitively intact, it seems reasonable to further evaluate the duct with additional tests, such as ERCP or MRCP, because this may change the grade of the injury and therefore the recommended treatment plan.
PICO Question 2: For adults with grade III/IV injury to the pancreas identified by CT scan (P), should operative intervention (I) or non-operative management (C) be performed?	We conditionally recommend operative management for grade III/IV pancreatic injuries diagnosed by CT scan. Although there was no statistically significant difference between groups for any single outcome, our group feels that there is a cumulative trend toward increased morbidity after non-operative management. Treatment failures after non-operative management occur regularly, and treatment delays likely contribute to morbid complications and death.
PICO Question 3: For adults undergoing an operation who are intra-operatively found to have a grade I/II pancreas injury (P), should resectional (I) or non-resectional management (C) be performed?	We conditionally recommend non-resectional management for operative management of grade I/II pancreatic injuries. Our pooled data analysis suggests that mortality from pancreas-related causes are generally low in this population and that there were significantly more intra-abdominal abscesses in the resection group.

(Continued)

Table 9.6.2 (Continued) Summary of EAST Evidence-Based Guidelines for Pancreatic Trauma

PICO Format	Recommendation
PICO Question 4: For adults undergoing an operation who are intra-operatively found to have a grade III/IV pancreas injury (P), should resectional (I) or non-resectional management (C) be performed?	We conditionally recommend resection for operative management of grade III/IV pancreatic injuries. Complications are frequent in both groups. In our pooled analysis, fistula development was associated with non-resection strategies. Pancreas-related mortality was higher in the non-resection group, but this finding was potentially confounded by incomplete mortality reporting and bias. Owing to the very low quality of available data, this is a conditional recommendation.
PICO Question 5: For adults with total destruction of the head of the pancreas (grade V) (P), should pancreaticoduodenectomy (I) or surgical treatment other than pancreaticoduodenectomy (C) be performed?	No recommendation is given. The literature on this topic is limited and dated. Surgical and resuscitation strategies have evolved significantly to include damage control procedures and early balanced resuscitations, making our ability to interpret the available literature limited. Grade V injury to the pancreas is extremely morbid, and the intra-operative and immediate post-operative rate of death is high.
PICO Question 6: For adults who have undergone an operation for pancreatic trauma (P), should routine octreotide prophylaxis (I) or no octreotide (C) be used?	We conditionally recommend *against* the routine use of octreotide for post-operative prophylaxis related to traumatic pancreatic injuries to prevent fistula. Data are limited, but pooled data show no difference in outcomes between groups. The subcommittee concluded that the less invasive (no medication) strategy would be preferable with no difference in outcomes.
PICO Question 7: For adults undergoing distal pancreatectomy for trauma (P), should routine splenectomy (I) or splenic preservation (C) be performed?	No recommendation is given. Existing data do not support either treatment modality, although splenic preservation was only considered for stable patients. If either the stability of the patient or the surgeon's ability to safely preserve the spleen is in doubt, a distal pancreatectomy with splenectomy is a reasonable choice.

REFERENCES AND RECOMMENDED READING

References

1. Degiannis E, Glapa M, Loukogeorgakis SP, Smith MD. Management of pancreatic trauma. *Injury*. 2008;**39**:21–9.
2. Bradley EL III, Young PR Jr, Chang MC, et al. Diagnosis and initial management of blunt pancreatic trauma: guidelines from a multi-institutional review. *Ann Surg*. 1998; **227**:861–9.
3. Leppaniemi A, Haapiainen R, Kiviluoto T, Lempinen M. Pancreatic trauma: acute and late manifestations. *Br J Surg*. 1988;**75**:165–7.
4. Biffl W. Injury to the duodenum and pancreas. In: Moore EE, Feliciano DV, Mattox KL, eds. *Trauma*, 8th ed. New York: McGraw-Hill Education, 2013: 621–38.
5. Takishima T, Sugimoto K, Hirata M, Asari Y, Ohwada T, Katika A. Serum amylase level on admission in the diagnosis of blunt injury to the pancreas: its significance and limitations. *Ann Surg*. 1997 Jul;**226**:70–6.
6. Ahkrass R, Kim K, Brandt C. Computed tomography: an unreliable indicator of pancreatic trauma. *Am Surg*. 1996 Aug;**62**:647–51.
7. Thomson DA, Krige JE, Thomson SR, Bornman P. The role of endoscopic retrograde pancreatography in pancreatic trauma: A critical appraisal of 48 patients treated at a tertiary institution. *J Trauma Acute Care Surg*. 2014 Jun; **76(6)**:1362–6. doi:10.1097/TA.0000000000000227.
8. Bret PM, Reinhold C. Magnetic resonance cholangiopancreatography. *Endoscopy* 1997 Aug;**29**:472–86.
9. Subramanian A, Dente CJ, Feliciano DV. The management of pancreatic trauma in the modern era. *Surg Clin N Am*. 2007 Dec; **87(6)**:1515–32, x. Review.
10. Hikida S, Sakamoto T, Higaki K, Hata H, Maeshiro K, Yamauchi K, et al. Intra-operative ultrasonography is useful for diagnosing pancreatic duct injury and adjacent tissue damage in a patient with penetrating pancreas trauma. *J Hepatobiliary Pancreat Surg*. 2004;**11**:272–5.

11. Moore EE, Cogbill TH, Malangoni MA, Jurkovich GJ, Shackford SR, Champion HR, et al. Organ injury scaling. II: Pancreas, duodenum, small bowel, colon, and rectum. *J Trauma*. 1990;**30**:272–5.

12. Kong Y, Zhang H, He X, Liu C, Piao L, Zhao G, et al. Endoscopic management for pancreatic injuries due to blunt abdominal trauma decreases failure of nonoperative management and incidence of pancreatic-related complications. *Injury*. 2014 Jan;**45(1)**:134–40. doi: 10.1016/j.injury.2013.07.017.

13. Wolf A, Bernhardt J, Patrzyk M, Heidecke CD. The value of endoscopic diagnosis and the treatment of pancreas injuries following blunt abdominal trauma. *Surg Endosc*. 2005 May;**19**:665–9.

14. Lin BC, Chen RJ, Fang JF, Hsu YP, Kao YC, Kao JL. Management of blunt major pancreatic injury. *J Trauma*. 2004 April;**56**:774–8.

15. Lin BC, Fang JF, Wong YC, Liu NJ. Blunt pancreatic trauma and pseudocyst: management of major pancreatic duct injury. *Injury*. 2007 May;**38**:588–93.

16. Velmahos GC, Tabbara M, Gross R, Willette P, Hirsch E, Burke P, et al. Blunt pancreatoduodenal injury: a multicenter study of the research consortium of New England Centers for trauma (ReCONECT). *Arch Surg*. 2009 May;**144**:13–9; discussion 419-20. doi: 10.1001/archsurg.2009.62.

17. DuBose JJ, Inaba K, Teixeira PG, Shiflett A, Putty B, Green DJ, et al. Pyloric exclusion in the treatment of severe duodenal injuries: results from the National Trauma Data Bank. *Am Surg*. 2008 Oct;**74**:925–29.

18. Fabian TC, Kudsk KA, Croce MA, Payne LW, Mangiante EC, Voeller GR, et al. Superiority of closed suction drainage for pancreatic trauma. A randomized prospective study. *Ann Surg*. 1990 Jun;**211**:724–8; discussion 728-30.

19. Feliciano DV, Martin TD, Cruse PA, Graham JM, Burch JM, Mattox KL, et al. Management of combined pancreatoduodenal injuries. *Ann Surg*. 1987 Jun;**205**:673–80.

20. Ginzburg E, Carrillo EH, Sosa JL, Hertz J, Nir I, Martin LC. Pyloric exclusion in the management of duodenal trauma: is concomitant gastrojejunostomy necessary? *Am Surg*. 1997 Nov;**63**:964–6.

21. Seamon MJ, Pieri PG, Fisher CA, Gaughan J, Santora TA, Pathak AS, et al. A ten-year retrospective review: does pyloric exclusion improve clinical outcome after penetrating duodenal and combined pancreaticoduodenal injuries? *J Trauma*. 2007 Apr;**62**:829–33.

22. Asensio JA, Petrone P, Roldán G, Kuncir E, Demetriades D. Pancreaticoduodenectomy: a rare procedure for the management of complex pancreaticoduodenal injuries. *J Am Coll Surg*. 2003 Dec;**197**:937–42.

23. Whipple A. Observations on radical surgery for lesions of the pancreas. *Surg Gynecol Obstet*. 1946;**82**:623.

24. Thompson CM, Shalhub S, DeBoard ZM, Maier RV. Revisiting the pancreaticoduodenectomy for trauma: a single institution's experience. *J Trauma Acute Care Surg*. 2013 Aug;**75**:225–8. doi: 10.1097/TA.0b013e31829a0aaf.

25. Krige JE, Navsaria PH, Nicol AJ. Damage control laparotomy and delayed pancreatoduodenectomy for complex combined pancreatoduodenal and venous injuries. *Eur J Trauma Emerg Surg*. 2016 April;**42**:225–30. doi: 10.1007/s00068-015-0525-9.

26. Krige JE, Kotze UK, Setshedi M, Nicol AJ, Navsaria PH. Management of pancreatic injuries during damage control surgery: An observational outcomes analysis of 79 patients treated at an academic Level 1 Trauma Centre. *Eur J Trauma Emerg Surg*. 2017 Jun;**43(3)**:411–420. doi: 10.1007/s00068-016-0657-6.

27. Walt AJ. Pancreatic trauma. In: Ivatury RR, Gayten CG eds. *The Textbook of Penetrating Trauma*. Baltimore Williams & Wilkins, 1996: 641–52.

28. Büchler M, Friess H, Klempa I, Hermanek P, Sulkowski U, Becker H, et al. Role of octreotide in the prevention of postoperative complications following pancreatic resection. *Am J Surg*. 1992 Jan;**163**:125–30; discussion 130-1.

29. McKay C, Baxter J, Imrie C. A randomized, controlled trial of octreotide in the management of patients with acute pancreatitis. *Int J Pancreatol*. 1997 Feb;**21**:13–19.

30. Naik-Mathuria BJ, Rosenfeld EH, Gosain A, Burd R, Falcone RA Jr., Takkar R, et al. Proposed clinical pathway for nonoperative management of high-grade pediatric pancreatic injuries based on a multicenter analysis: A Pediatric Trauma Society collaborative. *J Trauma Acute Care Surg*. 2017 Oct; **83(4)**:589–596. doi: 10.1097/TA.0000000000001576.

31. Ho VP, Patel NJ, Bokhari F, Madbak FG, Hambley JE, Yon JR, et al. Management of adult pancreatic injuries: A practice management guideline from the Eastern Association for the Surgery of Trauma. *J Trauma Acute Care Surg*. 2017 Jan; **82(1)**:185–99. doi: 10.1097/TA.0000000000001300.

32. Biffl WL, Moore EE, Croce M, Davis JW, Coimbra R, Karmy-Jones R, et al. Western Trauma Association critical decisions in trauma: management of pancreatic injuries. *J Trauma Acute Care Surg*. 2013;**75(6)**:941–6. doi: 10.1097/TA.0b013e3182a96572.

Recommended Reading

Biffl WL. Injury to the duodenum and pancreas. In Moore EE, Feliciano DV, Mattox KL, eds. *Trauma*, 8th ed. New York: McGraw-Hill Education, 2017: 621–38.

Phillips B, Turco L, McDonald D, Mause E, Walters RW. A subgroup analysis of penetrating injuries to the pancreas: 777 patients from the National Trauma Data Bank, 2010-2014. *J Surg Res*. 2018 May;**225**:131–141. doi: 10.1016/j.jss.2018.01.014.

9.7 The Duodenum

9.7.1 **Overview**

Duodenal injuries can pose a formidable challenge to the surgeon, and failure to manage them properly can have devastating results. The total amount of fluid passing through the duodenum exceeds 6 L per day, and a fistula in this area can cause serious fluid and electrolyte imbalance. A large amount of activated enzymes liberated into a combination of the retroperitoneal space and the peritoneal cavity can be life-threatening.

Both the pancreas and the duodenum are well protected in the superior retroperitoneum deep within the abdomen. Since these organs are in the retroperitoneum, they usually do not present with peritonitis, and are delayed in their presentation. Therefore, in order to sustain an injury to either one of them, there must be other associated injuries. If there is an anterior penetrating injury, the stomach, small bowel, transverse colon, liver, spleen, or kidneys are frequently also involved, whereas there needs to be a high index of suspicion with penetrating injury to the back, which can injure the duodenum leading to retroperitoneal contamination without peritonitis. If there is a blunt traumatic injury, there are frequently fractures of the lower thoracic or upper lumbar vertebrae. It requires a high level of suspicion and significant clinical acumen, as well as aggressive radiographic imaging, to identify an injury to these organs this early in the presentation.

Pre-operative diagnosis of isolated duodenal injury can be very difficult to make, and there is no single method of duodenal repair that eliminates the potential for dehiscence of the duodenal suture line. As a result, the surgeon is frequently confronted with the dilemma of choosing between several pre-operative investigations and many surgical procedures. A detailed knowledge of the available operative choices and when each one of them is preferably applied is important for the patient's benefit.[1]

9.7.2 **Mechanism of Injury**

9.7.2.1 PENETRATING TRAUMA

Penetrating trauma is the leading cause of duodenal injuries in countries with a high incidence of civilian violence. Because of the retroperitoneal location of the duodenum, and its proximity to several other viscera and major vascular structures, isolated penetrating injuries of the duodenum are infrequent. The need for abdominal exploration is usually dictated by associated injuries, and the diagnosis of duodenal injury is usually made in the operating room.

9.7.2.2 BLUNT TRAUMA

Blunt injuries to the duodenum are both less common and more difficult to diagnose than penetrating injuries, and they can occur in isolation or with pancreatic injury. These usually occur when crushing the duodenum between the spine and a steering wheel or handlebar, or when some other force is applied to the duodenum. These injuries can be associated with flexion/distraction fractures of the L1–L2 vertebrae – the Chance fracture. 'Stomping' and striking the mid-epigastrium are common. Less common in deceleration injury patterns are tears at the junction of the third and fourth parts of the duodenum. These injuries occur at the junction of free (intraperitoneal) parts of the duodenum with fixed (retroperitoneal) parts. A high index of suspicion based on the mechanism of injury and physical examination findings may lead to further diagnostic studies.

9.7.2.3 PAEDIATRIC CONSIDERATIONS

A recent multi-institutional investigation found that child abuse was consistently associated with duodenal injuries in children younger than 2 years; also, the most common mechanism causing duodenal injuries in children younger than 5 years was non-accidental trauma.

9.7.3 **Diagnosis**

9.7.3.1 CLINICAL PRESENTATION

The clinical changes in isolated duodenal injuries may be extremely subtle until severe, life-threatening peritonitis develops. In most of the retroperitoneal perforations, there is initially only mild upper abdominal tenderness with a progressive rise in temperature, tachycardia, and occasionally vomiting. After several hours, the duodenal contents may extravasate into the peritoneal cavity, with the development of peritonitis, or with posterior stab wounds, leak enteric contents from the wound. If the duodenal contents spill into the lesser sac, they are usually 'walled off' and localized, although they can occasionally leak into the general peritoneal cavity via the foramen of Winslow, with resultant generalized peritonitis.[2]

9.7.3.2 SERUM AMYLASE AND SERUM LIPASE

Theoretically, duodenal perforations are associated with a leak of amylase and other digestive enzymes, and it has been suggested that determination of the serum amylase concentration might be helpful in the diagnosis of blunt duodenal injury. However, the test lacks sensitivity. The duodenum is retroperitoneal, the concentration of amylase in the fluid that leaks is variable, and amylase concentrations often take hours to days to increase after injury. Although serial determinations of serum amylase are better than a single, isolated determination on admission, sensitivity is still poor, and necessary delays are inherent in serial determinations. If the serum amylase level is elevated on admission, a diligent search for duodenal rupture is warranted. The presence of a normal amylase level, however, does not exclude duodenal injury.[3]

Many institutions now use lipase as the marker pancreatic injury and studies suggest that it may be a more sensitive marker of pancreatic injury and abdominal injury than amylase, although its role in duodenal injury is unclear.

9.7.3.3 DIAGNOSTIC PERITONEAL LAVAGE/ULTRASOUND

The duodenum, like the pancreas, lies in the retroperitoneum, so that neither ultrasound nor diagnostic peritoneal lavage (DPL) will be reliable. If performed, the amylase level in the lavage fluid should be measured.

9.7.3.4 RADIOLOGICAL INVESTIGATION

9.7.3.4.1 Computed Tomography

CT scan is the method of choice for the investigation of subtle duodenal injuries.[4] It is very sensitive to the presence of small amounts of retroperitoneal air, blood, or extravasated contrast from the injured duodenum, especially in children;[5] however, in adults its reliability is

more controversial. The presence of periduodenal wall thickening or haematoma without extravasation of contrast material should be investigated with a gastrointestinal study using Meglumine (Gastrografin). If the result is normal, it should be followed by a barium study contrast, if the patient's condition allows this.

9.7.3.4.2 Radiological Contrast Studies

An upper gastrointestinal series using water-soluble contrast material can provide positive results in 50% of patients with duodenal perforations. Gastrografin should be administered, and the study should be done under fluoroscopic control with the patient in the right lateral position. If no leak is observed, the investigation continues with the patient in the supine and left lateral positions. If the Gastrografin study is negative, it should be followed by administration of barium to allow the detection of small perforations more readily. Upper gastrointestinal studies with contrast are also indicated in patients with a suspected intramural haematoma of the duodenum (see also Section 9.7.6.1), because they may demonstrate the classic 'coiled-spring' appearance of complete obstruction by the haematoma.[6]

9.7.3.5 DIAGNOSTIC LAPAROSCOPY

Unfortunately, diagnostic laparoscopy does not confer any improvement over more traditional methods in the investigation of the duodenum. In fact, because of its anatomical position, diagnostic laparoscopy is a poor modality to determine organ injury in these cases.[7]

9.7.4 Duodenal Injury Scale

Grading systems have been devised to characterize duodenal injuries (Table 9.7.1).[8]

9.7.5 Management

Exploratory laparotomy remains the ultimate diagnostic test if a high suspicion of duodenal injury continues in the face of absent or equivocal radiographic signs.[9]

Most duodenal injuries can be managed by simple repair. More complicated injuries may require more sophisticated techniques. 'High-risk' duodenal injuries are followed by a high incidence of suture line dehiscence, and their treatment should include duodenal diversion.

Table 9.7.1 Duodenum Injury Scale

Grade[a]	Type of Injury	Description of Injury
I	Haematoma Laceration	Involving a single portion of duodenum Partial thickness, no perforation
II	Haematoma Laceration	Involving more than one portion Disruption <50% of circumference
III	Laceration	Disruption 50%–75% of circumference of D2 Disruption 50%–100% of circumference of D1, D3 or D4
IV	Laceration	Disruption >75% of circumference of D2 Involving the ampulla or distal common bile duct
V	Laceration Vascular	Massive disruption of the duodenopancreatic complex Devascularisation of duodenum

Note: Duodenum injury scale (see also Appendix B).
Abbreviations: D1, first portion of duodenum; D2, second portion of duodenum; D3, third portion of duodenum; D4, fourth portion of duodenum.
[a] Advance one grade for multiple injuries up to grade III.

The management of all full-thickness duodenal lacerations should include adequate external periduodenal drainage. Pancreaticoduodenectomy is practised only if no alternative is available. 'Damage control' should precede the definitive reconstruction.

9.7.6 Surgical Approach

Although useful for research purposes, the specifics of the grading systems are less important than several simple aspects of the duodenal injuries:

- The anatomical relation to the ampulla of Vater.
- The characteristics of the injury (simple laceration versus destruction of duodenal wall).
- The circumference of the duodenum involved.
- Associated injuries to the biliary tract or pancreas, or major vascular injuries.

Timing of the operation is also very important as mortality rises from 11% to 40% if the time interval between injury and operation is more than 24 hours[7] (see also Section 9.6.7.2.7).

In addition to the Kocher manoeuvre to visualize the second part of the duodenum, a medial visceral rotation can be used to expose the entire transverse part of the duodenum. Alternatively, the fourth part of the duodenum can be mobilized by dividing the ligament of Treitz and gently dissecting with right index finger in the avascular plane behind the transverse duodenum. Combining this with the Kocher manoeuvre allows the index fingers to be brought together from both sides and thereby to exclude a posterior perforation of the transverse part of the duodenum.

From a practical point of view, the duodenum can be divided into one 'upper' portion that includes the first and second parts, and another 'lower' portion that includes the third and fourth parts. The 'upper' portion has complex anatomical structures within it (the common bile duct and the sphincter) and the pylorus. It requires distinct manoeuvres to diagnose injury (cholangiogram and direct visual inspection), and complex techniques to repair them. The first and second parts of the duodenum are densely adherent and dependent for their blood supply on the head of the pancreas; therefore, the diagnosis and management of any injury is complex, and resection, unless involving the entire 'C' loop and pancreatic head, is impossible. The 'lower' portion involving the third and fourth part of the duodenum can generally be treated like the small bowel, and the diagnosis and management of injury is relatively simple, including debridement, closure, resection, and anastomosis.

9.7.6.1 INTRAMURAL HAEMATOMA

This is a rare injury of the duodenum specific to patients with blunt trauma. It is most common in children with isolated force to the upper abdomen, possibly because of the relatively flexible and pliable musculature of the child's abdominal wall, and half of the cases can be attributed to child abuse.

The haematoma develops in the submucosal or subserosal layers of the duodenum. The duodenum is *not* perforated. Such haematomas can lead to obstruction. The symptoms of gastric outlet obstruction can take up to 48 hours to present. This is due to the gradual increase of the size of a haematoma as the breakdown of the haemoglobin makes it hyperosmotic, with resultant fluid shifts into it. The diagnosis can be made by double-contrast CT scan or upper gastrointestinal contrast studies that show the 'coiled spring' or 'stacked coin' sign.[6]

Management of the injury is usually considered non-surgical, and if associated injuries can be ruled out, best results are obtained by conservative treatment.[10] Gastric residual volume will slowly decrease, eventually allowing normal feeding. If there is no improvement, the patient should undergo laparotomy to rule out the presence of duodenal perforation or injury of the head of the pancreas, which may be an alternative cause of duodenal obstruction.

The treatment of an intramural haematoma that is found at early laparotomy is controversial. One option is to open the serosa, evacuate the haematoma without violation of the mucosa, and carefully repair the wall of the bowel. The concern is that this may convert a partial tear to a full-thickness tear of the duodenal wall. Another option is to carefully explore the duodenum to exclude a perforation, leaving the intramural haematoma intact and planning nasogastric decompression post-operatively.

9.7.6.2 DUODENAL LACERATION

The great majority of duodenal perforations and lacerations can be managed with simple surgical procedures. This is particularly true with penetrating injuries, when the time interval between injury and operation is normally short. On the other hand, the minority are 'high risk', for example with increased risk of dehiscence of the duodenal repair, increased morbidity, and sometimes mortality. These injuries are related to associated pancreatic injury, blunt or missile injury, involvement of more than 75% of the duodenal wall, injury of the first or second part of the duodenum, a time interval of more than 24 hours between injury and repair, and associated common bile duct injury. In these high-risk injuries, several adjunctive operative procedures have been proposed to reduce the incidence of dehiscence of the duodenal suture line.

Recently, further evidence has supported a more simplified surgical approach to these injuries with improved outcomes compared to complex technical solutions.[11] The methods of repair of the duodenal trauma as well as the 'supportive' procedures against dehiscence are described below.

9.7.6.3 REPAIR OF THE PERFORATION

Most injuries of the duodenum can be repaired by primary closure in one or two layers. The closure should be oriented transversely, if possible, to avoid luminal compromise. Excessive inversion should be avoided. Longitudinal duodenotomies can usually be closed transversely if the length of the duodenal injury is less than 50% of the circumference of the duodenum.

If primary closure would compromise the lumen of the duodenum, several alternatives have been recommended. Pedicled mucosal graft, as a method of closing large duodenal defects, has been suggested, using a segment of jejunum or a gastric island flap from the body of the stomach. An alternative to that is the use of a jejunal serosal patch to close the duodenal defect.[16] The serosa of the loop of the jejunum is sutured to the edges of the duodenal defect. Although encouraging in experimental studies, the clinical application of both methods has been limited, without beneficial results, and suture line leaks have been reported.[12]

9.7.6.4 COMPLETE TRANSECTION OF THE DUODENUM

The preferred method of repair is usually primary anastomosis of the two ends after appropriate debridement and mobilization of the duodenum. This is frequently the case with injuries of the first, third, or fourth part of the duodenum, where mobilization is technically not difficult. However, if a large amount of tissue is lost, approximation of the duodenum may not be possible without producing undue tension on the suture line. If this is the case and complete transection occurs in the first part of the duodenum, it is advisable to perform an antrectomy with closure of the duodenal stump and a Bilroth II gastrojejunostomy. When such injury occurs distal to the ampulla of Vater, closure of the distal duodenum and Roux-en-Y duodenojejunal anastomosis is appropriate.

Mobilization of the second part of the duodenum is limited by its shared blood supply with the head of the pancreas. A direct anastomosis to a Roux-en-Y loop sutured over the duodenal defect in an end-to-side fashion is the procedure of choice. This also can be applied as an alternative method of operative management of extensive defects to the other parts of the duodenum when primary anastomosis is not feasible.

External drainage should be provided in all duodenal injuries because it affords early detection and control of the duodenal fistula. The drain is preferably a simple, soft silicone rubber, closed system placed adjacent to the repair.

9.7.6.5 DUODENAL DIVERSION

In high-risk duodenal injuries, duodenal repair is followed by a high incidence of suture line dehiscence. In order to protect the duodenal repair, the gastrointestinal contents – with their proteolytic enzymes – can be diverted with a gastrojejunostomy; this is a practice that would also make the management of a potential duodenal fistula easier. The evidence for this procedure is equivocal, although there remains a role in selected cases.

9.7.6.6 DUODENAL DIVERTICULATION

This includes a distal Bilroth II gastrectomy, closure of the duodenal wound, placement of a decompressive catheter into the duodenum, and generous drainage of the duodenal repair. Truncal vagotomy and biliary drainage could be added. Resection of a normal distal stomach cannot be beneficial to the patient. This procedure is not recommended, and should not be considered unless there is a large amount of destruction and tissue loss, and no other course is possible.

9.7.6.7 TRIPLE TUBE DECOMPRESSION[14]

'Tube decompression' was the first technique, described in 1954, used for decompression of the duodenum and diversion of its contents to preserve the integrity of the duodenorrhaphy. To protect a duodenal repair, a tube duodenostomy can be used by inserting a tube through a separate incision through the lateral duodenal wall using the Witzel technique to ensure sealing of the hole after removing the tube. In trauma, the technique was introduced as a 'triple ostomy', which consists of a gastrostomy tube to decompress the stomach, a retrograde jejunostomy to decompress the duodenum, and an antegrade jejunostomy to feed the patient.

The initial favourable reports on the efficacy of this technique to decrease the incidence of dehiscence of the duodenorrhaphy have, however, not been supported by more recent reports.[13] The drawbacks of this technique are the formation of several new perforations in the gastrointestinal tract, the inefficiency of the jejunostomy tube to properly decompress the duodenum, and the common scenario of finding that the drains have fallen out or been removed by the patient. Establishment of enteral feeding preferably through a naso- or orojejunal tube placed at the surgical procedure is recommended at the final stage of damage control, when no further re-looks are planned.

9.7.6.8 PYLORIC EXCLUSION (SEE ALSO SECTION 9.6.7.2.7)

9.7.6.8.1 Pancreaticoduodenectomy (Whipple's Procedure)

This is a major procedure to be practised in trauma only if no alternative is available. Damage control with control of bleeding and of bowel contamination, and ligation of the common bile and pancreatic ducts, should be the rule.[14,15] Reconstruction should take place within 48 hours or when the patient is stable.

Extensive local damage of the intraduodenal or intrapancreatic bile duct injuries frequently necessitates a staged pancreaticoduodenectomy. Less extensive local injuries can be managed by intraluminal stenting, sphincteroplasty or reimplantation of the ampulla of Vater.

REFERENCES AND RECOMMENDED READING

References

1. Neal MD, Britt LD, Watson G, Murdock A, Peitzman AB. Abdominal injury – duodenum and pancreas. In: Peitzman AB, Rhodes M, Schwab SW, Yealy DM, Fabian TC eds. *The Trauma Manual: Trauma and Acute Care Surgery*. 4th Edn. Philadelphia: Lippincott Williams and Wilkins 2013: 374.
2. Carrillo EH, Richardson JD, Miller FB. Evolution in the management of duodenal injuries. *J Trauma*. 1996 Jun;**40(6)**:1037–45; discussion 1045-6. Review.
3. Takishima T, Sugimoto K, Hirata M, Asari Y, Ohwada T, Katika A. Serum amylase level on admission in the diagnosis of blunt injury to the pancreas: its significance and limitations. *Ann Surg*. 1997 Jul;**226**:70–6.

4. Kunin JR, Korobkin M, Ellis JH, Francis IR, Kane NM, Siegel SE. Duodenal injuries caused by blunt abdominal trauma: value of CT in differentiating perforation from haematoma. *Am J Roentgenol*. 1993 June;**160(6)**:1221–3.

5. Shilyansky J, Pearl RH, Kreller M, Sena LM, Babyn PS. Diagnosis and management of duodenal injuries. *J Paed Surg*. 1997 June;**32**:229–32.

6. Kadell BM, Zimmerman PT, Lu DSK. Radiology of the abdomen. In: Zimmer MJ, Schwartz SI, Ellis H, eds. *Maingot's Abdominal Operations*. Stanford, CT: Appleton & Lange, 1997: 3–116.

7. Brooks AJ, Boffard KD. Current technology: laparoscopic surgery in trauma. *Trauma*. 1999;**1**:53–60.

8. Moore EE, Cogbill TH, Malangoni MA, Jurkovich GJ, Shackford SR, Champion HR. Organ injury scaling, II: Pancreas, duodenum, small bowel, colon, and rectum. *J Trauma*. 1990 Nov;**30(11)**:1427–9.

9. Degiannis E, Boffard K. Duodenal injuries. *Br J Surg*. 2000 Nov;**87(11)**:1473–9. Review.

10. Toulakian RJ. Protocol for the nonoperative treatment of obstructing intramural duodenal haematoma during childhood. *Am J Surg*. 1983 Mar;**145**:330–4.

11. Ordoñez C, García A, Parra MW, et al. Complex penetrating duodenal injuries: Less is better. *J Trauma Acute Care Surg*. 2014;**76**:1177–83. doi: 10.1097/TA.0000000000000214.

12. Ivatury RR, Gaudino J, Ascer E, et al. Treatment of penetrating duodenal injuries. *J Trauma*. 1985 Apr;**25**:337–41.

13. Cogbill TH, Moore EE, Feliciano DV, Hoyt DB, Jurkovich GJ, Morris JA, et al. Conservative management of duodenal trauma: a multicentre perspective. *J Trauma*. 1990 Dec;**30(12)**:1469–75.

14. Kauder DR, Schwab SW, Rotondo MF. Damage control. In Ivantury RR, Cayten CG, eds. *The Textbook of Penetrating Trauma*. Baltimore: Williams & Wilkins, 1996: 717–25.

15. Feliciano DV, Martin TD, Cruse PA, Graham JM, Burch JM, Mattox KL, et al. Management of combined pancreato-duodenal injuries. *Ann Surg*. 1987 June;**205**:673–80.

Recommended Reading

Asensio JA, Demetriades D, Berne JD. A unified approach to surgical exposure of pancreatic and duodenal injuries. *Am J Surg*. 1997 July; **174(1)**: 54–60.

Phillips B, Turco L, McDonald D, Mause A, Walters RW. Penetrating injuries to the duodenum: An analysis of 879 patients from the National Trauma Data Bank, 2010 to 2014. *J Trauma Acute Care Surg*. 2017 Nov;**83(5)**:810–817. doi: 10.1097/TA.0000000000001604.

Ivatury RR, Nassoura ZE, Simon RJ, Simon RJ. Complex duodenal injuries. *Surg Clin North Am*. 1996 Aug;**76(4)**:797–812. Review.

9.8 The Urogenital System

9.8.1 Overview

Urogenital trauma refers to injuries to the kidneys, ureters, bladder and urethra, the female reproductive organs in the pregnant and non-pregnant state, and the penis, scrotum and testes.

Death from penetrating bladder trauma was mentioned in Homer's *Iliad*, as well as by Hippocrates and Galen, while Evans and Fowler in 1905 demonstrated that the mortality from penetrating intraperitoneal bladder injuries could be reduced from 100% to 28% with laparotomy and bladder repair. Ambroise Paré observed death following a gunshot wound of the kidney, with haematuria and sepsis, and it was only in 1884 that nephrectomy became the recommended treatment for renal injury.

Haematuria is the hallmark of urological injury, but may be absent even in severe trauma, and a high index of suspicion is then needed, based on the mechanism of injury and the presence of abdominal and pelvic injury.

9.8.2 Renal Injuries

Injury to the kidney is seen in up to 10% of patients with blunt or penetrating abdominal injuries; however, most cases involve blunt rather than penetrating injury. Serious renal injuries are frequently associated with injuries to other organs, with multi-organ involvement in 80% of patients with penetrating trauma and in 75% of those with blunt trauma.

Haematuria, defined as more than five red blood cells per high-power field, is present in over 95% of patients who sustain renal trauma; however, the absence of haematuria does not preclude significant renal injury.

9.8.2.1 DIAGNOSIS

The first investigation is to look for gross haematuria, followed by urinalysis to check for microscopic haematuria.

Pitfall

Up to 30% of patients with serious renal trauma will have no haematuria whatsoever, while most patients with significant abdominal trauma will have microscopic haematuria, often in the absence of relevant renal injury.

The haemodynamic status of the patient will then determine the subsequent steps, for both blunt and penetrating trauma.

9.8.2.1.1 Unstable Patient

The investigation of choice in unstable patients is immediate surgery.

9.8.2.1.2 Stable Patient

CT has replaced intravenous urography as the primary modality for the assessment of suspected renal injuries. The investigation of choice is the multiphase, double- or triple-contrast CT scan, but this can misgrade the renal injury. More commonly, however, it does allow grading of renal injuries, and forms the basis for non-operative treatment, possibly up to, and inclusive of, non-vascular grade IV injuries and blunt renal artery thrombosis.

It has been shown that the size of the haematoma can be related to the grade of renal injury, which is a useful correlation in suboptimal studies and where older machines are used.

Contrast-enhanced ultrasound can also allow the visualization of active intrarenal bleeds.

In addition, duplex Doppler ultrasound can allow visualization of arteriovenous fistulas and active intra-renal bleeds.

9.8.2.1.3 Penetrating Trauma

The individual trauma centre's accepted method of evaluation of penetrating torso trauma must be used,

the renal visualization being provided by an intravenous pyelogram (IVP)/tomogram, followed by angiography if suspicious, or multiphase contrast-enhanced CT scanning of the abdomen as a stand-alone investigation.

9.8.2.1.4 Blunt Trauma

Investigations as above are reserved for children irrespective of urinalysis, and adults with frank haematuria or a systolic blood pressure below 90 mm Hg.

9.8.2.2 RENAL INJURY SCALE

Table 9.8.1 outlines the renal injury scale, 2018 revision.[3]

9.8.2.3 MANAGEMENT

9.8.2.3.1 Unstable Patient

At laparotomy, it will become apparent whether the kidneys are the source of the shock. Should a large retroperitoneal haematoma be present in the region of the kidney, the options are to leave the kidney alone at first and perform a single shot on-table IVP, to assess the functionality of both kidneys, explore the injured kidney immediately, or pack the area around the kidney and get out, if in a damage control situation.

A 'single-shot' intravenous urogram can be performed in the emergency room (if the patient is too unstable for formal CT scan), by injecting 2 mL/Kg of radiographic contrast medium, followed by a single plain x-ray film of the abdomen, taken 10 minutes after the contrast was injected.

9.8.2.3.2 Stable Patient

9.8.2.3.2.1 *Non-Operative Management*

In recent years, it has been recognized that many renal injuries can be managed without operation, and angio-embolization is a worthwhile option, if the skills are readily available.

In a recent review, 97 patients sustained a kidney injury, 72 from blunt force trauma and 25 from penetrating injury. Of the 72 blunt trauma patients, only five patients (7%) underwent urgent nephrectomy, three (4%) had repair and/or stenting, and 89% were observed despite a 29% laparotomy rate for associated intra-abdominal injuries. Of the 25 patients with penetrating trauma, eight (31%) underwent a nephrectomy, one had a partial nephrectomy, and two underwent renal repairs. Nephrectomy was more likely to be required

Table 9.8.1 Renal Injury Scale 2018 Revision

AAST Grade	AIS Severity	Imaging Criteria (CT Findings)	Operative Goals	Pathologic Criteria
I	2	**Haematoma** Subcapsular haematoma and/or parenchymal contusion without laceration **Laceration** None	**Haematoma** Non-expanding subcapsular haematoma and/or parenchymal contusion without laceration **Laceration** None	**Haematoma** Subcapsular haematoma and/or parenchyrnal contusion without parenchymal laceration **Laceration** None
II	2	**Haematoma** Perirenal haematoma confined to Gerota's fascia **Laceration** Renal parenchymal laceration: ≤1 cm depth without urinary extravasation	**Haematoma** Subcapsular haematoma 10%–50% surface area Intraparenchymal haematoma <5 cm in diameter **Laceration** Renal parenchymal laceration: <1 cm depth without urinary extravasation	**Haematoma** Subcapsular haematoma 10%–50% surface area Intraparenchymal haematoma <5 cm in diameter **Laceration** Renal parenchymal laceration: <1 cm depth without urinary extravasation
III	3	**Laceration** Renal parenchymal laceration: >1 cm depth without collecting system rupture or urinary extravasation. **Vascular** Any injury in the presence of a kidney vascular injury or active bleeding contained within Gerota's fascia	**Laceration** Renal parenchymal laceration: >1 cm depth without collecting system rupture or urinary extravasation.	**Laceration** Renal parenchymal laceration: >1 cm depth without collecting system rupture or urinary extravasation.
IV	4	**Laceration** Parenchymal laceration extending into urinary collecting system with urinary extravasation **Disruption** Renal pelvis laceration and/or complete ureteropelvic disruption Segmental renal vein or artery injury Active bleeding beyond Gerota's fascia into the retroperitoneum or peritoneum Segmental or complete kidney infarction(s) due to vessel thrombosis without active bleeding	**Laceration** Parenchymal laceration extending into urinary collecting system with urinary extravasation **Disruption** Renal pelvis laceration and/or complete ureteropelvic disruption Segmental renal vein or artery injury Active bleeding beyond Gerota's fascia into the retroperitoneum or peritoneum Segmental or complete kidney infarction(s) due to vessel thrombosis without active bleeding	**Laceration** Parenchymal laceration extending into urinary collecting system **Disruption** Renal pelvis laceration and/or complete ureteropelvic disruption Segmental renal vein or artery injury Active bleeding beyond Gerota's fascia into the retroperitoneum or peritoneum Segmental or complete kidney infarction(s) due to vessel thrombosis without active bleeding

(Continued)

AAST Grade	AIS Severity	Imaging Criteria (CT Findings)	Operative Goals	Pathologic Criteria
V	5	**Vascular injury** Main renal artery or vein laceration or avulsion of the hilum Devascularized kidney with active bleeding **Disruption** Shattered kidney with loss of identifiable parenchymal anatomy	**Vascular injury** Main renal artery or vein laceration or avulsion of the hilum Devascularized kidney with active bleeding **Disruption** Shattered kidney with loss of identifiable parenchymal anatomy	**Vascular injury** Main renal artery or vein laceration or avulsion of the hilum Devascularized kidney with active bleeding **Disruption** Shattered kidney with loss of identifiable parenchymal anatomy

Table 9.8.1 (*Continued*) Renal Injury Scale 2018 Revision

Source: Kozar RA et al. *J Trauma Acute Care Surg*. 2018 December;85(6):1119–22.

Note: Vascular injury is defined as a pseudoaneurysm or arteriovenous fistula and appear, as a focal collection of vascular contrast that decreases in attenuation with delayed imaging.
Active bleeding from a vascular injury presents as vascular contrast, focal, or diffuse, which increases in size or attenuation in delayed phase.
Vascular thrombosis can lead to organ infarction.
Grade based on highest grade assessment made on imaging, at operation or on pathologic specimen.
More than one grade of kidney injury may be present and should be classified by the higher grade of injury.
Advance one grade for bilateral injuries up to Grade III.

after penetrating injury and was most likely in severely injured patients with ongoing haemorrhage.

An on-table IVP should be obtained even in the absence of a large haematoma to exclude renal artery thrombosis, followed by exploration with repair or nephrectomy in the persistently unstable patient.

Up to half of renal stab injuries, and up to one-third of gunshot in one series, can be treated non-operatively, provided excellent diagnostic methods can visualize the injuries.

In principle, management can be guided by the severity of injury, and many patients can be treated non-operatively.[1,2]

9.8.2.3.2.2 *Grades 1 and 2*

These comprise most renal injuries and can usually be treated non-operatively.

9.8.2.3.2.3 *Grade 3*

These comprise major lacerations through the cortex extending to the medulla or collecting system with or without urinary extravasation. Drainage may be necessary.

9.8.2.3.2.4 *Grade 4*

These are 'catastrophic' injuries and include multiple renal lacerations and vascular injuries involving the renal pedicle. These injuries often require surgery and may need nephrectomy. The most significant vascular injury following blunt trauma is thrombosis of the main renal artery, caused by deceleration with intimal tear and propagation of thrombus in the renal artery.

Partial nephrectomy should NOT be contemplated in the patient with competing injuries, or potential or actual haemodynamic instability.

9.8.2.3.2.5 *Grade 5*

Pelviureteric junction injuries are a rare consequence of blunt trauma, and are caused by sudden deceleration, which creates tension on the renal pedicle. The diagnosis may be delayed because haematuria is absent in one-third of patients. Pelviureteric junction injuries are classified into two groups: avulsion (complete transection) and laceration (incomplete tear). Nephrectomy is usually required.

9.8.2.4 SURGICAL APPROACH

Access should be by midline laparotomy, even if isolated renal injury is suspected, since the likelihood of other injuries is always present.

The kidneys are usually explored after dealing with the intra-abdominal emergencies. Ideally, control of the renal pedicle should be obtained before opening Gerota's fascia.

A direct approach to suspected peripheral penetrating injuries is advocated by some as being faster and equally safe. A left medial visceral rotation on the left, including

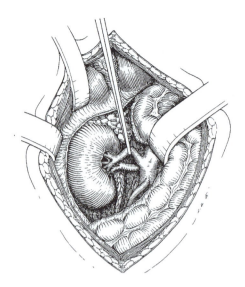

Figure 9.8.1 Access to the right kidney.

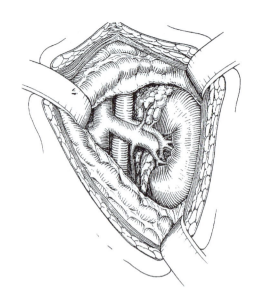

Figure 9.8.2 Access to the left kidney.

division of Gerota's fascia and medial rotation of the left kidney, or an extended Kocher's manoeuvre on the right can also afford good control of the aorta, inferior vena cava (IVC) and renal vessels, if required.

The right renal artery can be found by dissecting posteriorly between the aorta and the IVC (Figure 9.8.1). Dissection lateral to the IVC may lead to inadvertent isolation of a segmental branch of the right renal artery. The vessels are then controlled by loops to allow rapid occlusion should bleeding occur on opening Gerota's fascia. The right renal vein is easily controllable after reflection of the right colon and duodenum and must be mobilized to expose the artery. It always should be repaired if possible, because of the lack of collateral venous drainage.

The peritoneum over the aorta is opened, and the anterior wall of the aorta followed up to the left renal vein. After exposing the retroperitoneum from the right or the left, the left renal artery is identified by dissecting upwards on the lateral aspect of the aorta above the inferior mesenteric vein. The left renal vein crosses the aorta just below the level of the origin of the renal arteries (Figures 9.8.2 and 9.8.3).

Access to the left renal artery may also be improved by one of two manoeuvres:

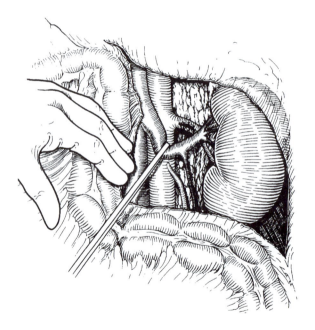

Figure 9.8.3 Access to the left renal vessels.

- Ligation of the adrenal, gonadal and lumbar tributaries of the left renal vein will enhance the mobilization of the vein to expose the renal artery.

- Ligation of the distal renal vein at the IVC can improve exposure of the origin of the renal artery. The collateral drainage via the lumbar gonadal and adrenal vessels will be sufficient to deal with the venous drainage on the left (Figure 9.8.4).

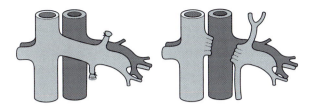

Figure 9.8.4 Division of the left renal vein.

After control of the renal pedicle has been obtained, Gerota's fascia can be opened or debrided as necessary. Care must be taken not to strip the renal capsule from the underlying parenchyma, as this may bleed profusely. The mobilized kidney now can be examined, debrided, trimmed, and sutured with drainage (Figure 9.8.5).

The kidney tolerates a single ischaemic event much better than repeated ischaemic times. However, the maximum warm ischaemic time that the kidney will tolerate is less than 1 hour, although this can be prolonged by ice packing.

With complete vascular isolation for up to 30 minutes, Gerota's fascia is then opened, and the injured kidney debrided by sharp dissection, and sutured or partially amputated. The renal pelvis collecting system should be closed with a running absorbable suture to provide a watertight seal. Nephrectomy will be required in less than 10% of stable patients.

Cover can then be effected using the renal capsule, omentum, meshes, etc., replacing the kidney within Gerota's fascia, and draining the area with a suction drain until it is draining minimally, and urine collections have been excluded.

Nephrostomy tubes or ureteric stents can be used either immediately or at some later time in cases of major renal trauma with extravasation.

9.8.2.5 ADJUNCTS

- *Pledgets*: The kidney does not hold sutures well. Care should be taken that the suture is not over-tightened, as it will cut though. The use of pledgets, though not essential, may be helpful.
- *Sealants*: Urine leakage is common. Tissue sealants can be a useful additional means of sealing the suture line.
- *Drains*: Whether a nephrectomy or a repair is performed, the high incidence of fluid (urine or blood) mandates the use of a suction drain.

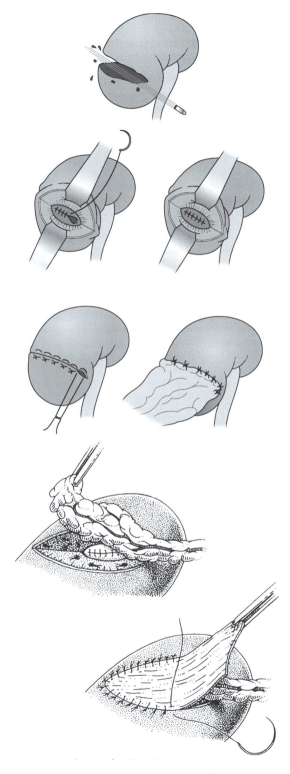

Figure 9.8.5 Techniques of renal repair.

9.8.2.6 POST-OPERATIVE CARE

Urinomas, infected urinomas, perinephric abscesses and delayed bleeding are the most common complications of conservative management, and are often amenable to imaging and percutaneous, transureteric, or angiographic management. Even when the kidney appears to be shattered into several pieces, drainage of the surrounding urinomas seems to encourage healing and avoid sepsis.

Hypertension (Page kidney) is a rare late complication.[4]

9.8.3 Ureteric Injuries

Significant ureteric injuries are often missed or not picked up until late, after the onset of complications or deterioration in renal function.

9.8.3.1 DIAGNOSIS

Patients with ureteric injury present without even microscopic haematuria in up to 50% of cases, and the injuries are mostly associated with penetrating trauma, although ureteric avulsion and rupture can happen in blunt trauma, especially in the paediatric population. Ureteric injuries may even be missed by high-dose IVP, and a high index of suspicion is essential. Intra-operative recognition may be facilitated by the intravenous or intra-ureteral injection of indigo carmine or methylene blue.

9.8.3.2 SURGICAL APPROACH

The procedures described for access to the retroperitoneal great vessels allow also perfect exposure to both ureters. Ureteric injuries are rare, usually due to penetrating trauma, so that local exploration and mobilization of part of the ascending or descending colon alone may be sufficient, depending on the site of injury. Minimal dissection of the periureteric tissues should take place, except at the precise level of injury, in order to preserve the delicate blood supply. Ureteric injuries close to the kidney are accessed by left or right medial visceral rotation as described above. Ureteric injuries near the bladder may be accessed by opening the peritoneal layer in the region and mobilizing the bladder.

9.8.3.2.1 Unstable Patients

Unstable patients require immediate surgery and exploration of the ureter after life-threatening injuries have been dealt with, ideally preceded by one-shot on-table IVP.

If the patient requires an abbreviated laparotomy, the ureteric injury can be safely left alone, stented or ligated until the patient returns to the operating theatre for definitive procedures; indeed, successful repair has frequently been affected after delayed or missed presentation. Percutaneous nephrostomy can be used as a post-operative adjunct for the ligated ureter.

In unstable patients with associated colonic injuries, especially those requiring colectomy, even nephrectomy can be justified.

9.8.3.2.2 Stable Patients

Stable patients with fresh injuries between the pelviureteric junction and the pelvic brim are treated by end uretero-ureterostomy with spatulation and interrupted suturing over a double-J stent (Figure 9.8.6).

The stent can be safely left *in situ* for 4–6 weeks. It has been suggested that stents can be omitted in injuries

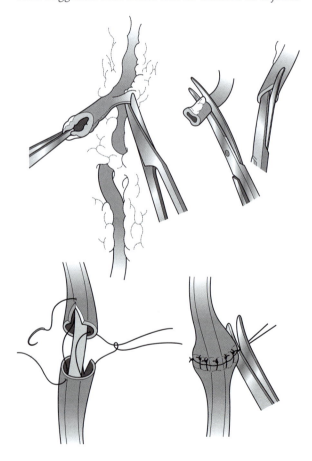

Figure 9.8.6 Technique of ureteric repair.

requiring minimal debridement, such as stab wounds, but not in gunshot wounds, where stenting results in significantly fewer leaks.

Injuries to the pelviureteric junction and its vicinity are treated in the same fashion, but a tube nephrostomy should be added.

Injuries around the pelvic brim are best treated by uretero-neocystostomy, with an antireflux reimplantation.

More advanced repair methods include the retrocolic transuretero-ureterostomy, and the creation of a Boari flap with attached uretero-neocystostomy.

In the case of loss of long segments where anastomosis to the contralateral ureter is not possible, an end-ureterostomy could be brought out, or nephrectomy done in rare cases of serious associated injuries in the area.

After surgery, the bladder is drained transurethrally, or ideally suprapubically, and closed suction drains can be placed retroperitoneally in proximity to the repaired ureter; these can be expected to drain for several days.

9.8.3.3 COMPLICATIONS

Complications comprise stricture with hydronephrosis, leakage from the anastomosis and infected urinomas, especially in late diagnosis, most of which are amenable to percutaneous management.

9.8.4 Bladder Injuries

Bladder injuries are mainly due to blunt trauma, and are found in about 8% of pelvic fractures. Penetrating trauma is due to gunshot, stabs, impalement, or iatrogenic injuries, mostly in relation to orthopaedic pelvic fixation.

9.8.4.1 DIAGNOSIS

Signs and symptoms vary from inability to void and frank haematuria, to vague abdominal or suprapubic tenderness without haematuria in a small percentage of cases.

Intraperitoneal injuries may be associated with a higher serum creatinine and urea, and low sodium, but this biochemical derangement takes some time to develop. Elevated serum creatinine levels are due to absorption of urine through the peritoneum.

Ultrasound and CT scanning can be of use to demonstrate free fluid in the abdomen, the presence of clots in the bladder, and a change in bladder filling and shape (with sonar probe compression). A CT cystogram can be done as part of an abdominal CT study, and can differentiate between intra- and extraperitoneal bladder injuries.

Retrograde cystography is the method of choice in the emergency room, as it is very accurate if a large enough volume of contrast (about 7 mL/kg) is instilled, and at least two separate projections (anteroposterior and lateral views) are obtained. Post-micturition films are essential. A minimum of 350 mL dilute contrast medium should be instilled.

Contrast extravasation will delineate loops of bowel and the peritoneal contours in intraperitoneal ruptures, while it will track along the pelvic bones, scrotum, obturator areas, etc., in extraperitoneal ruptures.

9.8.4.2 MANAGEMENT

Urgent operative treatment is indicated in all intraperitoneal, and some types of extraperitoneal, injuries, while others require delayed surgery upon failure of non-operative methods. Most penetrating injuries require immediate surgery.

9.8.4.2.1 Non-Operative Management

Urethral or suprapubic catheter drainage with a large-bore catheter, for up to 2 weeks, will allow most extraperitoneal injuries from blunt trauma to heal; surgery will be needed only if a cystogram at that stage shows ongoing leakage. Contraindications to non-operative management are bladder neck injury, the presence of bony fragments through the bladder wall, infected urine, and associated female genital injuries.

Extraperitoneal bladder repair during a laparotomy for other trauma is often easily accomplished, but may be dangerous if it requires opening into a tamponaded pelvic haematoma, and is inappropriate in the context of damage control.

9.8.4.3 SURGICAL APPROACH

Bladders can be repaired easily and with few complications with absorbable sutures.

All repairs should to be carried out through an intraperitoneal approach, from within the lumen of the bladder, after performing an adequate longitudinal incision on the anterior surface in order to avoid entering lateral pelvic haematomas. In cases of gunshot wound, *both* wounds to the bladder must be sought and identified. In some situations, it will be necessary to open the bladder widely, explore and repair from within. Single-layer mass suturing is indicated in extraperitoneal ruptures, but for intraperitoneal ruptures closure should be in separate layers.

Percutaneous suprapubic catheterization can be very difficult if the bladder is detached from the posterior urethra, and is not very full because of shock and partial emptying into the pelvic cavity. The recommended technique is to place a long intravenous catheter, such as a single lumen central line into the partially empty bladder under ultrasound (US) guidance, inflate the bladder with warm saline until very distended, and then insert the suprapubic catheter under US guidance.

The presence and patency of both ureteric orifices must be confirmed in all cases. If suturing in the vicinity, these should be cannulated with a size 5 feeding tube or ureteric catheter.

A large-bore transurethral or suprapubic catheter, or both, can be used, the latter being fed extraperitoneally into the bladder, and a drain left in the Retzius space. A cystogram will be done in most cases after 10 days to 2 weeks, followed by removal of the suprapubic catheter.

9.8.5 Urethral Injuries

Urethral injuries can have the most disastrous consequences of all genitourinary trauma, such as incontinence, long-lasting impotence, and strictures. They should be addressed as early as possible.

9.8.5.1 DIAGNOSIS

The mechanism of injury, a pelvic fracture, and blood at the meatus must alert the surgeon to the possibility of a urethral rupture, mainly of the posterior urethra from blunt trauma.

Rectal examination is mandatory before urethral catheter insertion, and a high-riding prostate will suggest that the urethra is disrupted. Rupture of the female urethra is, fortunately, very uncommon.

Once rupture is suspected, two completely different approaches are practised and acceptable:

- Retrograde urethrography is performed by placing a small Foley catheter in the fossa navicularis, with the patient in the oblique position.
- The preferable approach, however, is not to intervene with an emergency procedure at all. This is particularly important if a pelvic haematoma is present, due to the risk of effectively causing a compound injury.

It is preferable to place a suprapubic catheter (it will be necessary to allow the bladder to fill until it is palpable) prior to the insertion of the suprapubic catheter. A cystogram and, if necessary, cystoscopy can then be done under controlled circumstances at a later stage.

9.8.5.2 MANAGEMENT

9.8.5.2.1 Suprapubic Cystostomy

The mainstay of immediate treatment is the placement of a suprapubic catheter for urinary drainage. This can be done as an isolated open procedure, as an open procedure during a laparotomy, or using a percutaneous method. The isolated open method requires a lower midline laparotomy incision, and an intraperitoneal approach to the bladder to avoid entering a pelvic haematoma. Suprapubic placement during a laparotomy done for other reasons follows the same principles.

Percutaneous placement is done using specifically designed trochar and catheter kits.

The procedure requires a full bladder, as identified clinically or on ultrasound. If this is not the case, and the patient is not in a condition to produce a lot of urine, a small intravenous catheter can be placed under ultrasonic guidance using the Seldinger technique, and the bladder can then be distended with saline until a standard percutaneous method can be used.

9.8.5.3 RUPTURED URETHRA

Urethral injuries are most often associated with pelvic fractures, especially anterior arch fractures with displacement. Although blood at the urethral meatus, gross haematuria and displacement of the prostate are signs of urethral disruption, their absence does not exclude urethral injury.

The male urethra is divided into two portions:

- The *posterior urethra* is made up of the *prostatic* urethra and the *membranous* urethra, which courses between the prostatic apex and the perineal membrane.
- The *membranous urethra* is prone to injury from pelvic fracture because the puboprostatic ligaments fix the apex of the prostate gland to the bony pelvis, and shearing forces are applied to the urethra when the pelvis is disrupted.

- The *anterior urethra* is distal to that point. It is susceptible to blunt force injuries along its path in the perineum (such as from direct blows or fall astride injuries).

The conventional treatment for urethral injury is to divert the urinary stream with a suprapubic catheter and refer to a specialist centre for delayed reconstruction of the urethral injury. Early endoscopic realignment (within 1 week of injury) using a combined transurethral and percutaneous transvesical approach is advocated by some experts.

Anterior urethral trauma may present late, with symptoms of urethral stricture.

9.8.5.3.1 Urethral Repair

Immediate surgical intervention is recommended for the following conditions:

- All penetrating injuries of the posterior urethra and most of the anterior urethra.
- Posterior urethral injuries associated with rectal injuries and bladder neck injuries.
- Where there is wide separation of the ends of the urethra.
- Penile fracture.

Accurate approximation and end-to-end anastomosis are recommended for injuries to the anterior urethra, while for membranous urethra injuries, realignment and stenting over a Foley catheter for 3 or 4 weeks may be sufficient. This can be achieved by an open lower midline laparotomy and passage of Foley catheters from above and below, with ultimate passage into the bladder, or via flexible cystoscopy and manipulation.

Patients managed with a suprapubic catheter alone should have their definitive urethral repair after about 3 months from the injury.

> *Primary realignment may have better results than delayed repair, but delayed primary repair (day 8 to 10) is recommended when there is a large haematoma.*

9.8.6 **Injury to the Scrotum**

9.8.6.1 **DIAGNOSIS**

Ultrasound of the scrotum is indicated in evaluation of blunt trauma to the testicle, and can differentiate between torsion, disruption, and haematoma.

9.8.6.2 **MANAGEMENT**

The blood supply to the scrotum is so good that penetrating trauma usually can be treated by debridement and suturing.

If the tunica vaginalis of the testis is disrupted, the extruding seminiferous tubules should be trimmed off and the capsule closed as soon as possible, in order to minimize host reaction against the testis.

Loss of scrotal skin with exposed testicle, a well-described occurrence after burns and other trauma, often can be remedied by the creation of pouches in the proximal thigh skin and subsequent approximation, with little effect on the testicles.

9.8.7 **Gynaecological Injury and Sexual Assault**

Any evidence of gynaecological injury requires external and internal examination using a speculum, and exclusion of associated urethral and anorectal injuries. If rape is suspected or reported, the official sexual assault evidence collection kit should be used, and detailed clinical notes should be made. The patient must be counselled, and informed consent must, where possible, be obtained for *all* examinations.

Reporting of all cases of sexual assault should be carried out by the treating physician, in order to minimize underreporting by the already traumatized patient.

9.8.7.1 **MANAGEMENT**

Lacerations of the external genitalia and vagina can be sutured under local or general anaesthesia, and a vaginal pack left in for 24 hours to minimize the swelling.

Intrapelvic organs are dealt with at laparotomy by suturing, hysterectomy, or oophorectomy. Oxytocin is used to minimize uterine bleeding and colostomy to avoid soiling.

Additional supportive care for the psychological effects of sexual assault should be made available.

Antiretroviral treatment is more effective if instituted within 3 hours of injury, and sexually transmitted disease and pregnancy prophylaxis should be given according to standard protocols. Baseline blood tests required include human immunodeficiency virus (HIV) status, hepatitis B, full blood count, and liver and renal function; follow-up arrangements must be made to monitor medication and HIV status.

9.8.8 **Injury of the Pregnant Uterus**

Aggressive resuscitation of the mother and the foetus must be carried out in keeping with Advanced Trauma Life Support® recommendations. Midline laparotomy always should be used when surgery is necessary, but simple intrauterine death is best managed by induced labour at a later stage (see also Section 14.3).

REFERENCES AND RECOMMENDED READING

References

1. Armenakas NA, Duckett CP, McAninch JW. Indications for nonoperative management of renal stab wounds. *J Urol.* 1999 March;**161(3)**:768–71.

2. Velmahos GC, Demetriades D, Cornwell EE 3rd, Belzberg H, Murray J, Asensio J, et al. Selective management of renal gunshot wounds. *Br J Surg.* 1998 Aug;**85(8)**:1121–4.

3. Kozar RA, Crandall M, Shanmuganathan K, Zarzaur BL, Coburn M, Cribari C, et al. Organ injury scaling 2018 update: Spleen, liver and kidney. *J Trauma Acute Care Surg.* 2018 Dec;**85(6)**:1119–22. doi: 10.1097/TA.000000000000 2058.

4. Montgomery RC, Richardson JD, Harty JI. Posttraumatic renovascular hypertension after occult renal injury. *J Trauma.* 1998 Jul;**45(1)**:106–10.

Recommended Reading

Morey AF, Brandes S, Dugi DD 3rd, Armstrong JH, Breyer BN, Broghammer JA, et al. Urotrauma: AUA Guideline. American Urological Association Education and Research Inc 2014.

Santucci RA, Bartley JM. Urologic trauma guidelines: A 21st century update. *Nat Rev Urol.* 2010 Sep;**7(9)**:510–9. doi: 10.1038/nrurol.2010.119. Review.

Santucci RA, Wessells H, Bartsch G, Descotes J, Heyns CF, McAninch JW, et al. Evaluation and management of renal injuries: consensus statement of the Renal Trauma Subcommittee. *Br J Urol Int.* 2004 May;**93(7)**:937–54.

RENAL INJURIES

Hammer CC, Santucci RA. Effect of an institutional policy of non-operative treatment of grades I–IV renal injuries. *J Urol.* 2003 May;**169(5)**:1751–3.

Kim FJ, Da Silva RD. Genitourinary trauma. In Moore EE, Feliciano DV, Mattox KL Eds. *Trauma*, 8th edn. McGraw Hill Education, New York, 2017;669–708.

Velmahos GC, Constantinou C, Tillou A, Brown CV, Salim A, Demetriades D. Abdominal computed tomographic scan for patients with gunshot wounds to the abdomen selected for non-operative management. *J Trauma.* 2005 Nov;**59(5)**:1156–60; discussion 1160-61

URETERIC INJURIES

Armenakas NA. Current methods of diagnosis and management of ureteral injuries. *World J Urol.* 1999 April;**17**:78–83.

Velmahos GC, Degiannis E, Wells M, Souter I. Penetrating ureteral injuries: the impact of associated injuries on management. *Am Surg.* 1996 June;**62(6)**:461–8.

BLADDER

Haas CA, Brown SL, Spirnak JP. Limitations of routine spiral computerized tomography in the evaluation of bladder trauma. *J Urol.* 1999 July;**162(1)**:50–2.

Volpe MA, Pachter EM, Scalea TM, Macchia RJ, Mydlo JH. Is there a difference in outcome when treating traumatic intraperitoneal bladder rupture with or without a suprapubic tube? *J Urol.* 1999 April;**161(4)**:1103–5.

SCROTUM

Chang AJ, Brandes SB. Advances in diagnosis and management of genital injuries. *Urol Clin North Am.* 2013 Aug;**40(3)**:427–38. doi: 10.1016/j.ucl.2013.04.013. Epub 2013 May 29. Review.

Cline KJ, Mata JA, Venable DD, Eastham JA. Penetrating trauma to the male external genitalia. *J Trauma.* 1998 Mar;**44(3)**:492–4.

Munter DW, Faleski EJ. Blunt scrotal trauma: emergency department evaluation and management. *Am J Emerg Med.* 1989 Mar;**7(2)**:227–34.

Pelvic fractures may be due to low or high energy trauma, and consist of pelvic ring fractures and acetabular fractures, mainly due to blunt trauma. The likelihood of associated injuries in high energy trauma is 65%, usually involving the abdominal and pelvic viscera. In the haemodynamically unstable patient with severe pelvic fracture, there is a 90% risk of associated injury, a 50% risk of extra-pelvic bleeding, and a 30% risk of intra-abdominal bleeding.

The magnitude of pelvic bleeding as one of the 'hidden bleeding sources' is still underestimated, or missed completely. Mortality in the acute phase is largely due to exsanguination, and later to haemorrhage and pelvic soft tissue infections with related multiple organ failure. Overall mortality from pelvic fractures ranges from 5% to 16%, and rises to 30% in patients in hypovolaemic shock on admission. Open pelvic fractures are due to extreme forces and associated with a mortality rate of up to 50%. Severe pelvic fractures are often called 'killing fractures'.

Three questions need to be addressed:

- Is the patient in at high risk of massive bleeding?
- What are the sources of bleeding?
- What can be done to stop the bleeding?

Identification of a pelvic injury as bleeding source is a mandatory step in the primary survey of the ATLS®. Early eFAST and pelvic x-ray will guide the initial decision-making. The identification of an unstable pelvic ring fracture and the stabilization and/or compression of the pelvis by an external compression device ('reduce the pelvic volume') are potentially life-saving procedures that must be done in the emergency room. Severe pelvic injuries require a multidisciplinary team involving trauma-trained surgeons, anaesthesiologists, interventional radiologists, and orthopaedic surgeons. If adequate orthopaedic experience is unavailable, consideration should be given towards early transfer of this patient to an institution with the necessary expertise, as soon as the patient's condition allows. The decisions are made on an individual basis, considering the patient's status, the injury pattern, the available resources, and the experience in dealing with these complex injuries.

Formal treatment protocols for pelvic injuries have been shown to decrease mortality and should be developed in every hospital treating pelvic injuries.

10.1 **ANATOMY**

The surgical anatomy of the pelvis is the key to understanding pelvic injuries:

- The pelvic inlet is a circular structure that is immensely strong, but routinely gives way at more than one point should enough force be applied to it. Therefore, isolated fractures of the anterior or posterior pelvic ring are uncommon – look for the disruption of the opposite side of the pelvic ring as well.
- The forces required to fracture the pelvic ring do not respect the surrounding organ systems.
- The pelvic cavity is divided into the true and the false pelvis; the true pelvis refers to the space enclosed by the pelvic girdle below the pelvic brim and is located between the pelvic inlet and the pelvic floor.
- Most of the major pelvic bleeding originates in the true pelvis. External iliac vessels are in the false pelvis and may rarely cause major haemorrhage from iliac wing and acetabular fractures.
- The pelvis has a rich collateral blood supply, especially across the sacrum and posterior part of the ileum. The cancellous bone of the pelvis also has an excellent blood supply. More than 85% of pelvic haemorrhage is venous in origin, mainly from fracture sites. However, in the haemodynamically unstable patient with severe pelvic injury, arterial bleeding is frequent (>50%). Important for the treatment is

that the surgeon must deal with fractures, arterial bleeding, and venous bleeding.

- Post-mortem examination has shown that the pelvic peritoneum 'should' tamponade pelvic haematomas can accommodate more than 3000 mL. However, in case of severe pelvic fractures where the retroperitoneal compartment is disrupted, and the external bony barrier is not stable, haematoma may extend upwards towards the mediastinum ('chimney effect') or downwards into the medial thigh in case of rupture of the pelvic floor.
- All iliac vessels, the sciatic nerve roots, including the lumbosacral nerve, and the ureters cross the sacroiliac joint, and disruption of this joint may cause severe haemorrhage, and sometimes causes arterial and venous obstruction of the iliac vessels and nerve palsy. Fortunately, injuries to the ureters are rare.
- The pelvic organs (bladder, rectum, and female reproductive organs) as well as abdominal organs (parts of colon and small bowel in the false pelvis) are prone to shear and compression forces acting on the pelvis during the impact of injury.
- Apart from blunt compression injury, the bladder can also rupture owing to fracture penetration.
- The pelvis also features the acetabulum, a major structure in weight transfer to the leg. Failure to appreciate the injury or inappropriate treatment will lead to severe disability.

10.2 CLASSIFICATION

The two most used classification systems are mainly based on the direction and location of applied force (Young and Burgess), or fracture pattern allowing judgement on the stability of the pelvic ring (Tile). The different classification systems are all based on grade of fracture stability, and close correlation with risk of bleeding has been shown. However, no fracture pattern can exclude significant haemorrhage. In practice, no major differences have been shown between the two systems.[1]

10.2.1 Tile's Classification[2]

Tile's classification is one of the most used and classifies fractures into three main types (from A1 to C3). Pelvic ring fractures can be classified into three types, using the Tile classification, based on their severity.

10.2.1.1 TYPE A: COMPLETELY STABLE

Posterior pelvic integrity is intact. Rarely related to massive bleeding; however, severe wing fracture dislocation may cause bleeding in rare cases. This involves isolated fracture of the iliac wing or pubic rami, mostly caused by direct compression (Figure 10.1). These are stable fractures, to be treated conservatively (Figure 10.2).

10.2.1.2 TYPE B: VERTICALLY STABLE BUT ROTATIONALLY UNSTABLE

B-type fractures are subdivided into externally (B1) and internally (B2) rotated fractures (sometimes one side internal and other side external rotation may present same time – B3):

Type B1: This is the most common type of fracture, also known as an 'open book' fracture. There is horizontal (external rotational) instability owing to an anterior lesion (disruption of the symphysis and/or fracture of the superior and inferior pubic rami) combined with a posterior disruption of the anterior *or* posterior ligaments of the sacroiliac joint. The impact on the sacrum itself is small. It can result in bleeding in an enlarged pelvic cavity. Injury of the lower urogenital tract, rectum, and vagina and severe soft tissue damage owing to the rotation are frequently seen in these cases. Internal or external stabilization is required.

Type B2: This occurs less commonly, and is a lateral compression-type injury, which results in an intrinsically stable fracture of the pelvic ring, with an impression of the posterior complex in the sacral bone and mostly damage at the pubic arch. Perforation of the bladder can be caused by the anterior fracture, as can hypovolaemic shock owing to severe disruption of the soft tissues of the pelvic diaphragm; organ injury to the lower urogenital tract and rectum can be seen in these cases.

Type B3: This is a combined B1 and B2 injury.

10.2.1.3 TYPE C: WHOLLY UNSTABLE IN ROTATIONAL AND VERTICAL PLANES

There is complete horizontal and vertical instability, owing to anterior and posterior fractures and/or disruptions (complete sacroiliac disruption or displaced vertical sacral fracture). A fall from height, as well as anteroposterior shearing forces in a dashboard impact in a motor

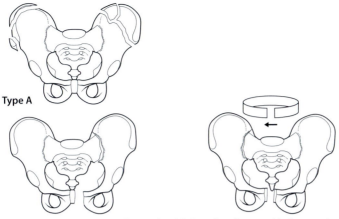

Type A

Type B1 Fracture ('unilateral open-book'). Rotationally unstable fracture (external rotation)

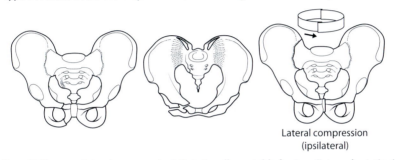

Lateral compression
(ipsilateral)

Type B2 Fracture (lateral compression). Rotationally unstable fracture (internal rotation)

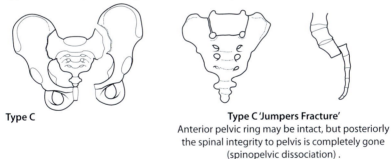

Type C

Type C 'Jumpers Fracture'
Anterior pelvic ring may be intact, but posteriorly
the spinal integrity to pelvis is completely gone
(spinopelvic dissociation) .

Figure 10.1 Tile classification of fractures of the pelvis.

vehicle crash, result in this type of fracture (disruption of symphysis pubis or fractures of rami combined with complete sacroiliac joint disruption or displaced vertical sacral/medial wing fracture). Type C fracture may involve one hemi-pelvis (C1 or C2) or both hemi-pelves (C3) and is the result of extensive mechanical force, and has the highest risk of major artery bleeding owing to shearing dislocation in the posterior pelvic ring. Type C fracture is most often the 'killing fracture' of all pelvic fractures. Major dislocations put pelvic organs at high risk of related injuries (bladder, urethra, rectum, vagina,

sciatic and femoral nerve). Extreme acceleration/deceleration forces also increase the risk of intra-abdominal and abdominal retroperitoneal shearing injuries (bowel, mesentery, kidney arteries).

10.2.1.4 A JUMPER'S FRACTURE

A 'jumper's fracture' is a special type of type C pelvic ring fracture. The posterior integrity of the pelvic ring, as well as integrity of lumbar spine to pelvis, is completely gone (also known as 'spinopelvic dissociation'). The

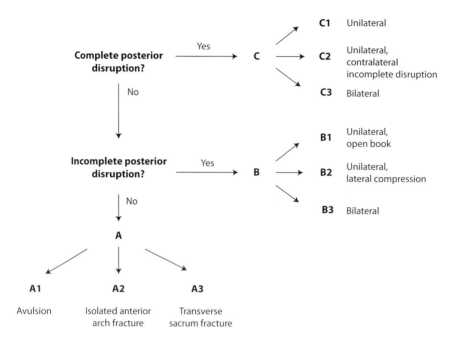

Figure 10.2 Summary of Tile classification of fractures of the pelvis.

phenomenal appearance of this injury is that there often is no disruption to the anterior pelvic ring, which makes it difficult to identify from plain x-rays. Jumper's fracture is due to landing on feet when falling from a height. The pelvis stops moving down when the feet contact the ground, but the rest of the body does not, resulting in spine and medial parts of sacrum (just below the lowest lumbar spine) being fractured and 'pushed' down into the pelvis (Figure 10.1). This injury may have bleeding and often affects sciatic and sacral nerves resulting in cauda equina syndrome. CT is required for accurate diagnosis.

10.2.1.5 ACETABULAR FRACTURES

Acetabular fractures do not involve the integrity of the posterior pelvic ring. However, some acetabular fractures may be easy to mistake and mix with pelvic ring injury, especially the ones involving major fracture of the medial iliac wing in close vicinity of the sacroiliac joint. Acetabular fracture-related major bleeding is rare and seldom involves the major internal iliac vessels. However, severe dislocation in acetabular fracture may also involve external iliac vessels, resulting in bleeding or blunt arterial distension injury with thrombosis.

10.2.1.6 FRACTURE COMBINATIONS

In some cases, there are combined pelvic fractures, involving both pelvic ring and acetabulum. There is no classification for these combined fractures, and both pelvic ring and acetabulum fractures are classified on an individual basis. Clinically, the most dislocated component results in the most likely source of bleeding.

10.2.2 Young and Burgess Classification[3]

This system is based primarily on the direction of the force causing the injury: anterior posterior compression (APC) types II and III, lateral compression (LC) type III and vertical shear (VS) fractures are characterized by major ligamentous disruption. VS fractures include the isolated vertical force vectors, and combined mechanism (CM) fractures include pelvic ring disruptions that do not fall into any single category.

10.2.2.1 ANTEROPOSTERIOR COMPRESSION (APC) (TYPE 1, 2, 3)

- *APC-1*: Stable injury pattern with 'sprain' of the pubic symphysis (<2.5 cm diastasis), no injury to the posterior elements.

- *APC-2*: Rotationally unstable injury pattern with complete disruption of pubic symphysis (>2.5 cm diastasis) and disruption of the anterior sacro-iliac ligament.
- *APC-3*: Rotationally and vertically unstable injury pattern with complete disruption of pubic symphysis (>2.5 cm diastasis) and complete disruption of the anterior and posterior SI ligaments (Figures 10.3 and 10.4).

10.2.2.2 LATERAL COMPRESSION (LC) (TYPE 1, 2, 3)

- *LC-1*: Stable injury pattern with transverse pubic rami fractures and stable impaction fracture of the ipsilateral sacrum. Minimal or no internal rotation deformity.
- *LC-2*: Rotationally unstable injury pattern with transverse pubic rami fractures, unstable posterior fracture/dislocation of the ipsilateral SI joint, and internal malrotation of the injured hemi-pelvis.

The 'classic' LC-2 pattern is reflected by a trans-iliosacral ('crescent') fracture dislocation.

- *LC-3*: Rotationally and vertically unstable injury pattern with ipsilateral and contralateral injury to the posterior elements ('windswept pelvis').

10.2.2.3 VERTICAL SHEAR

VS injury pattern consists of a complete disruption of the pubic symphysis (with or without associated pubic rami fractures) and a complete disruption of the SI joint (with or without associated fractures of the iliac wing and sacrum). The injured hemi-pelvis is externally rotated and vertically translated, resulting in a combined rotational and translation instability.

10.2.2.4 COMBINED MECHANISM

Any combination of any of the above, combined with haemodynamic instability.

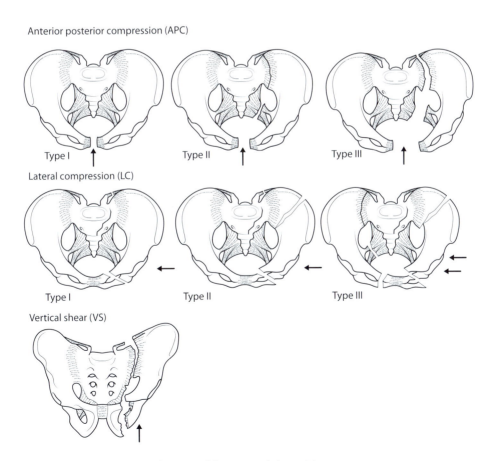

Figure 10.3 Young and Burgess classification of fractures of the pelvis.

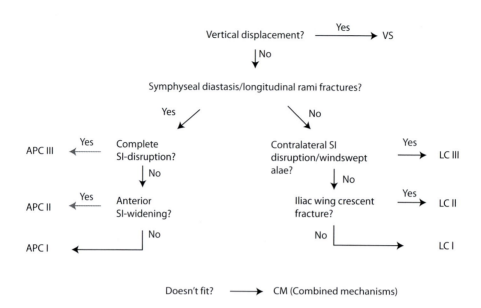

Figure 10.4 Summary of the Young and Burgess classification of fractures of the pelvis.

10.3 CLINICAL EXAMINATION AND DIAGNOSIS

Pelvic fractures should be easily identified if Advanced Trauma Life Support® (ATLS) guidelines are followed, (i.e. clinical palpation of the pelvic brim from the SI joint to pubic symphysis and a routine chest x-ray and pelvic x-ray for any blunt injury in a patient unable to walk). In the absence of x-ray facilities, a clinical examination can be performed with gentle bimanual palpation of the brim of the pelvis from the SI joints to the pubic symphysis. Difference of height of the superior anterior iliac spine can be found in type C injuries. Any palpable defect or boggy swelling is indicative of a pelvic disruption. In the absence of these signs, gentle bimanual lateral and antero-posterior compression (not distraction!) of the pelvis can be performed. Any instability felt indicates the presence of major pelvic instability, associated with life-threatening blood loss, requiring appropriate measures. The absence of clinical instability does not, however, preclude an unstable pelvic fracture. One-third of such trauma victims with pelvic ring fractures sustain circulatory instability on arrival. Extended focused abdominal sonography for trauma (eFAST) is needed to exclude intra-abdominal bleeding in these patients. Pelvic fracture-related intra-abdominal bladder rupture results in free fluid in the abdominal cavity. However, ultrasound does not have the sensitivity to tell the difference between blood and urine.

Inspection of the skin may reveal lacerations in the groin, perineum, or sacral area, indicating an open pelvic fracture, the result of gross deformation. Evidence of perineal injury or haematuria mandates radiological evaluation of the urinary tract from below upwards (retrograde urethrogram followed by cystogram or computed tomography [CT] cystogram, followed by an excretory urogram as appropriate) when the physiology allows. Inspection of the urethral meatus may reveal a drop of blood, indicating urethral rupture. There seems to be little evidence to support the fear of converting partial urethral rupture into a complete rupture by gently trying to insert a Foley catheter. Urological tract imaging is mandated if you cannot pass a catheter easily with the return of clear urine. Blood at the meatus, or a high riding prostate should have raised the alert and the most highly skilled person available should be utilized to insert an in-dwelling catheter with great care. Inability to pass the catheter easily mandates a cystourethrogram to define the suspected urethral injury. If there is resistance, the patient should have a suprapubic catheter inserted.

Inspection of the anus may reveal lacerations of the sphincter mechanism. Diligent rectal examination (and in females, a vaginal examination), may reveal blood in the rectum and/or discontinuity of the rectal wall, indicating a rectal laceration, and similarly in the vagina. In male patients, the prostate is palpated; a high-riding prostate indicates a complete urethral avulsion. A full neurological examination is performed of the perineal area, sphincter mechanism, and femoral and sciatic nerves.

The CT scanner is the diagnostic modality of choice in the haemodynamically stable patient, and CT angiography is particularly helpful.

10.4 **RESUSCITATION**

The priorities for resuscitating patients with pelvic fractures are no different from the standard. These injuries produce a real threat to the circulation, and management is geared toward controlling this. Management is based on haemodynamic status. Because of the capacity of the pelvis to continue to bleed, these patients require urgent control of haemorrhage. Most contemporary treatment protocols rely on pelvic stabilization and interventional radiology, alone or in combination. Other (damage control) options are needed for the unstable exsanguinating patient and when angiography is unavailable.

Since pelvic bleeding is commonly associated with traumatic coagulopathy, early blood and coagulation factor substitution is mandatory. Viscohaemostatic assays (VHA) should be routine in such patients. Volume resuscitation should be based on blood and blood products to prevent further dilutive coagulopathy.

10.4.1 **Haemodynamically Normal Patients**

There is usually an isolated injury possibly requiring external or internal (open) reduction and fixation to limit future instability and disability. The management is not critically urgent, and can be done either as immediate surgery in cases of isolated injury or in a delayed fashion with in the first week after trauma.

10.4.2 **Haemodynamically Stable Patients (Transient Responders)**

Patients responding to initial volume resuscitation need external stabilization of the pelvic ring. Several principal methods for external stabilization of the pelvic ring exist:

- External compression by circumferential wrap with standard hospital draw sheets or special devices as a sling or traumatic pelvic orthotic device (T-POD). Such devices are applied in the ER or in some trauma systems in a preclinical setting.

Pitfall

Do not place the compression device too low or too high over the abdomen itself. It is important to centre the compression at the level of the greater trochanters and internally rotate the legs before applying the compression. This will optimize the vector of compression force from the acetablular area to the middle of pelvis, and compress both the anterior and posterior part of the pelvic ring.

- External compression devices such as sheets or T-Pod are easy to place, however, they give less stability to the bony pelvis than an external fixator or a C-clamp. In addition, access to the abdomen or the femoral vessels is limited. Also, ICU nursing is hampered by such devices. Therefore, the surgeon should consider replacing the sheet or T-Pod in the OR with, for example, an external fixator.
- External fixators can be applied over the iliac crest or in the supra-acetabular region of the iliac bone. The latter may be technically more difficult to apply, however, it gives significantly more stability to the pelvic ring.
- The pelvic C-clamp, applied close to the level of the sacro-iliac joint, is most effective in providing pelvic compression. The application may be more difficult and cannot be performed in cases with dorsal iliac bone fractures. A pelvic x-ray needs to be done before application of a C-clamp to exclude an *os ilium* fracture at the insertion site of the clamp (Figure 10.5).

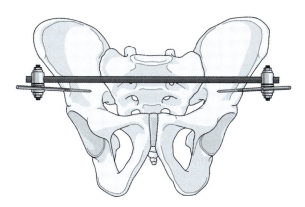

Figure 10.5 External fixation of the pelvis.

If patients continue to bleed after external fixation in the OR additional bleeding control needs to be done either by interventional angiography or pelvic packing (see Section 10.7 below).

10.4.3 **Haemodynamically Unstable Patients (Non-Responders)**

A severely disrupted pelvic fracture may present as the classical non-responder to any volume or blood restoration. These patients tend to exsanguinate rapidly, and immediate measures are required to control bleeding.

If the bleeding is considered possibly to be arterial in nature, especially with a blush on CT scan, there may be indication for REBOA as a temporising action until angioembolisation can be achieved (see also Section 16.4).

- The goal of the treatment is to decrease pelvic bleeding by temporary means and to find possible adjacent bleeding sites.
- Applying a pelvic binder or sheet, as described above, is the first step. In type C fractures, the C-clamp may be beneficial if available and can be applied quickly. However, the quickly and correctly applied pelvic binder is better than spending too much time on the C-clamp.[4]
- Pelvic x-ray will help working with the binder. It gives the idea of dislocation and needed reduction (compression) forces applied with the binder.
- Angioembolization or REBOA require access to the groin (common femoral artery). The pelvic binder will block this access initially, but may be repositioned. An unstable pelvic ring must not be left without stabilization during the procedure.
- Depending on the available resources, extraperitoneal pelvic packing (EPP) or interventional angioembolization is the next choice for bleeding control. Pelvic angioembolization is only a choice if there is no other urgent need for surgical interventions and it is available within a short timeframe. The full-scale resuscitation needs to be possible throughout the embolization process, therefore, remote or small angiography suites are not suitable for these patients.
- If the patient has undergone CT that reveals an arterial blush, the most effective management is angioembolization.
- Angioembolization should *precede* the pelvic packing if the haemodynamics are not improving. Every hour of delay counts in angioembolization.[5] Pelvic packing has little of effect on major arterial bleeding, but will reduce the pelvic volume and tamponade venous bleeding. Since 80%–90% of the venous, in almost all cases with arterial bleeding, there is concomitant venous bleeding.

- Angioembolization and pelvic packing are considered as complementary procedures.

Persistent bleeding after packing may require angioembolization and vice versa.

- In hemodynamically crushing patients ('patients in extremis'), the clamping of the thoracic aorta can temporarily support the haemodynamics, decrease the arterial pelvic bleeding, and buy time for both establishing and catching up with the fluid resuscitation.
- REBOA can be used for proximal bleeding control (zone III at the level of bifurcation) or both as resuscitative support and bleeding control (zone I at the level of thoracic aorta).
- REBOA may serve as a bridge to definitive hemostatic treatment after severe pelvic trauma.

Pitfall

REBOA, as well as clamping of the thoracic aorta, will *not* stop the bleeding but only buy time. The next step of the bleeding control has to be planned during REBOA deployment and executed promptly after that.

10.5 **EXTERNAL FIXATION**

Traditional external fixation cannot provide complete stability or compression. A force applied to a segment of a circle cannot stabilize defects outside of that segment, it can only do so in one dimension and will aggravate disruption outside of the segment across which it is applied. Generally, external fixators are best suited for APC and LC fractures, and pelvic C-clamps are best suited for VS types. Points of fixation include the following.

10.5.1 **Iliac-Crest Route**

This can be carried out without fluoroscopic imaging, and is the method of choice for ER external fixation; it is technically less demanding and faster for acute application, but is associated with a higher failure rate.

10.5.2 **Supra-acetabular Route**

This require more accurate pin placement under fluoroscopic guidance, C-arm, and a radio-transparent orthopaedic table. Its main benefits are a higher resistance to failure, since it is attached through a much stronger part of the bone, and normally only 1 pin is required.

10.5.3 **Pelvic C-clamp**

Pelvic C-clamps are applied close to the maximum diameter of the pelvis at the level of the sacro-iliac joint and should be more effective in providing pelvic compression. Their application may be more difficult, and not carried out in all trauma centres.

10.6 **LAPAROTOMY**

If the patient is exsanguinating or requires surgery for other injuries, or angiography is delayed or unavailable, it is prudent to perform a laparotomy to treat or exclude intra-abdominal bleeding. In such a case, the peritoneal incision should be limited at its lower end to few centimetres below the umbilicus, if feasible. If the major source of bleeding is the pelvis, consider extraperitoneal packing of the pelvis with intact peritoneum in the presence of a large or expanding pelvic haematoma, which should preferably be performed *first* (i.e. before the laparotomy). Packing of the pelvis will be most effective against a stabilized pelvic ring (external fixation). If pelvic bleeding persists, direct exploration with suturing or ligature of lacerations of major blood vessels may be required.

In the unstable patient, other sources of intra-abdominal bleeding must be excluded. Consider damage control surgery (DCS) (see also Chapter 6).

- Temporary closure of the abdominal wall is preferable, using a negative-pressure (sandwich) technique.
- Angiography should be performed after DCS for control of any remaining pelvic bleeding by embolization of the bleeding vessels. Extraperitoneal pelvic packing should be considered.

In the more stable patient, if bleeding persists, explore the pelvis and tamponade the area, with suturing or ligature of lacerations of the major blood vessels, repair of anatomical structures (bladder and rectum) where possible, and cystostomy and/or colostomy with rectal wash-out as required. If it is required and possible at this stage, undertake internal fixation of the pelvic ring in case of non-complex fracture types such as a symphyse-olysis. All complex type of fractures should be taken care of by external fixation.

After the initial haemorrhage has been controlled, general DCS principles apply to EPP, and the patient is returned to the operating room for definitive surgery when physiology has been restored (36–48 hours).

Pitfall

A caveat of pack removal is that the longer the packs are left in, the greater the risk of pelvic sepsis. Definitive internal fixation of the pelvis is ideally performed early, but timing will obviously depend on the physiology.

Formal treatment protocols for pelvic injuries have been shown to decrease mortality and should be developed in every hospital treating pelvic injuries.

Requirements for blood average 15 units for open pelvic fractures. To avoid dilutional coagulopathy, protocols for massive transfusion should be instituted. Volume replacement is ultimately only an adjunct to the treatment of haemorrhagic shock – stopping the bleeding. VHA is invaluable in monitoring and correcting any coagulopathies that may arise.

10.7 **EXTRAPERITONEAL PELVIC PACKING**

A total of 80%–90% of pelvic bleeding is venous, arising from the multiple venous plexuses around the pelvis. This bleeding is not controllable by arterial embolization. The properly performed EPP with a stabilized pelvic ring will be able to control venous and some arterial bleeding. In the most effective packing technique, the packing is done in the true pelvis.

EPP was first described in 1985 by Pohleman,[6] and the technique was further described by Ertel in 2001,[7] and Smith in 2005.[8] The original technique was more aggressive, but the current technique stops below or medial to the external iliac vessels at the pelvic brim.

World Society of Emergency Surgery (WSES) guidelines[9] recommend pelvic packing as first choice (although with a low level of recommendation), while the EAST guideline suggests the angioembolization a treatment of choice for the bleeding pelvis.[10] Comparative studies will not contribute further evidence to this debate. Therefore, the availability of the necessary resources in the local trauma system will influence the surgeon's decision in this context.

If the source of the bleeding is in doubt, or FAST or diagnostic peritoneal lavage (DPL) results are positive, it is wise to perform an exploratory laparotomy to treat or rule out intra-abdominal bleeding. In the presence of a large or expanding pelvic haematoma, extraperitoneal pelvic packing should be performed by grabbing the edges of the peritoneum and entering the preperitoneal space from the midline (Figure 10.6).

If other sources of bleeding have been ruled out, the EPP can be done without entering the abdomen via a lower midline suprapubic incision.

10.7.1 **Technique of Extraperitoneal Packing**[11,12]

- The patient is positioned supine, and, if necessary, to provide a firm surface to pack against, an anterior external fixator with bilateral single supra-acetabular pins and external fixator, or a C-clamp is applied.
- A 5 cm midline suprapubic incision is made, and the fascia anterior to the rectus muscle is exposed.
- The fascia is divided in the midline until the symphysis can be palpated directly (the preperitoneal plane has been reached), protecting against urinary bladder damage. From the symphysis, the pelvic brim is followed laterally and posterior to the sacro-iliac joint (first bony irregularity felt), first on the side of major bleeding (most often the side of sacro-iliac joint disruption).

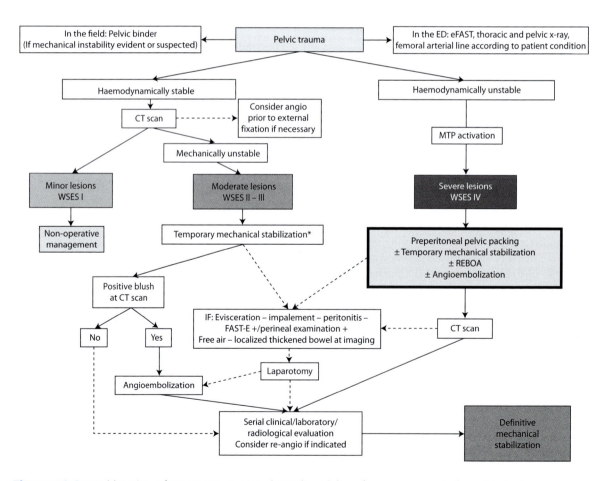

Figure 10.6 World Society of Emergency Surgery (WSES) guidelines for management of a pelvic fracture.

- The bladder and rectum are then held to the opposite side while the plane is opened bluntly down to the pelvic floor, avoiding injury to vascular and nerve structures in the area.
- The space is then packed with vascular or abdominal swabs, starting posteriorly and distal to the tip of the sacrum, and building the packs cranially and anteriorly.
- The procedure is then repeated on the opposite side.
- Packing a pelvis efficiently, implies also addressing arterial bleeding. This requires applying force while packing. In an unbroken pelvis with an intact pelvic floor, one should be able accommodate three large abdominal swabs on each side. In severe pelvic fractures, efficient packing might require much more (more than 10 packs not being unusual). The number of packs needed is defined by the available space and the appropriate force applied.
- Closure is by using standard DCS techniques, including negative pressure dressings.

As in the abdomen, the packs should be removed after 24–48 hours.

10.8 ASSOCIATED INJURIES

Associated injuries can only be managed once the patient is haemodynamically stable. In case of associated bleeding, the sequence of bleeding control interventions on pelvis and other bleeding sites depends on the individual choice of surgeon. Normally, the assumed most prominent bleeding is targeted first. Procedures for damage control may be the only available option.

10.8.1 Head Injuries

These are the most commonly associated major injuries. It is worthwhile remembering that 'C' precedes 'D' during resuscitation and management: the CT scan and neurosurgical procedures must wait for haemodynamic stability, and haemodynamic stability may be achieved only after DCS.

10.8.2 Intra-abdominal Injuries

These are frequently masked by pelvic pain. Retroperitoneal haematomas may break through into the peritoneal cavity, causing a false-positive result on eFAST or DPL. In the presence of a pelvic fracture, CT scanning is the diagnostic modality of choice in the stable patient. In all other patients, diagnostic ultrasound is preferred. If open diagnostic peritoneal lavage is performed, the entry point should be above the umbilicus to avoid entering extraperitoneal haematomas tracking up the anterior abdominal wall. A low threshold should be maintained for laparotomy because of associated intraperitoneal injury.

10.8.3 Bladder and Urethral Injuries (See also Section 9.8)

Bladder injuries are the most common accompanying injury of pelvic fractures. It is important to distinguish between extra peritoneal and intraperitoneal bladder injuries. While intraperitoneal bladder injuries demand primary surgical repair, extra peritoneal bladder injuries can be handled non-surgically (by suprapubic catheter).

10.8.4 Urethral Injuries (See Section 9.8)

Urethral injuries should be managed conservatively. Primary urethral repair by cystoperineal traction sutures results in minimal disability in the hands of experts when performed immediately in stable patients. For the majority, suprapubic cystostomy (preferably under ultrasonic guidance) and delayed urethral repair is required. If the patient needs to be taken to the operating theatre for extraperitoneal packing, it is usually very simple to railroad a catheter transurethrally into the damaged area and then pass it under vision into the bladder.

Endourological techniques with two cystoscopes can also allow early (2–7 days) primary realignment, which is accompanied by a significant decrease in stricture formation and need for further extensive surgery. Suprapubic cystostomy and delayed urethral repair may be needed if the patient is unstable but does not require surgery for other reasons. Septic complications with urethral injuries in the presence of pelvic fractures requiring fixation do not seem to be of concern.[13]

10.8.5 Anorectal Injuries[14]

Injuries of the anus and rectum are managed according to the degree of damage to the sphincters and anorectal mucosa. Injuries superficial to these require only debridement and dressings. Deep injuries require diversion colostomy and drainage.

Sphincter repair is best left for the experts, but repeated debridement and early approximation of mucosa to skin should limit infection and scarring.

10.8.6 Vaginal Injuries

All vaginal injuries should be explored under a general anaesthetic. Vaginal lacerations should be managed as follows:

- High lesions should be repaired and closed.
- Lower lesions should be packed and addressed after the patient is stable.

10.9 OPEN PELVIC FRACTURES

Complex pelvic fractures with open pelvic injury can be the most difficult of all injuries to treat. Initially, they can cause devastating haemorrhage and may later be associated with overwhelming pelvic sepsis and distant multiple organ failure.

10.9.1 Diagnosis

For those patients who present with compound pelvic fractures and are haemodynamically stable, diagnostic studies such as plain films of the pelvis, three-dimensional CT scans, and CT angiography should be rapidly carried out. The injuries to the rectum and vagina must be assessed.

10.9.2 Surgery

All patients with open (compound) pelvic fractures should be taken to the operating room as soon as the necessary diagnostic studies have been carried out. Control of pelvic bleeding can be temporarily achieved by packing the open wound and then making the decision of whether to obtain a pelvic arteriogram (which will be positive in 15% of cases), or to move rapidly to external fixation of the anterior pelvis and consideration for posterior stabilization as well. These decisions are made on an individual basis, considering the patient's status, the injury pattern, and the surgeon's experience in dealing with these complex injuries. Further diagnostics can then be carried on, keeping in mind that there is also high risk of internal pelvic bleeding and other associated pelvic area injuries.

Based on location of the injury, colostomy may be required in order to prevent contamination of the wound in the post-injury period. In general, all injuries involving the perineum and perianal area should have a diverting colostomy. However, in the damage control situation, contamination must be controlled (if necessary by temporary occlusion), but establishment of a colostomy should be postponed until the patient's physiology has returned to normal.

10.10 SUMMARY

A haemodynamically normal patient can be safely transferred for stabilization of unstable fractures within hours after injury and following control of the associated damage.

- Associated injuries should only be managed once the patient is haemodynamically stable.
- Procedures for damage control may be the only available option in the unstable patient.
- External stabilization of the pelvic ring is the basis of all treatments.
- Correction of coagulopathy and blood restoration using a massive transfusion protocol is the second step, and a prerequisite for the creation of a stable clot in the retroperitoneum.
- If necessary, further bleeding control can be achieved either by angioembolization or extraperitoneal packing.
- Extra peritoneal packing should be performed prior to opening the abdomen, where possible.
- Packing controls both venous and some arterial bleeding, while angioembolization only addresses arterial bleeders.

REFERENCES AND RECOMMENDED READING

References

1. Osterhoff G, Scheyerer MJ, Fritz Y, Bouaicha S, Wanner GA, Simmen HP, et al. Comparing the predictive value of the pelvic ring injury classification systems by Tile and by Young and Burgess. *Injury.* 2014 Apr;**45(4)**:742–7. doi: 10.1016/j.injury.2013.12.003.
2. Tile M. Acute pelvic fractures: causation and classification. *J Am Acad Orthop Surg.* 1996 May;**4(3)**:143–51.
3. Young JW, Burgess AR, Brumback RJ, Poka A. Pelvic fractures: Value of plain radiography in early assessment and management. *Radiology.* 1986 Aug;**160(2)**:445–51.
4. Bakhshayesh P, Boutefnouchet T, Tötterman A. Effectiveness of non-invasive external pelvic compression: a systematic review of the literature. *Scand J Trauma Resusc Emerg Med.* 2016 May;**24**:73. doi: 10.1186/s13049-016-0259-7.
5. Matsushima K, Piccinini A, Schellenberg M, Cheng V, Heindel P, Strumwasser A, et al. Effect of door-to-angioembolization time on mortality in pelvic fracture: Every hour of delay counts. *J Trauma Acute Care Surg.* 2018 Nov; **85(5)**:685–92. doi: 10.1097/TA.0000000000001803.
6. Pohleman T, Gänsslen A, Bosch U, Tscherne H. The technique of packing for control of haemorrhage in complex pelvic fractures. *Tech Orthop.* 1995;**9**:267–70.
7. Ertel W, Keel M, Eid K, Platz A, Trentz O. Control of severe haemorrhage using C-clamp and pelvic packing in multiply injured patients with pelvic ring disruption. *J Orthop Trauma.* 2001 Sep-Oct;**15(7)**:468–74.
8. Smith WR, Moore EE, Osborn P, Agudelo JF, Morgan SJ, Parekh AA, et al. Retroperitoneal packing as a resuscitation technique for haemodynamically unstable patients with pelvic fractures: report of two representative cases and a description of technique. *J Trauma.* 2005 Dec;**59**: 1510–14.
9. Coccolini F, Stahel PF, Montori G, Biffl W, Horer TM, Catena F, et al. Pelvic trauma: WSES classification and guidelines. *World J Emerg Surg.* 2017 Jan;**12(5)**. doi: 10.1186/s13017-017-0117-6. eCollection 2017. Review.
10. Cullinane DC, Schiller HJ, Zielinski MD, Bilaniuk JW, Collier BR, Como J, et al. Eastern Association for the Surgery of Trauma practice management guidelines for hemorrhage in pelvic fracture – update and systematic review. *J Trauma.* 2011 Dec;**71(6)**:1850–68. doi: 10.1097/TA.0b013e31823dca9a.
11. Filiberto DM, Fox AD. Preperitoneal pelvic packing: Technique and outcomes. *Int J Surg.* 2016 Sep;**33(Pt B)**: 222–24.
12. Burlew CC. Preperitoneal pelvic packing: A 2018 EAST Master Class Video Presentation. *J Trauma Acute Care Surg.* 2018 July;**85(1)**:224–8. doi: 10.1097/TA.0000000000001881.
13. Johnsen NV, Vanni AJ, Voelzke BB. Risk of infectious complications in pelvic fracture urethral injury patients managed with internal fixation and suprapubic catheter placement. *J Trauma Acute Care Surg.* 2018 Sep;**85(3)**:536–40. doi: 10.1097/TA.0000000000002012.
14. Fry RD. Anorectal trauma and foreign bodies. *Surg Clin N Am.* 1994 Dec;**74(6)**:1491–505.

Recommended Reading

HAEMORRHAGE

Costantini TW, Coimbra R, Holcomb JB, Podbielski JM, Catalano R, Blackburn A, et al. Current management of hemorrhage from severe pelvic fractures: Results of an American Association for the Surgery of Trauma multi-institutional trial. AAST Pelvic Fracture Study Group. *J Trauma Acute Care Surg.* 2017 Jun;**82(6)**:1030–38. doi: 10.1097/TA.0000000000001465.

Petersen DJ. Pelvic hematoma and hemodynamic instability in the absence of fracture; 2018; *J Trauma Acute Care Surgery.* 2018 Jul;**85(1)**:218–9. doi: 10.1097/TA.0000000000001900.

REBOA

Moore LJ, Martin CD, Harvin JA, Wade CE, Holcomb JB. Resuscitative Endovascular Balloon Occlusion of the Aorta (REBOA) for Control of Non-Compressible Truncal Hemorrhage in the Abdomen and Pelvis. *The American Journal of Surgery.* 2016 Dec;**212(6)**:1222–30. doi: 10.1016/j.amjsurg.2016.09.027.

Napolitano LM. Resuscitative Endovascular Balloon Occlusion of the Aorta: Indications, Outcomes, and Training. *Crit Care Clin.* 2017 Jan;**33(1)**:55–70. doi: 10.1016/j.ccc.2016.08.011. Review.

Pieper A, Thony F, Brun J, Rodière M, Boussat B, Arvieux C, et al. Resuscitative endovascular balloon occlusion of the aorta for pelvic blunt trauma and life-threatening hemorrhage: A 20-year experience in a Level I trauma center. *J Trauma Acute Care Surg.* 2018 Mar;**84(3)**:49–453. doi: 10.1097/TA.0000000000001794.

Extremity Trauma

11.1 OVERVIEW

Extremity injuries often look dramatic and occur in 85% of patients who sustain blunt trauma, but they rarely cause a threat to life or limb. However, in some circumstances, the relevance of such injuries assumes major importance.

Fractures of the bony skeleton may occur in isolation or as part of multiple injuries. Catastrophic external bleeding, mostly in the military setting due to gunshot wounds (GSW) and explosive devices, will lead directly to hypovolaemic shock. In the c-A-B-C concept, circulation control ('c') will be applied by a combat applied tourniquet (CAT) in the pre-hospital setting, even before airway control.

Multiple fractures, especially femoral shaft fractures, contribute to hypovolaemia as well. The possibility must be borne in mind when there are multiple long bone fractures associated with vascular damage, and non-visible, but ongoing bleeding is occurring. Where this is the case, and direct control of the bleeding is not possible, a timely and appropriately applied tourniquet may buy time to stabilize the patient and treat other life-threatening injuries.

11.2 MANAGEMENT OF SEVERE INJURY TO THE EXTREMITY

The primary survey and resuscitation must take priority.

Life saving:

- Notice ongoing external bleeding and control it (pressure bandage, tourniquet).
- Exclude of detect other bleeding sources.

Limb saving:

- Assess limb injuries, making careful note of distal perfusion.
- Involve the orthopaedic and plastic surgeons early.
- Perform fasciotomy.
- Restore impaired circulation.
- Cover open wounds with a sterile dressing and give tetanus toxoid and antibiotic prophylaxis.
- Debride non-viable tissue.
- Restore skeletal stability.
- Achieve temporary wound closure.
- Commence rehabilitation.

Pitfall

It is important to remember that a fracture is not a separate entity from the soft tissue damage that accompanies it – it is simply an extension of the soft tissue injury that involves bone, and the principles of management are the same.

A fracture is a soft tissue injury in which broken bone is present. (Unknown)

During the past two decades, a better understanding of the individual injuries, and technical advances in diagnostic evaluation and surgery (allowing revascularization of the extremity, stabilization of the complex fracture, and reconstruction of the soft tissues), medicine and rehabilitation have led to an increased frequency of attempts at limb salvage. In some of these patients, however, limb salvage may have subsequent deleterious results, being associated with a high morbidity and a poor prognosis, and often requiring late amputation (27%–70%), despite initial success. In these, early or primary ablation might even be beneficial. Especially in the elderly, significant co-morbidity (diabetes, pre-existent limb ischaemia, smoking) should be included in decision-making as well.

The management of the mangled limb remains a vexing problem, should be multidisciplinary, and involve the combined skills of the orthopaedic, vascular, plastic, and reconstructive surgeons, as well as the rehabilitation specialist. Poorly coordinated management often results in more complications, increased duration of treatment, and a less favourable outcome for the patient. Ultimately, the decision to amputate or repair is often a difficult one, and best shared, if possible, with a senior colleague. The cost of rehabilitation is often less – and the time shorter – if a primary amputation is performed, than if lengthy and repeated operations are undertaken, and persistent painful debility or an insensate or flail limb is still the outcome. A successful limb salvage is defined by the overall function and satisfaction of the patient.

11.3 MANAGEMENT OF VASCULAR INJURY OF THE EXTREMITY

Vascular injuries are present in 25%–35% of all penetrating trauma to the extremities. More recently, duplex scanning has been found to play a useful screening role. Except for inconsequential intimal injuries and distal artery injuries, most extremity vascular injuries should be repaired.

Extremity arterial injury after penetrating trauma is common in military conflict or civilian trauma centres. Most peripheral arterial injuries occur in the femoral and popliteal vessels of the lower extremity. Loss of distal pulse, and unilateral cool or pale extremities are the most significant hard signs of vascular impairment. It can be confirmed by Doppler-ultrasound and supported by lack of signal on pulse oximetry. In severe hypovolaemic shock (systolic blood pressure [SBP] <60 mm Hg), however, it is not always easy to evaluate vascular impairment in the acute phase. After primary survey and resuscitation, the extremity should be assessed again. Other more soft signs of vascular injury include an expanding or pulsating haematoma, a false aneurysm, continuous murmurs of arteriovenous fistulae, progressive swelling of an extremity, and unexplained ischaemia or dysfunction. A significant percentage of these patients have no physical findings suggesting vascular trauma; thus, routine further investigation has been advocated.

The most common cause of peripheral vascular injury is penetrating trauma, which includes a spectrum from simple puncture wounds to wounds resulting from high-energy missiles. Normal pulses do not rule out vascular injuries: 10% of significant and major vascular injuries have no physical findings. Penetrating trauma also includes iatrogenic injuries such as those following percutaneous catheterization of the peripheral arteries for diagnostic procedures, access for monitoring, or even REBOA. When a needle or catheter dislodges an arteriosclerotic plaque or elevates the intima, a vessel may thrombose, leading to acute ischaemia in a limb. The key, therefore, is to maintain a high index of suspicion based on the mechanism of injury and the proximity of vascular structures.

Recently, duplex scanning of blood vessels has been shown to be a useful adjunct in determining if an arteriogram is indicated. A positive duplex scan is valuable, but a negative one does not exclude vascular injury. A positive duplex scan, or an ankle-brachial index of less than 0.9 in a distal pulse, is a mandatory indication for arteriogram and possible operation.

The gold standard for confirming a suspected vascular injury remains the CT arteriogram. However, arteriography should not be performed in the patient who is unstable and needs emergency laparotomy or thoracotomy. The arteriogram should be delayed until after resuscitation and treatment of the life-threatening emergency.

If doubt exists, an angiogram should be obtained.

Blunt trauma also may cause peripheral vascular injuries, with shear injuries as the most common cause. Contusions or crushing injuries may produce transmural or partial disruption of arteries, resulting in elevation of the intima and the formation of intramural haematomas. Blunt trauma such as posterior dislocation of the knee may cause total disruption of a major vessel. Blunt trauma may also indirectly contribute to vascular occlusion by creating large haematomas in proximity to the vessel. These haematomas may lead to arterial spasm, distortion, or compartment syndromes that interfere with arterial flow.

In principle, it is wise to fix the bony skeleton before embarking on definitive vascular repair. However, this can be catastrophic if ischaemia is present. Shunting takes priority. The following protocol should be used:

- Initial assessment for ischaemia.
- Exploration of the vessels.
- Fasciotomy if required and in case of any doubt.
- Temporary stenting of the vein and artery.
- Temporary orthopaedic fixation of the skeletal damage.
- Definitive repair of the vascular damage.

> *Damage control of the extremity injury should take place in the same fashion as in the abdomen. If there is doubt regarding viability, the wound should not be closed.*

There are five options open to the surgeon when vascular damage is encountered: vessels may be repaired, replaced (grafted), ligated (and bypassed), stented, or shunted.

Intraluminal shunts may be manufactured out of intravenous tubing, nasogastric tubing, biliary T-tubes, or even chest drain tubing, depending on the size of the vessel to be shunted. Commercially made shunts (as used routinely in carotid surgery) are on the market, and others are now being made specifically for trauma. Essentially, the shunt is tied into the damaged vessel and ligated securely proximally and distally – there is no need for heparinization – and this allows time for other damage control procedures to take precedence while maintaining perfusion of the limb. Where possible, both artery and vein should be shunted if both are damaged. If not possible, the vein should be tied off. The shunts may safely be left in place for 24 hours and probably longer; there are no controlled trials reporting on this.

Some injury complexes should raise a specific suspicion of vascular damage, for example, a supracondylar fracture of the humerus, and posterior dislocation and high-energy impact periarticular fractures of the knee. The presence of palpable pulses does **not** exclude arterial injury, and a difference of 10% in the measured Doppler pressure compared with the opposite uninjured limb mandates urgent angiography. This is not hard to do, and the technique is well described elsewhere. An absent pulse mandates exploration if the level of injury is known, and angiography if it is not.

Repairs, particularly graft replacements of injured vessels, should only be attempted by those competent to do them, and only in limbs where the viability of the soft tissues is not in doubt (i.e. after fasciotomy). Ligation may be done as a measure of desperation in the exsanguinating patient, and limb survival is often surprising. Claudication pain may be dealt with later. Extra-anatomical bypass has no place in the setting of damage control and trauma surgery. Endovascular stenting is rapidly becoming a procedure of choice in some areas (e.g. traumatic aortic rupture), but requires facilities and expertise that may not always be available.

The Eastern Association for the Surgery of Trauma (EAST) first published guidelines for evaluation and treatment of such trauma in 2002. Since that time, there have been advancements in the management of penetrating lower extremity arterial trauma. The current guidelines are presented in Table 11.1.[1]

11.3.1 **Chemical Vascular Injuries**

The frequency of chemical injury to blood vessels has increased secondary to iatrogenic injury and the intra-arterial injection of illicit drugs. These agents may cause intense vasospasm or direct damage to the vessel wall, often associated with intense pain and distal ischaemia.

Chemical vascular injuries may be treated with intra-arterial or intravenous administration of 10,000 units heparin to prevent distal thrombosis. Reserpine (0.5 mg) also has been recommended, although its only effect experimentally has been to protect against the release of catecholamines from the vessel walls. Other vasodilators and thrombolytic enzymes have been tried, with variable results. A reliable combination is 5000 units heparin in 500 mL Hartmann's solution (Ringer's lactate) to which is added 80 mg papaverine to combat arterial spasm. This is administered in boluses of 20–30 mL intra-arterially every 30 minutes, or intravenously at the rate of 1100 units heparin per hour.

11.4 **CRUSH SYNDROME**

Badly injured limbs will all have an element of crush syndrome associated with them, unless one is dealing with a traumatic amputation by a sharp instrument such as a chainsaw or machete. As such, a watch must be kept for the development of a compartment syndrome and/or myoglobinuria.

Table 11.1 EAST Guidelines for the Management of Lower Extremity Arterial Injury

Level of Evidence	Recommendation
I	1. Computed tomographic angiography (CTA) may be used as a primary diagnostic study for evaluation of penetrating lower extremity vascular injury when imaging is required.
II	1. Patients with hard signs of arterial injury (pulse deficit, pulsatile bleeding, bruit, thrill, expanding haematoma) should be surgically explored. There is no need for arteriogram in this setting unless the patient has an associated skeletal or shotgun injury. Restoration of perfusion to an extremity with an arterial injury should be performed in less than 6 hours to maximize limb salvage.
	2. Patients (without hard signs of vascular injury) who have abnormal physical examination findings and/or ankle brachial index (ABI) of <0.9 should have further evaluation to rule out vascular injury.
	3. Patients with normal physical examination findings and an ABI >0.9 may be discharged (in the absence of other injuries requiring admission).
III	1. In cases of haemorrhage from penetrating lower extremity trauma in which manual compression is unsuccessful, tourniquets may be used as a temporary adjunct for haemorrhage control until definitive repair.
	2. The use of temporary intravascular shunts may be indicated to restore arterial flow in combined vascular orthopaedic injuries (Gustilo IIIC fractures) to facilitate limb perfusion during orthopaedic sterilization.
	3. Temporary intravascular shunts may be indicated in damage control situations to facilitate limb perfusion when the physiological status of the patient, or operative capabilities prevent definitive repair.
	4. There are no data to support the routine use of endovascular therapies following infra-inguinal trauma.
	5. Embolization of profunda branches tibial vessels is acceptable, and there are no data to support preferential use of coils or n-butyl-2-cyanoacrylate glue.
	6. The role of non-invasive Doppler pressure monitoring with duplex ultrasonography to confirm or exclude arterial injury is not well defined. There may be a role for these studies in patients with soft signs of vascular injury or with proximity injuries.
	7. Non-operative observation of asymptomatic non-occlusive arterial injuries is acceptable.
	8. Repair of occult and asymptomatic non-occlusive arterial injuries managed non-operatively league, and subsequently require repair, can be done without significant increase in morbidity.
	9. Simple arterial repairs fare better than grafts. If complete repair is required, vein graft seems to be the best choice. PTFE, however, is also an acceptable conduit.
	10. PTFE may be used in a contaminated field. Effort should be made to obtain soft tissue coverage.
	11. Tibial vessels may be navigated if there is no documented flow distally.
	12. Early four-compartment lower legs fasciotomy should be applied liberally when there is an associated injury, or where there has been prolonged ischaemia. If not performed, compartment pressures should be closely monitored.
	13. Arteriography for proximity is indicated only in patients with shotgun injuries.
	14. Completion arteriogram should be performed after arterial repair.
Unanswered questions	None

Source: Fox N et al. *J Trauma Acute Care Surg.* 2012;73(5) Supplement 4:S315–20.[1]

11.5 MANAGEMENT OF OPEN FRACTURES

Sepsis is a constant threat to the healing of open fractures. Risk factors for infection are:

- Severity of injury (especially the injury to the soft tissue envelope of a limb).
- Type of contamination.
- Delay from injury to surgical care (>6 hours).
- Failure to use prophylactic antibiotics.
- Inappropriate wound toilet.
- Lack of coverage of bony structures.
- Inappropriate wound closure (including primary wound closure) in contaminated and contused wounds.

11.5.1 Severity of Injury (Gustilo Classification)[2]

Table 11.2.

11.5.2 Sepsis and Antibiotics

Sepsis is a constant threat to healing, and the main risk factors include the severity of the injury, the delay from injury to surgical care, failure to use prophylactic antibiotics and inappropriate wound closure.

The early use of prophylactic antibiotics is important, but it must be recognized that antibiotics are an adjunct to appropriate wound care. The introduction of the Thomas splint and improved understanding of the need for surgical

Table 11.2 The Gustilo Classification of Injury	
Fracture Grade	**Description**
Grade I	Wound less than 1 cm with minimal soft tissue injury. Wound bed is clean. Bone injury is simple with minimal comminution.
Grade II	Wound is greater than 1 cm with moderate soft tissue injury. Wound bed is moderately contaminated. Fracture contains moderate comminution.
Grade III	Following fracture, automatically results in classification as type III: • Segmental fracture with displacement. • Fracture with diaphyseal segmental loss. • Fracture with associated vascular injury requiring repair. • Farmyard injuries or highly contaminated wounds. • High-velocity gunshot wound. • Fracture caused by crushing force from a fast-moving vehicle.
Grade IIIA	Wound greater than 10 cm with crushed tissue and contamination. Soft tissue coverage of bone is usually possible. Wound sepsis rate is ±4%.
Grade IIIB	Wound greater than 10 cm with crushed tissue and contamination; there is periosteal stripping and bone exposure, usually associated with contamination. Soft tissue injury is extensive – cover is inadequate and requires a regional or free flap. Wound sepsis rate is ±52%.
Grade IIIC	A fracture in which there is a major vascular injury requiring repair for limb salvage; major soft tissue injury is not necessarily significant. Wound sepsis rate ±42%. Fractures can be classified using the Mangled Extremity Severity Score. In some cases, it will be necessary to consider below-knee amputation.

Source: Gustilo RB et al. *J Trauma* 1984 August;24:742–6.[2]

wound care is credited with reducing the mortality rate for open fractures of the femur from 80% to 16% during the First World War.[3] During the Spanish Civil War, Truetta reported a septic mortality rate of 0.6% in 1069 open fractures with a policy of aggressive wound excision and debridement, reduction of the fracture, stabilization with plaster, and leaving the traumatic wound open.[4]

Secondary soft tissue management with coverage of the bone by reconstructive surgery, including free flaps, has the best results if completed within the first week.

Recent consensus guidelines (Eastern Association for the Surgery of Trauma Guidelines) recommend that antibiotics be discontinued 24 hours after wound closure for grade I and II fractures. For grade III wounds, the antibiotics should be continued for only 72 hours after the time of injury, or for not more than 24 hours after soft tissue coverage of the wound is achieved, whichever occurs first. Agents effective against *Staphylococcus aureus* appear to be adequate in fractures classified by Gustilo for grade I and II fractures; however, the addition of broader Gram-negative coverage may be beneficial for grade III injuries.[5]

11.5.3 **Venous Thromboembolism**

Deep venous thrombosis prophylaxis remains an integral part of management of patients with severe limb injury. Ideally, both mechanical and chemical prophylaxis should be used.[6]

11.5.4 **Timing of Skeletal Fixation in Polytrauma Patients**

Most comparative studies have shown a reduction in the risk of post-traumatic respiratory compromise after early, definitive fixation of fractures (within 48 hours) both for isolated injuries and for multisystem trauma. There is also evidence of reduction in mortality, duration of mechanical ventilation, thromboembolic events, and cost in favour of early fixation. There is no evidence that early fixation alters the outcome in those with concomitant head injury. The advantages of early fixation of fractures in patients with multiple injuries have been challenged.

EAST Guidelines make the following recommendation:

'In trauma patients with open or closed femur fractures, we suggest early (<24 hours) open reduction and internal fracture fixation. This recommendation is conditional, and the strength of the evidence is low. Early stabilization

of femur fractures shows a trend (statistically insignificant) toward lower risk of infection, mortality, and VTE. Therefore, the panel concludes that the desirable effects of early femur fracture stabilization probably outweigh the undesirable effects in most patients. Conditional recommendation (low quality of evidence)'.[7]

The acute stabilization by early external fixation as part of damage control orthopaedics may obviate some of the risks. In cases where damage control surgery is indicated, a phased approach by temporary fixation in the acute phase, followed by definitive reconstruction as a secondary procedure. Long bone fractures like femur, tibia, and humerus can be stabilized with a simple unilateral frame. Periarticular fracture can be treated initially with a bridging external fixation. Localization of pin placement is dictated by anatomy of relevant structures such as the radial nerve in case of a humeral shaft external fixation. The definitive care by internal fixation should be considered as well, pin placement should be as far as possible from the definitive approach.

11.5.4.1 RESPIRATORY INSUFFICIENCY[8]

Episodes of respiratory insufficiency often occur after orthopaedic injury. Extremity injury may occur as part of a multisystem insult, with associated head, chest, and other injuries. Hypoxia, hypotension, and tissue injury provide an initial 'hit' to prime the patient's inflammatory response; operative treatment of fractures constitutes a modifiable secondary insult. In addition, post-traumatic fat embolism has been implicated in the respiratory compromise that appears after orthopaedic injury, especially following intramedullary nailing.

In case of severe thoracic trauma, even in haemodynamically stable cases, damage control by external fixation should be considered.

11.5.4.2 HEAD INJURY

In approximately 5% of long bone fractures of the leg, the patient is physiologically unstable due to haemodynamic instability, raised intracranial pressure, or other problems. Temporary methods of fixation are attractive in this setting. Although some studies have suggested that early nailing of a femoral fracture may be harmful in patients with a concomitant head injury, there is no compelling evidence that early long bone stabilization in mildly, moderately, or severely brain injured patients enhances or worsens the outcome.[9] However, time-consuming procedures should be avoided and early transfer to intensive care unit (ICU) environment with a staged approach to the orthopaedic trauma should be considered.

11.6 MASSIVE LIMB TRAUMA: LIFE VERSUS LIMB

Certain skeletal injuries by their nature indicate significant forces sustained by the body and should prompt the treating surgeon to look for other associated injuries. Other limb injuries, presenting with crush injury with extensive soft tissue damage, concomitant vascular or nerve injury, and major bony disruption pose other threats to either life or limb, and it is on these that this topic concentrates.

Despite huge advances in the management of these injuries, and the resultant decrease in amputation rates associated with them, there remains a small group of patients who present with 'mangled limbs', produced by mechanisms of high-energy transfer or crush in which there is vascular disruption in combination with severe open comminuted fractures and moderate loss of soft tissue. These injuries most frequently affect healthy individuals during their prime years of gainful employment and can result in varying degrees of functional and emotional disability.

There are many ways to classify major limb injuries and their complications, and these scoring systems can be found towards the end of this chapter.

The salvage of severe lower extremity fractures can be extremely challenging. Even if the surgical team is successful in preserving the limb, the functional result may be unsatisfactory because of residual effects of injuries to muscle and nerve, bone loss, and the presence of chronic infection. Failed efforts at limb salvage consume resources and are associated with increased patient mortality and high hospital costs.

Many lower extremity injury severity scoring systems have been developed to assist the surgical team with the initial decision to amputate or salvage a limb.[10] Recent prospective studies have, however, sounded a note of caution about relying exclusively on a scoring system to make these important decisions.

11.6.1 Scoring Systems

11.6.1.1 MANGLED EXTREMITY SYNDROME INDEX (MESI)

Gregory et al.[11] proposed a Mangled Extremity Syndrome Index (MESI) (Table 11.3). The injury was

Table 11.3 Mangled Extremity Syndrome Index

Criterion	Score
Injury Severity Score	
<25	1
25–50	2
>50	3
Integument Injury	
Guillotine	1
Crush/burn	2
Avulsion/degloving	3
Nerve Injury	
Contusion	1
Transection	2
Avulsion	3
Vascular Injury	
Vein transected	1
Artery transected	1
Artery thrombosed	2
Artery avulsed	3
Bone Injury	
Simple	1
Segmental	2
Segmental comminuted	3
Bone loss <6 cm	4
Articular	5
Articular with bone loss >6 cm	6
Delay in time to operation	1 point per hour >6 hours
Age (Years)	
<40	0
40–50	1
50–60	2
>60	3
Pre-existing disease	1
Shock	2

Note: Score >20: functional limb salvage can be expected; Score >20: limb salvage is improbable.

categorized according to the integument, nerve, vessel, and bone injury. A point system quantified injury severity, delay in revascularization, ischaemia, age of the patient, pre-existing disease, and whether the patient was in shock.

11.6.1.2 PREDICTIVE SALVAGE INDEX SYSTEM

Howe et al.[12] proposed a predictive index incorporating the level of the arterial injury, degree of bony injury, degree of muscle injury, and interval for warm ischaemia time (Table 11.4). Variables such as additional injuries and the presence of shock were not felt to be predictive of amputation. Of the patients, 43% underwent amputation, infrapopliteal injuries being associated with the highest amputation rate (80%).

11.6.1.3 MANGLED EXTREMITY SEVERITY SCORE (MESS)

Johansen et al.[13] described the MESS (Table 11.5), which characterizes the skeletal and soft tissue injury, warm ischaemia time, presence of shock and age of the patient, as a means of solving the dilemma of which patient

Table 11.4 Predicted Salvage Index System

Criterion	Score
Level of Arterial Injury	
Suprapopliteal	1
Popliteal	2
Infrapopliteal	3
Degree of Bone Injury	
Mild	1
Moderate	2
Severe	3
Degree of Muscle Injury	
Mild	1
Moderate	2
Severe	3
Interval from Injury to Operating Room (hours)	
<6	0
6–12	2
>12	4

Note: Salvage: score <7; Amputation: score >8.

Table 11.5 Mangled Extremity Severity Score (MESS)

Factor	Score
Skeletal/Soft Tissue Injury	
Low energy (stab, fracture, civilian gunshot wound)	1
Medium energy (open or multiple fracture)	2
High energy (shotgun or military gunshot wound)	3
Very high energy (above plus gross contamination)	4
Limb Ischaemia	
Pulse reduced or absent but perfusion normal	1[a]
Pulseless, diminished capillary refill	2[a]
Patient is cool, paralysed, insensate, numb	3[a]
Shock	
Systolic blood pressure always >90 mm Hg	0
Systolic blood pressure transiently <90 mm Hg	1
Systolic blood pressure persistently <90 mm Hg	2
Age (Years)	
<30	0
30–50	1
>50	2

[a] Double the value if the duration of ischaemia is over 6 hours.
Note: Score >7 predicted amputation.

needs amputation. A MESS value greater than 7 predicted amputation.

In a further paper, 25 years on, the authors suggested that while a MESS >7 predicted amputation *at that time*, advances in care have meant that this number must be re-evaluated.[14]

11.6.1.4 NISSSA SCORING SYSTEM

McNamara et al.[15] and others have retrospectively evaluated the MESS. Attempts have been made to address criticisms of the MESS by including nerve injury in the scoring systems and by separating the soft tissue and skeletal injury components of the MESS. The result is the NISSSA (**n**erve injury, **i**schaemia, **s**oft tissue injury/contamination, **s**keletal injury, **s**hock/blood pressure, **a**ge) scoring system (Table 11.6), which is considered more sensitive and more specific than the MESS.

Pitfall

Scoring systems clearly have their limitations when the resuscitating surgeon is faced with an unstable polytrauma patient. Thus, these scoring systems are not universally accepted. They have shortcomings with respect to reproducibility, prognostic value, and treatment-planning in this context. These factors can lead to inappropriate attempts at limb salvage when associated life- and limb-threatening injuries might be overlooked if attention is focused mainly on salvage of the mangled limb, or to an amputation when salvage may have been possible. While experience with these scoring systems is generally limited, they may provide some objective parameters on which clinicians can base difficult decisions regarding salvage of life or limb, but it must be stressed that any recommendations derived from them must be judged in terms of available technology and expertise.

In summary, the decision of whether to amputate primarily or to embark on limb salvage and continue with planned repetitive surgeries is complex. Prolonged salvage attempts that are unlikely to be successful should be avoided, especially in patients with insensate limbs and predictable functional failures. Scoring systems should be used only as a guide for decision-making. The relative importance of each of the associated trauma parameters (apart from prolonged, warm ischaemia time or risking the life of a patient with severe, multiple organ trauma) is still of questionable predictive value. A good understanding of the potential complications facilitates the decision-making process in limb salvage versus amputation.

11.7 **COMPARTMENT SYNDROME**[16–18]

Compartment syndrome may occur after extremity injury, with or without vascular trauma. Increasing pressure within the closed fascial space of a limb compromises the blood supply of muscle. Early clinical

Table 11.6 NISSSA Scoring System

Factor	Score
Nerve Injury	
Sensate	0
Loss of dorsal	1
Partial plantar	2
Complete plantar	3
Ischaemia	
None	0
Mild	1[a]
Moderate	2[a]
Severe	3[a]
Soft Tissue Injury/Contamination	
Low	0
Medium	1
High	2
Severe	3
Skeletal Injury	
Low energy	0
Medium energy	1
High energy	2
Very high energy	3
Shock/Blood Pressure	
Normotensive	0
Transient hypotension	1
Persistent hypotension	2
Age (Years)	
<30	0
30–50	1
>50	2

[a] Double the value if the duration of ischaemia exceeds 6 hours.

Note: Score >11 predicted amputation.

diagnosis and treatment is important to prevent significant morbidity.

The 5Ps (pain, paraesthesia, paralysis, pallor, and pulselessness) are described as classical signs, but are unreliable and above all late parameters. Pain, pain at active movement, and pain at passive stretch of muscles should lead to awareness. In comatose or paralysed and sedated patients, one cannot monitor clinical signs at all.

Compartment syndrome occurs relatively commonly, following trauma or ischaemia to an extremity, with or without vascular injury. It is important to emphasize that reperfusion following vascular repair, plays a major role. As such, the classical clinical findings may be absent prior to vascular repair. Once the diagnosis of compartment syndrome is made, urgent fasciotomy is indicated. This applies to both upper and lower limbs.

The measurement of intra-compartment pressure[19] using devices like the Stryker® (Stryker, Kalamazoo, MI), is invaluable when doubt exists about the diagnosis. This can be particularly helpful in cases not accessible for physical examination, such as the unconscious patient and those in intensive care, sedated and ventilated. It must be emphasized that a pulse still may be palpable or recordable on the Doppler, even though a compartment syndrome exists. It is important that measurements be take on both lower legs, at the same place (e.g. in the tibialis anterior muscle 2 cm below and lateral to the tibial tubercle) for comparison.

The lower leg is the most common site but in crush injuries and high energy impact it can also occur the leg above knee and the upper extremity, especially the forearm.

11.8 FASCIOTOMY

Should there be doubt over whether the compartment syndrome is significant, a fasciotomy should be performed.

Fasciotomy must be performed *before* arterial exploration when an obvious arterial injury exists, or where there is a suspicion of high intra-compartmental pressures.

11.8.1 Lower Leg Fasciotomy

It is critically important that the fasciotomy is comprehensive and adequate, releasing all four lower limb compartments (Figure 11.1).

Several techniques have been described for the lower leg:

- Two incision, four compartment fasciotomies.
- One incision fasciotomy.
- Fibulectomy.
- Subcutaneous fasciotomy.

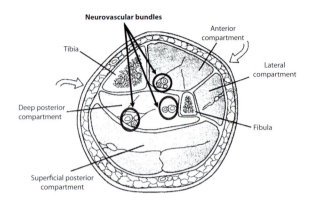

Figure 11.1 Cross section of lower leg, showing compartments.

Pitfall

In trauma, there is no place for single incision or subcutaneous fasciotomy, not fibulectomy.

11.8.1.1 TWO INCISION–FOUR COMPARTMENT FASCIOTOMY[20]

The skin must be opened widely, in order to allow a good view of the underlying fascia. It is critical that the fascia is split over its entire length, and this can only be done under direct vision. Care must be taken not to damage the saphenous veins, which may constitute the major system of venous return in such an injured leg. On the lateral side, the common peroneal nerve branches should be identified and preserved.

Two long incisions are made:

Lateral incision:

- The lateral incision starts anterolaterally over the fibula, 2–3 cm below the head.
- Retract skin.
- Make a transverse incision at mid-point across the septum (Figure 11.2).
- Cut the fascia on either side of the septum using curved scissors.

Pitfall

On the lateral side, the common peroneal nerve, running down the entire lateral side as far as 2 cm above the lateral malleolus should be identified and preserved.

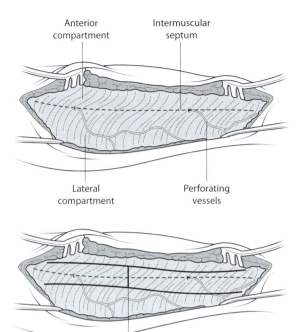

Figure 11.2 Technique of 'H' incision over lateral and anterior compartments.

Medial incision:

- A long posteromedial incision is made 2 cm medial to and below the tibial tuberosity, running down the entire lower leg, 2–3 cm behind the posterior border of the tibia, as far as 2 cm above the medial malleolus cm posterior to the medial border of the tibia.
- The subcutaneous tissue is pushed away by blunt dissection, and the superficial and deep posterior compartments are opened separately.

Pitfall

Care must be taken not to damage the saphenous veins medially, which may constitute the major system of venous return in such an injured leg.

11.8.1.2 SINGLE INCISION FASCIOTOMY

This is a longer procedure, and it is more difficult to do adequate decompression for major trauma.

It should not be practised in the trauma situation.

11.8.1.3 FIBULECTOMY

This is a difficult procedure, leading to extensive blood oozing, and may well result in damage to the peroneal artery.

It should not be practised in the trauma situation.

11.8.1.4 SUBCUTANEOUS FASCIOTOMY

It should not be practised in the trauma situation.

11.8.2 Upper Leg[21]

In the upper leg, compartments of quadriceps (ventral), hamstrings (dorsal), and adductors (medial) should be opened. Be aware that ongoing arterial bleeding can occur of branches of the profunda branches of the femoral artery, and selective angioembolization may be needed, or if not applicable, ligation of the profundal femoral artery.

11.8.3 Upper and Lower Arm[22,23]

In the upper arm, biceps (ventral) and triceps compartment (dorsal) can be at risk.

In the lower arm, the dorsal compartment of the extensors can be opened by direct approach. Ventral fasciotomy of the flexors should be completed with release of the carpal tunnel distally and division of the *lacertus fibrosis* in the elbow region proximally (Figure 11.3).

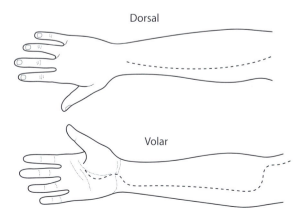

Figure 11.3 Fasciotomy incisions for the forearm.

Incision of the dorsal and volar compartment of the forearm:

- A long incision, anterolaterally, 2 cm anterior to the shaft of the fibula. The anterior and lateral fascial compartments are opened separately.
- A long posteromedial incision is made 2 cm posterior to the medial border of the tibia. The subcutaneous tissue is pushed away by blunt dissection, and the superficial and deep posterior compartments are opened separately.

11.9 COMPLICATIONS OF MAJOR LIMB INJURY

Table 11.7 outlines fracture complications.

In a review of 53 mangled lower extremities, Bondurant et al. compared primary with delayed amputation in terms of morbidity and cost.[24] Patients undergoing delayed ablation had longer periods of hospitalization (22.3 versus 53.4 days) and more surgical procedures (1.6 versus 6.9) at greater cost (US$28,964 versus US$53,462). Six patients with delayed amputation developed sepsis from the injured lower extremity and died, while no patient with a primary amputation developed sepsis or died.

The decision to amputate primarily is difficult. At the initial examination, the extent of the eventual loss of soft tissue can never be fully appreciated, distal perfusion is also difficult to assess (many patients are shocked), and the neurological evaluation is often unreliable (as a result of associated head injury or ischaemia and soft tissue disruption). Any thoughts of limb salvage should take conscience of Advanced Trauma Life Support® protocols, always maintaining the priority of life over limb, and thus minimizing systemic complications and missed injuries. In an attempt to facilitate this early decision-making, a number of guidelines have been devised providing management of injuries which might eventually require amputation.[25]

Table 11.7 Complications of Fractures	
Skin and soft tissue	Skin and tissue loss, wound slough, coverage failure.
Bone and fracture site	Compartment syndrome with necrosis of muscle/nerve injury. Deep infection – acute/chronic. Bone loss, delayed union, malunion/loss of alignment, non-union fixation problems – failure of hardware. Bone refracture.
Nerve	Direct injury or ischaemic damage. Reflex sympathetic dystrophy.
Vascular	Arterial occlusion, venous insufficiency. Deep vein thrombosis, compartment syndrome.
Joint motion	Associated joint surface fracture. Contracture, late arthritis.
Secondary	Ototoxicity, nephrotoxicity, myonecrosis from antibiotics. Secondary spread of infection, sepsis/multiple organ failure/death.
Psychosocial	Depression, loss of self-worth. Economic hardship, questionable employment status, marital problems.
Functional	Chronic pain. Disability – muscle strength/endurance. Decrease in activities of daily function. Loss of ability to return to work, inability to participate in recreational activities.
Cosmesis	Scars, bulky flaps.

11.10 SUMMARY

It seems preferable to perform early, definitive long bone stabilization in polytrauma patients. Recent consensus guidelines suggest that, for patients with dominant head or chest injuries, the timing of long bone stabilization should be individualized according to the patient's clinical condition. Damage control orthopaedics has a real place in limb salvage.[26]

REFERENCES AND RECOMMENDED READING

References

1. Fox N, Rajani RR, Bokhari F, Chie WC, Kerwin A, Seamon MJ, Skarupa D, Frykberg E. Evaluation and management of penetrating lower extremity arterial trauma: An Eastern Association for the Surgery of Trauma practice management guideline. *J Trauma Acute Care Surg.* 2012;**73(5) Supplement 4**: S315–20. doi: 10.1097/TA.0b013e31827018e.

2. Gustilo RB, Mendoza RM, Williams DN. Problems in the management of type III (severe) open fractures: a new classification of type III open fractures. *J Trauma.* 1984 Aug;**24**:742–6.

3. Gustilo RB, Anderson JT. Prevention of infection in the treatment of one thousand and twenty-five open fractures of long bones: retrospective and prospective analyses. *J Bone Joint Surg Am.* 2002 Apr;**84-A(4)**:682 only.

4. Truetta J. War surgery of extremities: treatment of war wounds and fractures. *Br Med J.* 1942;**1**:616.

5. Hoff WS, Bonadies JA, Cachecho R, Dorlac WC. EAST Practice Management Guidelines Work Group: update to Practice Management Guidelines for prophylactic antibiotic use in open fractures. *J Trauma.* 2011 Mar;**70(3)**:751–4. doi: 10.1097/TA.0b013e31820930e5. Available from www.east.org (accessed December 2018).

6. Rogers FB, Cipolle MD, Velmahos G, Rozycki G. Practice management guidelines for the management of venous thromboembolism (VTE) in trauma patients. *J Trauma.* 2002 July;**53(1)**:142–64. In *Eastern Association for the Surgery of Trauma. Practice Management Guidelines.* Available from www.east.org (accessed December 2018).

7. Gandhi RR, Overton T, Haut ER, Lau B, Vallier H, Rohs T, et al. Optimal timing of femur fracture stabilization in polytrauma patients: A practice management guideline from the Eastern Association for the Surgery of Trauma. *J Trauma.* 2014 Nov;**77(5)**:787–95.

8. Robinson CM. Current concepts of respiratory insufficiency syndromes after fracture. *J Bone Joint Surg.* 2001;**83B**: 781–91.

9. Scalea TM, Scott JD, Brumback RJ, et al. Early fracture fixation may be 'just fine' after head injury: no difference in central nervous system outcomes. *J Trauma.* 1999 May; **46(5)**:839–46.

10. Bosse MJ, MacKenzie EJ, Kellam JF, et al. A prospective evaluation of the clinical utility of the lower-extremity injury-severity scores. *J Bone Joint Surg.* 2001;**83A**:3–14.

11. Gregory RT, Gould RJ, Peclet M, Wagner JS, Gilbert DA, Wheeler JR, et al. The Mangled Extremity Syndrome (MES): a severity grading system for multisystem injuries of the extremities. *J Trauma.* 1985 Dec;**25(12)**:1147–50.

12. Howe HR Jr, Poole GV Jr, Hansen KJ, Clark T, Plonk GW, Koman LA, et al. Salvage of lower extremities following combined orthopedic and vascular trauma: a predictive salvage index. *Am Surg.* 1987 Apr;**53(4)**:205–28.

13. Johansen K, Daunes M, Howey T, Helfet D, Hansen ST Jr. Objective Criteria accurately predict amputation following lower extremity trauma. *J Trauma.* 1990 May;**30(5)**: 568–72; discussion 572-3.

14. Johansen K, Hansen ST Jr. MESS (Mangled Extremity Severity Score) 25 years on: Time for a reboot? *J Trauma Acute Care Surg.* 2015 Sep;**79(3)**:495–6. doi: 10.1097/ TA.0000000000000767.

15. McNamara MG, Heckman JD, Corley FG. Severe open fractures of the lower extremity: a retrospective evaluation of the Mangled Extremity Severity Score (MESS). *J Orthop Trauma.* 1994;**8(2)**:81–7.

16. Perron AD, Brady WJ, Keats TE. Orthopedic pitfalls in the ED: acute compartment syndrome. *Am J Emerg Med.* 2001 Sept;**19(5)**:413–16. Review.

17. Tiwari A, Haq AI, Myint F, Hamilton G. Acute compartment syndromes. *Br J Surg.* 2002 Apr;**89(4)**:397–412.

18. Schmidt AH. Acute Compartment Syndrome. *Orthop Clin North Am.* 2016 Jul;**47(3)**:517–25. doi: 10.1016/j. ocl.2016.02.001. Review.

19. Hammerberg EM, Whitesides TE Jr, Seiler JG 3rd. The reliability of measurement of tissue pressure in compartment syndrome. *J Orthop Trauma.* 2012 Sept;**26(9)**:e166; author reply e166. doi: 10.1097/BOT.0b013e3182673a3f.

20. Mubarak SJ, Owen CA. Double incision fasciotomy of the leg for decompression in compartment syndromes. *J Trauma.* 1977 Mar;**59(2)A**:184–7.

21. Ojike NI, Roberts CS, Giannoudis PV. Compartment syndrome of the thigh: a systematic review. *Injury.* 2010 Feb; **41(2)**:133–6. doi: 10.1016/j.injury.2009.03.016. Epub 2009 Jun 24.

22. Kalyani BS, Fisher BE, Roberts CS, Giannoudis PV. Compartment syndrome of the forearm: a systematic review. *J Hand Surg Am.* 2011 Mar;**36(3)**:535–43. doi: 10.1016/j.jhsa.2010.12.007.

23. Kistler JM, Ilyas AM, Thoder JJ. Forearm Compartment Syndrome: Evaluation and Management. *Hand Clin.* 2018 Feb;**34(1)**:53–60. doi: 10.1016/j.hcl.2017.09.006. Review.

24. Bondurant FJ, Cotler HB, Buckle R, Miller-Crotchett P, Browner BD. The medical and economic impact of severely injured lower extremities. *J Trauma.* 1988;**28**:1270–3.

25. Scalea TM, DuBose J, Moore EE, et al. Western Trauma Association critical decisions in trauma: management of the mangled extremity. *J Trauma Acute Care Surg.* 2012 Jan;**72(1)**:86–93. doi: 10.1097/TA.0b013e318241ed70.

26. Boulton CL. Damage Control Orthopaedics. *Orth Knowledge Online J.* 2013 **11(2)**: https://www.aaos.org/periodicalissue/?issue=OKOJ/vol11/issue2 (accessed online Dec 2018).

Recommended Reading

Harris AM, Althausen PL, Kellam J, Bosse MJ, Castillo R. Complications following limb-threatening lower extremity trauma. *J Orthop Trauma.* 2009 Jan;**23(1)**:1–6. doi: 10.1097/BOT.0b013e31818e43dd.

Helgeson MD, Potter BK, Burns TC, Hayda RA, Gajewski DA. Risk factors for and results of late or delayed amputation following combat-related extremity injuries. *Orthopedics.* 2010 Sept;**33(9)**:669. doi: 10.3928/01477447-20100722-02.

Head Trauma **12**

12.1 INTRODUCTION

Traumatic brain injury (TBI) is a leading cause of death and disability worldwide. Approximately 69 million individuals are estimated to suffer TBI from all causes each year, with the Southeast Asian and Western Pacific regions experiencing the greatest overall burden of disease.[1]

The incidence of TBI is increasing in low-income and middle-income countries, because of increased transport-related injuries, and young men are particularly affected. Ninety per cent of TBI-related deaths occur in these countries.[2] The elderly cohort is also increasing in most countries due to low-impact falls. On average, 39% of patients with severe TBI die from their injury, and 60% have an unfavourable outcome. Trauma patients with co-existing TBI have higher mean length of stay in hospital, higher hospital cost, and increased percentage of disability, compared with trauma victims without TBI.[3]

The mortality and morbidity of TBI is attributed to the **Primary Brain injury,** which includes diffuse axonal injury and intracranial haematomas, and the **Secondary Brain injury** due initially to hypoxia, hypotension, and cerebral ischaemia. Early evacuation of intracranial haematomas and the correction of secondary physiological derangements saves lives and improves outcome.

'**Damage control resuscitation**' aims to rapidly restore normal ventilation and oxygenation, correct hypovolaemia and hypotension, reverse hypothermia and correct coagulopathy. '**Hypotensive resuscitation**' may be used for penetrating trauma but the systolic blood pressure (SBP) should be kept above 90 mm Hg to maintain cerebral perfusion. Prompt imaging by computed tomography (CT), whenever possible, facilitates the treating team's immediate decisions.

12.2 INJURY PATTERNS AND CLASSIFICATION

TBIs are classified according to severity, mechanism of injury, and pathology. Knowledge of these classifications allows the trauma team to grade the severity, to suspect early the presence of intracranial pathology, and to initiate timely appropriate diagnostic procedures and treatment.

12.2.1 Severity

The **Severity of TBI** is assessed clinically with the Glasgow Coma Scale (GCS), which evaluates the neurological status of the patient (see Appendix B.2). It is essential to realize that GCS is not a single number and each of its three components has clinical value. Additional clinical signs and symptoms, such as focal neurological deficits, abnormal pupillary light reflexes, pupil inequality (anisocoria), and seizures contribute to the classification of TBI severity.

- **Mild TBI**: Brief loss of consciousness for a few seconds or minutes, post-traumatic amnesia (PTA) for less than an hour, normal brain imaging results, GCS score 13–15.
- **Moderate TBI**: Loss of consciousness for less than 24 hours, PTA for 1–24 hours, abnormal brain imaging findings, GCS score of 9–12.
- **Severe TBI**: Loss of consciousness or coma for more than 24 hours, PTA for more than 24 hours, abnormal brain imaging findings, GCS score of 3–8.

12.2.2 Pathological Classification of TBI

- **Focal brain injuries**: Impact forces acting directly on the head, create a wide range of focal lesions including

contusion, brain laceration, epidural or subdural haematoma, subarachnoid or intracerebral haemorrhage.
Contrecoup injury occurs when the brain impacts the
opposite side of the skull to the impact. Fast acquisition of brain imaging promotes early diagnosis and
prompt intervention that may critically affect patient
outcome. However, most patients with TBI do not
have a lesion suitable for neurosurgical intervention.

- **Diffuse brain injuries**: Sudden head movement,
  usually rapid deceleration often seen in motor vehicle
  accidents, results in **diffuse axonal injury (DAI)**. The
  CT scan shows diffuse cerebral oedema, multiple pete-
  chial haemorrhages, loss of grey white differentiation,
  loss of basal cisterns, and subarachnoid spaces and
  small ('slit') ventricles. DAI is frequently devastating for
  the patient and leads to extensive damage to the white
  matter and a variety of profound neurological deficits.[5]

The pathologies of TBI are frequently present in various combinations further complicating patient management and outcome prediction.

Both severity and type of TBI are directly associated
with the **mechanism** of injury and the forces applied to
the brain.

12.2.2.1 BLUNT HEAD TRAUMA

Blunt head trauma carries a high risk for secondary brain
damage, represents the main cohort of patients suffering from severe post-injury morbidity, and is the main
diagnostic target for a trauma team. The most frequent
causes of blunt head injury are motor vehicle collisions,
falls, and assaults, and result in scalp lacerations, scalp
haematomas, and skull fractures.

Fractures of the skull vault are classified as closed or
open (compound), linear, comminuted, or depressed. Skull
base fractures may result in periorbital haematomas and
CSF leaks from the nose or ears. The significance of skull
fractures should not be underestimated. A simple closed
linear skull fracture identified in a skull x-ray increases
chances of an intracranial haemorrhage by 400 times.
All open depressed skull fractures should be surgically
treated, especially if the underlying dura is damaged. A
closed depressed fracture may or may not require surgery.

12.2.2.2 PENETRATING HEAD TRAUMA

Penetrating injuries are caused mainly by bullets from
firearms, less commonly by knife or machete wounds,

and bomb blast fragments. A bullet causes a spreading
shock wave in the brain causing collateral brain damage
in addition to the primary track of the projectile. The
projectile may ricochet internally off the skull or perfo-
rate the skull and scalp in its path. Patients with penetrating cerebral injury require emergency craniotomy if
there is a significant mass effect from a haematoma or
projectile fragments. However, removal of bone or projectile fragments should not be pursued at the expense of
damaging normal brain tissue. Patients presenting with
GCS of 5 or less after resuscitation and CT findings of
bilateral brain injury have a particularly poor prognosis
for which conservative treatment may be indicated.

12.3 MEASURABLE PHYSIOLOGICAL PARAMETERS IN TBI

In addition to clinical assessment, three types of brain
monitoring are used in patients with severe TBI: intracranial pressure (ICP), cerebral perfusion pressure (CPP),
and advanced cerebral monitoring including brain oxygen ($PBrO_2$). Multimodality monitoring is available in
advanced countries, but it is unclear from the evidence
base how much this contributes to improved outcome.
In low and middle income countries (LMIC) these monitoring techniques are not usually available and decisions on management are made on a clinical basis with
the additional CT brain result, if available. The application of TBI guidelines may therefore not be applicable in
resource poor environments.

12.3.1 Mean Arterial Pressure

Mean arterial pressure (MAP) is defined as the average
arterial pressure during a single cardiac cycle and is an
indicator of the haemodynamic status in an injured
patient. It is represented mathematically by the formula:

$$\frac{SBP + 2DBP}{3}$$

where SBP is systolic blood pressure and DBP is diastolic
blood pressure.

12.3.2 Intracranial Pressure

ICP is the pressure inside the skull and is affected by
variations in cerebrospinal fluid volume, brain water,
cerebral blood volume, and venous return of the brain.

Normal ICP range is 7–15 mm Hg. Values persistently over 20 mm Hg are abnormal and may indicate the presence of an intracranial mass lesion, such as a haematoma or cerebral oedema that require surgical intervention.

12.3.3 Cerebral Perfusion Pressure

CPP is the net pressure gradient that drives cerebral blood flow to the brain. It can be calculated by the formula: MAP – ICP. The normal CPP range is 60 to 70 mm Hg in adults in the supine position.

12.3.4 Cerebral Blood Flow

Cerebral blood flow (CBF) represents the blood supply to the brain at any given time. Normal values are around 50–55 mL/min/100 g of brain tissue, which corresponds to 15% of the cardiac output in the adult. It is autoregulated tightly according to the brain's metabolic demands, blood pressure, the $PaCO_2$ and PaO_2 values, and shows significant derangement in severe TBI.

12.4 PATHOPHYSIOLOGY OF TRAUMATIC BRAIN INJURY[4]

The initial stages of cerebral injury are characterized by two main elements; direct tissue damage and impaired regulation of CBF and metabolism. This 'ischaemia-like' pattern leads to accumulation of lactic acid owing to anaerobic glycolysis, increased membrane permeability and consecutive oedema formation. On a cellular level, an excessive release of neurotransmitters takes place, along with an increase of free radicals and fatty acids, occurring from membrane degradation of cellular and vascular structures. These events lead to programmed cell death (apoptosis).

12.5 MANAGEMENT OF TBI

Current evidence-based Guidelines for the Management of Traumatic Brain Injury are published by the Brain Trauma Foundation.[5,6]

Time to treatment should be minimized to limit secondary brain injury. ATLS® principles are applied. An abbreviated neurological examination provides important baseline information. Maintenance of blood pressure and oxygenation are fundamental to TBI patient management:

- Maintain SBP at $\geq$100 mm Hg for patients 50 to 69 years old or at $\geq$110 mm Hg for patients 15 to 49 or >70 years old. This may decrease mortality and improve outcomes (level III evidence).
- Following restoration of blood volume, pressor support with noradrenaline may be required if the CPP is not maintained.
- Keep arterial blood oxygen saturation (SaO_2) >95%.
- Keep PaO_2 >80 mm Hg (>10.5 kPa).

Autoregulation: The normal brain maintains a constant CBF over a wide range of blood pressure. However, autoregulation is frequently deranged in severe TBI and the brain becomes more vulnerable to hypotension. Other systemic brain insults that aggravate secondary brain injury are:

- Anaemia (Hb <10 g/dL).
- Hyponatraemia (serum sodium <142 mmol/L).
- Hyperglyacemia (blood sugar >10 mmol/L).
- Hypoglycaemia (blood sugar <4.6 mmol/L).
- Fever (temperature >36.5°C).

Many intensive care units have developed basic care protocols for the management of severe TBI patients. A comprehensive example has been published recently.[7] An imaging and clinical examination (ICE) protocol has also been developed for managing severe TBI without ICP monitoring. This has been applied in resource poor countries, but has not yet been compared to the protocols which include ICP and CPP monitoring.

12.6 CEREBRAL PERFUSION PRESSURE THRESHOLD

An adequate CPP is achieved by optimizing blood pressure and minimizing ICP.[6] This will ensure the delivery of adequate blood flow and oxygenation to the brain. The CPP to aim for is 60 to 70 mm Hg. Whether 60 or 70 mm Hg is the optimal CPP threshold is unclear and may depend upon the patient's cerebral autoregulatory status. A level below 60 mm Hg may result in cerebral ischaemia and should be avoided (level IIB evidence).

CPPs maintained at >70 mm Hg should be avoided because the patient may develop fluid overload, pulmonary oedema, and respiratory failure (level III evidence).

> **To maintain adequate CPP (>70 mm Hg), blood pressure must be kept high and ICP low.**

12.7 INTRACRANIAL PRESSURE MONITORING AND THRESHOLD

Management of patients with severe TBI using information from ICP monitoring is recommended to reduce in-hospital and 2-week post-injury mortality[6] (level IIB evidence). Treating ICP >22 mm Hg is recommended because values above this level are associated with increased mortality[6] (level IIB evidence). A combination of ICP values and brain CT findings should be used to determine the need for treatment[6] (level III evidence). ICP monitoring is frequently not available in LMIC.

12.7.1 ICP Monitoring Devices

Measurement of ICP currently requires a burr hole or direct placement at craniotomy.

- **Intraventricular catheter**: This is the most accurate, cost-effective, and reliable ICP monitoring method. A hole is drilled through the skull and the catheter is inserted through the brain into the lateral ventricle. When the ICP is high, catheter placement can be challenging because the ventricles are compressed and may be shifted from their normal position.
- **Intraparenchymal catheter**: The calibration of these catheters may drift over several days and re-calibration may not be available. Some of the newer catheters can measure brain oxygen tension ($PBrO_2$) and temperature in addition to ICP.
- **Subarachnoid, subdural and epidural catheters**: These are unreliable.

12.7.1.1 CSF DRAINAGE

An external ventricular drain (EVD) can be used to drain CSF and assist with ICP reduction. An EVD system zeroed at the midbrain with continuous drainage of CSF may be considered to lower ICP burden more effectively

than intermittent use[6] (level III evidence). Use of CSF drainage to lower ICP in patients with an initial GCS <6 during the first 12 hours after injury may be considered[6] (level III evidence).

12.7.2 ICP Management – Do's and Don'ts

12.7.2.1 HYPERVENTILATION

Hyperventilation lowers $PaCO_2$, which causes cerebral vasoconstriction. This will reduce brain swelling and lower ICP; however, severe hyperventilation causes excessive vasoconstriction, and the local alkalosis that results will further interfere with oxygen delivery, resulting in cerebral ischaemia. Prolonged prophylactic hyperventilation with $PaCO_2$ of ≤ 35 mm Hg (<3 kPa) is not recommended. Hyperventilation is recommended as a temporizing measure for the reduction of elevated ICP, but hyperventilation should be avoided during the first 24 hours after injury when CBF often is reduced critically. If hyperventilation is used, jugular vein oxygen saturation (SjO_2) or $PBrO_2$ measurements are recommended to monitor oxygen delivery[6] (level IIB evidence).

12.7.2.2 OSMOTHERAPY (MANNITOL AND HYPERTONIC SALINE)

Although hyperosmolar therapy may lower intracranial pressure, the Brain Trauma Foundation Guidelines found insufficient evidence about effects on clinical outcomes to support a specific recommendation, or to support use of any specific hyperosmolar agent for patients with severe TBI.[6] Mannitol or hypertonic saline use prior to ICP monitoring should be restricted to patients with signs of transtentorial herniation (coning) or progressive neurological deterioration not attributable to extracranial causes. Mannitol is effective for control of raised ICP at doses of 0.25 to 1 g/kg body weight over 15 minutes. Arterial hypotension (systolic blood pressure <90 mm Hg) should be avoided. Repeated mannitol may lose its effect and aggravate cerebral oedema. A serum osmolality >320 mOsm/kg and a serum sodium >155 mmol/L should be avoided. Mannitol is the drug of choice for improving ICP, but bears a high risk of hypovolemia, arterial hypotension, and hypernatraemia. Hypertonic saline could reduce ICP without causing significant hypovolaemia, but its routine use remains controversial.

12.7.2.3 BARBITURATES AND PROPOFOL

High-dose barbiturate administration may be used to control elevated ICP refractory to maximum standard medical and surgical treatment. Haemodynamic stability is essential before and during barbiturate therapy.

Although propofol is recommended for the control of ICP, it is not recommended for improvement in mortality or 6-month outcomes. Caution is required as high-dose propofol can produce significant morbidity[6] (level IIB evidence).

12.7.2.4 STEROIDS

The use of steroids is *not* recommended for improving outcome or reducing ICP. In patients with moderate or severe TBI, high dose methylprednisolone is associated with increased mortality and is contraindicated[6] (level I evidence).

12.8 IMAGING

Skull x-rays are of limited use, unless a CT scan is not available, or a penetrating injury has occurred.

CT scan is the investigation of choice for TBI. All patients with moderate or severe TBI should have a head CT scan. Deteriorating neurological status, amnesia and focal neurological signs are additional criteria. According to the New Orleans criteria,[8] mild TBI patients with GCS 15 and normal neurological examination after blunt trauma should undergo CT if one of the following is present:

- Headache.
- Vomiting.
- Age over 60 years.
- Drug or alcohol intoxication.
- Short term memory deficit.
- Seizures.

> **For haemodynamically unstable patients requiring immediate non-cranial surgery, the imaging is postponed.**

12.9 INDICATIONS FOR SURGERY

Surgery aims to facilitate the insertion of ICP monitor, CSF drainage, the evacuation of significant space-occupying lesion and bony decompression.

Decision-making is primarily based on clinical assessment (drop in GCS, pupillary abnormality, focal neurological deficit), and CT scan findings. It must be emphasized that surgery to reduce ICP is only meaningful and safe if systemic haemodynamics and oxygenation are stable. Not all intracranial haematomas require removal; only those causing or have the potential to cause significantly raised ICP warrant surgery, (e.g. a large epidural haematoma should be evacuated quickly). A thin layer of acute subdural haematoma or traumatic subarachnoid haemorrhage may not need surgery.

Indications to perform emergency surgical treatment in the remote or rural setting are:

- Inability to perform head CT on a neurologically deteriorating patient.
- Transfer to the nearest neurosurgical unit is more than 2 hours away.
- A sizeable intracranial haematoma.

The remote general surgeon should contact the regional neurosurgeon for support and advice.

12.9.1 Burr Holes and Emergency Craniotomy

Rapidly expanding intracranial haematoma is a surgical emergency. These surgical interventions that can be performed by a non-neurosurgeon and avert progressive brain injury and death.

12.9.1.1 EMERGENCY BURR HOLE CRANIOTOMY[9]

Clear indications exist for performing a burr hole: GCS ≤8 with imaging evidence of an epidural haematoma causing midline shift and unequal pupils. In the absence of a head CT, a very high clinical suspicion (e.g. a palpable fracture, with an ipsilateral fixed dilated pupil, and deteriorating neurologic status) is the only exception for performing an emergency craniotomy without imaging. Otherwise, without imaging and/or with a GCS above 8, the craniotomy is contraindicated. Burr hole drilling sites are shown in Figure 12.1, relative to haematoma positions. The basic steps in burr hole technique are:

- Confirm the correct side and position of the haematoma.
- Shave the scalp.

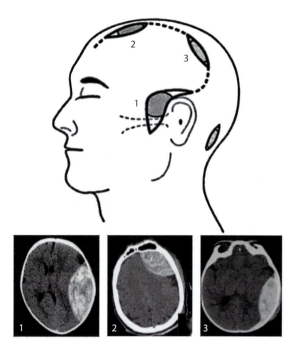

Figure 12.1 Diagram demonstrating position of standard burr holes, and frequent locations of epidural haematomas that are decompressed: (1) temporal (above the zygomatic arch), (2) frontal (over the coronal suture, approx. 10 cm cephalad and in line with the midpupillary line), (3) parietal (over the parietal eminence).

- Infiltrate the scalp with local anaesthetic (e.g. 0.5% bupivacaine (Marcaine®) and 1/2000 adrenaline).
- Make a 3 cm incision straight down to the bone.
- Push the periosteum with a knife/swab and insert the self-retaining retractor.
- If you are using the Hudson brace 'manual' burr holes, start drilling perpendicularly to the skull and simultaneously apply saline wash. (See Figure 12.2.)
- Stop when you feel a difference in tissue resistance.
- The perforator creates a conical opening and the burr converts this into a cylindrical opening.
- If the haematoma is epidural, dark blood clot will be identified and can be aspirated. If it is subdural, open the dura with a sharp knife.
- If no blood comes out review location and side, *without further delaying patient transfer.*
- If fresh blood continues to ooze from the wound, do NOT try to tamponade.

12.9.1.2 EMERGENCY CRANIOTOMY

This is a more complex surgical procedure that requires a non-neurosurgeon to have some training and familiarity. The scalp is raised as a myocutaneous flap, the burr holes are placed and then joined using the Gigli saw if a craniotome is unavailable. The frontotemporal craniotomy is the commonest type used in trauma (Figure 12.3).

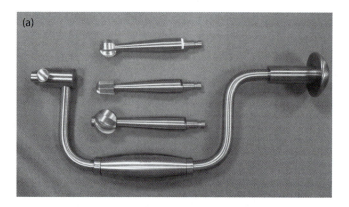

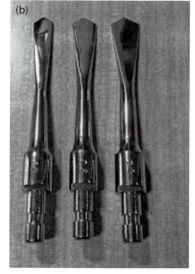

Figure 12.2 Hand driven burr hole craniotomy: (a,b) Hudson brace with a set of burrs and the 'V' shaped perforators.

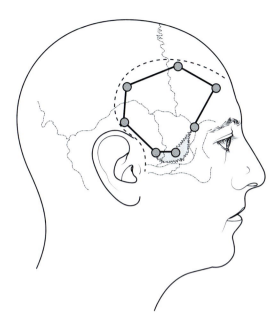

Figure 12.3 Diagram shows a frontotemporal craniotomy for evacuation of an intracranial haematoma. Note the line of the scalp incision, the position of the burr holes, and the removal of bone down to the floor of the middle cranial fossa.

12.9.1.2.1 Depressed Fractures

Depressed fractures should be elevated when the depth of the depression meets or exceeds the thickness of the adjacent skull table to alleviate compression of the underlying cortex. A burr hole is placed at the edge of the fracture in order to place an elevator beneath an impacted depressed fracture. Loose bone fragments and debris are removed, haemostasis obtained, and the dura underlying the fracture is repaired. Avoid elevating depressed fractures overlying the major venous sinuses.

12.9.1.2.2 Penetrating Cranial Injury

Patients with penetrating cerebral injury require emergency craniotomy/craniectomy to washout and debride the wound and to evacuate haematomas. Marked cerebral swelling frequently develops around the projectile track and a decompressive craniectomy is required to adequately decompress the brain. Removal of deep bone or projectile fragments should not be pursued at the expense of damaging normal brain tissue. Patients presenting with GCS score of ≤5 after resuscitation or CT

findings of bilateral brain injury have a poor prognosis and non-operative treatment may be indicated.

12.9.1.2.3 Decompressive Craniectomy

Removal of large segments of skull helps to control ICP. The commonest is the unilateral craniectomy or frontotemporoparietal flap, and is frequently used by neurosurgeons as a primary procedure in LMIC in the absence of ICP monitoring to evacuate acute haematomas and decompress the swollen brain. The technique has been described by Quinn et al.[10] The bifrontotemporal craniectomy is used mainly for bilateral diffuse swelling. In advanced countries, the craniectomy is used for acute subdural haematoma evacuation or as a secondary or salvage operation for intractable intracranial hypertension. Removal of the skull commits the patient to a second operation to replace the flap (cranioplasty).

12.10 ADJUNCTS TO CARE

12.10.1 Infection Prophylaxis

- IV antibiotics are administered for a trauma craniotomy at the induction of anaesthesia (cephalosporin or amoxicillin or flucloxacillin).
- Broad spectrum antibiotic prophylaxis is recommended for penetrating craniocerebral injuries (cephalosporin, amoxicillin/clavulanate).[11]

12.10.2 Seizure Prophylaxis

Seizure activity in the early post-traumatic period following TBI may cause secondary damage as a result of increased metabolic demands, raised intracranial pressure, and excess neurotransmitter release.

Anticonvulsants are indicated for patients who have had a seizure after TBI. The treatment regimen is also shown to decrease the incidence of early post-traumatic seizures (within seven days of injury) and is continued for six months to one year. Early seizures are not associated with a worse outcome.

Prophylactic use of phenytoin or valproate is not recommended for preventing late post-traumatic seizures (PTS). Phenytoin is recommended to decrease the incidence of early PTS (within 7 days of injury), when the overall benefit is thought to outweigh the complications associated with such treatment. However, early PTS have not been associated with worse outcomes. There is insufficient evidence to recommend levetiracetam compared with phenytoin regarding efficacy in preventing early post-traumatic seizures and toxicity[6] (level IIA evidence).

12.10.3 Nutrition

Patients should be fed (via a naso- or orogastric tube) to attain basal caloric replacement at the latest by day 5–7 post-injury and to decrease mortality[6] (level IIA evidence).

12.10.4 Deep Vein Thrombosis Prophylaxis

Low molecular weight (LMWH) or low-dose unfractioned heparin may be used in combination with mechanical prophylaxis (pneumatic calf compression stockings) until the patient is ambulant. However, there is an increased risk for expansion of intracranial haemorrhage.

In addition to compression stockings, pharmacological prophylaxis may be considered if the brain injury is stable and the benefit is considered to outweigh the risk of increased intracranial haemorrhage. There is insufficient evidence to support recommendations regarding the preferred agent, dose, or timing of pharmacological prophylaxis for deep vein thrombosis[6] (level III evidence).

The LMWH is usually commenced 48 hours after craniotomy if the patient is stable and the post-operative scan is satisfactory.

12.10.5 Steroids

The use of steroids is not recommended for improving outcome or reducing ICP. In patients with moderate or severe traumatic brain injury (TBI), high dose methyl prednisolone is associated with an increased mortality and is contraindicated[6] (level 1 evidence).

12.11 PAEDIATRIC CONSIDERATIONS

The approach for the paediatric TBI patient is like that followed in the adults. Preservation of SBP >90 mm Hg is critical. Young children and babies are more susceptible to hypovolaemia and anaemia from blood loss compared with adults.

12.12 PEARLS AND PITFALLS

- Always follow the ATLS® principles (avoid D before completing A-B-C's).
- Do not attribute a deterioration in level of consciousness to alcohol or drug abuse.
- Keep in mind the C-spine protection in presence of significant TBI.
- Control major bleeding from a scalp wound (especially in children).
- Closely monitor TBI patients to detect early clinical deterioration in neurological status, despite an early normal CT scan.
- GCS should not be used solely as a single number. It is calculated from three different parameters each of which has its own significance. The trend is important.
- Hypotensive resuscitation applies in combined TBI and systemic penetrating injury.
- ICP elevation is caused by various intracranial pathologies. Management of intracranial hypertension with conservative measures should not divert attention from identifying the specific cause, and its management including exploratory burr holes if CT is not available.
- Progressive bleeding within the cranial cavity causes death. Death is due to elevation of ICP, brain shift and herniation of brain that compresses and damages the brain stem.
- Proceed to emergency burr hole or craniotomy when indicated to avoid further harm to the patient. Preferably contact a neurosurgeon to discuss the case.

12.13 SUMMARY

Traumatic brain injuries are a major cause of mortality and morbidity. Primary treatment in TBI focuses on prevention of secondary brain injury, mainly through preservation of normovolaemia and adequate tissue oxygenation. Emergency burr holes or craniotomy may be required when there is delay reaching a neurosurgeon and the patient is deteriorating or likely to deteriorate further. Temporizing measures before surgery may include hyperventilation and hyperosmolar agents such as mannitol or hypertonic saline.

12.14 ANAESTHETIC CONSIDERATIONS

- Continue 'damage control resuscitation' – rapid sequence intubation is commonly used.
- If the patient is not already intubated, avoid the patient coughing and straining during and following intubation as this will increase the ICP.
- Take care of the neck during intubation and surgery.
- Insert an arterial line but if this is proving difficult, avoid delay, defer the arterial line, and allow the surgeons to commence the surgery.
- Monitor end-tidal CO_2 and avoid hyperventilation.
- Elevate the head end of the operating table tendegrees if BP is maintained.
- Maintain adequate intravenous fluids; correct hypothermia; maintain glycaemic control; insert a nasogastric tube if the anterior skull base has been cleared of fractures (otherwise insert an orogastric tube); be aware of blood loss and replace as required; replace clotting factors and platelets indicated.
- Time is of essence; only strictly needed procedures are allowed to delay CT-scan for diagnosis and potential neurosurgical treatment.
- For the TBI patient the aim is to reduce the secondary brain injury by improving the balance between oxygen demand and delivery.
- Oxygen delivery to the brain cells is improved by securing the airway, assuring proper ventilation and oxygenation, restoring adequate circulation, oxygen carrying capacity and perfusion pressure; and by aiming for reducing cerebral oedema by facilitating venous drainage (head up) and adequate serum sodium levels.
- Oxygen demand is reduced by proper sedation using anaesthetics that can reduce the $CMRO_2$ (cerebral metabolic rate of oxygen).
- (Not single TBI), a compromise of the above mentioned aims may often be required.
- Ketamine is safe in TBI patients and can be used in the acute setting until haemodynamics is under control. Thereafter, propofol is mostly used for short-term anaesthesia/sedation maintenance.

REFERENCES AND RECOMMENDED READING

References

1. Dewan MC, Rattani A, Gupta S, Baticulon RE, Hung YC, Punchak M, et al. Estimating the global incidence of traumatic brain injury. *J Neurosurg*. 2018 Apr;**1**:1–18. doi: 10.3171/2017.10.JNS17352.

2. Rosenfeld JV, Maas AI, Bragge P, Morganti-Kossmann MC, Manley GT, Gruen RL. Early management of severe traumatic brain injury. *Lancet*. 2012;**380(9847)**:1088–98. doi: 10.1016/S0140-6736(12)60864-2.

3. Centers for Disease Control (CDC). Traumatic brain injury and concussion. *Get the facts*. 2017. Available from: http://www.cdc.gov/traumaticbraininjury/get_the_facts.html (accessed online January 2019).

4. McGinn MJ, Povlishock JT. Pathophysiology of Traumatic Brain Injury. *Neurosurg Clin N Am*. 2016 Oct;**27(4)**:397–407. doi: 10.1016/j.nec.2016.06.002.

5. Carney N, Totten AM, O'Reilly C, Ullman JS, Hawryluk GW, Bell MJ, et al. Guidelines for the Management of Severe Traumatic Brain Injury, Fourth Edition. *Neurosurgery* 2017 Jan 1;**80(1)**:6–15. doi: 10.1227/NEU.0000000000001432.

6. Guidelines for the Management of Severe Traumatic Brain Injury. 4th Edn. *The Brain Trauma Foundation*. 2016; Available from: https://braintrauma.org/guidelines/guidelines-for-the-management-of-severe-tbi-4th-ed#/ (accessed online January 2019).

7. Chesnut RM, Temkin N, Dikmen S, Rondina C, Videtta W, Petroni G, et al. A Method of Managing Severe Traumatic Brain Injury in the Absence of Intracranial Pressure Monitoring: The Imaging and Clinical Examination Protocol. *J Neurotrauma*. 2018 Jan 1;**35(1)**:54–63. doi: 10.1089/neu.2016.4472.

8. Bouida W, Marghli S, Souissi S, Ksibi H, Methammem M, Haguiga H, et al. Prediction value of the Canadian CT head rule and the New Orleans criteria for positive head CT scan and acute neurosurgical procedures in minor

head trauma: A multicenter external validation study. *Ann Emerg Med.* 2013 May;**61(5)**:521–7. doi: 10.1016/j.annemergmed.2012.07.01.

9. Wilson MH, Wise D, Davies G, Lockey D. Emergency burr holes: "How to do it". *Scand J Trauma Resusc Emerg Med.* 2012 Apr 2;**20**:24. doi: 10.1186/1757-7241-20-24.

10. Quinn TM, Taylor JJ, Magarik JA, Vought E, Kindy MS, Ellegala DB. Decompressive craniectomy: technical note. *Acta neurologica Scandinavica.* 2011 Apr;**123(4)**:239–44. doi: 10.1111/j.1600-0404.2010.01397.x.

11. Bayston R, de Louvois J, Brown EM, Johnston RA, Lees P, Pople IK. Use of antibiotics in penetrating craniocerebral injuries. "Infection in Neurosurgery" Working Party of British Society for Antimicrobial Chemotherapy. *Lancet.* 2000 May 20;**355(9217)**:1813–7.

Recommended Reading

Joseph B, Friese RS, Sadoun M, et al. The BIG (brain injury guidelines) project: defining the management of traumatic brain injury by acute care surgeons. *J Trauma Acute Care Surg.* 2014;**76(4)**:965–9.

Maas AI, Dearden M, Teasdale GM, Braakman R, Cohadon F, Iannotti F, et al. EBIC-guidelines for management of severe head injury in adults. *European Brain Injury Consortium. Acta Neurochir (Wien).* 1997;**139(4)**:286–94.

Rosenfeld JV. *Practical Management of Head and Neck Injury.* Elsevier, Churchill Livingstone. 2012. ISBN 978-0-7295-3956-2.

Rosenfeld JV, Bell RS, Armonda R. Current concepts in penetrating and blast injury to the central nervous system. *World journal of surgery.* 2015;**39(6)**:1352–62.

Burns 13

13.1 OVERVIEW

Globally, burns are a serious public health problem. There are over 300,000 deaths each year from fires alone, with more deaths from scalds, electrical burns, and other forms of burns. Fire-related deaths alone rank among the 15 leading causes of death among children and young adults aged 5–29 years. Over 95% of fatal fire-related burns occur in low and middle income countries. Southeast Asia alone accounts for just over one-half of the total number of fire-related deaths worldwide, and females in this region have the highest fire-related burn mortality rates globally.[1]

High-income countries have made considerable progress in lowering rates of burn-related death and disability, through combinations of proven prevention strategies and improvements in the care of burn victims. Most of these advances in prevention and care have been incompletely applied in low and middle income countries.[2]

Burns are common, often disfiguring, disruptive to families and work, financially burdensome, and painful. The concept of near-total early wound excision cannot be overstated for large burns and the clock starts ticking for the wound and the patient from the moment of injury. Delay to resuscitation and operation is harmful. Major burns cause massive tissue destruction and result in activation of a cytokine-mediated inflammatory response that leads to dramatic pathophysiological effects at sites local and distant from the burn.

13.2 BURNS PATHOPHYSIOLOGY

The early (ebb) phase of a major burn injury is characterized by decreased cardiac output, and decreased blood flow to all organs. The decreased cardiac output is due to loss of intravascular volume, direct myocardial depression, increased pulmonary and systemic vascular resistance (PVR and SVR, respectively), and haemoconcentration, and can lead to metabolic acidosis and venous desaturation ($\downarrow$SVO$_2$). Decreased urine flow results from decreased glomerular filtration, and elevated aldosterone and antidiuretic hormone (ADH) levels. Oxygenation and ventilation problems can occur due to inhalation injury and the systemic effects of burns including adult respiratory distress syndrome (ARDS). Compartment syndrome ensues if there is a circumferential burn that does not undergo escharotomy to release the constriction. Compartment syndrome can also occur in the abdomen, extremities, or orbits without local or circumferential burns. Mental status can be altered because of psychological stress, hypoxia, hypotension, inhaled toxins, and administered drugs (Figure 13.1).

At 48–72 hours, the hypermetabolic-hyperdynamic (flow) phase starts, characterized by increased oxygen consumption, carbon dioxide production, and cardiac output, with enhanced blood flow to all organs including skin, kidney (glomerular filtration rate [GFR]) and liver, and decreased SVR. Increased venous oxygen saturation ($\uparrow$SVO$_2$) is related to peripheral arteriovenous shunting. The markedly decreased SVR mimics sepsis. Lungs and airways may continue to be affected because of inhalation injury and ARDS, and pulmonary oedema can occur due to redistribution of resuscitation fluids and resultant hypervolemia. The altered mental status may be related to continued systemic inflammatory response syndrome (SIRS) and continued drug therapy. Release of catabolic hormones and insulin resistance leads to muscle protein catabolism and hyperglycaemia (Figure 13.2).

13.3 ANATOMY

Apart from simple erythema (sunburn), all other burns constitute an open wound of greater or lesser severity. To create a dramatic analogy, a burn is like an evisceration with exposed bowel. In the case of the burn, it is the

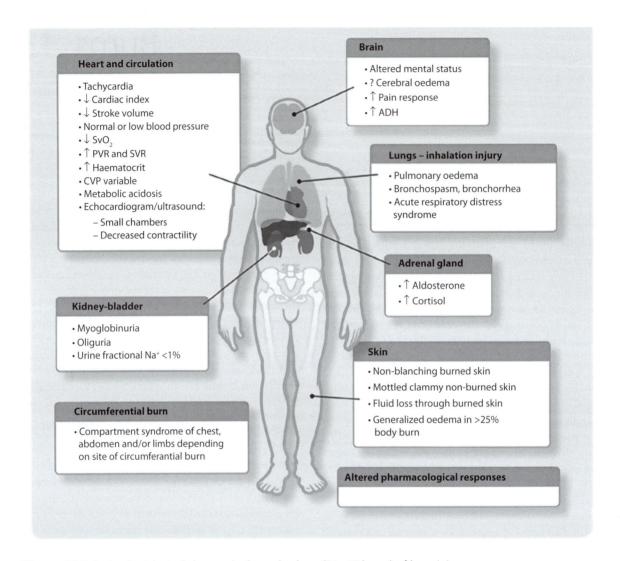

Heart and circulation

- Tachycardia
- ↓ Cardiac index
- ↓ Stroke volume
- Normal or low blood pressure
- ↓ SvO$_2$
- ↑ PVR and SVR
- ↑ Haematocrit
- CVP variable
- Metabolic acidosis
- Echocardiogram/ultrasound:
  - Small chambers
  - Decreased contractility

Brain

- Altered mental status
- ? Cerebral oedema
- ↑ Pain response
- ↑ ADH

Lungs – inhalation injury

- Pulmonary oedema
- Bronchospasm, bronchorrhea
- Acute respiratory distress syndrome

Adrenal gland

- ↑ Aldosterone
- ↑ Cortisol

Kidney-bladder

- Myoglobinuria
- Oliguria
- Urine fractional Na$^+$ <1%

Skin

- Non-blanching burned skin
- Mottled clammy non-burned skin
- Fluid loss through burned skin
- Generalized oedema in >25% body burn

Circumferential burn

- Compartment syndrome of chest, abdomen and/or limbs depending on site of circumferantial burn

Altered pharmacological responses

Figure 13.1 Pathophysiological changes in the early phase (24–48 hours) of burn injury.

dermis (Figure 13.1) that is exposed to a lesser or greater extent, resulting in significant losses of fluid from the body, along with loss of the bacterial barrier, leaving the path open for infection, as well as loss of heat by convection and conduction (Figure 13.3).

In physiological terms, there is a significant loss of protein – primarily albumin – and electrolytes, and haemoconcentration, along with a massive increase in energy requirements to heal the wound.

The burn wound is divided into three areas (Figure 13.4):

- The zone of coagulation.
- The zone of stasis.
- The zone of hyperaemia.

Inadequate resuscitation or the inappropriate use of ice or iced water to cool the burn may lead to deepening the burn due to vasoconstriction in the zone of stasis, extending the zone of coagulation.

13.4 SPECIAL TYPES OF BURN

13.4.1 Chemical Burns

First aid should be extended for chemical burns to 30 minutes of washing. Alkali goes deep as it dissolves fat, but acid can 'tan' the skin and be surprisingly

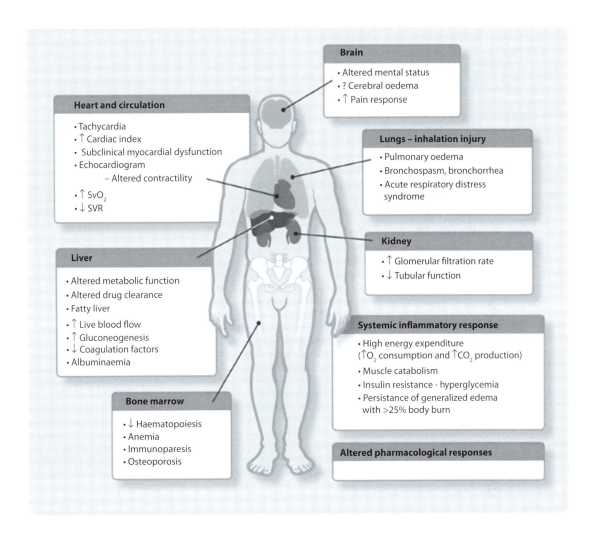

Figure 13.2 Pathophysiological changes during hypermetabolic/hyperdynamic phase of burn.

shallow although diagnosis of depth for these chemicals is just plain difficult. Time, however, does tell.

Hydrofluoric acid will continue to injure until the fluorine is chelated. Extreme pain is the hallmark as nerves are irritated. Neuropathic pain is common for months afterwards. After washing the area, the next step is to introduce cations to the injury front. Ca++ and Mg++ are used. Techniques include:

- Calcium added to gel and applied topically.
- Calcium gluconate solution added to dimethyl sulfoxide (DMSO) and especially useful for soaking fingertips.
- Intra-arterial infusion of calcium.

- Bier's block with calcium gluconate.
- Hypocalcaemia can result from small areas burned with concentrations >10%. The amount of calcium that may need to be intravenously infused is staggering. Beware!

13.4.2 Electrical Injury

Electrical burns are always more extensive than the surface wound indicates. This is especially so for high voltage (>1000 volts) injuries. Low voltage domestic current injury is often seen on the fingers and thumb. The wound frequently extends down to joints and so the operator

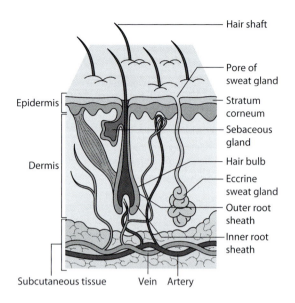

Figure 13.3 Layers and structures of the skin.

should be ready to create flap coverage at the time of excision.

Cardiac arrhythmias can result. Loss of consciousness is a prime indicator of this. A 12 lead ECG, a rhythm strip, cardiac-specific troponin levels are the minimum investigations. If normal and no loss of consciousness, no further cardiac specific investigation or management is needed. Otherwise, cardiac monitoring, echocardiography, and cardiology input are indicated.

High voltage electrical injuries are associated with devastating injuries, both burn and musculoskeletal. Posterior dislocation of the shoulder, compression fractures of the spine, trauma from being thrown – rib/

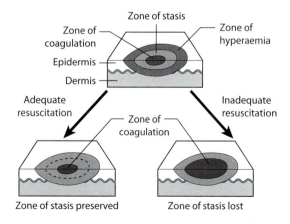

Figure 13.4 Zones of a burn.

chest/long bone, and head trauma should be sought and excluded. The nature of the injury is different to other burn aetiology including low voltage. The body is a volume conductor, therefore narrower diameter areas accumulate heat. The current runs up periosteum, nerves, and vessels while effecting muscle cells also. Electroporation of cell walls particularly injures myocytes, with cell necrosis increasing over 5 days; if the muscle looks abnormal at first, it is destined to die. Early release with fasciotomy full length of the compartments should be performed and re-looks planned. There will always be more to do. In the upper limb, carpal tunnel and Guyon's canal releases should be incorporated in the extensile incisions. Remember, the deep muscles such as pronator quadratus and rotator cuff will be most affected.

Early excision of obviously dead tissue combined with fasciotomy is performed immediately with planned take-backs at regular intervals for further debridement.

13.5 **DEPTH OF THE BURN**

Burns have been traditionally divided into first, second, and third degree, but the terms 'partial thickness' (superficial and deep) and 'full-thickness' are more informative and will be used here. There is also a group of 'indeterminate' thickness burns, which represent a separate challenge.

13.5.1 **Superficial Burn (Erythema)**

'Sunburn' is painful, dry, is not blistered, and will fade on its own within 7 days. It requires no debridement and is not counted in the calculation of percentage of total burn surface area (TBSA). Simple oral analgesics and anti-inflammatory agents are usually all that is needed.

13.5.2 **Superficial Partial Thickness**

These involve the entire epidermis down to the basement membrane and no more than the upper third of the dermis. Rapid re-epithelialization occurs in 1–2 weeks. Because of the large number of remaining epidermal cells and the good blood supply, there is a very small zone of injury or stasis beneath the burn eschar (Figure 13.5).

A superficial partial thickness (SPT) burn is wet, often blistered, intensely painful and red or white (including in

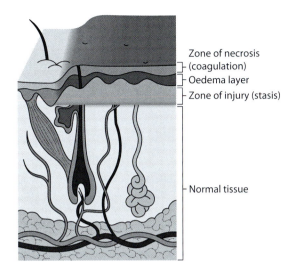

Figure 13.5 Superficial partial thickness burn.

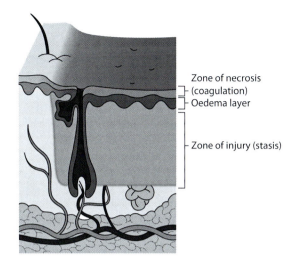

Figure 13.6 Deep partial thickness burn.

darker-skinned patients), blanches on pressure, and will generally heal without split-skin grafting (SSG), usually within 10–14 days. The hairs remain attached when they are pulled. The skin still feels elastic and supple. These burns are often caused by hot water and steam. They do not scar.

13.5.3 Deep Partial Thickness

Destruction of the epidermis occurs down to the basement membrane plus the middle third of the dermis. Re-epithelialization is much slower (2–4 weeks) due to fewer remaining epidermal cells and a lesser blood supply. More collagen deposition will occur, especially if the wound has not been excised and grafted within 3 weeks. The depth of the wound has a significant risk of conversion. The zone of stasis is much larger than in the SPT injury because of the lower blood flow and greater initial injury to the remaining epidermal cells (Figure 13.6).

A deep partial thickness (DPT) burn is often a mixture of wet and dry. The drier it is, the deeper. Sensation is variable but is still present to touch, although often less painful. The skin texture is thicker and more rubbery. Red patches do not blanche on pressure but exhibit 'fixed skin staining' due to capillary stasis. The hairs will come out readily when pulled. If not excised, these burns take 4–6 weeks to heal and scar badly. The function of a re-epithelialized DPT burn is poor due to fragility of the epidermis and the rigidity of the scar-laden dermis.

13.5.4 'Indeterminate' Partial Thickness Burns

Indeterminate burns are usually a mixture of SPT and DPT burns and may exhibit the clinical features of both. The history may help in deciding which is the predominant element and enable management decision-making.

13.5.5 Full Thickness

Full-thickness burns involve the entire epidermis and at least two-thirds of the dermis, leaving very few dermis and epidermal cells to regenerate. Spontaneous healing is very slow, over 4 weeks. Sharp debridement is needed to remove the eschar. Scarring is usually severe if the wound is not skin-grafted, and there is a high risk of infection.

Full-thickness burns are thick, dry, insensate, leathery, and usually black or yellow. Thrombosis is often visible in the surface vessels. The hairs have been burned off. Escharotomies and fasciotomies may be indicated for circumferential full-thickness burns. If left, these burns will contract, become infected, and scar badly. They require early excision and grafting. All electrical burns are full thickness, as are many flame and chemical burns.

13.6 TOTAL BODY SURFACE AREA BURNED

For the purposes of calculating the total body surface area (TBSA) burned as a percentage of the entire body surface area, only SPT and DPT burns, along with

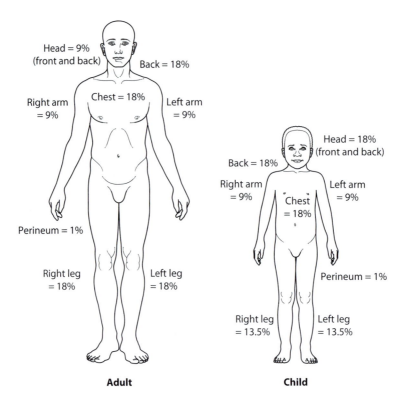

Head = 9%
(front and back)
Back = 18%
Chest = 18%
Right arm = 9%
Left arm = 9%
Perineum = 1%
Right leg = 18%
Left leg = 18%

Adult

Head = 18%
(front and back)
Back = 18%
Right arm = 9%
Left arm = 9%
Chest = 18%
Perineum = 1%
Right leg = 13.5%
Left leg = 13.5%

Child

Figure 13.7 Body surface area.

full-thickness burns, are included in the calculation. Erythema – simple 'sunburn' – alone is ignored.

All units involved in the management of burns should have a clearly established protocol, and this should include the use of a burns resuscitation chart that also shows TBSA affected, in diagrammatic form (traditionally the 'rule of nines' in the adult, and the Lund and Browder chart in the child; Figure 13.7). The patient's palm, including the fingers, represents approximately 1% TBSA and is useful when calculating patchy burns.

It must be emphasized that TBSA calculation is only a starting point for working out a plan of management. Subsequent management is dictated by the patient's response – not by calculated numbers!

13.7 MANAGEMENT

13.7.1 Safe Retrieval

As with all trauma, this will follow the usual Advanced Trauma Life Support® protocols of 'Airway, Breathing, Circulation', etc. – the ABCDEs.

However, it may, in addition, include removing the casualty from the source of burning without concomitant risk to the rescuer. This may mean that electrical power supplies must be switched off, chemical and fuel spillages contained, and fires extinguished to allow rescuers access to the casualty. Burning clothing must be removed, and caustic substances washed off as much as possible, but little time should be spent at the scene.

Pitfall

Do not forget that a burned patient is still a trauma patient and may well have suffered other major injuries in addition to the burn.

13.7.2 First Aid

Do: Cool the burn with *lukewarm* running water. If a tap is not available, use a bucket and jug. Continue for at least 20–30 minutes; this provides analgesia and limits burn size. Remember to monitor body temperature. In intubated patients this process should not exceed 30 minutes.

Don't: Use ice or iced water as these may extend the depth of burn. Do not let the patient get cold; removing burning clothing and leaving the patient exposed to the elements will very quickly result in hypothermia.

> **The principle is to cool the burn but to keep the patient warm.**

Any burn produces inflammation and associated swelling and capillary leakage. The greater the TBSA affected, the greater the inflammatory response, so that any burn of over 20% TBSA will produce a total body systemic reaction with resultant systemic inflammatory response syndrome (SIRS). This is unavoidable and should be anticipated.

13.7.3 Initial Management

13.7.3.1 AIRWAY

A rapid assessment of the circumstances of the burn may well alert the medical team to the potential for an airway burn. Fires in an enclosed space (such as house fires) with combustible material and a prolonged extrication time will clearly represent a significant risk.

The inability to make a high-pitched sound ('eeee'), redness, blisters, or smoke inside the teeth mean the upper airway has been injured. Endoscopy or laryngoscopy, with liberal application of local anaesthesia can help judge the severity of injury and guide the need for intubation.

Aspiration of caustic substances may produce a chemical pneumonitis, and steam inhalation from boiling water may cause significant airway injury. Where obvious signs of airway injury exist, including stridor, obvious airway burns, redness and swelling of the uvula and pharynx, and wheezing breath sounds or respiratory distress, not only should supplemental oxygen by administered, but early intubation should be accomplished before swelling closes the upper airway.

> **When in doubt, INTUBATE.**
> **It is easier to subsequently extubate a stable patient who has been intubated early, than to try a late intubation on a patient whose airway is swollen, distorted and burnt.**

Pitfall

Use the biggest tube possible, as narrow tubes become clogged with thick, sooty secretions and DO NOT CUT THE TUBE SHORT. The amount of swelling is startling!

Carbon monoxide intoxication most often presents with coma or obtundation, rarely the oft-described cherry red appearance and is best diagnosed with carboxyhaemoglobin (COHb) levels on blood gas analysis. Treatment is high dose oxygen.

13.7.3.2 ANALGESIA

Partial thickness burns are intensely painful and usually require repeated doses of intravenous opiates, titrated against the pain. Analgesia must always be given, even if the child or adult cannot communicate with you. However, the deeper the burn gets, the fewer nerve endings survive, to the point where full-thickness burns are insensate. Providing early, adequate pain relief will reduce stress to the patient and attending medical staff alike, and should be a priority in management after airway control.

13.7.3.3 INTRAVENOUS ACCESS

Intravenous access, (preferably central access) should be initiated (if necessary, through the burn itself), and at the same time, blood samples taken for full blood count, electrolytes, blood type and screen, and glucose. If possible, arterial blood gases with an assessment of carboxyhaemoglobin should be obtained, and a note made of the fraction of inspired oxygen (FiO_2), so that the degree of pulmonary shunting can be calculated. This may be helpful if subsequent ventilation is required.

In patients with a greater than 50% burn, it is likely that a consumption coagulopathy may develop; therefore, a thromboelastogram should be performed, or a conventional coagulation screen.

Pitfalls

- Where possible, central lines should be used in larger burns, as with oedema, other lines may not remain in the vein. The lines should be sutured in place, as dressings will not hold them.
- Central lines are best placed above the diaphragm initially as abdominal pressure can rise so severely that fluid will not flow. The earlier fluid resuscitation is commenced the less mortality and morbidity from acute kidney injury, wound progression, and early and late infection of wound and lung.

13.7.3.4 EMERGENCY MANAGEMENT OF THE BURN WOUND

Coverage of the burn wound in the emergency setting is best accomplished with large quantities of 'clingfilm', which has been shown to be sterile and is available in industrial quantities. Clingfilm reduces pain by covering exposed nerve endings, and contains and reduces fluid losses, while still allowing proper inspection of the burn wound. The old practice of 'mummifying' the patient in swathes of gauze and crepe bandages (with or without the addition of underlying silver creams) is unhelpful, painful for the patient, messy, time-consuming, inefficient for nursing staff, and obstructive to the clinician.

13.7.3.5 FLUID RESUSCITATION

All burns over 20% constitute 'major burns'. All of these will require intravenous fluid replacement, a urinary catheter to monitor output, a nasogastric tube for early feeding, and at least high-care nursing. Lesser percentage burns may be treated by aggressive oral rehydration, but particularly in infants it is better to err on the side of caution, and some units still routinely resuscitate those under 12 years who have a greater than 10% TBSA burn with intravenous fluids.

Pitfalls

- All fluid replacement formulae are only *guidelines* to resuscitation. Adequacy of resuscitation is based on urine output rather than slavishly following a formula such as the Parkland formula for fluid requirements.
- Fluid losses start at the time of burn, and fluid replacement is calculated *from the time of burn*, and not from the time of admission to hospital.

The Parkland formula is traditionally used to work out requirements for the first 24 hours:

$$\text{TBSA (\%) burned} \times 4\,\text{mL} \times \text{mass in kg}$$
$$= \text{requirement in first 24 hours (mL)}$$
$$(\text{If BSA} > 60\%, \text{use } 3\,\text{mL/kg})$$

The first half of the total requirement is given in the first 8 hours, and the other half over the following 16 hours; this is given as Ringer's lactate. There is limited evidence that changing to a colloid solution in the next 24 hours will reduce capillary leakage. Urine output should be maintained at no more than 0.5–1.0 mL/kg per hour for adults, and 1.0–2 mL/kg per hour for infants and children. If too much fluid is given, capillary leakage will increase, producing 'fluid creep' and increasing oedema as the fluid shifts into the 'third space', increasing the likelihood of SIRS and adult respiratory distress syndrome (ARDS).[3] The exception would be if there were myoglobinuria, as in electrical burns, where an output over 1.0 mL/kg per hour would be required for an adult.

Pitfalls

- It is imperative to not bolus patients secondary to burn shock hypotension.
- *Antibiotics are not indicated for early burns* within 72 hours of injury, as the burn is still essentially sterile.
- If the patient is hypotensive on admission, it is wrong to attribute signs of shock to the burn until all other sources of shock have been ruled out. Burn shock does not usually develop in the first 24 hours post-burn.

13.7.3.6 ASSOCIATED INJURIES

It is easy to focus on the burn alone and miss any associated injuries. A careful history will give clues to not only the type and depth of the burn, but also the possibility of the associated injuries. A full examination is essential once analgesia is adequate, intravenous lines (which may have to transgress a burned area of skin) are running, oxygen is being administered, and the burn has been covered.

Any other injuries found during examination of the patient must be dealt with according to clinical need. Injuries that are bleeding take priority, and the normal principles of resuscitation, including damage control, apply. Most orthopaedic injuries may be deferred for definitive treatment until the resuscitation phase of the burn injury is over. This is usually within the first 48 hours. However, if the patient requires early tangential excision and SSG, and the patient's physiology is not compromised, it may be appropriate to attend to orthopaedic conditions at the same time.

The clinician must be alert to the possibility of deliberate abuse, especially in children, where the nature and distribution of the burn is inconsistent with the story given by the parent or caregiver. The pattern of burn and an unacceptably late presentation may further clues to a deliberate, 'punishment' burn. Where suspicion exists, it is important to document the burn injury meticulously, with photographs if possible. Other signs of abuse should be looked for, and social services contacted if appropriate.

13.7.4 Escharotomy and Fasciotomy

In any trauma resuscitation, the purpose is to combat shock, defined as tissue hypoxia inadequate to the needs of that tissue's survival. Burns are no different, but they present with some special challenges, particularly when the airway is compromised, or when circumferential full-thickness burns with a thick, unyielding eschar produce a tourniquet effect. This can occur around the chest, neck or limbs, producing a slow asphyxiation or critical limb ischaemia. Recognition of the need for escharotomy is vital and needs to be acted upon, usually within the emergency department. An escharotomy is indicated for relief of pressure in a limb or torso to allow vascular supply or ventilation. Circumferential deep limb burns with large overall burn area requiring large volume fluid resuscitation is the commonest scenario. The eschar does not expand to accommodate, and so fluid accumulates, and pressure rises. This process takes some time to reach a crescendo – some 6–8 hours. In an awake patient, the same symptoms and signs as a tight plaster cast are complained of: increasing, unbearable, deep aching pain, loss active muscle movement, extreme pain with forced stretching of muscle groups, cool digits, slowed capillary refill, and loss of digital Doppler signal. The feel of a limb that needs escharotomy can be likened to squeezing an apple- no give. It is common for limbs to be firm, but if there is 'give', escharotomy is not (yet) indicated. If pulses are lost and there is still 'give' to palpation, first check another limb and the blood pressure. Hypovolaemia may be the cause.

*An escharotomy (skin) is not necessarily
a fasciotomy (fascia).*

The technique is simple. An operating room is not required for performance of an escharotomy but good lighting, instruments to achieve haemostasis, and preferably an assistant are. In an awake patient, local anaesthetic injected proximally and into areas of partial thickness burn makes the procedure quite possible. A full thickness burn is insensate. A scalpel, artery forceps, sutures, and ligatures should be at hand; diathermy is a good alternative in the ventilated patient.

Incisions are made in the axial planes. The upper limb wishes to be in a pronated position when oedematous, so must be forced into full supination otherwise the incisions can easily cross flexure creases leading to division of longitudinal structures and contracture. An antimicrobial cream should be applied to the wounds and a non-stick absorbent dressing loosely bandaged.

Pitfall

If the procedure has been delayed, efflux of metabolites will cause hypotension and hyperkalaemia. Be ready!

Linear incisions are made to allow the escharotomy wounds to gape apart, relieving the tension. The escharotomy wounds must be extensive enough to reach normal tissue. Although a scalpel is usually adequate to achieve this, diathermy may be necessary.

Figure 13.8 shows the main incision lines for the release of eschar causing constriction. Escharotomy should be a largely painless procedure as it is only transgressing devitalized tissue, except at its limits where it may encroach upon living tissues which will be normally sensate, or even hypersensate. This will not only alert the

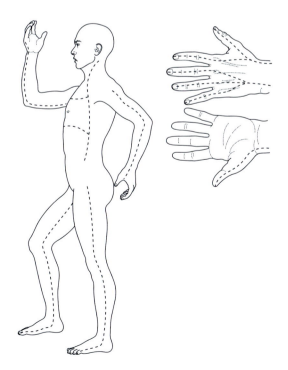

Figure 13.8 Escharotomy sites.

clinician to stop but ensures that constriction rings of dead eschar are not left at the limits of the escharotomy.

Pitfall

Despite escharotomy release, some tissues – especially in limbs – may remain ischaemic, particularly where there has been an electrical burn, which is always full thickness and frequently produces significant myonecrosis. In these cases, it may be necessary to extend the escharotomy into a fasciotomy to release the compartment syndrome. Fasciotomy is usually accompanied by profuse bleeding if the tissue within is still viable, and it is as well to be prepared for this.

13.7.5 Definitive Management

13.7.5.1 'CLOSING' THE BURN WOUND

Burns are not static wounds: they are 'pathology-in-evolution'. The longer the burn remains uncovered by either the patient's own skin or an effective biological alternative, the longer it remains a significant breech of the skin's antibacterial barrier and a significant source of heat and fluid loss to the body, analogous to bowel evisceration.

From about 72 hours post-burn, surface bacteria migrate into the remaining deep dermis and below, rendering topical antiseptics and antibiotics ineffective, and increasing the chances of systemic septicaemia. For these reasons, there has been a move towards early excision of the wound and SSG where necessary. Clearly, not all burns require grafting. Hot water and scalds from steam will often heal on their own within 10 days, despite their dramatic initial appearances. It is wise to wait for this time before deciding to operate. The SSG rate for these burns has been almost halved by such an approach. However, *all* burns should undergo an initial cleaning and debridement under anaesthesia as soon as possible after admission, preferably within the first 48 hours. The reasons for this are fourfold:

- This cleans the wound thoroughly and enables an appropriate choice of dressing, as clingfilm is difficult to secure for more than 48 hours.
- It allows a proper inspection of the burn and removal of blisters, because it is not unusual for the area of the burn to be underestimated in the emergency room, and a 9% burn may turn out to be 16%, putting

it into the 'major burn' category, with all its attendant requirements.

- It is often (wrongly) assumed that blistered burns are always SPT burns. Blistered skin should be removed, unless it is slack, so that the clinician can be sure there is no deeper burn beneath. It is safer to excise the blister and assess the depth of the burn beneath, as it may turn out to be DPT or even full thickness.
- If it is seen that excision and SSG are required, this may be accomplished at the same surgical procedure.

13.7.5.2 TECHNIQUE OF EXCISION AND SPLIT SKIN GRAFTING

Both these techniques can be accomplished by using either the Humby knife (or a modification of it) or an electric dermatome. The 'set' of the blade (depth of cut) will need to be greater for excision than for the harvesting of skin for SSG.

13.7.5.3 TUMESCENT TECHNIQUE

Blood loss can be significant in both procedures, but may be minimized by using tourniquets for the limbs, or the 'tumescent technique' on the torso:

- The technique uses 2 mL 1:1000 adrenaline (epinephrine) +40 mL 0.5% plain bupivacaine added to 1000 mL of warm normal saline.
- Take a 19-gauge 3.5 inch spinal needle, and attach a giving set to the bag, which is placed in a pressurized infusion device and the injection given subdermally.
- The raised skin should feel cold (and look white in Caucasian races).
- Once the skin has been harvested or the burn excised, adrenaline-soaked abdominal packs (5 mg in 1000 mL normal saline) can be applied to the wound bed, with a significant reduction in blood loss.

SSGs are secured by skin clips, tissue glue or sutures, depending on the site, and then covered with several layers of paraffin gauze to prevent movement, followed by dry gauze and bandaging.

If infection has been a problem, activated nanocrystalline silver (e.g. Acticoat® – Smith and Nephew, London, UK) may be applied and secured in place with water-soaked gauze and bandages. The dressing will remain bacterially active for up to 4 days and may also have anti-inflammatory properties.

The choice of site for harvesting skin depends on the site that is burned (e.g. back or eyelids), and what skin is available:

- Neck skin is good for eyelids.
- Inner arm skin is good for the face.
- Wherever possible, match the colour, texture and hair growth.
- When skin substitutes are not an option, re-harvesting donor sites is usually possible within 10–14 days.
- Scalp skin is thicker, usually of good quality, and regenerates faster. When all else fails, it will provide an extra source.

13.7.5.4 WOUND COVERAGE

Wound coverage can be a dilemma. In the first instance, for burns >30% TBSA, a temporary cover with Biobrane® (Mylan, Canonsburg PA USA) – a bilaminate biosynthetic skin substitute composed of nylon mesh, coated with porcine collagen peptides bonded to a silicon membrane, serves to seal the excised wound, and in the case of debrided partial thickness burn, may well be its final coverage with the wound healing.[4] It also serves the principle of not extending the wound area. For excised full thickness burns, Biobrane® has a short life span if applied to fat but longer on fascia. It does need to be replaced by more permanent wound coverage before it goes 'sour', which is characterized by loss of adherence then fluid accumulation, which then turns to pus in a few days.

Smaller deep burns are autografted at this stage, with the meshed versus unmeshed debate being beyond the scope of this piece. All agree that less or no mesh expansion gives better cosmesis, especially in people with any skin colour, more frequent seroma/haematoma formation, and less area coverage.

Permanent wound coverage for a large or massive burn usually becomes a patchwork quilt of different applications. Dermal replacement template, widely expanded (1:4) meshed autograft with Zimmer or using a MEEK (Humeca, Woodstock, GA) technique with narrow meshed allograft overlay (torso), or unmeshed autograft (face/hands).[8] Originally designed by Cicero Meek, from the University of South Carolina, the technique, compared with the mesh graft technique has the following advantages:

- The Meek method provides true expansion up to 9:1.
- Small graft remnants can be utilized.

- Grafting of full thickness burns up to 70%–75% TBSA becomes possible with one harvest of the donor sites.
- The reliability of graft take is equal or better.
- Epithelialization is achieved within 3 to 4 weeks depending on the expansion ratio.

Versajet II (Smith & Nephew plc, London, UK) debridement is frequently used for mid-dermal burns prior to application of Biobrane® and for multiple applications with children.[5] It is a hydrodissector that works in some way similar to a pressure washer combined with suction. It is excellent for preservation of live dermis and as such, early facial excision and unmeshed allograft has obviated the need for autografting in all but the worst facial burns.

13.7.5.5 BURN WOUND EXCISION AND CLOSURE

The larger the burn, the more quickly it should be removed. In massive burns, operation should proceed as soon as the patient has regained normothermia, is passing urine appropriately, and coagulation corrected. Blood loss is much decreased if excision takes place within the first 24 hours.

General issues that need to be attended before commencing a large wound excision include:

- A clear predetermined operative plan that encompasses the initial and subsequent procedures, including donor site usage: What is going where, mesh expansion ratio along with which coverage is temporary and which permanent.
- Large and secure venous access.
- An operating room warmed so that the air surrounding the patient is at least 32°C and preferably much above that figure (latent heat of evaporation from the moist wound will come from the atmosphere rather than the patient).
- Regular 'checking-in' with the anaesthetic team.
- Multiple surgical teams operating simultaneously.
- Frequent use of TEG/RoTEM.
- Availability of blood and blood products in large quantities.
- Pre-set 'bail-out' endpoints and methods.
- Cold electrolyte rich drinks for the OR staff!

Small burns can be dealt with in fairly routine operating room set-up as long as the patient is being kept warm.

The following protocol is an example:

- Appropriate antibiotic prophylaxis is used routinely.
- Hair is clipped.
- The wounds are washed with warmed antiseptic solution (aqueous chlorhexidine).
- Normal saline with 1 ampoule of 1:1000 adrenalin is injected subdermally with a 19-gauge needle and Pitkin self-loading syringe. Do not go deeply, as subcutaneous vessels can be severed with loss of the accompanying fat lobule and graft loss.
- Tourniquets are used on limbs with appropriate padding and timekeeping. If the area for tourniquet application is burned, excision of the wound after injection occurs first.
- Excision is effected by either sequential, tangential excision using a hand, or powered dermatome or with diathermy in massive and very deep burns. Living dermis is white and live fat is glistening yellow.
- It is important to finish one small area at a time before moving on, as any bleeding will obscure the detail by staining. Further unnecessary tissue removal may follow.
- Wounds are covered with 1:200,000 adrenalin soaked dressings, with limbs being wrapped in aqueous chlorhexidine soaked sponges/lap pads and bandaged.
- Let the tourniquet down!

13.7.6 Assessing and Managing Airway Burns

13.7.6.1 UPPER AIRWAY

Suspicion is the watchword, with early intervention before the opportunity to protect the airway by intubation has been lost. Listening to the respiration is vital, and dyspnoea with hoarse, coarse breathing or stridor should prompt immediate action.

Upper airway burns to the larynx and trachea may be suspected by the history (e.g. a steam valve blew into the face) or by inspection of the mouth, tongue, and oropharynx, which may be red, injected, and swollen. These burns usually require intubation but generally resolve within 36 hours. It is important to remember that the burn is 'pathology-in-evolution' and that the early signs will get worse in the next 24 hours.

13.7.6.2 LOWER AIRWAY

The deep, 'alveolar' burn is much more difficult to detect or predict. The rate of onset is slower, and it may only manifest itself 3–5 days after the burn. Some indication that a lower airway burn is present may come from the history of prolonged smoke exposure and raised carboxyhaemoglobin levels. Blood gases should be taken whenever possible, and the ventilation–perfusion shunt worked out by plotting the FiO_2 against the PaO_2 (partial pressure of oxygen in arterial blood).

13.7.6.3 INHALATIONAL TOXICITY

This third component of airway burns may present first as the effects of carbon monoxide poisoning are immediate.

Remember that the peak level of carbon monoxide is present at the scene, and not at first measurement in the hospital.

Any carbon monoxide level of over 10% is regarded as toxic, and 100% oxygen should be given until the carbon monoxide level has fallen to below 5%.

Pitfall

Pulse oximetry may be unreliable if high levels of carbon monoxide are present, as the haemoglobin is saturated with carbon monoxide and not oxygen.

13.7.7 Tracheostomy

Early tracheostomy should be considered, especially if the area of the burn includes the neck. It is quite acceptable to place a tracheostomy through the site of a burn. Once the oedema has occurred, placement of a tracheostomy is far more difficult and hazardous. The tracheostomy should be well secured, as if it is displaced, replacement may prove very difficult.

13.8 SPECIAL AREAS

The face, hands, perineum, and feet are special areas that need special attention to obtain a good outcome.

13.8.1 Face

Biobrane® is very useful for SPT burns of the face. It needs to be held in place firmly with compression for 48 hours to 'bond'. This may be accomplished by crepe bandaging, which is then removed after 2 days. Biobrane® reduces pain and may be left in place until it begins to separate by itself after about 10 days, leaving new epithelium that does not need to be grafted.

13.8.2 Hands

Function is the priority for burned hands. Wrapping up in boxing glove-type dressings will rapidly result in stiff, contracted hands, so wherever possible leave the hands exposed or with minimal dressings. The practice of smothering burned hands in silver sulphadiazine cream and then placing them in plastic bags is not recommended. Superficial partial thickness burns can be covered with copious amounts of mupirocin ointment to combat staphylococcal and streptococcal infection, keep the burn supple, and allow the occupational therapist the freedom to work without restriction. Deeper burns to the hand may be covered with a biosynthetic dressing such as Biobrane®.

If escharotomy is needed, it is important to try to preserve the 'pinch grip' between finger and thumb. For this reason, the incisions should be on the ulnar side of the thumb, and the radial side of the fingers. It may be necessary to splint the hand at night to prevent contracture. This must be done in the 'intrinsic-plus' or 'position of function', with the wrist slightly dorsiflexed, the metacarpophalangeal joints at a right angle and the fingers in full extension (Figure 13.9).

The splint is best applied from the palmar surface and wrapped gently around the edges of the index and little fingers to stop them falling off the splint platform. It is important to place paraffin gauze between the fingers on

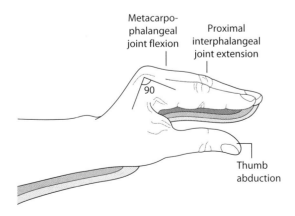

Figure 13.9 Functional position of the hand.

the splint to prevent adherence to each other, with the potential for later syndactyly.

13.8.3 Perineum

Early catheterization is recommended, as is nursing by exposure as much as possible. Nappies/diapers coated with silver sulphdiazine cream are comfortable and practical, for both adults and children. A temporary colostomy for faecal diversion should be considered.

13.8.4 Feet

Apart from preventing syndactyly, as mentioned previously, the importance of burns to the feet is the ability to be able to weight-bear, and to prevent foot-drop during the recovery period. Splints will be needed to maintain the ankle joint at a right angle.

Weight-bearing on an SSG will rapidly result in destruction of the graft. If a full thickness burn of the sole of the foot is present, it may take the skills of a reconstructive plastic surgeon to embark on lengthy cross-leg flap procedures to obtain adequate coverage that will withstand body weight. In resource-constrained countries, a below-knee amputation may seem a drastic measure, but frequently returns the patient to work and their family quicker.

13.9 ADJUNCTS IN BURN CARE

13.9.1 Nutrition in the Burned Patient[6]

A dietitian is an essential member of the burns team. All patients with a major burn (>20% TBSA) should have a nasogastric tube or fine-bore feeding tube for early enteral nutrition. This should ideally be started within 18 hours of the burn. Not only does this help in the early replacement of fluids, but it also protects against gut bacterial translocation and systemic sepsis. The best way to determine calorie requirement is by indirect calorimetry performed on a regular basis while in a post-absorptive state. Oxygen consumption and carbon dioxide production are measured, and a formula produces resting energy expenditure, thereby enabling nutritional supplementation to be accurately delivered to the individual as they progress through the post-burn state.

Estimating the nutritional needs of burn patients is essential to the healing process.[7] The Harris-Benedict equation is designed to calculate the calorie needs of adults, and the Galveston formula is used for children. The Curreri formula addresses the needs of both. There is no single formula that can accurately determine how many calories a patient needs, so it is important to monitor a patient's nutritional condition closely.

Good enteral nutrition may in addition protect against the development of the rare Curling's ulcer.[8]

Protein requirements generally increase more than energy requirements, and appear to be related to the amount of lean body mass. The body loses protein through the burn, and this will be reflected in a significant drop in serum albumin level over the first week, which will take at least a month to recover despite assiduous nutritional care. However, most increased protein requirements come from muscle breakdown for use in extra energy production. Providing an increased intake of protein does not stop this obligatory breakdown; it simply provides the materials needed to replace lost tissue.

Carbohydrates provide the majority of calorie intake under most conditions, including the stress of burns. Providing adequate calories from carbohydrates spares incoming protein from being used for fuel. The body breaks down carbohydrates into glucose that the body then uses for energy.

Fat is needed to meet essential fatty acid requirements and provide needed calories. Common recommendations include giving 30% of calories as fat, although this can be higher if needed. Excess fat intake has been implicated in decreased immune function, and intake levels should be monitored carefully. Vitamins and trace elements are also necessary.

13.9.1.1 PAEDIATRIC BURN NUTRITION

Providing adequate calories and nutrients is a difficult task when treating burn injuries. This task becomes even more difficult when the patient is a child.

13.9.2 **Ulcer Prophylaxis[9] (See Table 17.2 S)**

In the presence of good nutritional policies, sucralfate should be used for prophylaxis. H_2 receptor-blockers and protein pump inhibitors should be reserved for therapy, and not used for prophylaxis, especially in the ventilated

patient where nosocomial and candida ventilator associated pneumonia (VAP) is a major risk factor.

13.9.3 **Venous Thromboembolism Prophylaxis[7,10] (See Table 17.2 R)**

Patients with major burns are at high risk of venous thromboembolism. Venous thromboembolic prophylaxis is often forgotten. Sequential compression devices can be placed over burns and grafts with impunity and fractionated heparin is needed in startlingly high dose. Anti-factor Xa levels can be used to titrate the dose to achieve 0.2–0.4 U/mL.[11] A range of 30–80 mg every 12 hours is required.

13.9.4 **Vitamin C**

Vitamin C infusion does carry level 2 and 3 evidence as support, although it is not universally accepted.[12]

- Consider a continuous ascorbic acid (vitamin C) infusion (66 mg/kg/h for 24 hours) in burn patients sustaining injury ≥30% TBSA.
- Infusion should be begun within 6 hours of burn injury.
- The fluid volume associated with the ascorbic acid infusion should be included in the total volume of fluid resuscitation calculated according to the Parkland formula.
- Total fluid volume infused with rate adjusted to maintain a urine output in adults of 50–100 mL/h.
- Point of care glucose testing becomes inaccurate during and after vitamin C infusion and therefore serum glucose levels are required.

13.9.5 **Antibiotics**

Antibiotic prophylaxis is NOT routinely used for burns, however the great difficulty with burns patients is differentiating inflammation from infection. There is no substitute for good wound care, hand-washing, and infection control measures, including good microbiological surveillance and when treatment is deemed appropriate it should be, where possible, goal directed and of short duration. Tissue excised during tangential excision should be sent for culture, and when skin-grafting, cultures (sometimes obtained by local punch biopsy) should again be sent. The risk of fungal infection is high in these patients and this should be taken into consideration with those patients who are not responding to broad therapy antibiotic treatment.

13.9.6 Other Adjuncts

- Bowel management is mundane but germane. Evacuation of hard stool, instillation of aperients such as sorbitol 30 mL every 8 hours until a liquid stool is forthcoming, followed by insertion of a faecal management system has made everyone's life easier and decreases the amount of faecal wound contamination considerably.
- Preventing pressure on burned ears is a constant battle, but imperative as cosmetic defects result from pressure necrosis. Foam covered with plastic with a central cut-out when side-rolled helps.
- Tube security is problematic when facial burns are present. The tie will cause pressure and an unsightly line of scar in partial thickness wounds.
- Propranolol, a non-selective beta blocker, binds to beta receptors on skeletal muscle and fat cells and decreases proteolysis and lipolysis. This treatment is particularly efficacious in the young and is dosed to an endpoint of a decrease in heart rate of 25% below resting. Four times daily administration is often needed for children, as the burn response leads to much shortened half-life.
- Use of oxandrolone, an anabolic steroid, is also well supported by evidence.[13] Decreased time to donor-site healing, decreased weight and nitrogen loss, and additional gain in lean body mass are all significant. A dose of 0.1 mg/kg/day in divided doses has been established.

13.10 SUMMARY

Burns are a huge problem worldwide, with the majority occurring in countries that are ill-equipped to deal with them as resources are few, transport is lacking, and cultural influences militate against early referral to modern facilities. Education is the cornerstone of prevention, and up to 95% of burns in developing countries are preventable.

Burn care remains a 'team effort', and no amount of highly skilled grafting in the operating room will be rewarded by a happy and functional outcome if the feeding, nursing, intensive care, physiotherapy, or occupational therapy is lacking.

REFERENCES AND RECOMMENDED READING

References

1. Vos T, Abajobir AA, Abate KH, Abbafati C, Abbas KM, Abd-Allah F, et al. Global, regional, and national incidence, prevalence, and years lived with disability for 328 diseases and injuries for 195 countries, 1990-2016: a systematic analysis for the Global Burden of Disease Study. 2016. *The Lancet.* 2017;**390(10100)**:1211–59. doi: 10.1016/S0140-6736(17)32154-2.

2. Haagsma JA, Graetz N, Bolliger I, Naghavi M, Higashi H, Mullany EC, et al. The global burden of injury: incidence, mortality, disability-adjusted life years and time trends from the Global Burden of Disease study 2013. *Inj Prev.* 2016;**22(1)**:3–18. doi: 10.1136/injuryprev-2015-041616.

3. Rogers AD, Karpelowsky J, Millar AJW, Argent A, Rode H. Fluid creep in major paediatric burns. *Eur J Pediatr Surg.* 2010;**20**:133–8. doi: 10.1055/s-0029-1237355.

4. Tan H, Wasiak J, Paul E, Cleland H. Effective use of Biobrane® as a temporary wound dressing prior to definitive slit-skin graft in the treatment of severe: A retrospective analysis. *Burns.* 2015;**41(5)**:969–76. doi: 10.1016/j.burns.2014.07.015.

5. Smith and Nephew Versajet. Details available from: http://www.smith-nephew.com/key-products/advanced-wound-management/versajet/ (accessed online January 2019).

6. Jacobs DO, Kudsk KA, Oswanski MF, Sacks GS, Sinclair KE. Practice management guidelines for nutritional support of the trauma patient. In: *Eastern Association for the Surgery of Trauma. Practice Management Guidelines.* Available from www.east.org (accessed January 2019).

7. Burn nutrition calculator. Available from: http://www.surgicalcriticalcare.net/Resources/burn_nutrition.php (accessed online January 2019).

8. Muir IFK, Jones PF. Curling's ulcer: a rare condition. *Br J Surg.* 1976;**63**:60–6.

9. Guillamondegui OD, Gunter OL Jr, Bonadies JA, Coates JE, Kurek SJ, De Moya MA et al. Practice management guidelines for stress ulcer prophylaxis. EAST Practice Management Guidelines Workgroup. Available from www.east.org (accessed online December 2014).

10. Rogers FB, Cipolle MD, Velmahos G, Rozycki G. Practice management guidelines for the management of venous thromboembolism (VTE) in trauma patients. *J Trauma.* 2002;**53**:142–64. Available from Eastern Association for the Surgery of Trauma. Practice Management Guidelines Workgroup. Available from www.east.org (accessed December 2014).

11. Lin H, Faraklas I, Cochran A, Saffle J. Enoxaparin and anti-factor Xa levels in acute burn patients. *J Burn Care Res.* 2011;**31(1)**:1–5. doi: 10.1097/BCR.0b013e318204b34.

12. Guidelines on the Use of Ascorbic Acid in Burns. Available from: http://www.surgicalcriticalcare.net/Guidelines/ascorbic%20acid%202013.pdf (accessed online January 2019).

13. Li H, Guo Y, Yang Z, Roy M, Guo Q. The efficacy and safety of oxandrolone treatment for patients with severe burns: A systematic review and meta-analysis. *Burns.* 2016;**42(4)**:717–27. doi: 10.1016/j.burns.2015.08.023.

Recommended Reading

Greenwood JE. Development of patient pathways for the surgical management of burn injury. *A NZ J Surg* 2006; **76**:805–11.

Herndon D, Ed. *Total Burn Care.* 3rd Edition. 2007. Saunders Elsevier. Philadelphia PA, USA.

Special Patient Situations **14**

14.1 PAEDIATRIC TRAUMA

14.1.1 Introduction

Unintentional injury is the most common cause of death in children throughout the world. In most countries, blunt trauma, often caused by falls or traffic-related accidents, constitute more than 90% of injuries. Many will be treated in a hospital with limited expertise in paediatric trauma care. Paediatric anatomy and physiology have potential clinical implications and the need for referral should be considered as soon as the patient will tolerate safe transfer to an appropriate facility.

14.1.2 Injury Patterns

Certain injury patterns of paediatric trauma are well recognized.[1]

- Lap belt complex.
- Pancreatic and duodenal injury.
- Chance fracture of the lumbar spine.
- Horizontal contusion on the abdominal wall from the lap belt component.
- Pedestrian–vehicle crash (PVC) complex.
- Leg and head injuries.
- Forward-facing infant complex.
- Flexion fracture of the cervical spine.
- Liver and spleen injury.
- The common cycle scenarios:
  - Handlebar in the epigastrium, and splenic or liver or pancreatic injury.
  - The fall astride with urethral or perineal injury.
- Non-accidental injury.

Injury patterns suggestive of non-accidental injury are very well known. The most vulnerable group with the highest mortality rates is infants. The presence of a severe head injury in an infant without a clear history of a fall from a significant height or a vehicle collision should always arouse suspicion.

14.1.3 Pre-Hospital

Pre-hospital interventions should be limited to basic life support with airway and ventilatory support, securing haemostasis of external bleeding, and basic attempts to secure vascular access. Extensive unsuccessful roadside resuscitative procedures are a common cause of morbidity and mortality. The younger the child and the more unstable his or her condition, the greater the tendency should be to 'scoop and run' to the nearest **appropriate** facility.

If a child is treated at an interim facility prior to transfer for definitive care, then care should be taken to avoid unnecessary imaging without immediate therapeutic consequence, particularly CT scanning, to avoid delay in reaching definitive care.

14.1.4 Resuscitation Room

14.1.4.1 AIRWAY

The indications for airway control are identical to those in the adult patient. The routine administration of oxygen and the stepwise system of management according to severity of airway compromise are the cardinal features of paediatric airway management. Orotracheal intubation without force, done by an experienced anaesthesiologist, will minimize the post-extubation stridor that can result from a traumatic intubation. A surgical airway is seldom necessary. If it is required, a tracheostomy should be performed.

Pitfalls

- The danger of tube dislodgement, commonly owing to failure to secure the tube adequately, or the endotracheal tube may be too small.
- The airway of the obligate nasal breather (the neonate or infant) must not be compromised with a nasogastric tube.

The c-spine in children can be cleared by a combination of the National Emergency X-Radiography Utilization Study (NEXUS) low-risk criteria and the Canadian C-Spine Rule. Caution is advised for non-verbal and/or unconscious children. In these children, plain radiographs should be performed. If these images are inadequate or show hints suggesting bony injury, a computed tomography (CT) of the c-spine should be considered.

14.1.4.2 VENTILATION

Hypoventilation is a prominent cause of hypoxia in the injured child. Because the child depends primarily on diaphragmatic breathing, one must be particularly cautious of conditions that impair diaphragmatic movement (tension pneumothoraces, diaphragmatic rupture, and severe gastric dilatation) and treat expeditiously.

14.1.4.3 CIRCULATION

Frequent assessment of circulatory status is important. Children have effective mechanisms for compensating for blood loss, depending predominantly on an adequate heart rate. Tachycardia, peripheral vasoconstriction, and signs of inadequate central nervous system perfusion predominate. Hypotension is a late sign of blood loss, reflecting a class IV shock with greater than 40% blood volume loss.[2]

The practitioner must recognize and treat shock aggressively. The primary management of bleeding is surgical haemostasis. Rapid vascular access is obtained, tailored to the severity of the child's shock and the practitioner's experience: central lines are reserved for the larger child and the more experienced physician. Although most children respond rapidly to crystalloid resuscitation, early use of blood products in a child with hypovolaemic shock and ongoing bleeding is indicated.[3]

Do not delay the transfer of the unstable child to the operating room – establish good access and the anaesthesiologist can resuscitate while the surgeon stops the bleeding. NEVER transfer a haemodynamically unstable patient to the CT scanner. Hypothermia is critical and must be avoided. The urinary output is an invaluable aid to determine the adequacy of resuscitation after the initial phase.

14.1.4.4 DISABILITY

Make a quick neurological assessment including the Glasgow Coma Scale score, pupils, and movements of all extremities. In general, children have a lower incidence of intracranial mass lesions requiring surgical drainage after blunt injury compared with adults. Signs of sudden neurological deterioration must prompt urgent neurosurgical evaluation and CT scan that supersedes all other priorities except the management of the airway and the treatment of hypovolaemic shock.[4]

14.1.4.5 CARDIAC ARREST

In children, cardiac arrest usually is not caused by ventricular fibrillation, and is often heralded by bradycardia, pulseless electrical activity, or asystole. The primary objective of resuscitation should be to correct the underlying cause (such as tension pneumothorax, hypovolaemia, hypothermia, or hypoxia). If return of spontaneous circulation is not achieved, resuscitative thoracotomy is indicated, however, the success rate in patients with cardiac arrest after blunt trauma is low.

14.1.5 Specific Organ Injury

14.1.5.1 HEAD INJURY

Head injury remains the leading cause of traumatic death in children. CT is the most accurate imaging modality to evaluate paediatric patients with a suspected head injury. Diffuse brain injury occurs commonly in children. Techniques to improve cerebral monitoring have evolved considerably but their clinical application remains difficult. Decompressive craniectomy should be considered in patients who display evidence of sustained, refractory intracranial hypertension in the absence of signs of a dismal prognosis.

14.1.5.2 THORACIC INJURY

Young children have a more flexible thoracic cage than adults. Rib fractures in children are uncommon and indicate major injury. Pulmonary contusion is the most common injury to the chest and is commonly seen in the absence of rib fractures. Contusions are typically delayed in appearance on chest x-ray. If pathological findings (of pulmonary contusion) are visible on the admission chest x-ray, then the contusion is severe, and hypoxia should be expected to worsen over the next 1–2 days.

14.1.5.3 ABDOMINAL INJURY[5]

Abdominal injuries must be suspected after high-energy trauma. The upper abdominal organs have little protection from the rib cage and musculature. Not surprisingly, the spleen and the liver are the most frequently injured intra-abdominal organs in children. Most children with abdominal injuries from blunt trauma can be treated safely non-operatively. For the trauma surgeon, the challenge is to identify expeditiously those patients who require surgical intervention. Patients with haemoperitoneum and haemodynamic instability not responding to resuscitation, those with clear signs of peritonitis or bowel injury as evidenced by free intraperitoneal air, should be explored urgently. Diaphragmatic rupture and intraperitoneal bladder rupture are other early indications for surgery.

Hollow viscus injuries are relatively rare, and symptoms can be vague in the early stage after trauma. Repeated examination remains essential in the early diagnosis of these injuries. Free fluid in the absence of solid organ injury on a CT scan in a patient with an appropriate injury mechanism (e.g. lap belt injury) is highly indicative of an intestinal lesion.

Pancreatic injuries are rare, and diagnosis often is delayed. Contusions can be treated non-operatively, whereas operative treatment is most often recommended in patients with transection through the gland.

Duodenal injuries are uncommon, diagnosis often being delayed and associated with serious complications. In the absence of significant trauma, a duodenal injury in a child under 2 years should arouse suspicions of child abuse.

14.1.5.4 GENITOURINARY INJURY

The hallmark of genitourinary tract injury is haematuria. However, the degree of haematuria does not correlate with injury severity, and the absence of blood in the urine does not exclude significant urological injury. The kidneys are most commonly involved. Less than 5%

of children with renal injuries will need operative treatment. A CT scan of the abdomen is highly sensitive and specific, although it does not reliably exclude bladder rupture unless dedicated cystography views with bladder distension are obtained.

14.1.5.5 PELVIC INJURY

Pelvic fracture is a rare cause of exsanguination in children, and most fractures are treated non-operatively.

14.1.5.6 SUSPECTED NON-ACCIDENTAL INJURY

Successful management of the abused child requires recognition at the level of treating providers, as well as institutional support and resources for the provision of the appropriate medical, social, and psychological support. It is critical for physicians to feel the moral responsibility of being mandatory reporters of such injuries in abused children, as well as being willing to discharge the often onerous legal duties that such cases usually entail. In the ideal circumstances, physicians do not have to accuse any party of deliberate injury to the child but merely raise the alarm on its possibility so that the case can be satisfactorily investigated.

14.1.6 Analgesia

For children, an age-appropriate pain scale should be taken and be repeated. For each age group there are observational, behavioural, and self-reporting pain scales available ranging from neonatal to 12 year olds. A very prevalent fear of providing children with appropriate analgesia needs to be overcome.

Opiates are appropriate for acute pain and should be offered to the paediatric trauma patient to reduce pain and anxiety.

Adequate titrated doses of morphine are 0.1 mg/kg 4 hourly or when required.

Such an approach will facilitate resuscitation and assessment, and does not mask important clinical signs. Careful monitoring of respiratory and haemodynamic status, and level of consciousness is essential. Ketamine remains a useful alternative or second agent and can be given via several routes and carries less respiratory side-effects. For hospitalized patients, multimodal approaches, including locoregional techniques, non-opiate analgesics, and behavioural therapies are suggested. It is important to ensure that opioid analgesia is used in a judicious manner at discharge with a limit on the number of tablets provided for home use and a focus on multimodal treatment. Generous opioid-based home analgesia regimens have been recently associated with high rates of development of dependency and adverse effects.[6]

14.2 TRAUMA IN THE ELDERLY

14.2.1 Definition of 'Older' and Susceptibility to Trauma

Population ageing is a global phenomenon.[7] In 2017, there were an estimated 960 million people worldwide aged 60 years and over: approximately 13% of the total global population. By 2050, all regions (Africa aside), will have nearly a quarter of their populations aged above 60 years. Twenty-five per cent of Europe's present population is already aged 60 years and over. The number of persons aged 80 years and over will triple globally from 137 million in 2017 to 425 million in 2050. More older persons will mean more 'older trauma'.

What defines an 'older patient'? It depends on the context. In 2001, WHO's Africa Minimum Data Set Project collaborators adopted the age of 50 years as 'old' in sub-Saharan Africa.[8] Accepted practice in the UK is to classify any patient over 75 years as 'older'. But it is wise to be pragmatic and make a judgement based on the perceived interplay of chronological, local geographic, socio-economic, and biological factors. In current trauma scoring systems, the break-point for an age-linked increased risk of complication and mortality ranges from 45 to 55 years of age. In the United States, the 12.5% of the population over the age of 65 accounts for almost one third of all deaths from injury. The UK Trauma Audit Research Network records a linear increase in post-trauma mortality with age.[9] Older people seem to be both more susceptible to trauma and to experience higher mortality rates and complications.[10]

Certain medications (e.g. zopiclone, benzodiazepines) are prescribed more commonly and for longer among the older generations, yet by impairing reactions render them more susceptible to road traffic accidents and head injury.[11]

14.2.2 Access to Trauma Care

Despite pre-hospital trauma triage criteria, older trauma patients are less likely to be transported to a major trauma service and they have, unsurprisingly, poorer outcomes than younger trauma patients, and can attract greater costs and length of stay, which may increase with age and injury severity. Yet, with active intervention, the outcomes for older trauma patients may be substantially better than preconceptions might suggest, resulting not only in better clinical outcomes, but also cost and time savings.

14.2.3 Physiology

The older person's response to bodily insult, whether disease or trauma, may be atypical or even masked, in part due to the ageing process, and in part due to existing comorbidity and medication. Ageing is a risk factor for microvascular dysfunction and hyperpermeability. Apart from age-related remodelling of the vascular wall, endothelial barrier integrity and function in the periphery and at the blood-brain barrier declines with age. Under oxidative stress there are age-related increases of inflammatory markers and of apoptotic signalling. Oxidative stress can impact negatively in all forms of major surgery including trauma surgery; this is particularly so in older persons. As a result of the interplay of the above, the older trauma patient may present not only with vague and misleading clinical signs, but also tip precipitously into 'extremis'.

The following potential age-related changes should also be borne in mind.

14.2.3.1 RESPIRATORY SYSTEM

- Decreased lung elasticity; decreased pulmonary compliance.
- Alveolar collapse and loss of surface area available for gas exchange.
- Atrophy of bronchial epithelium, leading to a decrease in clearance of particulate foreign matter.
- Chronic bacterial colonization of the upper airway.

14.2.3.2 CARDIOVASCULAR SYSTEM

- Diminished pump function; lower cardiac output.
- Inability to mount an appropriate response to both intrinsic and extrinsic catecholamines.

- Reduced flow to vital organs.
- Commonly prescribed medications may blunt normal physiological responses.

14.2.3.3 NERVOUS SYSTEM

- Decline in cerebral and cognitive functions.
- Hearing and visual impairment.
- Proprioceptive impairment.
- Gait impairment; loss of muscle bulk/strength.
- Blunted baroreceptor function (predisposes to postural hypotension).
- Decreased cerebral blood flow (exacerbated by atherosclerosis).

14.2.3.4 RENAL

- Decline in renal mass.
- Normal serum creatinine no longer implies normal renal function.
- Increased vulnerability to nephrotoxic agents (e.g. NSAIDs and ACE inhibitors).

14.2.3.5 MUSCULOSKELETAL

- Osteoporotic fractures with minimal energy transfer.
- Diminution of vertebral body height.
- Decrease in muscle mass.

14.2.3.6 INFLUENCE OF COMORBID CONDITIONS

In addition to the physiological changes listed above, the onset of age-related disorders may predispose to an impaired response to injury. These can include any chronic degenerative disease, and especially disease in any major organ, or bodily system (e.g. metabolic disorder; obesity etc.), which might occur in isolation or in any combination.

14.2.4 Multiple Medications – Polypharmacy

A clear correlation exists between the number of medications taken and the likelihood of drug induced complications. As ageing advances, the rates of drug metabolism diminish. Drug accumulations with associated unwanted interactions become more likely. In turn

a misleading clinical picture may emerge which may mask vital changes in signs.

14.2.5 Analgesia

Older persons need appropriate and adequate analgesia in any given trauma context. Adequate analgesia allows for an improvement in physiological variables such as neuroendocrine stress responses and pulmonary function.[12] This, in turn, renders the older patient potentially more suitable for a major surgical procedure and allows for more rapid recovery.

Suggested guiding principles include:

- Mindful of the patient's physical state and co-existing medication, utilize the most appropriate category of analgesic.
- Opioids should not be avoided.
- Start analgesia from a low dose and titrate as required.
- Consider a multimodal approach to pain treatment to reduce total dosages.
- An analgesic regimen which augments an effective afferent block (regional analgesia) may be effective and medication sparing.

14.2.6 Decision to Operate

Mortality data and survival curves for major abdominal surgery in the octogenarian population indicate it is safer than previously thought to operate. These data enable risk stratification and prediction of outcomes.

With age-related increase in mortality, the surgeon should:

- Recognize the risk from decreased physiological reserve.
- Seek and address comorbid disease.
- Rationalize polypharmacy.
- Consider atypical manifestations with masked signs for any given clinical situation.
- Seek subtle changes in function with careful monitoring.
- Assume any mental status changes are associated with brain injury, and only accept age-related change after exclusion of injury.
- Be aware of the distinction between aggressive care and futile care.

14.2.7 **Anaesthetic Considerations in the Elderly**[13]

- Elderly trauma patients must be diagnosed and treated aggressively owing to their limited reserve capacities. 'Halfway is no way' for the elderly. This principle should be followed until/unless treatment is seen as futile.

- Age-related reduction in cardiac output is linked to reduced medication effect. Patience and careful monitoring is required in order to avoid undesirable effects of overdose. Doses of anesthetics might often need to be reduced.

- While endotracheal intubation is easily performed in most trauma patients, this becomes more complicated in the elderly (especially with limited neck and jaw movement).

- Consider NIV (non-invasive ventilation) early if no contraindication in order to support the patient thus avoiding endotracheal intubation.

- If an epidural or other regional anesthesia techniques are indicated, these should be performed as soon as possible other contraindications allowing (night shift work, do not delay until the next day).

- Be aware of a markedly increased susceptibility to pressure sores and skin injury in the unconscious elderly trauma patient.

- Be cautious in the use of anticoagulants and platelet inhibitors, which might exacerbate traumatic bleeding thus requiring this effect to be 'counteracted'. On the other hand, excessive bleeding is a possible signal of underlying problems that might not benefit from uncritical procoagulant therapy.

Source: Banks SE, Lewis MC. *Anesthesiol Clin.* 2013 March;31(1):127–39.

14.3 **TRAUMA IN PREGNANCY**[14]

Trauma in pregnancy remains a challenge with the need for multidisciplinary management and the fact that, when the pregnancy is at a viable stage (usually around 22–26 weeks), one is dealing with TWO patients. Engage gynaecology early in the process. The ABCDE basics apply in the same way as in the non-pregnant patient, but there are anatomical and physiological changes that require consideration. These include a baseline respiratory alkalosis (leading to falsely normal blood gases in shock), generalized oedema, and gastric reflux.

In the pregnant patient, always check for vaginal haemorrhage.

Pitfall

The risk of hypotension from the enlarged uterus occluding the inferior cava is a common but avoidable pitfall.

14.3.1 **Evaluation**

- Early maternal resuscitation, ultrasound evaluation of the foetal heart, and the use of cardiotocography are recommended in the evaluation of these patients.

- Suppression of premature labour may be required.
- Undertake necessary imaging but using non-ionizing methods if possible.[15]
- Administration of RhoGAM® anti-D antibody (Kedrion Biopharma Inc, Melville, NY) in cases of maternal Rh-negative status and steroids for foetal lung maturation are important considerations.
- Damage control surgery may include the need to deliver the foetus urgently through caesarean section (especially in cases with massive maternal abdomino-pelvic trauma), or maternal cardiac arrest.

14.4 **NON-BENEFICIAL (FUTILE) CARE**

In every environment, there are circumstances where the provision of adequate healthcare may not alter the outcome. In providing this care, there may be a significant drain on the resources available, and denial to others of adequate care as a result. This 'rationing' of healthcare may be the result of operating theatres being in use, and consequently not available, inadequate numbers of intensive care unit beds, or financial restrictions.

All patients are entitled to an aggressive initial resuscitation and careful comprehensive diagnosis. The magnitude of their injuries should be assessed within their wider health context, and only then can the appropriateness and aggression required in their care be determined. In providing this care, optimal treatment of one patient might represent too heavy a burden on the resources available, and denial to others of adequate care as a result.

Inevitably, occasions arise in the management of older patients (as in any age group), when it is abundantly clear to the clinician that intervention is no longer beneficial. Prolongation of obviously futile care should prompt ethical considerations and discussions independently of resources available.

Sometimes, continued treatment can be justified by the wish to prolong the life until relatives arrive at the hospital. Local and national legislation needs to be adhered to. The clinician must be guided by basic ethical principles and it is essential to be humane, not to prolong life without definite and realistic therapeutic goals, nor without realistic expectations of any possibility of a positive outcome. Opting to allow the patient a death that is comfortable and dignified may be more positive as an outcome than a futile surgical intervention.[16]

REFERENCES AND RECOMMENDED READING

References

PAEDIATRIC TRAUMA

1. Tracya ET, Englumb BR, Barbasb AS, Foleyc C, Riced HE, Shapiro ML. Pediatric injury patterns by year of age. *J Pediatr Surg.* 2013 June;**48(6)**:805–11. doi: 10.1016/j.jpedsurg.2013.03.041.

2. Nystrup KB, Stensballe J, Bøttger M, Johansson PI, Ostrowski SR. Transfusion therapy in paediatric trauma patients: a review of the literature. *Scand J Trauma Resusc Emerg Med.* 2015 Feb 15;**23**:21. doi: 10.1186/s13049-015-0097-z.

3. Eckert MJ, Wertin TM, Tyner SD, Nelson DW, Izenberg S, Martin MJ. Tranexamic acid administration to pediatric trauma patients in a combat setting: the pediatric trauma and tranexamic acid study (PED-TRAX). *J Trauma Acute Care Surg.* 2014 Dec;**77(6)**:852–8; discussion 858. doi: 10.1097/TA.0000000000000443.

4. Figaji AA, Graham Fieggen A, Mankahla N, Enslin N, Rohlwink UK. Targeted treatment in severe traumatic brain injury in the age of precision medicine. *Childs Nerv Syst.* 2017 Oct;**33(10)**:1651–61. doi: 10.1007/s00381-017-3562-3.

5. Letton RW, Worrell V; APSA Committee on Trauma Blunt Intestinal Injury Study Group. Delay in diagnosis and treatment of blunt intestinal injury does not adversely affect prognosis in the pediatric trauma patient. *J Pediatr Surg* 2010 Jan;**45(1)**:161–5; discussion 166. doi: 10.1016/j.jpedsurg.2009.10.027.

6. Harbaugh CM, Lee JS, Hu HM, McCabe SE, Voepel-Lewis T, Englesbe MJ, et al. Persistent Opioid Use Among Pediatric Patients After Surgery. *Pediatrics.* 2018 Jan;**141(1)**.pii: e20172439. doi: 10.1542/peds.2017-2439.

TRAUMA IN THE ELDERLY

7. Ageing. *The United Nations Report.* 2017. Available from: http://www.un.org/en/sections/issues-depth/ageing/ (accessed online January 2018).

8. Peachey K, Kowal P. Indicators for the Minimum Data Set Project on Ageing: A Critical Review in sub-Saharan Africa. *WHO.* 2001 June; Available from https://www.who.int/healthinfo/survey/ageing_mds_report_en_daressalaam.pdf (accessed online January 2019).

9. Herron J, Hutchinson R, Lecky F, Bouamra O, Edwards A, Woodford M, et al. The Trauma Audit & Research Network 2017 (Manchester Academic Health Science Centre, University of Manchester). Major Trauma in Older People. *Bone Joint J.* 2017 Dec;**99-B(12)**:1677–80. doi: 10.1302/0301-620X.99B12.BJJ-2016-1140.R2.

10. Kozar RA, Arbabi S, Stein DM, Shackford SR, Barraco RD, Biffl WL, et al. Injury in the aged: Geriatric trauma care at the crossroads. *J Trauma Acute Care Surg.* 2015 Jun;**78(6)**:1197–209. doi: 10.1097/TA.0000000000000656.

11. Gustavsen I, Bramness JG, Skurtveit S, Engeland A, Neutel I, Mørland J. Road traffic accident risk related to prescriptions of the hypnotics zopiclone, zolpidem, flunitrazepam and nitrazepam. *Sleep Med.* 2008;**9(8)**:818–22.

12. Richardson J, Bresland K. The management of postsurgical pain in the elderly population. *Drugs Aging.* 1998 Jul;**13(1)**:17–31.

13. Banks SE, Lewis MC. Trauma in the elderly: considerations for anesthetic management. *Anesthesiol Clin.* 2013 Mar;**31(1)**:127–39. doi: 10.1016/j.anclin.2012.11.004.

TRAUMA IN PREGNANCY

14. Mendez-Figueroa H, Dahlke JD, Vrees RA, Rouse DJ. Trauma in pregnancy: an updated systematic review. *Am J Obstet Gynecol.* 2013;**209(1)**:1–10. doi: 10.1016/j.ajog.2013.01.021.

15. Gilet AG, Dunkin JM, Fernandez TJ, Button TM, Budorick NE. Fetal radiation dose during gestation estimated on an anthropomorphic phantom for three generations of CT scanners. *AJR Am J Roentgenol.* 2011 May;**196(5)**:1133–7. doi: 10.2214/AJR.10.4497.

NON-BENEFICIAL CARE

16. Ardagh M. Futility has no utility in resuscitation medicine. *J Med Ethics. J Med Ethics.* 2000 Oct;**26(5)**:396–9.

Recommended Reading

PAEDIATRIC TRAUMA

The Paediatric Trauma Manual. Royal Children's Hospital, Melbourne, Australia. Available from: https://www.rch.org.au/trauma-service/manual/. (accessed online January 2019).

TRAUMA IN THE ELDERLY

Bonne S, Schuerer DJ. Trauma in the older adult: epidemiology and evolving geriatric trauma principles. *Clin Geriatr Med.* 2013 Feb;**29(1)**:137–50. doi: 10.1016/j.cger.2012.10.008. Review.

Adams SD, Holcomb JB. Geriatric trauma. *Curr Opin Crit Care.* 2015 Dec;**21(6)**:520–6. doi: 10.1097/MCC.0000000000000246. Review.

TRAUMA IN PREGNANCY

Wallis LA, Reynolds T (Eds), Trauma in the pregnant patient. Chapter 281, pp. 732–733. In: *AFEM Handbook of Acute and Emergency Care.* Oxford University Press, Cape Town 2013.

NON-BENEFICIAL CARE

Deborah L Kasman MD,MA. When Is Medical Treatment Futile? A Guide for Students, Residents, and Physicians. *J Gen Intern Med.* 2004 Oct;**19(10)**:805–11. doi: 10.1111/j.1525-1497.2004.40134.x.

Part 4

Modern therapeutic and diagnostic technology

Minimal Access Surgery in Trauma **15**

Minimally invasive access techniques, laparoscopy, and thoracoscopy have yet to be widely adopted by trauma surgeons. However, selective indications for the use of these techniques are emerging rapidly in both adult and paediatric fields, especially in post-operative surveillance after non-operative management (NOM).

15.1 LAPAROSCOPY

Laparoscopy is now regarded as an acceptable alternative to laparotomy in both penetrating and blunt abdominal trauma.[1,2] However, the decision to utilize laparoscopy is highly dependent on the laparoscopic skills of the attending surgeon and the laparoscopic capabilities of the surgical unit.

The following definitions apply when discussing laparoscopy in trauma.

15.1.1 Screening Laparoscopy

This is trauma laparoscopy in its simplest form. The laparoscope is purely used to ascertain whether the *peritoneum* has been breached in penetrating trauma. In abdominal stab wounds, laparoscopy can prevent an unnecessary laparotomy in one half to more than 80% of the cases, in an equivocal wound by assessment of breach of the peritoneal cavity.

Although initially laparoscopy appeared to be a poor screening tool after blunt trauma (16% incidence of missed intra-abdominal injuries in one series), the sensitivity and specificity of laparoscopy have in detecting blunt small bowel injuries has improved considerably over recent years. However, sensitivity remains problematic for hollow viscus injury. Indirect signs, or injection of dyes or air through gastrointestinal tubes are sometimes useful adjuncts.

15.1.2 Diagnostic Laparoscopy

A systematic inspection is performed of the peritoneal cavity as well as the retroperitoneal organs as necessary. The findings at diagnostic laparoscopy will govern decision-making regarding further surgical management.

15.1.3 Non-Therapeutic Laparoscopy

Laparoscopy is regarded as a non-therapeutic procedure where no injuries are identified, or injuries are identified that do not require repair.

15.1.4 Therapeutic Laparoscopy

Laparoscopy is regarded as therapeutic when an advanced manoeuvre is performed to repair an identified injury. Simple manoeuvres such as organ mobilization or evacuation of a clot should not be considered therapeutic. Therapeutic laparoscopy should be abandoned in favour of exploratory laparotomy if haemodynamic instability arises, extensive bleeding or complex injuries are encountered, visibility is poor, or equipment fails.

15.1.5 Technique

Correct positioning and preparation of the patient for trauma laparoscopy are essential.

- The patient is placed supine (dorsal decubitus), legs spread apart, on a beanbag and firmly strapped, because adequate abdominal organ exposure relies on dependency obtained with table rotation and tilting, rather than with retractors.

- Skin prep and draping should allow for rapid conversion to a complete laparotomy if necessary.
- Appropriate laparoscopic instruments and well as those for a traditional trauma laparotomy (and vascular surgery) must be available.
- One or more (flat) high-resolution screens should be placed opposite each surgeon. Monitors should be mobile and moved accordingly so that the surgeon always has the screen in front of their eyes without turning their head.
- The operating table should be adapted to the height of the surgeon's arms to ensure proper ergonomics for exploration as well as for advanced techniques of haemostasis and suturing. The surgeon can stand between the legs of the patient ('French' position), or opposite the target organ once this is recognized.
- Insertion of a bladder catheter is advised.
- Pneumoperitoneum should be:
  - Obtained with low flow to allow timely detection of a tension pneumothorax, leading to immediate stopping in insufflation and insertion of a thoracic drain.
  - Maintained at low pressures (8–12 mm Hg) to avoid gas embolism if a large vein is injured.
- Trocar insertion should avoid all previous scars (incisions or drainage sites).
  - The first trocar should always be inserted with an open technique. Ideally, the trocar set up should allow for triangulation; the optic should ideally be placed midway between the working trocars (equal azimuth angles). When performed for diagnostic purposes in a patient with an unclear abdomen, the optic trocar should be in the centre of the abdomen, that is, at the level of the navel.
  - Next, two trocars should be inserted along the anterior axillary line in either flank: on the right slightly above the navel line and on the left slightly lower, so that both the upper and lower abdomen can easily be accessed.
  - Port positioning is governed by the indication for the operation and monitors must be in direct line of view.
  - In specific indications, the trocars are located according to the organ involved as determined by appropriate pre-operative imaging.
- A straight or 30° 10 mm scope can be used according to the surgeon's preferences. Ten millimetre scopes are better than 5 mm, as blood absorbs white light and darkens the optical field. Adequate tissue handling requires 5 mm atraumatic bowel graspers.

15.1.6 **Risks**

Laparoscopy in abdominal trauma entails four specific risks:

- Missed injuries, mainly intestinal, with their attending high morbidity and mortality.
- Gas embolism, supposedly higher when mesenteric and hepatic (venous) lesions have occurred, but apparently as rare as in any laparoscopic procedure today.
- Impeded venous return (because of elevated intra-abdominal pressure).
- Increased intracranial pressure.

> **Pitfall**
>
> - These last two make physiological instability and severe head injury absolute contraindications to the creation of the pneumoperitoneum, necessary for most minimally invasive techniques.
> - Caution is warranted as well, in the presence of abdominal compartment syndrome or diaphragmatic tears.[6] While laparoscopy may rarely detect and treat the cause of the former, the risk of tension pneumothorax if there is a co-existing diaphragmatic tear requires that a large-bore needle, or better still, a chest tube, be inserted into the thorax.

15.1.7 **Applications**

15.1.7.1 BOWEL INJURY

Laparoscopic examination for penetrating injury of the bowel requires diligent and rigorous exploration in order not to miss occult or small lesions. Different techniques have been described to best run the bowel. One of these is the hand-over-hand technique, with care taken to use atraumatic graspers and routinely explore both sides. Laparoscopy can be successfully employed to repair small bowel injuries, and to raise a colostomy to defunction the lower intestinal tract in colorectal injuries.[3]

15.1.7.2 SPLENIC INJURY

Although laparoscopic splenic preservation or partial splenectomy have been reported after trauma using fibrin glue, argon beam coagulator, and by splenic-wrapping with mesh, the role of minimal access techniques is limited in splenic injury. Independent of injury grade on CT scan, stable patients should be treated non-operatively. Laparoscopy is contraindicated in the unstable patient who should be treated per trauma laparotomy. Although rarely indicated, laparoscopy can be entertained in the patient with splenic trauma treated non-operatively with ongoing oozing requiring blood transfusions. Successful autotransfusion of haemoperitoneum aspirated from the peritoneum has also been reported. Laparoscopy might also be an excellent approach for secondary treatment of post-traumatic localized splenic infarcts or pseudocysts, or even post-traumatic splenic artery pseudoaneurysm.

15.1.7.3 LIVER INJURY

Patients failing a trial of non-operative management for hepatic injury have been managed successfully using minimally invasive surgery, including laparoscopic application of fibrin glue as a haemostatic agent.[4] Haemoperitoneum may be drained, and biliary leaks, with or without peritonitis, can be controlled via the laparoscope usually combined with endoscopic retrograde cholangiopancreatography (ERCP).[5]

15.1.7.4 AFTER NON-OPERATIVE MANAGEMENT

After NOM (especially after embolization), laparoscopy can check the abdominal cavity in case of suspicion of organ ischaemia/perforation, persistent abdominal signs in stable patients (after blunt trauma), and perform washouts in case of poor tolerance of biloperitoneum, haemobiloperitoneum, or persistent occult bleeding. It can also be used to treat intraperitoneal bladder rupture or release an abdominal compartment syndrome.[6]

15.1.7.5 DIAPHRAGMATIC INJURY

In asymptomatic patients with stab wounds of the *left* thoraco-abdominal area (ribcage below the fifth intercostal space), the risk of an occult diaphragmatic injury is about 7%.

Since imaging cannot reliably demonstrate a diaphragmatic defect (where no herniation has occurred), suspected diaphragmatic injury owing to either or both blunt or penetrating injury can be diagnosed by direct inspection. Either video-assisted thoracoscopic surgery (VATS) or laparoscopy may be employed in this setting. If there is no indication for exploration of the pleural cavity, most surgeons prefer laparoscopy, while VATS is preferable when there is a specific indication for it, such as a chest collection which needs to be evacuated simultaneously. If VATS is employed, there must be no suspicion of intra-abdominal injuries needing laparoscopy or laparotomy.

Laparoscopy is especially helpful to exclude occult diaphragmatic injury in a setting where non-operative management of penetrating thoraco-abdominal injuries is employed.[11,12] After a period of observation, if the patient has no abdominal signs of concern, laparoscopy can be performed with the diaphragm as main focus, whereas if laparoscopy is employed in the acute setting, a complete diagnostic laparoscopy needs to be performed and identified intra-abdominal injuries need to be dealt with either laparoscopically or via exploratory laparotomy.

Diaphragmatic injuries can be repaired laparoscopically or thoracoscopically. It is theoretically easier to repair the diaphragm from above (i.e. on the convex side of the muscle); however, it is imperative to place one's working ports in such a position as to facilitate easy access to the injury. The ribs are not pliable and do not allow working at acute angles without great difficulty.

Finally, repair of longstanding post traumatic diaphragmatic herniation may be possible with either laparoscopy or VATS.

> **Pitfall**
>
> All the above assume significant laparoscopic experience on the behalf of the operator, as unfamiliarity with the anatomy and techniques required lead to missed injury, sometimes with catastrophic results.

15.2 VIDEO-ASSISTED THORACOSCOPIC SURGERY[7]

Thoracic injuries may be managed by VATS in lieu of thoracotomy in selected circumstances (see below).

15.2.1 Technique

Double lumen endotracheal intubation is essential, to facilitate lung collapse on the operative side. Positioning depends on the indication for the procedure; for most cases, a lateral position (injured side up) is appropriate with either a sandbag under the chest or the table broken to facilitate splaying of the ribs and allowing easy access to the intercostal spaces. The arm is secured overhead, and the patient is secured to the table. The first port is placed via the open technique and further ports are placed as appropriate. Ports are positioned in such a way as to triangulate towards the working area, with the monitor directly in line.

> ### Pitfall
>
> Care must be taken not to accidentally place ports below the diaphragm.

15.2.2 Applications

In the acute trauma setting in stable patients, VATS may be employed to:

- Pinpoint and manage persistent, non-exsanguinating haemorrhage (>300 cc within 3 hours).[8,9]
- Perform a pericardial window in suspected penetrating cardiac trauma.[10]

In the post-acute or semi-elective setting, VATS can be utilized for the following:

- Evacuation of a clotted haemothorax.
- Direct visualization and stapling of persistent or recurrent air leaks, with aspiration of associated haemothorax.
- To ligate (rare) thoracic duct injuries (when conservative medical management fails to reduce chyle leakage).
- Foreign body extraction.

15.2.3 Summary

Although minimally invasive surgery still plays a minor role in trauma surgery relative to general surgery, it is being employed ever increasingly. Surgeons should be encouraged to incorporate laparoscopy and VATS into their trauma protocols and gain familiarity and expertise with their use. It should, however, in the light of current knowledge, still be regarded as suitable only for carefully selected stable patients.

15.3 RESUSCITATIVE ENDOVASCULAR BALLOON OCCLUSION OF THE AORTA (REBOA)

The use of modern endovascular bleeding treatment modalities started with the treatment of aortic aneurysmal disease and has since spread into trauma care. The evolvement in modern endovascular devices (embolization and endografts), as well as improved diagnostic tools (CT, ultrasound, angiography), have resulted in wide increase in endo-vascular resuscitation and trauma management (EVTM). The use of endovascular tools alone or in combination with open surgery (hybrid procedures) is now part of standard treatment for trauma. In the last few years, there has been an increasing interest in resuscitative endovascular balloon occlusion of the aorta (REBOA), which, by definition, is an endovascular tool in hybrid or endovascular procedures to achieve temporarily haemodynamic stability.[13] REBOA is one of the most actively researched fields in EVTM and has been implemented in clinical use in several institutes as an adjunct for *temporary* control of massive non-compressible torso haemorrhage. REBOA is a balloon catheter for proximal aorta flow control, which is usually inserted into the aorta via the common femoral artery, but can be used through other vessels, such as the brachial, axillar, or iliac vessels, or even the aorta directly.

> ### Pitfall
>
> REBOA does not stop bleeding and is only a bridge to definitive treatment.

15.3.1 Anatomy

In REBOA placement, the aorta is divided into three zones. Zone I (supracoeliac) is from the ascending thoracic aorta to the level of coeliac axis. Zone II (pararenal) is the abdominal aorta from coeliac axis to renal vessels and is considered as a no-go zone for balloon occlusion. Zone III (infrarenal) is from the infrarenal aorta down to bifurcation.

A REBOA balloon can be placed in zone I (supracoeliac), zone II (pararenal), or zone III (infrarenal), areas of the aorta (see Figure 15.1), or in the iliac arteries. The method can also be used for flow control in other vessels, such as the subclavian artery or the inferior vena cava (but is not then referred to as REBOA).

Zone I REBOA has been gaining acceptance as a feasible and less invasive resuscitation alternative to resuscitative thoracotomy and aortic clamping.[14]

Zone III REBOA is used to control pelvic haemorrhage.

REBOA can be used for total occlusion, partial occlusion or intermittent occlusion, and can be modified actively to control the haemodynamic status and organ perfusion in unstable patients.

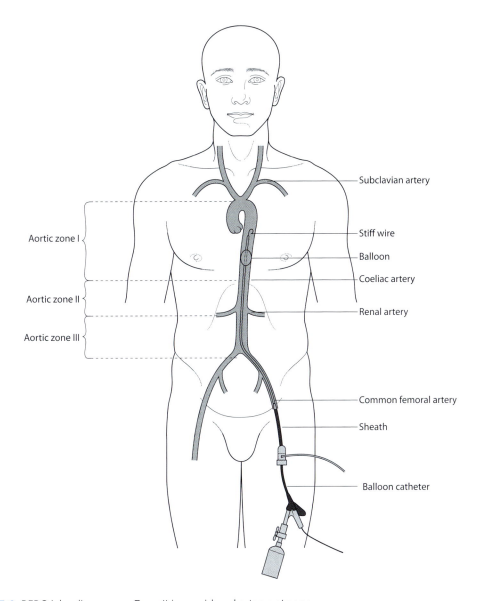

Subclavian artery

Stiff wire

Balloon

Coeliac artery

Aortic zone I

Renal artery

Aortic zone II

Aortic zone III

Common femoral artery

Sheath

Balloon catheter

Figure 15.1 REBOA landing zones. Zone II is considered a 'no go' zone.

Pitfalls

- REBOA does not stop bleeding and is not a bleeding control procedure as such.
- REBOA requires a simultaneous plan for definitive bleeding control.
- REBOA can buy time for the team to stabilize the patient and catch up with resuscitation.
- Despite rapidly expanding use of REBOA in trauma and other non-traumatic bleedings, the solid evidence of the indications, methods, or benefits has still to be clarified.

15.3.2 **Physiology**

Aortic occlusion will increase the central systolic blood pressure proximal to the occlusion resulting in increased blood flow to coronary and cerebral arteries and is used in critical cases as a part of the resuscitation. Blood pressure elevation of around 20%–40% is often observed but is heavily dependent on the REBOA level (zone I versus zone III), cardiac output, total remaining blood volume, resuscitation volumes versus blood product infusions, and vasoconstrictor effects.[15]

The effects are highly dynamic and depend on the REBOA method used (as partial REBOA, described later in this chapter). In addition to a resuscitative support, aortic occlusion will decrease the arterial bleeding distal to the occlusion; however, tissues with poor perfusion before balloon occlusion will become almost completely non-perfused. Liver and kidneys are the most vulnerable, but also the spinal cord poorly tolerates extended thoracic aortic occlusion, increasing the risk of paraplegia. In zone III occlusion (infrarenal aorta), the effect on central blood pressure is relatively small but has an impact on pelvic bleeding as a proximal control. It is important to remember that REBOA affects arterial pressure and bleeding, and does not have a *direct* effect on venous bleeding.

The REBOA occlusion time needs to be limited as short as needed preferably not more than 30 minutes in zone I and 60 minutes in zone III.

In reperfusion after the balloon is deflated, there is a sudden decrease of blood volume due to arterial blood flow distribution to the previously closed area. Also, the reperfusion results in a large challenge of cold, acidotic, and hyperkalaemic venous blood back to heart and circulation. This has a sudden direct effect on the cardiac output, but will also have a later effect on capillary leakage and increase the risk of multi organ failure.

Occlusion will not stop arterial back bleeding or venous bleeding, even though it might decrease perfusion pressure to visceral organs and thereby decrease bleeding pressure. Depending on level of occlusion, organ ischaemia will follow an occlusion time of some length (even 10–20 minutes), and ischaemia-reperfusion reaction will always follow to some degree. Acidosis and ischaemic metabolism with systemic effects will follow even if a short occlusion time is used due to the metabolic acidosis that has already affected the trauma patient.

It is very important to communicate with the anaesthesia team during REBOA use, since the patient will receive parallel massive transfusion, and to prevent a hypertensive state during late resuscitation.

15.3.3 Insertion Technique

The main limiting stage is vascular arterial access, which can be achieved by ultrasound (the method of choice), surgical cut-down, or using anatomical landmarks. Modern REBOA catheters need sheaths of around 7–8

French gauge (FG) for insertion, and proper sheath insertion is essential to the whole REBOA procedure. The change to smaller catheters (from former 12–14 FG to 7–8 FG) has made the method simpler to use, and results in fewer complications.

REBOA should be used in zone I or III, but can be used for short periods in zone II (although not recommended). Before insertion of the REBOA balloon, one can measure the length to zone I or III using external body landmarks (mid-sternum for zone I, or umbilicus for zone III) or use fluoroscopy (or other techniques as described in the *Top Stent Manual* – see Recommended Reading). In general, with blunt trauma and an unclear bleeding source, zone I is used first while different methods should be applied to minimize ischaemia time. REBOA can be changed to zone III if the source of bleeding is pelvic, for example.

Femoral artery cannulation should be done in experienced hands, as part of the EVTM concept, already on arrival and during the primary survey if possible. Once the needle is in the vessel, a guidewire is inserted and then a sheath of the proper size (7–8 FG), followed by the REBOA balloon (Figure 15.2). A femoral arterial line (4–5 FG) might be upgraded to a proper sheath and used for REBOA (different types exist). The intraluminal location and proper function of the sheath must be verified by ultrasound and/or aspiration. It can be used as a distal arterial line parallel to the REBOA line.

In patients *in extremis,* parallel bilateral arterial access (venous at times) might be beneficial. Vascular access should not delay any other life-saving procedure.

On insertion, the REBOA catheter is carefully advanced (no resistance to wire or catheter) and positioned. When at its designated location, slow inflation of the balloon follows, with careful monitoring of central pressure if available, carotid pulses or contralateral femoral pressure via the sheath, when using partial occlusion (pREBOA) or intermittent occlusion (iREBOA) (see also Section 15.3.5). In general, it can be claimed that if blood pressure is not elevated when using REBOA, there are three main reasons:

- The REBOA is not in the aorta.
- The balloon is damaged/malfunctioning.
- The patient has died.

15.3.4 Monitoring

There are several ways to follow the haemodynamic effects of REBOA. The most obvious is measurement of central pressure, radial/brachial/subclavian artery

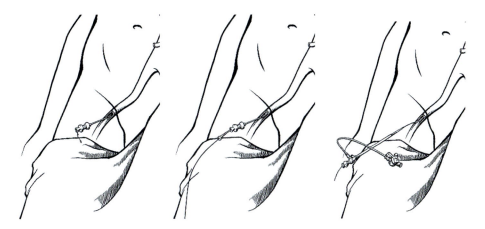

Figure 15.2 Puncture of the femoral artery, followed by guide wire and sheath. These are the basic steps to be followed by the REBOA catheter. Puncture by ultrasound to be preferred, but depends on the experience of the operator.

pressure, carotid pulse, and possibly end-tidal CO_2, which decreases with total occlusion of the aorta. It is highly important to follow the clinical effects of REBOA and the simultaneous surgical management and adjust them during resuscitation, as well as in the direct post-operative period. Owing to coagulopathy followed by massive transfusions and coagulation factors, thrombosis might occur, especially in the iliac-femoral vessels and lower extremities. It may occur during resuscitation or in the direct post-operative period.

15.3.5 Total, Partial, and Intermittent Occlusion, and Targeted Blood Pressure

Balloon occlusion can be *total* (no flow below the balloon – tREBOA), or *partial* (balloon is not inflated totally, resulting in partial flow below the balloon – pREBOA). Intermittent REBOA (iREBOA), done by alternately inflating and deflating the balloon, results in intermittent partial flow below the balloon. In a critically unstable patient the occlusion is normally total at the start, but as soon as some stability has been gained, there should be attempts to transfer into partial or intermittent occlusion. This is done in balance with the haemodynamic stability and the tolerance to balloon deflation. The goal is to minimize the occlusion time. It also is possible to continuously work with the partial balloon inflation volume and aim for some targeted blood pressure. This prevents blood pressure peaks that are too high and allows some distal perfusion.

15.3.6 Perioperative and Post-operative Care

The vascular access and REBOA catheter should always be held by the REBOA operator, since it is a 'living entity', and can and should be modified to the haemodynamic need and situation of the patient. When the REBOA balloon is deflated (slowly, due to possible circulatory collapse), one should consider if it will be needed again. It might be best to leave the sheath for some time (6–12 hours), using a saline flush to prevent clotting.

> **Pitfall**
>
> All REBOA procedures should be considered as invasive, with the potential to cause thrombosis of the femoral artery. Accordingly, distal lower extremity status must be controlled during the first 24 hours on an hourly basis. REBOA might also cause aorta or iliac intimal damage, so vascular and distal clinical and radiological evaluation after its use is crucial.

Removal of the sheath can be done by manual compression, open cut-down and suture, or closure devices. The choice depends heavily on the experience of the operator.

15.3.7 Indications

The main, most used, and obvious indication is blunt trauma with non-compressible torso bleeding. It could be visceral organ bleeding, but the most documented and recognized indication is traumatic (blunt) pelvic bleeding. It should be noted that REBOA has been used successfully for penetrating trauma, even during cardiopulmonary resuscitation. In general, a hypotensive patient (with a systolic blood pressure of less than 80 mm Hg), or a non-responsive bleeder, might benefit from REBOA as a bridge to definitive care. In this sense, it is a form of intraluminal aorta clamping, which should be used carefully to increase and maintain an acceptable blood pressure, preferably by partial or intermitted occlusion of the aorta. The main advantage of REBOA use in these situations is to avoid opening another cavity for aortic clamping.

At times, REBOA has been used very late when the patient has been in deep shock for a long time, a factor to be considered when evaluating survival of these patients and well known in ruptured abdominal aorta patients. REBOA has been used as a time-winning tool in an austere environment, when there are no appropriate resources available, in transport, or in multiple casualty scenarios. REBOA has been used successfully in military and pre-hospital scenarios, but there is much to investigate regarding its use and indications.

15.3.8 Contraindications

The peak increase in blood pressure after REBOA balloon deployment can be hazardous in case of intracranial, thoracic bleeding, or neck bleeding, and are commonly considered as contraindications for REBOA. In case of blunt thoracic aortic injury, the expanding balloon itself or sudden peak increase in blood pressure may deliver too much tension on the injured aortic wall resulting in catastrophic consequences. The widened mediastinum and suspicion of blunt aortic injury is contraindication for REBOA.

15.3.9 Complications[16,17]

Even being minimally invasive, REBOA has risks of potentially devastating complications. The vascular access is usually done via the common femoral artery (CFA) and there is a risk of intimal injury resulting in thrombus and inferior extremity ischaemia. The modern balloon catheters are compatible with smaller sheath size and thus carry a relatively lower risk of thromboembolic complications. Blind catheter deployment carries the risk of wrong landing zone. Also, when deploying

in zone I balloon, the unnoticed balloon migration may lead to faulty positioning.

15.3.10 Summary

REBOA is a minimally invasive procedure that might be useful as a bridge to definitive treatment in a bleeding trauma patient. It is no substitute for excellent surgical care but might assist surgical, hybrid, or endovascular procedures. It should be regarded as part of the EVTM toolbox and used wisely. Great care should be taken to use it on patients who might benefit from its use and to avoid complications.[18] Current evidence-based recommendations are shown in Table 15.1.

Table 15.1 Evidence-Based Recommendations for REBOA

Level of Evidence	Reccomendations
I	None
II	None

III	• Consider early placement of a common femoral artery catheter in the hypotensive trauma patient (SBP <90 mm Hg) to facilitate rapid upsizing to a 7-French sheath to accommodate a REBOA catheter if necessary.
	• REBOA should be considered in patients with ahemorrhagic shock and the following:
	  ○ Penetrating or blunt abdominopelvic trauma patients who are hypotensive (SBP <90 mm Hg).
	  ○ Transient responders to fluid resuscitation, or receiving a massive transfusion protocol (MTP).
	  ○ Positive focused assessment by sonography for trauma (FAST) examination.
	  ○ Suspected pelvic or lower extremity trauma with hemorrhage.
	• The REBOA device may also be considered for the following alternative indications:
	  ○ Prophylactic use in women undergoing surgery for abnormal placentation.
	  ○ Severe gastrointestinal bleeding.

15.4 **ANAESTHETIC CONSIDERATIONS**

- Severe head injury mandates special attention and communication between surgeons and anaesthesiologists during the creation of the pneumoperitoneum. Monitoring of intracranial pressure (ICP) (or at least pupil reactivity) during the operation, possibly insufflating the abdomen at a lower pressure (10 instead of 14–15) and repeating the CT scan after the operation are just a few of the precautions to be recommended in patients with head trauma.
- REBOA, especially deployed in zone I, will have a major impact on the need of ventilation. The perfused tissue volume will decrease dramatically when closing the aorta, meaning that if the respirator settings are not adjusted to the new circulated and perfused blood volume, will that result in severe hyperventilation.
- The dramatically increased perfused volume after the balloon deflation will result in hypoventilation if no ventilator adjustment is done. This must not happen, especially in combined head injury patients, and rewards close communication and cooperation between surgeons and anaesthesiologists.
- Owing to coagulopathy followed by massive transfusions and coagulation factors, the coagulation status changes quickly, and monitoring with Visco-Haemostatic Assays (Section 5.4.6.2) is very helpful.
- **REBOA will cause an increase in bleeding from the liver, owing to increased intrathoracic pressure with occlusion in zone I, and back-bleeding. Eighty-five per cent of bleeding from the liver is venous, and this will therefore be substantially increased. REBOA is contraindicated in liver injuries.**

REFERENCES AND RECOMMENDED READING

References

LAPAROSCOPY

1. Bain K, Meytes V, Chang GC, Timoney F. Laparoscopy in penetrating abdominal trauma is a safe and effective alternative to laparotomy. *Surg Endosc.* 2018 September 12. doi: 10.1007/s00464-018-6436-1.
2. Koto MZ, Mosai F, Matsevych OY. The role of laparoscopy in blunt abdominal trauma: diagnostic, therapeutic or both? *S Afr J Surg.* 2017 Jun;**55(2)**:60.
3. Mathonnet M, Peyrou P, Gainant A, Bouvier S, Cubertafond P. Role of laparoscopy in blunt perforations of the small bowel. *Surg Endosc.* 2003 Apr;**17**:641–5.
4. Chen RJ, Fang JF, Lin BC, Hsu YB, Kao JL, Kao YC, et al. Selective application of laparoscopy and fibrin glue in the failure of nonoperative management of blunt hepatic trauma. *J Trauma.* 1998 Apr;**44**:691–5.
5. Griffen M, Ochoa J, Boulanger BR. A minimally invasive approach to bile peritonitis after blunt liver injury. *Am Surg.* 2000;**66**:309–12.
6. Ivatury RR, Sugerman HJ, Peitzman AB. Abdominal Compartment Syndrome: recognition and management. *Advances in Surgery.* 2001;**35**:251–69.

THORACOSCOPY

7. Lowdermilk GA, Naunheim KS. Thoracoscopic evaluation and treatment of thoracic trauma. *Surg Clin North Am.* 2000 Oct;**80(5)**:1535–42. Review.

8. Lang-Lazdunski L, Mouroux J, Pons F, Grosdidier G, Martinod E, Elkaim D, et al. Role of videothoracoscopy in chest trauma. *Ann Thorac Surg.* 1997 Feb;**63**:327–33.
9. Freeman RK, Al-Dossari G, Hutcheson KA, Huber L, Jessen ME, Meyer D, et al. Indications for using video-assisted thoracoscopic surgery to diagnose diaphragmatic injuries after penetrating chest trauma. *Ann Thorac Surg.* 2001 Aug;**72**:342–7.
10. Morales CH, Salinas CM, Henao CA, Patino PA, Munoz CM. Thoracoscopic pericardial window and penetrating cardiac trauma. *J Trauma.* 1997 Feb;**42(2)**:273–5.

DIAPHRAGM

11. Mjoli M, Oosthuizen G, Clarke D, Madiba T. Laparoscopy in the diagnosis and repair of diaphragmatic injuries in left-sided penetrating thoracoabdominal trauma: laparoscopy in trauma. *Surg Endosc.* 2015;**29(3)**:747–52. doi: 10.1007/s00464-014-3710-8.
12. Friese RS, Coln E, Gentilello L. Laparoscopy is sufficient to exclude occult diaphragmatic injury after penetrating abdominal trauma. *J Trauma.* 2005 Apr;**58(4)**:789–92.

REBOA

13. Horer T. Resuscitative endovascular balloon occlusion of the aorta (REBOA) and endovascular resuscitation and trauma management (EVTM): a paradigm shift regarding hemodynamic instability. *Eur J Trauma Emerg Surg.* 2018 Aug;**44(4)**:487–9. doi: 10.1007/s00068-018-0983-y.
14. Brenner M, Inaba K, Ailofi A, DuBose JJ, Fabian T, Bee T, et al. Resuscitative Endovascular Balloon Occlusion of the Aorta and Resuscitative Thoracotomy in select patients

with Haemorrhagic shock: Early results from the American Association for the Surgery of Trauma's Aortic Occlusion in Resuscitation for Trauma and Acute Care Surgery Register. *J Am Coll Surg*. 2018 May;**226(5)**:730–40. doi: 10.1016/j.jamcollsurg.2018.01.044.

15. Qasim ZA, Sikorski RA. Physiologic Considerations in Trauma Patients Undergoing Resuscitative Endovascular Balloon Occlusion of the Aorta. *Anesth Analg*. 2017;**125(3)**: 891–4. doi: 10.1213/ANE.0000000000002215.

16. Manzano-Nunez R, Orlas CP, Herrera-Escobar JP, Galvagno S, DuBose J, Melendez JJ, et al. A meta-analysis of the incidence of complications associated with groin access after the use of resuscitative endovascular balloon occlusion of the aorta in trauma patients. *J Trauma Acute Care Surg*. 2018 Sep;**85(3)**:626–34. doi: 10.1097/TA.0000000000001978.

17. Davidson AJ, Russo RM, Reva VA, Brenner ML, Moore LJ, Ball C, et al. The pitfalls of resuscitative endovascular balloon occlusion of the aorta: Risk factors and mitigation strategies. *J Trauma Acute Care Surg*. 2018 Jan;**84(1)**:192–202. doi: 10.1097/TA.0000000000001711.

18. Resuscitative Endovascular Occlusion of the Aorta (REBOA) Evidence based guidelines for use. Aug 2018. Available from: http://www.surgicalcriticalcare.net/Guidelines/REBOA%202018.pdf (accessed January 2019).

Recommended Reading

LAPAROSCOPY

Cirocchi R, Birindelli A, Inaba K, Mandrioli M, Piccinini A, Tabola R, et al. Laparoscopy for Trauma and the Changes in its Use From 1990 to 2016: A Current Systematic Review and Meta-Analysis. *Surg Laparosc Endosc Percutan Tech*. 2018 Feb;**28(1)**:1–12. doi: 10.1097/SLE.0000000000000466.

Hajibandeh S, Hajibandeh S, Gumber AO, Wong CS. Laparoscopy versus laparotomy for the management of penetrating abdominal trauma: A systematic review and meta-analysis. *Int J Surg*. 2016;**34**:127–36. doi: 10.1016/j.ijsu.2016.08.524.

Li Y, Xiang Y, Wu N, Wu L, Yu Z, Zhang M, et al. A Comparison of Laparoscopy and Laparotomy for the Management of Abdominal Trauma: A Systematic Review and Meta-analysis. *World J Surg*. 2015;**39(12)**:2862–71. doi: 10.1007/s00268-015-3212-4.

THORACOSCOPY

Wu N, Wu L, Qiu C, Yu Z, Xiang Y, Wang M, et al. A comparison of video-assisted thoracoscopic surgery with open thoracotomy for the management of chest trauma: a systematic review and meta-analysis. *World J Surg*. 2015 Apr;**39(4)**:940–52. doi: 10.1007/s00268-014-2900-9.

REBOA

Brenner M, Bulger EM, Perina DG, Henry S, Kang CS, Rotondo MF, et al. Joint statement from the American College of Surgeons Committee on Trauma (ACS COT) and the American College of Emergency Physicians (ACEP) regarding the clinical use of Resuscitative Endovascular Balloon Occlusion of the Aorta (REBOA). *Trauma Surg Acute Care Open*. 2018 Jan 13;**3(1)**:e000154. doi: 10.1136/tsaco-2017-000154.

Brenner M, Perina DG, Bulger EM, Winchell RJ, Kang CS, Henry S, et al. Response to letter to the editor from Dubose and colleagues regarding the Joint statement from the American College of Surgeons Committee on Trauma (ACS COT) and the American College of Emergency Physicians (ACEP) regarding the clinical use of Resuscitative Endovascular Balloon Occlusion of the Aorta (REBOA). *Trauma Surg Acute Care Open*. 2018 Mar 2;**3(1)**:e000170. doi: 10.1136/tsaco-2018-00017.

Brenner M, Inaba K, Aiolfi A, DuBose J, Fabian T, Bee T, et al. Resuscitative Endovascular Balloon Occlusion of the Aorta and Resuscitative Thoracotomy in Select Patients with Hemorrhagic Shock: Early Results from the American Association for the Surgery of Trauma's Aortic Occlusion in Resuscitation for Trauma and Acute Care Surgery Registry. *J Am Coll Surg*. 2018 May;**226(5)**:730–40. doi: 10.1016/j.jamcollsurg.2018.01.044.

DuBose JJ, Rasmussen TE, Davis MR. Letter to the editor regarding the joint statement from the American College of Surgeons' Committee on Trauma (ACS-COT) and the American College of Emergency Physicians (ACEP) regarding the clinical use of resuscitative endovascular balloon occlusion of the aorta (REBOA). *Trauma Surg Acute Care Open*. 2018 Mar 2;**3(1)**:e000167. doi: 10.1136/tsaco-2018-000167.

Hörer TM MJ, DuBose JJ, Reva VA, Matsumoto J, Matsumura Y, Falkenberg M, et al. Top Stent Manual, The art of EndoVascular hybrid Trauma and bleeding Management. The REBOA Manual. 1st ed. Hörer T, editor. Örebro, Sweden: Örebro University Hospital; 2017. Available from: http://www.jevtm.com/top-stent/ (accessed online Jan 2019).

Imaging in Trauma 16

16.1 INTRODUCTION

In the emergency room (ER), traditionally, a series of conventional x-rays were performed. Today, examination of the c-spine is replaced by computed tomography (CT). Anteroposterior (AP) imaging of the thorax and pelvis are, while still widely available and used, increasingly replaced by trauma CT. Supine chest and pelvic x-rays have a relatively low sensitivity for injuries, and clinical examination combined with CT provides a more accurate diagnosis.

An additional imaging method in the ER is, where available, focused assessment by sonography for trauma (FAST), which indicates the presence of pericardial effusions, and largely replaces diagnostic peritoneal lavage (DPL) as the method of choice to find intra-abdominal bleeding. Extended FAST (eFAST) may, in addition, show pneumothoraces and pleural effusions.

However, in many modern trauma centres, the trauma bay is near the CT, which enables transient responders who used to bypass CT to go through imaging first. Modern CTs are very fast, and the time-consuming moment today is transportation and the positioning of the patient on the CT table, along with dealing with tubes, lines, monitoring equipment, and other external devices.

Pitfalls

- Patients who are haemodynamically unstable despite resuscitation may be directed to the operating room (OR) for immediate operative treatment after the initial workup in the ER. Radiology should never delay an emergency procedure.
- Patients who are mentally alert, not intoxicated and do not show signs of other than minor injuries do **not** benefit from CT and may be managed with repeated clinical evaluation combined with specific CT exams if needed.

- The use of any imaging technique, including ultrasound, should never delay the definitive treatment; for this reason, any algorithm should start from the physiology of the patient and not from ultrasound (US) findings.

Multi-detector computed tomography (MDCT) will allow for a fast diagnosis of injuries and comprehensively show the most compelling bleeding source. The patient may then be evaluated for surgery or for non-operative management (NOM), with or without interventional radiology (IR). NOM is increasingly applied to patients who used to go to the OR, which places heavy demands on quick and adequate radiological assessment. Every trauma centre needs close cooperation between radiologists, interventionists, and surgeons, who all must be well acquainted with the available options at their hospital. Facilities may vary, and the workup depends on what equipment and expertise is available.[1]

In patients who need surgery, a CT before the procedure will help the surgeon to decide what injuries need attention first. If the patient is eligible for IR, a CT angiogram (CTA) is mandatory before going to the angiography or hybrid suite and may avoid the need for either.

MDCT is more comprehensive, sensitive, and specific than clinical examination, plain films, or ultrasound in identifying injury, and is the standard of care in stable patients with severe injuries. If local logistics allow, CT should be considered for transient responders as well. If there is a decision to go for MDCT, this should not be delayed by plain films and/or FAST.

16.2 RADIATION DOSES AND PROTECTION FROM RADIATION

Ionizing radiation affects the human cells. In high doses or with repeated exposure, it may be harmful. Trying to estimate morbidity and mortality owing to medical imaging is extremely difficult and should be accompanied by estimates of the benefits of the procedures.

There is no evidence to suggest at which exact dose the harmful effects begin; they are stochastic. Therefore, healthcare normally acts from the assumption that there is no safe threshold dose.

All efforts must be made to minimize the effect of ionising radiation on the human body.
Dose: As Low as Reasonably Achievable (ALARA)

'Any decision that alters the radiation exposure situation should do more good than harm'. ICRP (International Committee for Radiation Protection)

The basic dose or radiation absorbed by the tissues is the Grey (Gy) – 1 joule/kg of tissue.

The Siewert (Sv) is used in setting radiological protection standards and contains 1000 milliSieverts (mSv).

The World Health Organisation and the IRCP recommend a maximum annual radiation dose.[2]

- Average annual natural background radiation worldwide is 2.4 mSv, ranging from 1–20 mSv, mainly owing to terrestrial and airborne radiation, and radiation from building materials. (In 250 flying hours, aircrew receive 50 mSv per year.)
- Maximum annual dose for radiation workers is 20 mSv average over 5 years, not exceeding 50 mSv per year.
- The current maximum *whole-body dose* is recommended not to exceed 50 mSv per annum.
- For therapeutic oncological radiation of single organ targets, the dose may reach 500 mSv (see Table 16.1).

Table 16.1 Dose Examples of Common Diagnostic Radiological Procedures

Examination	Effective Dose (mSv)
Chest x-ray, bedside AP view	0.02–0.1
Chest CT	6–10
Whole body CT (WBCT = brain, face, neck, torso including pelvis, proximal femur)	20–40
Chest x-ray	2
Pelvic x-ray	5

Modern CTs will customize radiation according to the density and size of the patient. The transfer itself, as well as the neck collar and the headrest of the CT will add to the dose required. The dose will also vary widely with the equipment; the dose examples are estimations.

The younger the patient, the greater the risk of a radiation induced malignancy owing to the impact on proliferating cells and the longer life expectancy. In these cases, observation and repeated clinical exams combined with specific CT exams should be considered as an option.

With pregnant patients, the health of the mother is always first priority. If possible, specific CT scans instead of whole body CT scan (WBCT) may be discussed. If local criteria for WBCT are fulfilled, however, this should be performed. A hospital physicist can calculate the foetus dose after the examination.

The 64-MDCT scanner is the most dose-efficient machine when the foetus is outside the direct scan volume, as in the case of pulmonary angiograms. For abdominal examinations, the 64-MDCT scanner imparted the highest foetal dose.[3]

2% of all malignant disease now being recorded in the USA and Australia can be attributed directly to medical radiation.

It is therefore important not to overuse the ionizing radiological diagnostic and therapeutic techniques available to us, unless benefits available exceed the risks incurred.[4]

Pitfall

A correct diagnosis is vital in the care of polytrauma patients and fear of radiation should not prevent adequate imaging.

16.3 PRINCIPLES OF TRAUMA IMAGING

- A short but comprehensive medical history on the referral will facilitate correct imaging and speed up reading.
- If the patient is positioned off centre on the trauma transfer, the images may be incomplete, and the patient may not fit into the gantry. Repositioning is time consuming.

- Artefacts from external devices as well as from arms positioned beside the body may impede correct diagnosis of injuries mainly to the liver and the spleen. Lifting the arms above the head or securing them on a pillow in front of the torso and removing as many objects like draining and monitoring devices as possible from the scan field will therefore help to optimize image quality and may even reduce the radiation dose.
- A trauma protocol should be robust and fast, and as far as possible eliminate the need for additional CTs because the first one was inadequate. For severely injured patients who need a WBCT, this means:
  - Always scan thorax and abdomen – the impact of the trauma doesn't stop at the diaphragm.
  - Never scan only the vertebral column – if there is risk of a vertebral injury, there may well be injuries to the abdomen and thorax as well.
  - There is seldom need for additional plain films of the pelvis,[5] or proximal extremities – these may be included in the scan, and CT offers better imaging than plain films.
- Intravenous (IV) contrast is essential for diagnosing injury to solid organs and vessels.

Sometimes, the question about impaired kidney function arises. If a trauma patient needs an emergency examination, it must never be delayed waiting for a creatinine level – postponing the CT or diverging from the contrast protocol may cause greater harm than the contrast itself.[6] In patients who require repeated CTs during their hospital stay, however, it is important to monitor the creatinine level. Repeated IV contrast administration in a short time span may be harmful, especially in patients with impaired kidney function.

- If needed, the protocol can be adjusted to look for vessel injuries or distal extremity fractures; however, all adjustments will add to the time spent in the radiology department.
- Specific examinations, such as triple contrast CT for intestinal evaluation, or contrast infusion to examine the urine bladder are, in many trauma centres, performed at a later stage and not part of the initial workup.

Communicate with the radiologist to set up for the best possible protocol and speedy examination, reading and reporting.

16.4 PITFALLS AND PEARLS

- If it is not possible to insert an IV needle, the contrast may be given in an intra-osseous (IO) needle. High pressure is needed, and power injection is possible, although very little studied. Humeral placement is the preferred site of access. The procedure is painful, and a local anaesthetic should be given if the patient is not sedated. The arm must be kept still when the humeral IO needle is in place and must therefore not be lifted above the head.
- Use external wound markers for all visible entry sites (e.g. vitamin E-capsules, paper clips) to facilitate wound tracking and to enhance the speed of the reading of images. In the case of gunshot wounds, counting entry and exit wounds and projectiles will also help to localize any missing bullets.
- Use the planning overview image (also known as the scout image) to look for foreign bodies, fractures, and large pneumo- and haemothoraces.
- Notoriously difficult areas include the diaphragm and the oesophagus; a negative examination does not exclude injury even with modern MDCT.
- CT after damage control surgery is an entity that involves the most badly wounded, unstable patients who go to the OR before CT, and needs special attention. It can be difficult to differentiate between traumatic injuries and post-operative findings. Vessels may be ligated, organs removed, bowels stapled, and foreign objects such as packings and thrombus generating cellulose (e.g. Surgicel®) may cause confusion.
- It is of great value to practise trauma management regularly. Ideally, this is done together with the other departments who are involved in trauma care. In addition to initial resuscitation and radiological procedures, safe transportation and transfer of the patient also need to be practised regularly. This includes making sure the anaesthetic team is well acquainted with the surroundings and limited space in the CT lab.
- Quality is improved by regular multidisciplinary morbidity and mortality conferences, where all involved disciplines discuss trauma cases together.
- Dual energy imaging is a relatively new CT application, which may facilitate the diagnosis of bleeding, metal fragments, bone oedema, and injuries to the bowel wall.

Key success factors in trauma management include:

- A well-known trauma routine which is practised regularly.
- A robust protocol for WBCT.
- Communication, evaluation, and feedback.

16.5 TRAUMA ULTRASOUND

After introduction of FAST (focused assessment by sonography for trauma) in the 1990s, ultrasound (US) has rapidly become not only an available technique, but a tool coupled with clinical evaluation for the assessment and management of trauma patients. Ultrasound can be clinically integrated into the A-B-C-D-E primary survey and secondary survey of any trauma patient, helping to answer to specific clinical issues.

In the perspective of a clinically integrated US, questions to be answered are simple and often require binary answers (yes/no). For the same reasons, US in trauma is always a rapid exam, and the use by non-radiologists (surgeons, emergency physicians, intensivists) who are in charge of the patient is essential. The findings must be interpreted together with the mechanism of trauma, the physiology of the patient, and the anatomy of the injuries.

Appropriately trained surgeons have been demonstrated to have equal or superior accuracy to radiologists in performing clinical US.

16.5.1 Extended Focused Assessment by Sonography for Trauma

The basic application of US in trauma is extended focused assessment by sonography for trauma (eFAST), which aims to answer the following simple questions:

- Is there free fluid (blood) in abdomen, pleural spaces and pericardium?
- Is there free air (pneumothorax) in pleural cavities?

Four areas of the abdomen are scanned for the detection of free fluid (the FAST protocol):

- Pericardial.
- Perihepatic.
- Perisplenic.
- Pelvic.

The cranial extension of the perihepatic and perisplenic views, obtained by simply sliding the probe upwards, allows a check for haemothorax.

Parasternal sagittal views on the anterior thoracic wall are used for searching the physiologic sliding of the visceral pleura (the so-called 'sliding lung'). The absence of the sliding lung and the recognition of the contact of the lung with the thoracic wall ('lung point') are US signs of pneumothorax. Lung point is not detectable in complete pneumothorax.

Sensitivity and specificity of US in the detection of haemothorax are similar to portable chest x-rays. Sensitivity of US for the detection of pneumothorax in the supine position is twice that of chest x-rays and approximates that of CT.

eFAST is not organ-specific, so organ injuries (liver, spleen, etc.) are not the goal and must not be included in the eFAST protocol.

eFAST is non-invasive and repeatable. Whenever the physical assessment and/or the physiology of the patient require, eFAST could be used to answer clinical questions.

Repeated scans have been shown to increase sensitivity for abdominal views in haemodynamically normal patients. Repetition of eFAST is even more important where no further diagnostic investigations are available.

The amount of free fluid detected can be estimated according to some available scores in the abdomen, and at glance in the thorax. In the abdomen, immediate and easy detection of fluid in all three views means more than 800 mL of blood is present in 85% of cases.

Correlation with potential or already established injuries and with the physiological status allows the best clinical decision (observation, definitive treatment, further investigation) to be made rapidly.

- eFAST should be performed:
  - During the primary survey in physiologically unstable patients.
  - At the end of primary survey in normal and stable patients.
  - During the secondary survey and whenever needed by changes in patient clinical status.
- eFAST refers to steps B and C of the primary survey.

16.5.2 Indications and Results

16.5.2.1 PENETRATING ABDOMINAL TRAUMA

There is no role for US in hypotensive patients with abdominal penetrating trauma, except for those with thoraco-abdominal injuries, when eFAST could help in prioritizing the surgical approach (thorax versus abdomen first).

A positive FAST after penetrating injury in a haemodynamically normal patient is a strong predictor of significant injury (high positive predictive value). If negative, a different approach (additional diagnostic studies, clinical observation, diagnostic laparoscopy) may be required to rule out occult injury.

16.5.2.2 BLUNT ABDOMINAL TRAUMA

Even if a positive FAST exam is defined by the detection of fluid in one or more views, the meaning of positivity depends on the clinical setting, mechanism of trauma, and associated lesions. FAST significantly shortens time to definitive treatment.

A small amount of fluid in the perisplenic view in a hypotensive patient suggests other sources of shock (retroperitoneal, pelvic, thoracic, or long bone bleeding; tension pneumothorax; neurogenic shock). The same small amount of free fluid in a normotensive trauma patient with a seat belt sign, entails a high index of suspicion for hollow viscus injury.

In other words, a negative or slightly positive FAST gives information for the decision-making process, which may be as useful as a grossly positive one, according to the clinical status.

16.5.2.3 PELVIC TRAUMA

Ultrasound plays a relevant role in hypotensive patient with haemorrhagic pelvic fractures. A grossly positive exam is a marker of intraperitoneal bleeding and associated abdominal injuries and mandate surgical exploration. A negative or slightly positive FAST exam suggests pelvic bleeding in the major cause of shock. These two findings allow for the better therapeutic strategy, according to institutional resources.

16.5.2.4 BLUNT THORACIC TRAUMA

Accuracy of US in detection of haemothorax and pneumothorax is well established. Detection of occult 'small' pneumothorax by US has similar accuracy than CT and can anticipate the need for drainage in mechanically ventilated patients.

16.5.2.5 PENETRATING THORACIC TRAUMA

Detection of pneumothorax and haemothorax by US cannot not delay obvious indications for immediate thoracic drainage or surgery.

Ultrasound (subxiphoid or parasternal view) has replaced pericardiocentesis for the diagnosis of pericardial effusion. Penetrating precordial or transthoracic wound suspicious for cardiac injury demonstrated accuracy in the detection of pericardial fluid of more than 97%. If it is decided that a pericardiocentesis is required, either as a bridge to surgery, or for monitoring, US can help in performing a safer and easier procedure.

16.5.3 Other Applications of Ultrasound in Trauma

- In an A-B-C-D-E sequence, US could be used for assessing proper orotracheal intubation (tracheal and lung views), to speed recognition of landmarks for cricothyroidotomy or tracheostomy, and for assessing presence and evolution of pulmonary contusions.
- Inferior vena cava diameter and collapsibility helps in evaluation of volume status and shock management, together with the subxiphoid assessment of cardiac chambers repletion and contractility.[7]
- Bone fractures edges can be easily detected by US (sternum, ribs, long bones).
- A more advanced applications of US is contrast enhanced US (CEUS), which could be used both for the detection of solid organ injuries in selected groups of patients (for instance, haemodynamically normal paediatric patients sustaining blunt abdominal trauma) and for the follow-up of non-operative management of parenchymatous organs (liver, spleen, kidney).

16.5.4 Training

Ultrasound, like any technical skill, is operator dependent. Formal training is needed for getting competence in acquisition and interpretation of US findings. Hands-on courses and proctored practice are needed. Owing to its clinical value and relative ease of learning, e-FAST training still represents the suggested first step for beginners.

Pitfalls

- Subcutaneous emphysema makes undetectable deep structures and is a contraindication to the use of US.
- Organ injuries are in general out of the scope of clinical US in trauma patients (except CEUS-FAST).

Diagnosis of bowel injury, diaphragmatic rupture, retroperitoneal lesions and haematomas, and solid organ injury could be considered based on direct/indirect B-mode US findings but need to be assessed with other methods when suspected.

- Free abdominal fluid is not always blood. When in doubt, aspiration under US guidance can enhance the decision-making process (i.e. enteric/bile aspiration in suspected hollow viscus injury, urine in stable patients with pelvic fracture).

16.5.5 Summary

The use of US in trauma has extended from FAST to a comprehensive US-enhanced management. eFAST remains the basic diagnostic application.

- FAST is a good initial screening tool for blunt abdominal injury and shortens time to definitive treatment in hypotensive patients.
- Ultrasound is the best method for detecting haemothorax and pneumothorax in trauma patients.
- Many procedural manoeuvres could be realized under US guidance, increasing decisional process and safety.
- The clinically integrated use of US in trauma requires specific training.

REFERENCES AND RECOMMENDED READING

References

1. Huber-Wagner S, Lefering R, Qvick LM, Körner M, Kay MV, Pfeifer KJ, et al. Effect of whole-body CT during trauma resuscitation on survival: a retrospective, multicentre study. *Lancet.* 2009 Apr 25;**373(9673)**:1455–61. doi: 10.1016/S0140-6736(09)60232-4.

2. International Commission for Radiological Protection (ICRP) publication 103: The 2007 recommendations of the International Committee for Radiation Protection. Available from: Radiologyinfo.org (accessed online January 2019).

3. Gilet AG, Dunkin JM, Fernandez TJ, Button TM, Budorick NE. Fetal radiation dose during gestation estimated on an anthropomorphic phantom for three generations of CT scanners. *Am J Roentgenol.* 2011 May;**196(5)**:1133–7. doi: 10.2214/AJR.10.4497.

4. Linder F, Mani K, Juhlin C, Eklöf H. Routine whole body CT of high energy trauma patients leads to excessive radiation exposure. *Scand J Trauma Resusc Emerg Med.* 2016 Jan;27;**24**:7. doi: 10.1186/s13049-016-0199-2.

5. Soto JR, Zhou C, Hu D, Arazoza AC, Dunn E, Sladek P. Skip and save: utility of pelvic x-rays in the initial evaluation of blunt trauma patients. *Am J Surg.* 2015 Dec;**210(6)**:1076–9; discussion 1079-81. doi: 10.1016/j.amjsurg.2015.07.011.

6. Aycock RD, Westafer LM, Boxen JL, Majlesi N, Schoenfeld EM, Bannuru RR. Acute kidney injury after computed tomography: a meta-analysis. *Ann Emerg Med.* 2018 Jan;**71(1)**: 44–53.e4. doi: 10.1016/j.annemergmed.2017.06.041.

7. Stawicki, SP, Adkins EJ, Eiferman DS, Evans DC, Ali NA, Njoku C, et al. Prospective evaluation of intravascular volume status in critically ill patients: does inferior vena cava collapsibility correlate with central venous pressure? *J Trauma Acute Care Surg,* 2014 Apr;**76(4)**:956–63; discussion 963-4. doi: 10.1097/TA.0000000000000152.

Recommended Reading

International Commission for Radiological Protection (ICRP) Publications. Available from: http://www.icrp.org/page.asp?id=5 (accessed online January 2019).

Royal College of Radiologists. Standards of practice and guidance for trauma radiology in severely injured patients. 2015; Available from: https://www.rcr.ac.uk/system/files/publication/field_publication_files/bfcr155_traumaradiol.pdf (accessed online January 2019).

Part 5

Specialised aspects of total trauma care

Critical Care of the Trauma Patient 17

17.1 INTRODUCTION

Most trauma mortality in the intensive care unit (ICU) occurs during the first few days of admission, primarily as a result of severe traumatic brain injury, hypoxaemic respiratory failure, or refractory haemorrhagic shock, all of which are largely non-preventable deaths. Trauma ICU care is best provided by a multidisciplinary team focused on resuscitation, monitoring, and life support.

The fundamental goals are early restoration and maintenance of tissue oxygenation, diagnosis and treatment of occult injuries, prevention and treatment of infection and multiple organ failure, and early optimization to achieve the best possible outcome. In the ICU, those who take care of a patient admitted with lethal brain injury play a vital role in the support and maintenance of potential organ donors.

17.2 PHASES OF ICU CARE

17.2.1 Resuscitative Phase (First 24 Hours Post-Injury)[1]

Management is focused on haemostatic resuscitation, and the goal of treatment is the maintenance of adequate tissue oxygenation. Simultaneously, occult life-threatening or limb-threatening injuries are carefully sought, and should be addressed.

Inadequate tissue oxygenation must be recognized and treated immediately. Deficient tissue oxygen delivery in the acutely traumatized patient is usually caused by impaired perfusion, severe hypoxaemia, or impaired oxygen delivery. Although several different types of shock can be present, inadequate resuscitation from hypovolaemia and blood loss is most common.

After major trauma, some patients experience considerable delay before organ perfusion is fully restored, despite apparently adequate systolic blood pressure and apparently normal urine output. This phenomenon has been called 'occult hypoperfusion'.[2] A clear association has been identified between occult hypoperfusion or persistent hypovolaemia after major trauma and increased rates of infections, length of stay, days in surgical/trauma intensive care unit, hospital charges, multiple organ dysfunction/failure and mortality.[3] Rapid control of bleeding and early identification and aggressive resuscitation aimed at correcting hypovolemia has been shown to improve survival and reduce complications in severely injured trauma patients.

An elevated fluid balance alone is an independent risk factor for acute respiratory distress syndrome (ARDS) and multiple organ failure (MOF). Currently, a more balanced approach utilizes an initial restricted or controlled volume resuscitation (systolic blood pressure [SBP] approximately 90 mm Hg) until surgical bleeding is controlled (see also Chapter 6).

17.2.1.1 'TRADITIONAL' END POINTS OF RESUSCITATION

These include the following:

- Clinical examination.
- Base deficit and lactic acidosis – failure to clear in a 24 hour period is an ominous sign.
- Non-invasive haemodynamic monitoring.
- Gastric tonometry – largely obsolete.

Pitfall

Blood pressure, central venous pressure, heart rate, arterial partial pressure of oxygen (PaO_2), etc., may not identify occult hypoperfusion.

17.2.1.2 POST-TRAUMATIC ACUTE LUNG INJURY

Aetiology:

- Chest trauma.
- Fluid overload.

- Distributive shock.
- Aspiration.
- Fat embolism syndrome.
- Acute insult with pre-existing respiratory disease.

17.2.1.3 RESPIRATORY ASSESSMENT AND MONITORING

Work of breathing:

- Respiratory rate.
- Arterial blood gases – including repeat measurement of base deficit (BD) and lactate.
- Oxygen delivery and consumption.
- Bronchoscopy.

Ventilatory support should be instituted earlier rather than later; select a mode of ventilation tailored to the patient's need using appropriate tidal volumes and amounts of positive end-expiratory pressure (PEEP):

- Pressure support ventilation (PSV) – poorly tolerated following severe injury.
- Lung protective ventilation (LPV) with low volume and low peak pressures is frequently not possible early in resuscitation due to severe hypoxia and low compliance, use adequate volumes despite the frequent requirement for higher pressures.
- High positive end-expiratory pressure PEEP (>10 up to 20–25 cm H_2O may be required) to recruit alveoli.
- ECMO (extracorporeal membrane oxygenation) may be considered where appropriate (see also Section 17.3).
- Non-invasive ventilatory support in selected cases only.

A safe strategy is to maintain a driving pressure (plateau pressure – PEEP) of <15 cm water while accounting for lung injury.[4]

17.2.2 Early Life Support Phase (24–72 Hours Post-Injury)

During this phase, treatment is focused on the management of post-traumatic respiratory failure and progressive intracranial hypertension in patients suffering from severe head injury. Usually, the diagnostic evaluation for occult injuries is now complete. Evidence of early multiple organ failure may become apparent during this time.

Problems that may develop at this time include intracranial hypertension, systemic inflammatory response syndrome (SIRS), early multiple organ dysfunction

syndrome (MODS) and continued respiratory insufficiency. The main priorities of the early life support phase are the maintenance of tissue oxygenation, the control of intracranial hypertension, an ongoing search for occult injuries, and the institution of nutritional support and withdrawal or replacement of trauma resuscitation lines or devices that may have been placed in less than ideal conditions. Further establishment of the medical history or events of the injury is also completed.

17.2.2.1 PRIORITIES

- Gas exchange and ventilatory support.
- Haematological parameters.
- Fluid and electrolyte balance.
- Intracranial pressure (ICP) monitoring and control.
- Occult injuries.
- Delayed intracranial haematoma formation.
  - Follow-up computed tomography (CT) scan of the head.
- Intra-abdominal injuries.
  - Follow-up CT or ultrasound of the abdomen.
- Spinal injury.
  - Completion of the radiographic survey and clinical examination if possible.
  - Thoracic and lumbar spine injury.
- Extremity injury: hands and feet.
- Nerve injuries.

17.2.3 Prolonged Life Support (>72 Hours Post-Injury)

The duration of the prolonged life support phase depends on the severity of the injury and its associated complications. Many of those who are critically injured can be successfully weaned from life support early, while the more seriously injured enter a phase in which ongoing life support is necessary to prevent organ system failure. Predominant clinical concerns that arise include infectious complications that may lead to the development of late multiple organ failure or death.

The main objective of the management of patients developing MODS is to provide support for failing organ systems while attempts are made to isolate and eliminate inflammatory foci that could be perpetuating the organ system failure. In addition, prolonged immobility can cause problems with muscle wasting, joint contractures and skin compromise in pressure areas. Physiotherapy should be commenced early, with the proper use of splints, early exercise and ambulation when possible. ECMO has an increasing role[6] (see also Section 17.4).

17.2.3.1 RESPIRATORY FAILURE

- Unexplained respiratory failure – look for occult infection or necrotic tissue.
  - Consider early tracheostomy.

17.2.3.2 INFECTIOUS COMPLICATIONS

- Nosocomial pneumonia.[5]
  - Perform Gram stain of sputum and microbiological culture.
- Lung abscess and empyema.
- Surgical site infection.
  - Superficial incisional surgical site, for example, wound infection.
  - Deep incisional surgical site infection.
  - Organ/space surgical site infection, for example, intra-abdominal abscess.
- Intravenous catheter-related sepsis.
- Bloodstream infections.
- Urinary tract infection.
- Acalculous cholecystitis.
- Sinusitis and otitis media.
- Ventriculitis and meningitis.

Pitfalls

- Antibiotic therapy should ideally be of limited spectrum and directed toward cultures.
- Antibiotic stewardship: duration of antibiotics as short as possible.
- De-escalation strategy when cultures available.
- Remember the risk of antibiotic-associated colitis.

17.2.3.3 NON-INFECTIOUS CAUSES OF FEVER

- Metabolic response.
- Drugs.
- Pulmonary embolus (PE).
- Deep venous thrombosis (DVT).

17.2.3.4 PERCUTANEOUS TRACHEOSTOMY[6]

Percutaneous tracheostomy has been shown to have fewer perioperative and post-operative complications compared with conventional tracheostomy and is now the technique of choice in critically ill patients.

Various techniques are described, with dilation by forceps or multiple or single dilators. Patient selection is important.

Pitfalls

- Percutaneous tracheostomy should not be attempted if the procedure is non-elective, the landmarks are obscure in the neck or the patient has a coagulopathy.
- Caution should be exercised if the patient has a known cervical spine injury.
- Confirmation of correct placement by fibreoptic bronchoscopy is valuable and should be available, though not essential is end-tidal CO_2 is monitored.
- Ultrasound scanning of the neck and routine endoscopy during the procedure appear to reduce early complications.
- Percutaneous tracheostomy is not suitable for children.

17.2.3.5 WEANING FROM VENTILATORY SUPPORT

During the recovery phase, the most important transition made is that from mechanical ventilation to unassisted breathing, known as weaning. Weaning begins as soon as the causes of respiratory failure have resolved.

17.2.3.6 EXTUBATION CRITERIA ('SOA2P')

S – Secretions – minimal.
O – Oxygenation – good.
A – Alert.
A – Airway: without injury or compromise.
P – Pressures or parameters: measurements of tidal, volume, vital capacity, negative inspiratory force, etc.

17.2.4 Recovery Phase (Separation from the ICU)

During the recovery phase, the patient is weaned from full ventilatory support until breathing spontaneously and invasive monitoring devices can be removed. The patient and family are prepared for the transition from the ICU to general patient or intermediate care unit, and plans for further convalescence and rehabilitation are developed (see Table 17.1).[7]

Table 17.1 ICU Liberation ABCDEF Bundle			
Symptoms	**Monitoring Tools**	**Care**	**Done**
Pain	Critical-Care Pain Observation Tool (CCPOT) Numeric Rating Scale (NRS) Behavioural Pain Scale (BPS)	A: Assess, Prevent, and Manage Pain	☐
Agitation	Richmond Agitation-Sedation Scale (RASS) Sedation-Agitation Scale (SAS)	B: Both Spontaneous Awakening Trials (SAT) and Spontaneous Breathing Trials (SBT)	☐
Delirium	Confusion Assessment Method for the Intensive Care Unit (CAM-ICU) Intensive Care Delirium Screening Checklist	C: Choice of Analgesia and Sedation	☐
		D: Delirium: Assess, Prevent, and Manage	☐
		E: Early Mobility and Exercise	☐
		F: Family Engagement and Empowerment	☐
Source: Ely EW. *Crit Care Med.* 2017 February;45(2):321–30.			

17.3 EXTRACORPOREAL MEMBRANE OXYGENATION[8-10]

17.3.1 Overview

Extracorporeal membrane oxygenation, also known as 'lung rescue', is not a novel therapy in the true sense of the word. The first case report appeared in 1972. Thereafter, the first randomized, prospective study of ECMO in severe acute respiratory failure was published in 1979, with only four patients in each group surviving. The author's conclusion at the time, was that ECMO could support respiratory gas-exchange, but did not increase the probability of survival for severe ARDS.

ECMO is an expensive therapy, so outcomes should be unequivocally improved to justify its use. It is a technology that has been shown to be efficient in improving oxygenation but has substantial cost implications and limited evidence of survival benefit, depending on patient selection. It is envisaged, however, that as ECMO is more frequently employed and expertise is improved, new indications and exclusions may become apparent. This is a living science that will develop along with new technical developments.

17.3.2 Modes of ECMO

Currently, there are three types of ECMO available.

17.3.2.1 VENO-VENOUS ECMO (VV-ECMO)

Blood is extracted from the vena cava/right atrium and returned to the right atrium.

- Primary ARDS with refractory hypoxaemia.
- Pneumonia (particularly viral, but any pneumonia without multiple organ failure).
- Pulmonary contusion, gas inhalation, aspiration, smoke inhalation.
- Status asthmaticus or reversible airway obstruction not able to be ventilated conventionally.
- Pulmonary embolism (if haemodynamically stable).
- Hypoxaemic respiratory failure PaO_2/FiO_2 ratio <100 mm Hg despite optimum ventilator settings (tidal volume/PEEP/I:E ratio).
- Berlin consensus document – ARDS suggest ECMO if P/F ratio <70.
- Hypercapnoeic respiratory failure with pH <7.2.
- Ventilatory support as a bridge to lung transplantation.
- Cardiac/circulatory failure/refractory cardiogenic shock.
- Massive pulmonary embolism.
- Cardiac arrest.

17.3.2.2 VENO-ARTERIAL ECMO (VA-ECMO)

Blood is extracted from the right atrium and returned to the arterial system.

It allows haemodynamic support and is indicated for cardiac failure, with or without respiratory failure.

- Weaning from cardiopulmonary bypass after cardiac surgery.
- As a bridge to cardiac transplantation.
- Acute myocarditis.
- Pulmonary hypertension (after pulmonary endarterectomy or following surgery on congenital heart defects).

17.3.2.3 ARTERIO-VENOUS ECMO (AV-ECMO)

Facilitates gas exchange, especially carbon dioxide removal, by using the patient's own arterial pressure to pump blood through the circuit. The latter is sometimes referred to as an extracorporeal carbon dioxide removal (ECCO2R) system, as it is more efficient at CO_2 removal than it is at correcting hypoxaemia. Low-flow VV-ECMO may also be used primarily for ECCO2R.

The potential for improvement in oxygenation with VV-ECMO is less than that with VA-ECMO and is due to an increase in the central venous oxygen saturation, such that the shunted blood elevates overall arterial saturation despite a potential increase in shunt fraction from loss of hypoxic pulmonary vasoconstriction. This mode may, however, reduce pulmonary pressures and right ventricular strain through a similar mechanism. VV-ECMO also has a lower risk of thromboembolic complications, and because the lung is perfused, in contrast to VA-ECMO, pulmonary endocrine function remains normal. This allows for extracorporeal removal of carbon dioxide while providing lung rest, avoiding ventilator-induced lung injury. In addition, the dual-chamber cannula (Avalon Laboratories, Rancho Dominguez, CA, USA) drains the inferior and superior vena cava, returning the blood to the region of the tricuspid valve without significant re-recirculation (drainage of oxygenated blood injected by the return cannula when dual-catheter systems are utilized) and allowing better patient mobilization.

> **ECMO for respiratory failure results are better if instituted within 7 days of intubation.**

17.3.3 Exclusions

It is recommended that the following should be overall exclusions for ECMO:

- Non-availability of a trained multidisciplinary team with access to a specialized intensive care and cardiothoracic and vascular surgical services.
- Multiple-organ failure from severe sepsis or a systemic inflammatory response syndrome.
- Severe co-morbid illness that will impact significantly on life expectancy, for example, severe neurological injury, or overwhelming sepsis or any pre-existing condition that is incompatible with recovery.
- Pulmonary oedema from myocardial dysfunction, unless ECMO is a holding measure before transplantation, or the patient has acute myocarditis and likely to recover.
- Exacerbations of chronic obstructive pulmonary disease with respiratory failure.
- Inadequate recruitment and/or diuresis/dialysis in the presence of fluid overload.
- Technical difficulty associated with the procedure.
- Where systemic anticoagulation is contraindicated.
- Immunosuppression not likely to recover rapidly.
- Patients mechanically ventilated for longer than 7 days as underlying lung damage might be irreversible.
- Age >75 years.

Pitfall

Despite VA-ECMO improving oxygenation more than VV-ECMO, and the fact that there is no loss of hypoxic pulmonary vasoconstriction, there are increased risks associated with this method. The technique requires arterial cannulation with large catheters and therefore has the potential for limb ischaemia, and if blood is returned to a femoral artery, brain oxygenation cannot be guaranteed.

17.4 COAGULOPATHY OF MAJOR TRAUMA[11–13] (See also Chapter 5)

Trauma patients are susceptible to the early development of coagulopathy, and the most severely injured patients are coagulopathic on hospital admission. The coagulopathy is worsened by:

- *Haemodilution*: Dilutional thrombocytopenia is the most common coagulation abnormality in trauma patients.
- Consumption of clotting factors.

- *Hypothermia*: Causes platelet dysfunction and a reduction in the rate of the enzymatic clotting cascade.
- *Acidosis*: Metabolic derangements (especially acidosis), which also interfere with the clotting mechanism.

More recently in trauma, the focus has shifted from a disseminated intravascular coagulation (DIC) type coagulopathy without microthrombi, to extensive tissue trauma in combination with reduced perfusion in which the endothelium shows an increased expression of thrombomodulin, thus binding thrombin.

With the reduced levels of thrombin, there is a reduced production of fibrin. The thrombin–thrombomodulin complex activates protein C. The activated protein C inactivates co-factors V and VIII, causing anticoagulation. Activated protein C also inactivates plasminogen activator inhibitor type 1 increasing fibrinolysis. The thrombin–thrombomodulin complex also binds thrombin-activated fibrinolysis inhibitor (TAFI), reducing the inhibition of fibrinolysis. In trauma-induced coagulopathy, the shifting balance between the binding of protein C and TAFI may be the cause of the different clinical presentations. Long-standing hypotension, acidosis, and ischaemia give a release of a tissue plasminogen activator. Together with reduced liver function, the consumption of coagulation factors, activated plasmin, and fibrin degradation products, haemostasis is compromised.

Platelet survival is so short that severe thrombocytopenia is common. There is a consumptive deficiency of coagulation factors.

Excess plasmin generation is reflected by reduced plasma levels of fibrin and elevated levels of fibrin degradation products, with abnormal concentrations being found in 85% of patients. In addition, Tranexamic acid may have a major role in clot stabilization[14] and reversal of the coagulopathy if given early within three hours of injury. Despite the increased use of tranexamic acid, the gathering and validity of the data has been called into question in a major trauma centre environment. In addition, a recent study indicated that most severely injured patients have a fibrinolysis shutdown, and therefore, tranexamic acid may have no effect.[15] In major trauma centres, goal-directed haemostasis using visco haemostatic assays (VHA) is appropriate.

17.4.1 **Management**

The management of diffuse bleeding after trauma relies on haemorrhage control, active re-warming, and replacement of blood products using a haemostatic resuscitation ischaemia. Clinically, it is difficult to identify the entities of the coagulopathy of major trauma described above. The condition will not resolve until the underlying cause has been corrected; while this is being achieved, component therapy is indicated.

Among patients who require active correction of haemorrhagic coagulopathy, use of a red cells:plasma:platelets ratio of 1:1:1 results in more rapid haemostasis and decreased mortality (the PROPPR trial).[16]

17.5 **HYPOTHERMIA**

While hypothermia may itself cause cardiac arrest, it is also protective to the brain through a reduction in metabolic rate and thus reduced oxygen requirements. Oxygen consumption is reduced by 50% at a core temperature of 30°C. The American Heart Association guidelines recommend that the hypothermic patient who appears dead should not be considered so until a near-normal body temperature is reached. However, hypothermia is on balance extremely harmful to trauma patients, especially by virtue of the way it alters oxygen delivery. Therefore, the patient must be warmed, and further heat loss minimized at all costs.

Primary hypothermia is common after immersion injury. Re-warming must take place with intensive monitoring. Patients who have spontaneous respiratory effort and whose hearts are beating, no matter how severe the bradycardia, should not receive unnecessary resuscitation procedures. A hypothermic heart is resistant to both electrical and pharmacological cardioversion, especially if the core temperature is below 29.5°C, and cardiopulmonary resuscitation should be continued if necessary. Patients are at high risk of ventricular arrhythmias, but recent studies have not shown any increase in ventricular arrhythmias with rapid rewarming. Survival from posttrauma hypothermia with a core temperature if less than 32°C is unusual.

Resuscitation should not be abandoned while the core temperature is subnormal, since it may be difficult to distinguish between cerebro-protective hypothermia and hypothermia resulting from brainstem death.

Secondary hypothermia occurs secondary to the metabolic derangements from trauma and for this group of patients rapid re-warming is far more important for haemostasis. The same methods are used, however, these must be more aggressive, while controlling haemorrhage and securing the airway, giving warmed blood products, and preparing for surgical intervention.

External measures

- Removal of wet or cold clothing and drying of the patient.
- Infrared (radiant) heat.
- Electrical heating blankets.
- Warm air heating blankets.

Pitfall

In the presence of hypothermia, 'space blankets' are ineffective, since there is minimal intrinsic body heat to reflect.

Internal measures

- Heated, humidified respiratory gases to 42°C.
- Intravenous fluids warmed to 37°C.
- Gastric lavage with warmed fluids (usually saline at 42°C).
- Continuous bladder lavage with water at 42°C.
- Peritoneal lavage with potassium-free dialysate at 42°C (20 mL/kg every 15 minutes).
- Intrapleural lavage.
- Extracorporeal (ECMO) rewarming.

17.6 MULTISYSTEM ORGAN DYSFUNCTION SYNDROME (MODS)

MODS is a clinical syndrome characterized by the progressive failure of multiple and interdependent organs. The 'dysfunction' identifies a phenomenon in which organ function is not capable of maintaining homeostasis, so it occurs along a continuum of progressive organ failure, rather than absolute failure. The lungs, liver, and kidneys are the principal target organs; however, failure of the cardiovascular and central nervous system may be prominent as well. The main inciting factors in trauma patients are haemorrhagic shock and infection. As life support and resuscitation techniques have improved, so the incidence of MODS has increased.

MODS/MOF develops because of local inflammation with activation of the innate immune system, and a subsequent uncontrolled or inappropriate systemic inflammatory response to inciting factors such as severe tissue injury (e.g. brain, lung, or soft tissue), hypoperfusion, or infection. Two basic models have emerged: the 'one-hit' model involves a single insult that initiates a SIRS, which may result in progressive MODS, whereas the 'two-hit' model involves sequential insults that may lead to MODS. The initial insult may prime the inflammatory response such that a second insult (even a modest one) results in an exaggerated inflammatory response and subsequent organ dysfunction.

The early development of MODS (<3 days post-injury) is usually a consequence of shock or inadequate resuscitation, while late onset is usually a result of severe infection (see also Chapter 4).

Specific therapy for MODS is currently limited, apart from providing adequate and full resuscitation, treatment of infection, and general ICU organ supportive care. Strategies to prevent MODS include adequate fluid resuscitation to establish and maintain tissue oxygenation, debridement of devitalized tissue, early fracture fixation and stabilization, early enteral nutritional support when possible, the prevention and treatment of nosocomial infections, and early mobility and resumption of exercise.

17.7 SYSTEMIC INFLAMMATORY RESPONSE SYNDROME (See also Chapter 4)

Fifty per cent of patients with 'sepsis' are abacteraemic. It is also recognized that the aetiology in these abacteraemic patients may be burns, pancreatitis, significant soft tissue and destructive injuries to tissue, particularly when associated with shock. The common theme through all these various injuries and types of sepsis is that the inflammatory cascade has been initiated and runs amok. Once the inflammatory response has been initiated, it leads to systemic symptoms that may or may not be beneficial or harmful.

Patients who have one or more primary components are thought to have SIRS. The primary components associated with SIRS include:

- Temperature <36°C or >38°C.
- Heart rate >90 beats per minute.
- Respiratory rate >20 breaths per minute.
- Deranged arterial gases: partial pressure of carbon dioxide ($PaCO_2$) <32 mm Hg (4.2 kPa).
- White blood count >12.0 × 10^9/L or <4.0 × 10^9/L or 0.10% immature neutrophils.

17.8 SEPSIS

17.8.1 Definitions

International consensus definitions for sepsis and septic shock were suggested in 2016,[17] and reviewed in 2018.[18]

17.8.1.1 SEPSIS

Sepsis is SIRS plus documented infection.

17.8.1.2 SEVERE SEPSIS

Severe sepsis is sepsis plus organ dysfunction, hypoperfusion abnormalities, or hypotension.

17.8.1.3 SEPTIC SHOCK

Septic shock is defined as sepsis-induced hypotension despite fluid resuscitation. For surgical patients, however, the new definitions do not reliably cover the abacteraemic group and are not universally accepted.[19]

One of the corollary concepts that has grown out of our understanding of SIRS is that the inflammatory cascade is not to be interpreted as harmful. It is only when dysregulation occurs that it is a problem in patient management. The second concept is that cytokines are messengers, and that we must not kill the messenger. Whether or not we can control them by either up-regulation or down-regulation remains to be proven by careful human studies.

17.8.2 Surviving Sepsis Guidelines

Updated 'Surviving Sepsis Campaign: International Guidelines for Management of Severe Sepsis and Septic Shock' were published in 2004, 2008, 2012,[20] and 2016.[21]

A full summary of the guidelines are given in Table 17.2.

17.9 ANTIBIOTICS

The goal of antibiotic treatment is to improve survival; however, preventing the emergence of antibiotic resistance is also important.

There must be a clear distinction between prophylaxis and treatment.

There is good evidence to limit the use of antibiotics in the critically ill trauma patient.[22]

There is conflicting evidence regarding the need for routine antibiotics with tube thoracostomy. For thoraco-abdominal injuries requiring operation, a single dose of broad-spectrum antibiotics is indicated. Prolonged courses of antibiotics, extending beyond 24 hours, are not currently indicated in most patients.[23]

For patients with hollow viscus injuries or closed space infections, with major contamination, once the patient has surgical source control obtained, antibiotics can be limited to a short course.[24]

Patients with open fractures are frequently treated with both Gram-negative and Gram-positive prophylaxis for long periods. There is no evidence for this practice, nor for whether management should be any different from that for torso injury.[25,26]

Patients in the ICU on mechanical ventilation, with or without known aspiration, have *no indication* for antibiotics to prevent pneumonia. In fact, this practice has hastened the onset of antibiotic resistance worldwide.

According to the Centers for Disease Control, a diagnosis of pneumonia must meet the following criteria:

- Rales or dullness to percussion AND any of the following:
  - New purulent sputum or a change in sputum.
  - Culture growth of an organism from blood or tracheal aspirate, bronchial brushing, or biopsy.
  - Radiographic evidence of new or progressive infiltrate, consolidation, cavitation, or effusion.

AND any of the following:

- Isolation of virus or detection of viral antigen in respiratory secretions.
- Diagnostic antibody titres for pathogen.
- Histopathological evidence of pneumonia.

For ventilator-associated pneumonia (VAP) there are new guidelines.[27]

The VAP diagnosis interventions considered most appropriate for inclusion in the care bundle were as follows:

- Early chest x-ray with expert interpretation within 1 hour.
- Immediate reporting of respiratory secretion Gram-stain findings, including cells.

Table 17.2 Surviving Sepsis Guidelines 2016[21]

A. **Initial Resuscitation – Goals**

Sepsis-induced hypoperfusion is defined as hypotension persisting after initial fluid challenge or a blood lactate of ≥4 mmol/L.

1. Sepsis and septic shock are medical emergencies, and we recommend that treatment and resuscitation begin immediately (BPS).
2. We recommend that, following initial fluid resuscitation, additional fluids be guided by frequent reassessment of haemodynamic status (BPS).
3. We recommend further haemodynamic assessment (such as assessing cardiac function) to determine the type of shock if the clinical examination does not lead to a clear diagnosis (BPS).
4. We recommend that, in the resuscitation from sepsis-induced hypoperfusion, at least 30 mL/kg of IV crystalloid fluid be given within the first 3 hours (strong recommendation, low quality of evidence).
5. We suggest that dynamic over static variables be used to predict fluid responsiveness, where available (weak recommendation, low quality of evidence).
6. We recommend an initial target mean arterial pressure (MAP) of 65 mm Hg in patients with septic shock requiring vasopressors (strong recommendation, moderate quality of evidence).
7. We suggest guiding resuscitation to normalize lactate in patients with elevated lactate levels as a marker of tissue hypoperfusion (weak recommendation, low quality of evidence).
   - Central venous pressure (CVP) 8–12 mm Hg.
   - Mean arterial pressure (MAP) ≥65 mm Hg.
   - Urine output ≥0.5 mL/kg.
   - Central venous oxygen saturation ≥70% or arterial saturation ≥90%.

B. **Screening for Sepsis and Performance Improvement**

1. We recommend that hospitals and hospital systems have a performance improvement programme for sepsis, including sepsis screening for acutely ill, high-risk patients (BPS).
   - Cultures should be taken within 45 minutes of initial diagnosis, and *before* initiation of appropriate antibiotic therapy.

C. **Diagnosis**

1. We recommend that appropriate routine microbiologic cultures (including blood) be obtained before starting antimicrobial therapy in patients with suspected sepsis or septic shock if doing so results in no substantial delay in the start of antimicrobials (BPS).
   Remarks: Appropriate routine microbiologic cultures always include at least two sets of blood cultures (aerobic and anaerobic):
   - Through intravenous device.
   - Percutaneous.
   - Identify source through imaging studies.
   - Draw procalcitonin level (PCT) – preferable to C reactive protein (CRP).

D. **Antimicrobial Therapy**

1. We recommend that administration of IV antimicrobials be initiated as soon as possible after recognition and **within one hour** for both sepsis and septic shock (strong recommendation).
2. We recommend that dosing strategies of antimicrobials be optimized based on accepted pharmacokinetic/pharmacodynamic principles and specific drug properties in patients with sepsis or septic shock (BPS).
3. If combination therapy is initially used for septic shock, we recommend de-escalation with discontinuation of combination therapy within the first few days in response to clinical improvement and/or evidence of infection resolution. This applies to both targeted (for culture-positive infections) and empiric (for culture-negative infections) combination therapy (BPS).
4. We recommend daily assessment for de-escalation of antimicrobial therapy in patients with sepsis and septic shock (BPS).

(Continued)

Table 17.2 (*Continued*) Surviving Sepsis Guidelines 2016[21]

5. We recommend that empiric antimicrobial therapy be narrowed once pathogen identification and sensitivities are established and/or adequate clinical improvement is noted (BPS).
6. We recommend **against** sustained systemic antimicrobial prophylaxis in patients with severe inflammatory states of non-infectious origin (e.g. severe pancreatitis, burn injury) (BPS).
7. We recommend empiric broad-spectrum therapy with one or more antimicrobials for patients presenting with sepsis or septic shock to cover all likely pathogens (including bacterial and potentially fungal or viral coverage) (strong recommendation, moderate quality of evidence; grade applies to both conditions).
8. We recommend against combination therapy for the routine treatment of neutropenic sepsis/bacteraemia (strong recommendation, moderate quality of evidence).
9. We suggest empiric combination therapy (using at least two antibiotics of different antimicrobial classes) aimed at the most likely bacterial pathogen(s) for the initial management of septic shock (weak recommendation, low quality of evidence).
10. We suggest that combination therapy not be routinely used for ongoing treatment of most other serious infections, including bacteraemia and sepsis without shock (weak recommendation, low quality of evidence).
    Remarks: This does not preclude the use of multidrug therapy to broaden antimicrobial activity.
11. We suggest that an antimicrobial treatment duration of 7–10 days is adequate for most serious infections associated with sepsis and septic shock (weak recommendation, low quality of evidence).
12. We suggest that longer courses are appropriate in patients who have a slow clinical response, undrainable foci of infection, bacteraemia with *S. aureus*, some fungal and viral infections, or immunological deficiencies, including neutropenia (weak recommendation, low quality of evidence).
13. We suggest that shorter courses are appropriate in some patients, particularly those with rapid clinical resolution following effective source control of intra-abdominal or urinary sepsis and those with anatomically uncomplicated pyelonephritis (weak recommendation, low quality of evidence).
14. We suggest that measurement of procalcitonin levels can be used to support shortening the duration of antimicrobial therapy in sepsis patients (weak recommendation, low quality of evidence).
15. We suggest that procalcitonin levels can be used to support the discontinuation of empiric antibiotics in patients who initially appeared to have sepsis, but subsequently have limited clinical evidence of infection (weak recommendation, low quality of evidence).
    - Antibiotic therapy should ideally consist of an extended spectrum beta-lactam, and a fluoroquinolone (for *Pseudomonas*) or a macrolide (for *Streptococcus* or *Klebsiella*).
    - Duration of therapy should be 7–10 days, and antibiotics should be discontinued guided by low procalcitonin, taken at days 3, 5, 7, or 10.
    Remarks: It is important to note that procalcitonin and all other biomarkers can provide only supportive and supplemental data to clinical assessment. Decisions on initiating, altering, or discontinuing antimicrobial therapy should never be made solely based on changes in any biomarker, including procalcitonin.

E. **Source Control**

1. We recommend that a specific anatomic diagnosis of infection requiring emergent source control be identified or excluded as rapidly as possible in patients with sepsis or septic shock, and that any required source control intervention be implemented as soon as medically and logistically practical after the diagnosis is made (BPS).
2. We recommend prompt removal of intravascular access devices that are a possible source of sepsis. (BPS).
3. We recommend selective oral decontamination using oral chlorhexidine gluconate should be used throughout, to reduce the risk of ventilator associated pneumonia.is or septic shock after other vascular access has been established (BPS).

(Continued)

Table 17.2 (*Continued*) Surviving Sepsis Guidelines 2016[21]

F. **Fluid Therapy**
1. We recommend that a fluid challenge technique be applied where fluid administration is continued if haemodynamic factors continue to improve (BPS).
2. We recommend **against** using hydroxyethyl starches (HESs) for intravascular volume replacement in patients with sepsis or septic shock (strong recommendation, high quality of evidence).
3. We recommend crystalloids as the fluid of choice for initial resuscitation and subsequent intravascular volume replacement in patients with sepsis and septic shock (strong recommendation, moderate quality of evidence).
4. We suggest using either balanced crystalloids or saline for fluid resuscitation of patients with sepsis or septic shock (weak recommendation, low quality of evidence).
5. We suggest using albumin in addition to crystalloids for initial resuscitation and subsequent intravascular volume replacement in patients with sepsis and septic shock when patients require substantial amounts of crystalloids (weak recommendation, low quality of evidence).
6. We suggest using crystalloids over gelatins when resuscitating patients with sepsis or septic shock (weak recommendation, low quality of evidence).

G. **Vasoactive Medications**
1. We recommend **against** using low-dose dopamine for renal protection (strong recommendation, high quality of evidence).
2. We recommend norepinephrine (noradrenaline) as the first-choice vasopressor (strong recommendation, moderate quality of evidence).
3. We suggest adding either vasopressin (DDAVP) (up to 0.03 U/min) (weak recommendation, moderate quality of evidence) or epinephrine (adrenaline) (weak recommendation, low quality of evidence) to norepinephrine with the intent of raising MAP to target or adding vasopressin (up to 0.03 U/min) (weak recommendation, moderate quality of evidence) to decrease norepinephrine dosage.
4. We suggest using dopamine as an alternative vasopressor agent to norepinephrine **only** in highly selected patients (e.g. patients with low risk of tachyarrhythmias and absolute or relative bradycardia) (weak recommendation, low quality of evidence).
5. We suggest using dobutamine in patients who show evidence of persistent hypoperfusion despite adequate fluid loading and the use of vasopressor agents (weak recommendation, low quality of evidence). A trial of dobutamine infusion up to 20 µgm/kg/min may be administered in the presence of:
   - Myocardial dysfunction (elevated cardiac filling pressures and low cardiac output.
   - Ongoing signs of hyperperfusion, despite adequate volume and MAP.
   - Do NOT use a strategy to increase cardiac index to supranormal levels.
     Remarks: If initiated, vasopressor dosing should be titrated to an end point reflecting perfusion, and the agent reduced or discontinued in the face of worsening hypotension or arrhythmias.
6. We suggest that all patients requiring vasopressors have an arterial catheter placed as soon as practical if resources are available (weak recommendation, very low quality of evidence).
   - Vasopressor therapy can be used to achieve a minimum MAP of 65 mm.
   - Phenylephrine is NOT recommended except in the presence of serious arrhythmias, cardiac output is known to be high, and blood pressure is consistently low, and where other measures have failed.

H. **Corticosteroids**
1. We suggest **against** using IV hydrocortisone to treat septic shock patients if adequate fluid resuscitation and vasopressor therapy can restore haemodynamic stability. If this is not achievable, we suggest IV hydrocortisone at a dose of 200 mg per day, preferably by infusion. In treated patients, hydrocortisone should be tapered when vasopressors are no longer required (weak recommendation, low quality of evidence).

(Continued)

Table 17.2 (*Continued*) Surviving Sepsis Guidelines 2016[21]

I. **Blood Product Administration**

1. Once tissue hypoperfusion has been resolved, and in the absence of extenuating circumstances (e.g. active haemorrhage, myocardial ischaemia), transfusion should ONLY take place if the haemoglobin is <7.0 Gm/dl, to achieve a target of 7–9 G/dl.

2. Fresh frozen plasma (FFP) should NOT be used to correct clotting abnormalities in the absence of active bleeding or planned invasive procedures.

3. Use TEG or RoTEM goal-directed maintenance of coagulation parameters.

4. In patients with severe sepsis, administer platelets:
   - In the absence of bleeding ONLY when counts are less than 10,000/mm³.
   - If risk of bleeding, administer platelets when count is >20,000/mm³.
   - If actively bleeding, administer platelets for a minimum of >50,000/mm³.

5. We recommend that RBC transfusion occur only when haemoglobin concentration decreases to <7.0 g/dL in adults in the absence of extenuating circumstances, such as myocardial ischaemia, severe hypoxemia, or acute haemorrhage (strong recommendation, high quality of evidence).

6. We recommend **against** the use of erythropoietin for treatment of anaemia associated with sepsis (strong recommendation, moderate quality of evidence).

7. We suggest **against** the use of fresh frozen plasma to correct clotting abnormalities in the absence of bleeding or planned invasive procedures (weak recommendation, very low quality of evidence).

8. We suggest prophylactic platelet transfusion when counts are <10,000/mm³ (10 × 109/L) in the absence of apparent bleeding and when counts are <20,000/mm³ (20 × 109/L) if the patient has a significant risk of bleeding. Higher platelet counts (≥50,000/mm³ [50 × 109/L]) are advised for active bleeding, surgery, or invasive procedures (weak recommendation, very low quality of evidence).

J. **Immunoglobulin Administration**

1. We suggest against the use of IV immunoglobulins in patients with sepsis or septic shock (weak recommendation, low quality of evidence).

K. **Blood Purification**

1. We make no recommendation regarding the use of blood purification techniques.

L. **Anticoagulants**

1. We recommend against the use of antithrombin for the treatment of sepsis and septic shock (strong recommendation, moderate quality of evidence).

2. We make no recommendation regarding the use of thrombomodulin or heparin for the treatment of sepsis or septic shock.

M. **Mechanical Ventilation of Sepsis-Induced ARDS**

1. We recommend that mechanically ventilated sepsis patients be maintained with the head of the bed elevated between 30° and 45° to limit aspiration risk and to prevent the development of VAP (strong recommendation, low quality of evidence).

2. We recommend using spontaneous breathing trials in mechanically ventilated patients with sepsis who are ready for weaning (strong recommendation, high quality of evidence).

3. We recommend using a target tidal volume of 6 mL/kg predicted body weight (PBW) compared with 12 mL/kg in adult patients with sepsis-induced ARDS (strong recommendation, high quality of evidence).

4. We recommend **against** the routine use of the PA catheter for patients with sepsis-induced ARDS (strong recommendation, high quality of evidence).
   Remark: PA catheters have been generally replaced with cardiac output computed data.

5. We recommend using an upper limit goal for plateau pressures of 30 cm H_2O over higher plateau pressures in adult patients with sepsis-induced severe ARDS (strong recommendation, moderate quality of evidence).

(Continued)

Table 17.2 (*Continued*) Surviving Sepsis Guidelines 2016[21]

6. We recommend against using high-frequency oscillatory ventilation (HFOV) in adult patients with sepsis-induced ARDS (strong recommendation, moderate quality of evidence).
7. We recommend using prone over supine position in adult patients with sepsis-induced ARDS and a PaO_2/FIO_2 ratio <150 (strong recommendation, moderate quality of evidence).
8. We recommend a conservative fluid strategy for patients with established sepsis-induced ARDS who do not have evidence of tissue hypoperfusion (strong recommendation, moderate quality of evidence).
9. We recommend **against** the use of β-2 agonists for the treatment of patients with sepsis-induced ARDS without bronchospasm (strong recommendation, moderate quality of evidence).
10. We suggest using higher PEEP (8–12 cm H_2O) over lower PEEP in adult patients with sepsis-induced moderate to severe ARDS (weak recommendation, moderate quality of evidence).
11. We suggest using recruitment manoeuvres in adult patients with sepsis-induced, severe ARDS (weak recommendation, moderate quality of evidence).
12. We suggest using neuromuscular blocking agents (NMBAs) for ≤48 hours in adult patients with sepsis-induced ARDS and a PaO_2/FIO_2 ratio <150 mm Hg (weak recommendation, moderate quality of evidence).
13. We recommend using a weaning protocol in mechanically ventilated patients with sepsis-induced respiratory failure who can tolerate weaning (strong recommendation, moderate quality of evidence).
    - A weaning protocol be in place and mechanically ventilated patients undergo spontaneous breathing trials regularly to evaluate weaning potential. The patient MUST satisfy the following criteria:
    a. Patient must be arousable.
    b. Patient must be haemodynamically stable without vasopressors.
    c. No new potentially serious conditions.
    d. Low ventilatory requirements:
        i. PEEP <8 cm H_2O.
        ii. Pressure support <10 cm H_2O.
        iii. Rate <8 bpm.
    e. Low FiO_2 requirements (≤0.4) which can safely be delivered by face mask.
    f. Extubate when successful and safe.
14. We suggest using lower tidal volumes over higher tidal volumes in adult patients with sepsis-induced respiratory failure without ARDS (weak recommendation, low quality of evidence).
15. We make no recommendation regarding the use of non-invasive ventilation (NIV) for patients with sepsis-induced ARDS.

N. Sedation and Analgesia
1. We recommend that continuous or intermittent sedation be minimized in mechanically ventilated sepsis patients, targeting specific titration end points (BPS).

O. Glucose Control
1. We recommend that blood glucose values be monitored every 1–2 hours until glucose values and insulin infusion rates are stable, then every 4 hours thereafter in patients receiving insulin infusions (BPS).
2. We recommend that glucose levels obtained with point-of-care testing of capillary blood be interpreted with caution because such measurements may not accurately estimate arterial blood or plasma glucose values (BPS).
3. We recommend a protocolized approach to blood glucose management in ICU patients with sepsis, commencing insulin dosing when two consecutive blood glucose levels are >6 mmol/dL (180 mg/dL). This approach should target an upper blood glucose level ≤6 mmol/L, (180 mg/dL) rather than an upper target blood glucose level ≤4 mmol/L (110 mg/dL) (strong recommendation, high quality of evidence).
4. We suggest the use of arterial blood rather than capillary blood for point-of-care testing using glucose meters if patients have arterial catheters (weak recommendation, low quality of evidence).

(Continued)

Table 17.2 (*Continued*) Surviving Sepsis Guidelines 2016[21]

P. **Renal Replacement Therapy (RRT)**
  1. We suggest that either continuous RRT (CRRT) or intermittent RRT be used in patients with sepsis and acute kidney injury (weak recommendation, moderate quality of evidence).
  2. We suggest using CRRT to facilitate management of fluid balance in haemodynamically unstable septic patients (weak recommendation, very low quality of evidence).
  3. We suggest against the use of RRT in patients with sepsis and acute kidney injury for increase in creatinine or oliguria without other definitive indications for dialysis (weak recommendation, low quality of evidence).

Q. **Bicarbonate Therapy**
  1. We suggest **against** the use of sodium bicarbonate therapy to improve haemodynamics or to reduce vasopressor requirements in patients with hypoperfusion-induced lactic acidaemia with pH ≥ 7.15 (weak recommendation, moderate quality of evidence).

R. **Venous Thromboembolism (VTE) Prophylaxis**
  1. We recommend pharmacological prophylaxis (unfractionated heparin [UFH] or low-molecular-weight heparin [LMWH]) against VTE in the absence of contraindications to the use of these agents (strong recommendation, moderate quality of evidence).
  2. We recommend LMWH rather than UFH for VTE prophylaxis in the absence of contraindications to the use of LMWH (strong recommendation, moderate quality of evidence).
  3. We suggest combination pharmacological VTE prophylaxis and mechanical prophylaxis, whenever possible (weak recommendation, low quality of evidence).
  4. We suggest mechanical VTE prophylaxis when pharmacologic VTE is contraindicated (weak recommendation, low quality of evidence).

S. **Stress Ulcer Prophylaxis**
  1. We recommend that stress ulcer prophylaxis be given to patients with sepsis or septic shock who have risk factors for gastrointestinal (GI) bleeding (strong recommendation, low quality of evidence).
  2. We recommend **against** stress ulcer prophylaxis in patients without risk factors for GI bleeding (BPS).
     • Patients with no risk factors need no prophylaxis.
     • Trauma patients should receive Sucralfate, to minimize the risk of VAP.
     • High risk patients with bleeding risk should receive protein pump inhibitors.
  3. We suggest using either proton pump inhibitors (PPIs) or histamine-2 receptor antagonist (H$_2$RAs) when stress ulcer prophylaxis is indicated (weak recommendation, low quality of evidence).

T. **Nutrition**
  1. We recommend against the administration of early parenteral nutrition alone or parenteral nutrition in combination with enteral feedings (but rather initiate early enteral nutrition) in critically ill patients with sepsis or septic shock who can be fed enterally (strong recommendation, moderate quality of evidence).
  2. We recommend **against** the administration of parenteral nutrition alone or in combination with enteral feeds (but rather to initiate IV glucose and advance enteral feeds as tolerated), over the first 7 days in critically ill patients with sepsis or septic shock for whom early enteral feeding is not feasible (strong recommendation, moderate quality of evidence).
  3. We recommend **against** the use of IV selenium to treat sepsis and septic shock (strong recommendation, moderate quality of evidence).
  4. We recommend **against** the use of glutamine to treat sepsis and septic shock (strong recommendation, moderate quality of evidence).
  5. We recommend **against** the use of omega-3 fatty acids as an immune supplement in critically ill patients with sepsis or septic shock (strong recommendation, low quality of evidence).
  6. We suggest the early initiation of enteral feeding rather than a complete fast or only IV glucose in critically ill patients with sepsis or septic shock who can be fed enterally (weak recommendation, low quality of evidence).

(Continued)

Table 17.2 (*Continued*) Surviving Sepsis Guidelines 2016[21]

7. We suggest either early trophic/hypocaloric or early full enteral feeding in critically ill patients with sepsis or septic shock; if trophic/hypocaloric feeding is the initial strategy, then feeds should be advanced according to patient tolerance (weak recommendation, moderate quality of evidence).
8. We suggest the use of prokinetic agents in critically ill patients with sepsis or septic shock and feeding intolerance (weak recommendation, low quality of evidence).
9. We suggest against routinely monitoring gastric residual volumes (GRVs) in critically ill patients with sepsis or septic shock (weak recommendation, low quality of evidence).
10. However, we suggest measurement of gastric residuals in patients with feeding intolerance or who are at high risk of aspiration (weak recommendation, very low quality of evidence).
    Remarks: This recommendation refers to non-surgical critically ill patients with sepsis or septic shock.
11. We suggest placement of post-pyloric feeding tubes in critically ill patients with sepsis or septic shock with feeding intolerance or who are at high risk of aspiration (weak recommendation, low quality of evidence).
12. We suggest **against** the use of arginine to treat sepsis and septic shock (weak recommendation, low quality of evidence).
13. We make no recommendation about the use of carnitine for sepsis and septic shock.
    - Administer enteral feeds within 48 hours.
    - Avoid full mandatory caloric feeding during the first week, or on inotropes.
    - Use nutrition with NO immuno-modulation supplementation in severe sepsis.

U. Setting Goals of Care
1. We recommend that goals of care and prognosis be discussed with patients and families (BPS).
2. We recommend that goals of care be incorporated into treatment and end-of-life care planning, utilizing palliative care principles where appropriate (strong recommendation, moderate quality of evidence).
3. We suggest that goals of care be addressed as early as feasible, but no later than within 72 hours of ICU admission (weak recommendation, low quality of evidence).

BPS: Best Practice Statement	Appropriate when benefit or harm is unequivocal	
Recommendations:	Strong	'We recommend'
	Weak	'We suggest'
Quality of Evidence:	High	
	Moderate	
	Weak	

Source: Rhodes A et al. *Crit Care Med.* 2017;45:486–552.

The VAP treatment interventions considered most appropriate for inclusion in the care bundle were as follows:

- Immediate treatment after microbiological sampling.
- Empirical therapy based on a knowledge of local pathogens and an assessment of risk factors.
- De-escalation of antibiotics in responding patients once culture results are available.
- Assessment of response to treatment within 72 hours.
- Short-therapy duration (8 days) if the patient is on an appropriate regimen and not infected by a multidrug-resistant pathogen.

Given the variations in antibiotic susceptibility profiles of VAP pathogens, both in location and with respect to changes over time, it is inappropriate to specify the use of specific antibiotic regimens.

17.10 ABDOMINAL COMPARTMENT SYNDROME (ACS)

17.10.1 Introduction

Raised intra-abdominal pressure (IAP) has far-reaching consequences for the physiology of the patient. There have been major developments in our understanding of IAP and intra-abdominal hypertension (IAH). The syndrome that results when organs fail as a result is known as 'abdominal compartment syndrome' (ACS). Increasingly, it is being recognized that ACS is not uncommon in trauma patients, and failure to consider its prevention, detect it in a timely fashion, and treat it aggressively results in a high mortality.

The formation of the World Society of the Abdominal Compartment Syndrome[28] has been a major advance, with the production of consensus definitions, the formation of a research policy, multicentre trials and the publication of the consensus guidelines on ACS. The first World Congress on ACS was held in 2004 and an internal consensus agreement relating to definitions, updated in 2009 and 2013. Various aspects were defined (see Table 17.3).[29]

17.10.2 Definition of ACS

The concept of IAP measurement and its significance is increasingly important in the ICU and is rapidly becoming part of routine care. Patients with raised IAP require close and careful monitoring, aggressive resuscitation, and a low index of suspicion for the requirement of surgical abdominal decompression.

- *Primary ACS* develops owing to conditions associated with injury or illness in the abdominopelvic region. This includes conditions requiring emergency surgical or angioradiological intervention, including damage control laparotomy, bleeding pelvic fractures, massive retroperitoneal haematomas, and failed non-operative management of solid organ injuries, and following disease processes such as severe acute pancreatitis.
- *Secondary ACS* develops from causes originating outside the abdomen, such as sepsis, capillary leak, major burns, and over-enthusiastic fluid resuscitation.

17.10.3 Pathophysiology

The incidence of IAH in post-operative trauma patients ranges from 20% to 50%. It is common after many forms of emergency surgery. The causes of acutely increased IAP are usually multifactorial (see Table 17.4). Raised IAP occurs commonly with over-enthusiastic fluid resuscitation.[30] In addition to the direct causes shown, hypothermia, acidosis, and overall injury severity will further exacerbate the problem.

17.10.4 Effect of Raised IAP on Individual Organ Function

17.10.4.1 CARDIOVASCULAR

Increased IAP reduces cardiac output as well as increasing central venous pressure, systemic vascular resistance, pulmonary artery pressure and pulmonary artery wedge pressure. Cardiac output is affected mainly by a reduction in stroke volume, secondary to a reduction in preload and an increase in afterload. This is further aggravated by hypovolaemia. Paradoxically, in the presence of hypovolaemia, an increase in IAP can be temporarily associated with an increase in cardiac output. It has been identified that venous stasis occurs in the legs of patients with abdominal pressures above 12 mm Hg. In addition, recent studies of patients undergoing laparoscopic cholecystectomy show up to a fourfold increase in renin and aldosterone levels.

17.10.4.2 RESPIRATORY

In association with increased IAP, there is diaphragmatic splinting, exerting a restrictive effect on the lungs, with a reduction in ventilation, decreased lung compliance, an increase in airway pressures, and a reduction in tidal volumes.

In critically ill ventilated patients, the effect on the respiratory system can be significant, resulting in reduced lung volumes, impaired gas exchange, and high ventilatory pressures. Hypercarbia can occur, and the resulting acidosis can be exacerbated by simultaneous cardiovascular depression as a result of raised IAP. The effects of raised IAP on the respiratory system in ICU can sometimes be life-threatening, requiring urgent abdominal decompression. Patients with true ACS undergoing abdominal decompression demonstrate a remarkable change in their intra-operative vital signs.

17.10.4.3 VISCERAL PERFUSION

There is an association between IAP, and visceral perfusion as measured by gastric pH. This has recently been

Table 17.3 Final 2013 Consensus Definitions of the World Society of Abdominal Compartment Syndrome[29]

2006 Consensus Statements	
Definition 1	Intra-abdominal pressure (IAP) is the steady-state pressure concealed within the abdominal cavity.
Definition 2	The reference standard for intermittent IAP measurement is via the bladder with a maximal instillation volume of 25 mL of sterile saline.
Definition 3	IAP should be expressed in mm Hg and measured at end-expiration in the complete supine position after ensuring that abdominal muscle contractions are absent and with the transducer zeroed at the level of the mid-axillary line.
Definition 4	Normal IAP is approximately 5–7 mm Hg in critically ill adults.
Definition 5	IAH is defined by a sustained or repeated pathological elevation of IAP $\geq$12 mm Hg.
Definition 6	ACS is defined as a sustained IAP $\geq$20 mm Hg (with or without an abdominal perfusion pressure (APP) <60 mm Hg) that is associated with new organ dysfunction/failure.
Definition 7	IAH is graded as follows: • Grade I: IAP 12–15 mm Hg. • Grade II: IAP 16–20 mm Hg. • Grade III: IAP 21–25 mm Hg. • Grade IV: IAP >25 mm Hg.
Definition 8	Primary ACS is a condition associated with injury or disease in the abdominopelvic region that frequently requires early surgical or interventional radiological intervention.
Definition 9	Secondary ACS refers to conditions that do not originate from the abdominopelvic region.
Definition 10	Recurrent ACS refers to the condition in which ACS redevelops following previous surgical or medical treatment of primary or secondary ACS.
Definition 11	Abdominal perfusion pressure (APP) = Mean arterial pressure (MAP) – Intra-abdominal pressure (IAP).
2013 New Definitions Accepted by the Consensus Panel	
Definition 12	A polycompartment syndrome is a condition where two or more anatomical compartments have elevated compartmental pressure.
Definition 13	Abdominal compliance is a measure of the ease of abdominal expansion, which is determined by the elasticity of the abdominal wall and diaphragm. It should be expressed as the change in intra-abdominal volume per change in IAP.
Definition 14	The open abdomen is one that requires a temporary abdominal closure due to the skin and fascia not being closed after laparotomy.
Definition 15	Lateralization of the abdominal wall is the phenomenon where the musculature and fascia of the abdominal wall, most exemplified by the rectus abdominus muscles and their enveloping fascia, move laterally away from the midline with time.

Source: Malbrain ML et al. *Intensive Care Med.* 2006 November;32(11):1722–32.
Abbreviations: ACS, Abdominal compartment syndrome; APP, Abdominal perfusion pressure; IAH, Intra-abdominal hypertension; IAP, Intra-abdominal pressure; MAP, Mean arterial pressure.

Table 17.4 Causes of Raised Intra-Abdominal Pressure (IAP)
Massive resuscitation
Major intra-abdominal and retroperitoneal haemorrhage
Tissue oedema secondary to insults such as ischaemia and sepsis
Secondary to generalized oedema, for example, from burns resuscitation
Paralytic ileus
Ascites

confirmed in 18 patients undergoing laparoscopy in whom a reduction of between 11% and 54% in blood flow was seen in the duodenum and stomach, respectively, at an IAP of 15 mm Hg. Animals studies suggest that the reduction in visceral perfusion is selective, affecting intestinal blood flow before, for example, adrenal blood flow. Early decreases in visceral perfusion are related to levels of IAP as low as 15 mm Hg.

17.10.4.4 RENAL

The most likely direct effect of increased IAP is an increase in the renal vascular resistance, coupled with a moderate reduction in cardiac output.[31] Pressure on the ureter has been ruled out as a cause, as investigators have placed ureteric stents with no improvement in function. Other factors that may contribute to renal dysfunction include humeral factors and intraparenchymal renal pressures.

The absolute value of IAP that is required to cause renal impairment is probably in the region of 15 mm Hg. Maintaining adequate cardiovascular filling pressures in the presence of increased IAP also seems to be important.

17.10.4.5 INTRACRANIAL PRESSURE

Raised IAP can have a marked effect on intracranial pathophysiology and cause severe rises in intracranial pressure.

17.10.5 Measurement of IAP

The gold standard for IAP measurement involves using a urinary catheter. The patient is positioned flat on the bed. A standard Foley catheter is used. The size of the urinary catheter does not matter. Elevation of the catheter and measuring the urine column provides a rough guide and is

simple to perform. A T-piece bladder pressure device connected to a pressure transducer on-line to the monitoring system can be used. The pressure transducer is placed in the mid-axillary line and the urinary tubing is clamped. If the patient is not lying flat, IAP can be measured from the pubic symphysis. Approximately 25 mL isotonic saline is inserted into the bladder via a three-way stopcock. After zeroing, the pressure on the monitor is recorded. Commercial direct transducers are available.

Pitfalls

- A strict protocol and staff education on the technique and interpretation of IAP is essential.
- Very high pressures (especially unexpected ones) are usually caused by a blocked urinary catheter and should be repeated.

Increasingly, it is recognized that IAP is not a static condition and should be measured continuously. In addition, whether IAP is measured intermittently or continuously, consideration should be given to abdominal perfusion measurement.

17.10.5.1 MEASUREMENT OF APP

As with the concept of cerebral perfusion pressure, calculation of the 'abdominal perfusion pressure', which is defined as mean arterial pressure minus IAP, assesses not only the severity of IAP present, but also the adequacy of the patient's abdominal blood flow.

APP has been studied as a resuscitation end point in four clinical trials. These demonstrated statistically significant differences in APP between survivors and non-survivors with IAH/ACS. Cheatham et al.,[32] in a retrospective trial of surgical and trauma patients with IAH (mean IAP 22 ± 8 mm Hg), concluded that an APP of greater than 50 mm Hg optimized survival based upon receiver operating characteristic curve analysis. Abdominal perfusion pressure was also superior to global resuscitation end points such as arterial pH, base deficit, arterial lactate and hourly urinary output in its ability to predict patient outcome.

Malbrain et al.[33,34] suggested that 60 mm Hg represented an appropriate resuscitation goal. A persistence of IAH and a failure to maintain an APP of 60 mm Hg or more by day 3 following the development of IAH-induced acute renal failure was found to discriminate between survivors and non-survivors.

17.10.6 Management

17.10.6.1 PREVENTION

To avoid ACS developing in the first place, in the emergency department, concepts of damage control resuscitation, coupled with adequate pre-hospital information will help identify patients at high risk even before they arrive in the emergency room, and avoiding excessive fluid resuscitation is an important factor in reducing the risk of developing subsequent ACS. In patients undergoing damage control laparotomy, it is mandatory to leave the abdomen open to prevent ACS and in anticipation of a second operation.

17.10.6.2 TREATMENT

There are several key principles in the management of patients with potential ACS:

- Regular appropriate monitoring of IAP in the ICU.
- Optimization of systemic perfusion, circulating volume and organ function in the patient with IAH grade I and grade II (i.e. ≤20 mm Hg).
- Institution of specific medical procedures to reduce IAP and the end-organ consequences of IAH/ACS, including diuretics, and removing excess ascites if present by percutaneous puncture.
- In patients with grade III–IV IAH (IAP >20 mm Hg) with evidence of new-onset organ failure not responding to non-operative management, a decompressive laparostomy performed as soon as possible.

The decompressed abdomen should be closed using a low-vacuum sandwich technique.

17.10.6.3 REVERSIBLE FACTORS

The second aspect of management is to correct any reversible cause of ACS, such as intra-abdominal bleeding. Massive retroperitoneal haemorrhage is often associated with a fractured pelvis, and consideration should be given to measures that would control haemorrhage, such as pelvic fixation or vessel embolization. In some cases, severe gaseous distension or acute colonic pseudo-obstruction can occur in ICU patients. This may respond to drugs such as neostigmine, but if it is severe, surgical decompression may be necessary. A common cause of a raised IAP in ICU is related to the ileus. There is little that can be actively done in these circumstances apart from optimizing the patient's cardiorespiratory status and serum electrolytes, and inserting a nasogastric tube.

Remember that ACS is often only a symptom of an underlying problem. In a prospective review of 88 post-laparotomy patients, Sugrue et al., found that those with an IAP of 18 mm Hg had an increased odds ratio for intra-abdominal sepsis of 3.9 (95% confidence interval 0.7–22.7).[35] Abdominal evaluation for sepsis is a priority, and this should obviously include a rectal examination as well as investigations such as ultrasound and CT scanning. Surgery is the obvious mainstay of treatment in patients whose rise in IAP is due to postoperative bleeding.

17.10.7 Surgery for Raised IAP

There are few guidelines for exactly when surgical decompression is required in the presence of raised IAP. Some studies have stated that abdominal decompression is the only treatment and that it should be performed early in order to prevent ACS. This is an overstatement and not supported by level 1 evidence. The indications for abdominal decompression are related to correcting pathophysiological abnormalities as much as achieving a precise and optimum IAP.

In general, temporary abdominal closure is superior to conventional techniques for dealing with intra-abdominal sepsis. Indications for performing temporary abdominal closure include:

- Abdominal decompression.
- When re-exploration is planned.
- To facilitate re-exploration in abdominal sepsis.
- Inability to close the abdomen.
- Prevention of ACS.

Many different techniques have been used to facilitate a temporary abdominal closure, including intravenous bags, Velcro, silicone, and zips. Whatever technique is used, it is important that effective decompression be achieved with adequate incisions.

17.10.7.1 TIPS FOR SURGICAL DECOMPRESSION FOR RAISED IAP

- There should be early investigation and correction of the cause of raised IAP.
- Ongoing abdominal bleeding with raised IAP requires urgent operative intervention.
- Reduction in urinary output is a late sign of renal impairment. Gastric tonometry may provide earlier information on visceral perfusion.

- Abdominal decompression requires a full-length abdominal incision.
- The surgical dressing should be closed using a sandwich technique using two suction drains placed laterally to facilitate fluid removal from the wound.

17.10.8 Management Algorithm

Suggested management of intra-abdominal hypertension (IAH) and abdominal compartment syndrome (ACS) including medical management algorithms are given in Figures 17.1 and 17.2.[36]

17.11 ACUTE KIDNEY INJURY[37]

While the frequency of acute kidney injury (AKI) is relatively low, injured patients are at high risk of its development. Several indicators of the severity of physiological injury, including the lowest body temperature, the highest lactate level and the need for packed red blood cell and cryoprecipitate transfusions, were independently associated with a higher risk of developing AKI.

Other factors included tissue damage and necrosis, hypotension, rhabdomyolysis, and pre-existing conditions such as diabetes. The development of AKI complicates the ICU management of a patient, increases the length of stay, and is associated with a mortality of approximately 60%. Approximately one-third of acute post-traumatic AKI cases are caused by inadequate resuscitation, while the remainder seem to develop as part of MODS.

The clinician should look for and manage these common causes:

- Hypovolaemia.
- Rhabdomyolysis.
- Abdominal compartment syndrome.
- Obstructive uropathy.
- Avoid nephrotoxic dyes where possible. There is evidence that CT contrast is unlikely to be harmful.[38]

17.12 METABOLIC DISTURBANCES

Disturbances in acid–base and electrolyte balance can be anticipated in patients in shock, those who have received massive transfusions and the elderly with co-morbid conditions.

Typical abnormalities may include:

- Acid base disorders.
- Electrolyte disorders.
  - Hypokalaemia.
  - Hyperkalaemia.
  - Hypocalcaemia.
  - Hypomagnesaemia.
  - Hypophosphataemia.

In acid–base disorders, one must identify and correct the aetiology of the disturbance, for example, metabolic acidosis caused by hypoperfusion secondary to occult pericardial tamponade.

> **Pitfall**
>
> Sodium bicarbonate is contraindicated for correction of acidosis in acute trauma, as this is usually respiratory in origin.

17.13 NUTRITIONAL SUPPORT[39,40]

Trauma patients are hypermetabolic and have increased nutritional needs owing to the immunological response to trauma and the requirement for accelerated protein synthesis for wound healing. Early enteral feeding has been shown to reduce postoperative septic morbidity after trauma. A meta-analysis of several randomized trials has demonstrated a twofold decrease in infectious complications in patients treated with early enteral nutrition compared with total parenteral nutrition.

Traumatic brain injury (TBI) patients appear to have similar outcomes whether fed enterally or parenterally. A Cochrane review has confirmed that early (either parenteral or enteral) feeding is associated with a trend towards better outcomes in terms of survival and disability compared with later feeding.[41] Patients with a TBI exhibit protein wasting and gastrointestinal dysfunction, which may be risk factors for a septic state. However, standard nutritional support may not allow restoration of the nutritional state of TBI patients.[42]

Enteral nutrition should be used when the gut is accessible and functioning. Enteral nutrition is not invariably safer and better than parenteral nutrition, but a mix of the two modalities can be used safely.

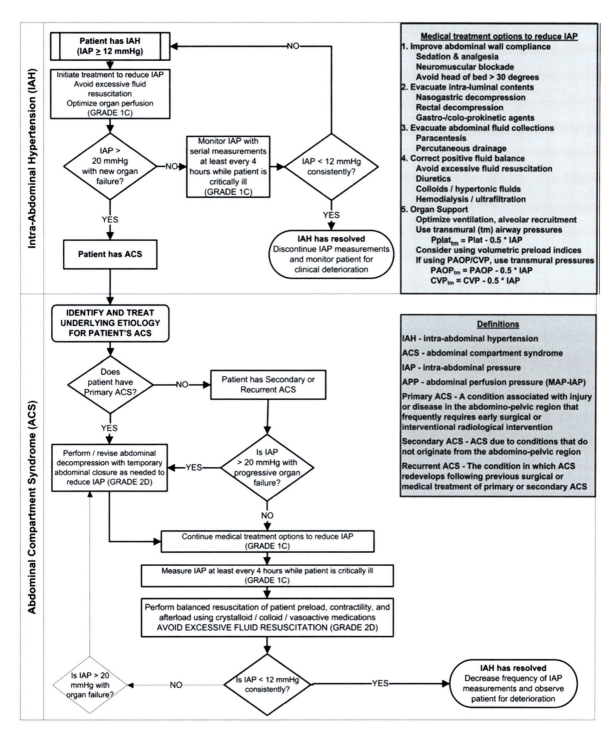

Figure 17.1 Intra-abdominal hypertension (IAH) and abdominal compartment syndrome (ACS) Management Algorithm. (From Cheatham ML et al. *Recomm Intensive Care Med.* 2007 June;33(6):951–62.)

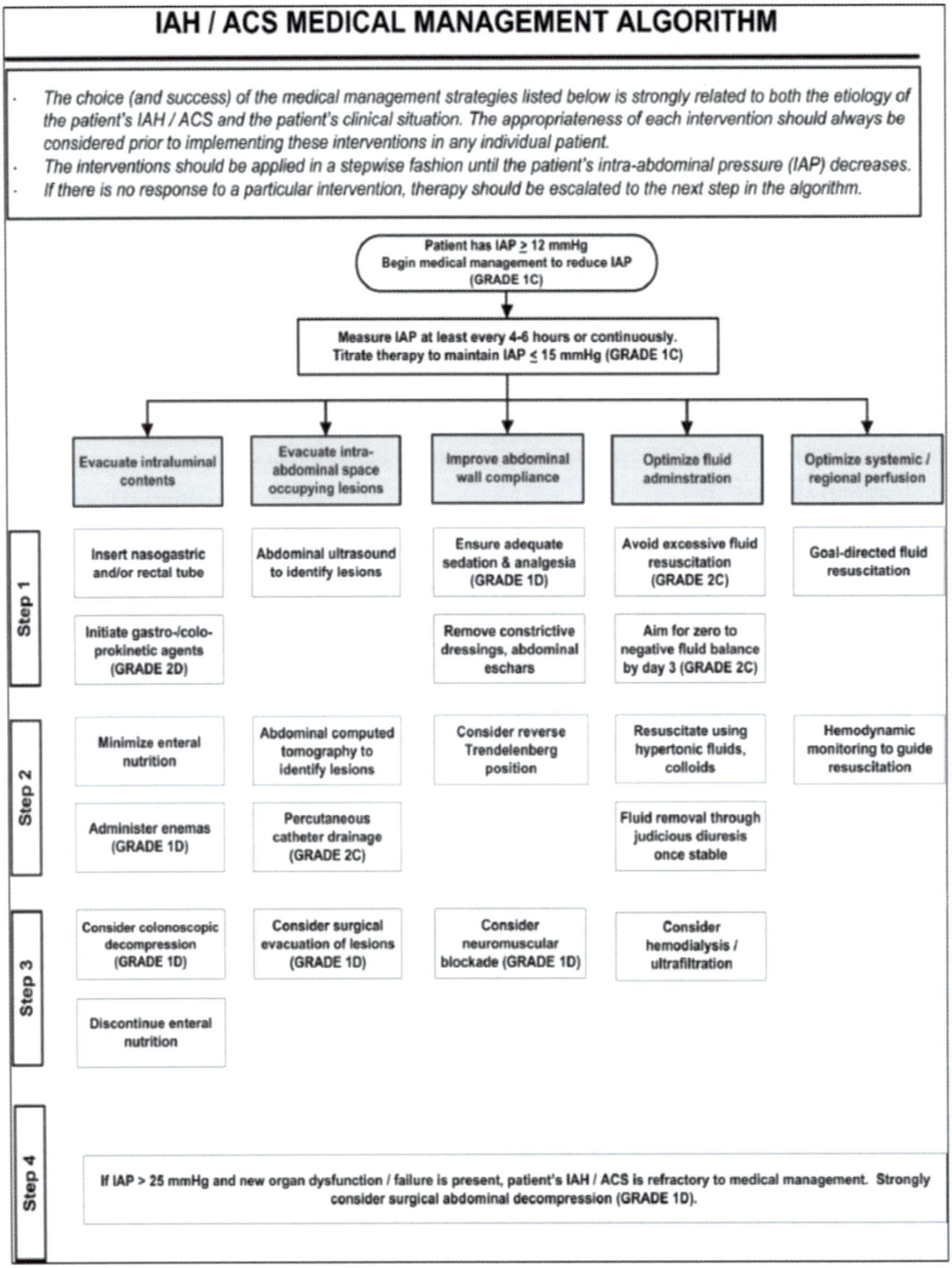

IAH / ACS MEDICAL MANAGEMENT ALGORITHM

- The choice (and success) of the medical management strategies listed below is strongly related to both the etiology of the patient's IAH / ACS and the patient's clinical situation. The appropriateness of each intervention should always be considered prior to implementing these interventions in any individual patient.
- The interventions should be applied in a stepwise fashion until the patient's intra-abdominal pressure (IAP) decreases.
- If there is no response to a particular intervention, therapy should be escalated to the next step in the algorithm.

Patient has IAP ≥ 12 mmHg
Begin medical management to reduce IAP
(GRADE 1C)

Measure IAP at least every 4-6 hours or continuously.
Titrate therapy to maintain IAP ≤ 15 mmHg (GRADE 1C)

Evacuate intraluminal contents	Evacuate intra-abdominal space occupying lesions	Improve abdominal wall compliance	Optimize fluid adminstration	Optimize systemic / regional perfusion

Step 1

| Insert nasogastric and/or rectal tube | Abdominal ultrasound to identify lesions | Ensure adequate sedation & analgesia (GRADE 1D) | Avoid excessive fluid resuscitation (GRADE 2C) | Goal-directed fluid resuscitation |
| Initiate gastro-/colo-prokinetic agents (GRADE 2D) | | Remove constrictive dressings, abdominal eschars | Aim for zero to negative fluid balance by day 3 (GRADE 2C) | |

Step 2

| Minimize enteral nutrition | Abdominal computed tomography to identify lesions | Consider reverse Trendelenberg position | Resuscitate using hypertonic fluids, colloids | Hemodynamic monitoring to guide resuscitation |
| Administer enemas (GRADE 1D) | Percutaneous catheter drainage (GRADE 2C) | | Fluid removal through judicious diuresis once stable | |

Step 3

| Consider colonoscopic decompression (GRADE 1D) | Consider surgical evacuation of lesions (GRADE 1D) | Consider neuromuscular blockade (GRADE 1D) | Consider hemodialysis / ultrafiltration | |
| Discontinue enteral nutrition | | | | |

Step 4

If IAP > 25 mmHg and new organ dysfunction / failure is present, patient's IAH / ACS is refractory to medical management. Strongly consider surgical abdominal decompression (GRADE 1D).

Figure 17.2 Intra-abdominal hypertension/abdominal compartment syndrome medical management algorithm.

Patients at risk include those with:

- Major trauma.
- Burns.

It is critical to:

- Determine energy and protein requirements.
- Determine and establish a route of administration.
- Set a time to begin nutrition support.

17.13.1 Access for Enteral Nutrition

17.13.1.1 SIMPLE

- Nasogastric tube.
- Nasoduodenal tube.
- Nasojejunal tube.

Most critically ill trauma patients should be started on early enteral nutrition. The majority do not require prolonged feeding (beyond 10–14 days). For patients who have prolonged tube-feeding requirements, nasoenteric tubes are inconvenient, as they tend to dislodge, worsen aspiration, and are uncomfortable.

17.13.1.2 MORE COMPLICATED

- *Percutaneous endoscopic gastrostomy (PEG)*: This does not interfere with swallowing, is easy to nurse and has target feeding rates that are more likely to be achieved compared with nasoenteric tubes. However, it is an invasive procedure with some risk.
- *Jejunostomy*: Jejunostomy can be placed endoscopically or during laparotomy. Rates of major complications should be less than 5%.[43]

17.14 PROPHYLAXIS IN THE ICU

17.14.1 Stress Ulceration[44]

Stress ulceration and associated upper gastrointestinal bleeding has been on the decline in most ICUs. This is, in great part, due to the improved resuscitation efforts in the pre-hospital environment, emergency department, and operating room. Additionally, the use of acid-blocking and cytoprotective therapies has become commonplace.

Those patients at greatest risk for stress ulcer development are those with a previous history of ulcer disease, those requiring mechanical ventilation and those with a coagulopathy, regardless of whether it is intrinsic or chemically induced, and patients on steroids. Burn patients have also been labelled as high risk in historical studies.

Proton pump inhibitors may have replaced H_2 blockade as the mainstay of therapy. Intravenous H_2-receptor blockade therapy (e.g. ranitidine) to some degree blocks the production of stomach acid. Most studies demonstrating its efficacy in stress ulcer prevention do not attempt to neutralize gastric pH.

Cytoprotective agents (e.g. sucralfate) as a preventive measure have been shown to be the most cost-effective by statistical analysis in several trials. However, the marked decrease in the rate of development of ventilator-associated pneumonia seen in the sucralfate population does make this therapeutic option quite attractive.[14]

Perhaps the simplest and safest method of stress ulcer prevention is adequate resuscitation and early intragastric enteric nutrition. During the early resuscitative phase and while vasoactive drugs to elevate blood pressure are in use, it is not always prudent to provide nutrition enterally. It is in these circumstances that the use of acid blockade, cytoprotective agents, or both is necessary.

17.14.2 Deep Venous Thrombosis and Pulmonary Embolus[45]

Pulmonary embolus from DVT continues to be a leading preventable cause of death in the injured patient. Recognizing the risk factors for the development of DVT and instituting an aggressive management regimen can reduce this risk from DVT in the ICU with little added morbidity. The incidence of DVT in trauma patients is 12%–32% and those at highest risk of fatal PE include those with spinal cord injuries, weight-bearing pelvic fracture, and combined long bone fracture/TBI or long bone fracture/pelvic fracture.

There is a separate guideline for paediatric patients.[46]

Recent evidence in trauma suggests reduction in DVT and PE with weight-based prophylaxis, rather than standard doses across the board.[47] The anti Xa levels in larger patients may be inadequate and should be monitored.[48]

A high index of suspicion in these severely injured patients should result in preventative therapy and diagnostic screening measures to be taken in the ICU. Unless haemorrhagic TBI or spinal cord epidural haematoma precludes the use of subcutaneous heparin therapy, these patients should all receive fractionated low molecular weight subcutaneous heparin. Unfractionated heparin does not appear to be as effective in this severely injured population. Similarly, unless extremity injury precludes their use, graded pneumatic compression devices should be used on all such patients. Foot pumps may also be of some benefit.

Screening for the presence of DVT, which, if present, would necessitate more aggressive anticoagulant therapy, should also be implemented in these patients. The easiest and safest screening tool is venous Doppler ultrasound or duplex scanning. This is a portable, readily available, repeatable and cost-effective procedure with no side effects for the patient. These modalities are, however, operator-dependent and can fail to diagnose DVT in the deep pelvic veins, but contrast ultrasound trials to overcome this weakness are now being conducted. This screening should be performed whenever clinical suspicion of DVT arises, within 48 hours of admission, and each 5–7 days thereafter if the patient remains in the ICU.

In the highest risk patients previously mentioned, consideration for prophylactic placement of an inferior vena cava (IVC) filter may be made However, prophylactic IVC filter placement has been associated with an increased incidence of DVT (OR = 1.83; 95% CI, 1.15–2.93). Further, prophylactic IVC filter placement has not been effective in reducing trauma patient mortality.[49] The combination of aggressive prevention measures, screening by duplex and VTE chemoprophylaxis can result in a fatal PE rate of significantly less than 1% of the trauma ICU population.

17.14.3 Tetanus Prophylaxis

In patients with any open wounds from trauma, it is imperative that the tetanus immunization status of the patient is addressed. For those patients immunized within the previous 5 years, no additional treatment is generally needed, while booster tetanus toxoid should be administered to those who have previously received the initial tetanus series but have not been re-immunized in the preceding 5–10 years. Tetanus immune globulin should be administered to those patients who lack any previous history of immunization.

Patients undergoing splenectomy require immunization for *Haemophilus influenza* type B, meningococcus and pneumococcus (see also Section 9.5). Debate continues regarding the timing of administration of these vaccines in trauma patients, but adult patients do not benefit from the antibacterial chemoprophylaxis needed in paediatric patients, post-splenectomy. Owing to the multiple strains of each organism, the immunizations are not foolproof in preventing overwhelming post-splenectomy infection (OPSI). Therefore, patients must be carefully counselled to seek medical attention immediately for high fevers, and healthcare providers must be aggressive in the use of empirical antibiotics in patients who may have overwhelming post-splenectomy infection upon presentation in the outpatient setting.

17.14.4 Line Sepsis

Thrombophlebitis and sepsis from intravenous cannulae are significant considerations as these intravenous lines are frequently placed under less than optimal circumstances and technique in the field and in the resuscitation areas. Removal and replacement of all such lines as early as possible, but in every instance in less than 24 hours, is paramount to avoid these infectious complications.

17.15 PAIN CONTROL

If the patient can cooperate, visual analogue pain scores may be helpful. Several adverse consequences result when pain is inadequately treated. These include increased oxygen consumption, increased minute volume demands, psychic stress, sleep deprivation, and impaired lung mechanics with associated pulmonary complications. Subjective pain assessment is best documented objectively and, after initiation of treatment, requires serial re-evaluation. Inadequate pain relief can be determined objectively by the failure of the patient to achieve adequate volumes on incentive spirometry, persistently small radiographic lung volumes, or a reluctance to cough and cooperate with chest physiotherapy.

Early pain control in the ICU is primarily achieved using intravenous opiates, although there is emerging evidence for the use of ketamine infusion as an opiate-sparing option. Other techniques are employed and tailored to the individual patient and injury:

- Bolus analgo-sedation opiates and non-opiates.
  - Morphine, fentanyl or ketamine equivalent titrated intravenously.
- Patient-controlled analgesia (PCA).
- Epidural or paraspinal analgesia (patient-controlled epidural analgesia).
- Intrapleural anaesthesia.
- Extrapleural analgesia.

- Intercostal nerve blocks.
- Catheter techniques for peripheral nerve blocks, for example, femoral nerve, brachial plexus, popliteal nerve and paravertebral nerve blocks.

Delirium is a recognized complication in patients on the ICU. A breakdown of treatment strategies is beyond the scope of this chapter, but identification of causative factors, re-establishing day/night rhythm, and medical strategies should be attempted.

17.16 ICU TERTIARY SURVEY[50]

The tertiary survey is a complete re-examination of the patient, plus a review of the history and all available results and imaging. Missed injuries are a potent cause of morbidity, and the majority will be identified by a thorough tertiary survey. A tertiary trauma survey has much to recommend it in minimizing the delay in the ultimate diagnosis of missed injury. Nevertheless, it is not a complete solution, and an ongoing analysis of errors should be undertaken at any major trauma centre.

17.16.1 Evaluation for Occult Injuries

Factors predisposing to missed injuries:

- Mechanism of injury – re-verify the events surrounding the injury.

High-priority occult injuries:

- Brain, spinal cord and peripheral nerve injury.
- Thoracic aortic injury.
- Intra-abdominal or pelvic injury.
- Vascular injuries to the extremities.
- Cerebrovascular injuries – occult carotid/vertebral artery injury.
- Cardiac injuries.
- Aerodigestive tract injuries – ruptured bowel.
- Occult pneumothorax.
- Compartment syndrome – foreleg, thigh, buttock or arm.
- Eye injuries (remember to remove the patient's contact lenses).
- Other occult injuries – hands, feet, digits or joint dislocations.
- Vaginal tampons.

17.16.2 Assess Co-Morbid Conditions

- Medical history (including drugs and alcohol).
- Contact the patient's personal physicians.
- Check pharmacy records.

17.16.3 ICU Summary

Complete a **FAST HUGS BID** protocol for all patients (Table 17.5).[51]

Table 17.5 FAST HUGS BID Medical Mnemonic for a Surgical Patient

	Medical Patient	Surgical Patient
F	Feeding	Feeding (*NPO*, enteral, TPN)
A	Analgesia	Analgesia (VAS score)
S	Sedation	Sensorium (GCS/Ramsay sedation score)
T	Thromboprophylaxis	Thromboprophylaxis/temperature/tubes
H	Head-up position	Head-up position/haemodynamics
U	Ulcer prophylaxis	Ulcer prophylaxis/urine output
G	Glycaemic control	Glycaemic control
B	Bowel movement	Bowel (ileus/gastroparesis/distension/movement)
I	Indwelling catheter	Indwelling lines (catheter, A-line, CVC, epidural, Foley Imbalance (electrolyte/cumulative fluid)
D	Drug de-escalation	Drugs (de-escalation, delirium, number of days)

Abbreviation: **TPN**, Total Parenteral Nutrition; **VAS**, Visual Analog Scale; **GCS**, Glasgow Coma Scale; **NIV**, Nin-invasive ventilation; **CVC**, Central Venous Catheter, **NPO**, *Nil per os* (Nil by mouth).

17.17 **FAMILY CONTACT AND SUPPORT (See also Chapter 19)**

It is very important to establish early contact and maintain ongoing relationships with family members in an open, honest, clear, and completely transparent manner, by using simple language that is understandable when describing the injuries, clinical condition, and prognosis of the patient. This provides family members with essential information and establishes a relationship between the ICU care team and the family. Administrative facts, such as ICU procedures, visiting hours, and available services, should also be explained. With the elderly, the identifying the existence of living wills or other predetermination documents is important. Patient and their families should be familiar with multidisciplinary approach to patient care in the ICU as well.

REFERENCES AND RECOMMENDED READING

References

1. Hardcastle TC, Maier R, Muckart DJ. Ventilation in trauma patients – the first 24 hours is different! *World J Surg.* 2017 May;**41(5)**:1153–58. doi: 10.1007/s00268-016-3530-1.

2. Claridge JA, Crabtree TD, Pelletier SJ, Butler K, Sawyer RG, Young JS. Persistent occult hypoperfusion is associated with a significant increase in infection rate and mortality in major trauma patients. *J Trauma.* 2000 Jan;**48(1)**:8–14.

3. Blow O, Magliore L, Claridge JA, Butler K, Young JS. The golden hour and the silver day: detection and correction of occult hypoperfusion within 24 hours improves outcome from major trauma. *J Trauma.* 1999 Nov;**47(5)**:964–9.

4. Amato MB, Meade MO, Slutsky AS, Brochard L, Costa EL, Schoenfeld DA, et al. Driving pressure and survival in the acute respiratory distress syndrome. *N Engl J Med.* 2015 Feb;**19**:747–55. doi: 10.1056/NEJMsa1410639.

5. Garner JS, Jarvis WR, Emori TG, Horan TC, Hughes JM. CDC definitions for nosocomial infections, 1988. *Am J Infect Control.* 1988 Jun;**16(3)**:128–40.

6. Mallick A, Bodenham AR. Tracheostomy in critically ill patients. *Eur J Anaesthesiol.* 2010 Aug;**27(8)**:676–82. doi: 10.1097/EJA.0b013e32833b1ba0. Review.

7. Ely EW, The ABCDEF Bundle: Science and Philosophy of How ICU Liberation Serves Patients and Families. *Crit Care Med.* 2017 Feb;**45(2)**:321–30. doi: 10.1097/CCM.0000 000000002175.

8. Zonies D, Merkel M. Advanced extracorporeal therapy in trauma. *Curr Opin Crit Care.* 2016 Dec;**22(6)**:578–83. Review.

9. Zonies D. ECLS in Trauma: Practical Application and a Review of Current Status. *World J Surg.* 2017 May;**41(5)**: 1159–64. doi: 10.1007/s00268-016-3586-y.

10. Swol J, Brodie D, Napolitano L, Park PK, Thiagarajan R, Barbaro RP, et al. Extracorporeal Life Support Organization (ELSO). *J Trauma Acute Care Surg.* 2018 Jun;**84(6)**:831–837. doi: 10.1097/TA.0000000000001895.

11. Tieu BH, Holcomb JB, Schreiber MA. Coagulopathy: its pathophysiology and treatment in the injured patient. *World J Surg.* 2007 May;**31(5)**:1055–64. Review.

12. Ganter MT, Pittet JF. New insights into acute coagulopathy in trauma patients. *Best Pract Res Clin Anaesthesiol.* 2010 Mar;**24(1)**:15–25. Review.

13. Geeraedts LMG Jr, Kaasjager HAH, van Vugt AB. Exsanguination in trauma: a review of diagnostics and treatment options. *Injury.* 2009 Jan;**40(1)**:11–20. https://doi.org/10.1016/j.injury.2008.10.007.

14. CRASH-2 Trial Collaborators. Effects of tranexamic acid on death, vascular occlusive events, and blood transfusion in trauma patients with significant haemorrhage (CRASH-2): a randomised, placebo-controlled trial. *Lancet.* 2010;**376**: 27–32.

15. Moore HB, Moore EE, Gonzales E, Chapman MP, Chin TL, Silliman CC, Banerjee A, Sauiaia A. Hyprinofibrinolysis, physiologic fibrinolysis, and fibrinolysis shutdown: The spectrum of post injury fibrinolysis and relevance to antifibrinolytic therapy. *J Trauma Acute Care Surg.* 2014 Dec;**77(6)**:811–7.

16. Holcomb JB, Tilley BC, Baraniuk S, Fox EE, Wade CE, Podbielski JM, et al. Transfusion of plasma, platelets, and red blood cells in a 1:1:1 vs a 1:1:2 ratio and mortality in patients with severe trauma: the PROPPR randomized clinical trial. *JAMA.* 2015 Feb 3;**313(5)**:471–82. doi: 10.1001/jama.2015.12.

17. Singer M, Deutschman CS, Seymour CW, Shankar-Hari M, Annane D, Bauer M, et al. The Third International Consensus Definitions for Sepsis and Septic Shock (Sepsis-3). *JAMA.* 2016;**315(8)**:801–10. doi: 10.1001/jama. 2016.0287.

18. Napolitano LM. Sepsis 2018: Definitions and Guideline Changes. *Surg Infect. (Larchmt).* 2018 Feb/Mar;**19(2)**:117–125. doi: 10.1089/sur.2017.278.

19. Sartelli M, Kluger Y, Ansaloni L, Hardcastle TC, Rello J, Watkins RR, et al. Raising concerns about the Sepsis-3 definitions. *World J Emerg Surg.* 2018;**13**:6 doi: 10.1186/s13017-018-0165-6.

20. Dellinger RP, Levy MM, Rhodes A, Annane D, Gerlach H, Opal SM, et al. Surviving Sepsis Campaign: International Guidelines for Management of Severe Sepsis and Septic Shock: 2012. *Critical Care Medicine.* 2013;**41(2)**: 580–637.

21. Rhodes A, Evans LE, Alhazzani W, Levy MM, Massimo A, Ferrer R, et al. Surviving sepsis campaign: International guidelines for management of sepsis and septic shock 2016. *Critical Care Medicine*. 2017;**45**:486–552. Available from: http://journals.lww.com/ccmjournal/Fulltext/2017/03000/Surviving_Sepsis_Campaign___International.15.aspx (accessed online January 2019).

22. Sartelli M, Chichom-Mefire A, Labricciosa FM, Hardcastle T, Abu-Zidan FM, Adesunkanmi AK, et al. The management of intra-abdominal infections from a global perspective: 2017 WSES guidelines for management of intra-abdominal infections. *World J Emerg Surg*. 2017;**12**:29. doi: 10.1186/s13017-017-0141-6 and Erratum in: *World J Emerg Surg*. 2017 Aug 2;12:36.

23. Sawyer RG, Claridge JA, Nathens AB, Rotstein OD, Duane TM, Evans HL, et al. Trial of short-course antimicrobial therapy for intraabdominal infection. *N Engl J Med*. 2015 May 21;**372(21)**:1996–2005. doi: 10.1056/NEJMoa1411162.

24. Velmahos GC, Toutouzas KG, Sarkisyan G, Chan LS, Jindal A, Karaiskakis M, et al. Severe trauma is not an excuse for prolonged antibiotic prophylaxis. *Arch Surg*. 2002 May; **137(5)**:537–41.

25. Hoff WS, Bonadies JA, Cachecho R, Dorlac WC. Eastern Association for the Surgery of Trauma. *Eastern Association for the Surgery of Trauma*. Practice Management Guidelines Workgroup: Update to practice management guidelines for prophylactic antibiotic use in open fractures. *J Trauma*. 2011 Mar;**70(3)**:751–4. doi: 10.1097/TA.0b013e31820930e5. Available from www.east.org (accessed online January 2019).

26. Hauser CJ, Adams CA Jr, Eachempati SR. Council of the Surgical Infection Society. Surgical Infection Society Guidelines: prophylactic antibiotic use in open fractures: an evidence-based guideline. *Surg Infect*. (Larchmt) 2006 Aug;**7(4)**:379–405.

27. Rello J, Paiva JA, Baraibar J, Barcenilla F, Bodi M, Castander D, et al. International Conference for the Development of Consensus on the Diagnosis and Treatment of Ventilator-associated Pneumonia. *Chest*. 2001 Sep;**120(3)**:955–70.

28. Abdominal Compartment Syndrome. *World Society for Abdominal Compartment Syndrome*. Available from www.wsacs.org (accessed online January 2019).

29. Malbrain ML, Cheatham ML, Kirkpatrick A, Sugrue M, Parr M, De Waele J, et al. Results from the International Conference of Experts on Intra-abdominal Hypertension and Abdominal Compartment Syndrome. I. Definitions. *Intensive Care Med*. 2006 Nov;**32(11)**:1722–32.

30. Balogh Z, McKinley BA, Cocanour CS, Kozar RA, Valdivia A, Sailors RM, et al. Supranormal trauma resuscitation causes more cases of abdominal compartment syndrome.

31. Sugrue M, Jones F, Deane SA, Bishop G, Bauman A, Hillman K. Intra-abdominal hypertension is an independent cause of postoperative renal impairment. *Arch Surg*. 1999 Oct;**134(10)**:1082–5.

32. Cheatham ML, White MW, Sagraves SG, Johnson JL, Block EF. Abdominal perfusion pressure: a superior parameter in the assessment of intra-abdominal hypertension. *J Trauma*. 2000 Oct;**49(4)**:621–6; discussion 626-7.

33. Malbrain ML, Chiumello D, Pelosi P, Wilmer A, Brienza N, Malcangi V, et al. Prevalence of intra-abdominal hypertension in critically ill patients: a multicentre epidemiological study. *Intensive Care Med*. 2004 May;**30(5)**:822–9.

34. Malbrain ML, Chiumello D, Pelosi P, Bihari D, Innes R, Ranieri VM, et al. Incidence and prognosis of intraabdominal hypertension in a mixed population of critically ill patients: a multiple-centre epidemiological study. *Crit Care Med*. 2005 Feb;**33(2)**:315–22.

35. Sugrue M, Buist MD, Hourihan F, Deane S, Bauman A, Hillman K. Prospective study of intra-abdominal hypertension and renal function after laparotomy. *Br J Surg*. 1995 Feb;**82(2)**:235–8.

36. Cheatham ML, Malbrain ML, Kirkpatrick A, Sugrue M, Parr M, De Waele J, et al. Results from the International Conference of Experts on Intra-abdominal Hypertension and Abdominal Compartment Syndrome: II. Recommendations *Intensive Care Medicine* 2007 Jun;**33(6)**:951–962.

37. Bihorac A1, Delano MJ, Schold JD, Lopez MC, Nathens AB, Maier RV, et al. Incidence, clinical predictors, genomics, and outcome of acute kidney injury among trauma patients. *Ann Surg*. 2010 Jul;**252(1)**:158–65. doi: 10.1097/SLA.0b013e3181deb6bc.

38. Aycock RD, Westafer LM, Boxen JL, Majlesi N, Schoenfeld EM, Bannuru RR. Acute Kidney Injury After Computed Tomography: A Meta-analysis. *Ann Emerg Med*. 2018 Jan; **71(1)**:44–53.e4. doi: 10.1016/j.annemergmed.2017.06.041.

39. Jacobs DO, Kudsk KA, Oswanski MF, Sacks GS, Sinclair KE. Practice management guidelines for nutritional support of the trauma patient. In: *Eastern Association for the Surgery of Trauma. Practice Management Guidelines. J Trauma*. 2004 Sep;**57(3)**:660–78; discussion 679. Available from www.east.org (accessed online January 2019).

40. Kreymann KG, Berger MM, Deutz NE, Hiesmayr M, Jolliet P, Kazandjiev G, et al. ESPEN (European Society for Parenteral and Enteral Nutrition). ESPEN Guidelines on Enteral Nutrition: intensive care. *Clin Nutr*. 2006 April;**25(2)**:210–23.

41. Perel P, Yanagawa T, Bunn F, Roberts I, Wentz R, Pierro A. Nutritional support for head-injured patients. *Cochrane Database Syst Rev*. 2006 Oct 18;**(4)**:CD001530. Review.

Arch Surg. 2003 Jun;**138(6)**:637–42; discussion 642-3.

42. Cook AM, Peppard A, Magnuson A. Nutrition considerations in traumatic brain injury. *Nutr Clin Pract*. 2008 Dec-2009 Jan;**23(6)**:608–20. doi: 10.1177/0884533608326060

43. Holmes JH 4th, Brundage SI, Yuen P, Hall RA, Maier RV, Jurkovich GJ. Complications of surgical feeding jejunostomy in patients. *J Trauma* 1999 Dec;**47(6)**:1009–12.

44. Guillamondegui OD, Gunter OL Jr, Bonadies JA, Coates JE, Kurek SJ, De Moya Mae, et al. Practice management guidelines for stress ulcer prophylaxis. In: *Eastern Association for the Surgery of Trauma. Practice Management Guidelines*. Available from https://www.east.org/education/practice-management-guidelines/stress-ulcer-prophylaxis (accessed online December 2018).

45. Rogers FB, Cipolle MD, Velmahos G, Rozycki G. Practice management guidelines for the management of venous thromboembolism (VTE) in trauma patients. *J Trauma* 2002 Jul;**53(1)**:142–64. In: *Eastern Association for the Surgery of Trauma. Practice Management Guidelines*. Available from www.east.org (accessed online December 2018).

46. Mahajerin A, Petty JK, Hanson SJ, Thompson AJ, O'Brien SH, Streck CJ, et al. Prophylaxis against venous thromboembolismin pediatric trauma: A practice management guideline from the Eastern Association for the Surgery of Trauma and the Pediatric Trauma Society. *J Trauma Acute Care Surg*. 2017 Mar;**82(3)**:627–636. doi: 10.1097/TA.0000000000001359.

47. Kay AB, Majercik S, Sorensen J, Woller SC, Stevens SM, White T, et al. Weight-based enoxaparin dosing and deep vein thrombosis in hospitalized trauma patients: A double-blind, randomized, pilot study. *Surgery*. 2018 Apr 23. pii: S0039-6060(18)30094-1. doi: 10.1016/j.surg.2018.03.001.

48. Malinoski D, Jafari F, Ewing T, Ardary C, Conniff H, Baje M, et al. Standard prophylactic enoxaparin dosing leads to inadequate anti-Xa levels and increased deep venous thrombosis rates in critically Ill trauma and surgical patients. *Journal of Trauma*. 2010 Apr;**68(4)**:874–80. doi: 10.1097/TA.0b013e3181d32271.

49. Haemmila MR, Osborne NH, Henke PK, Kepros JP, Patel SG, Cain-Nielsen AH, et al. Prophylactic Inferior Vena Cava Filter Placement Does Not Result in a Survival Benefit for Trauma Patients. *Ann Surg*. 2015 Oct;**262(4)**:577–85. doi: 10.1097/SLA.0000000000001434.

50. Janjua KJ, Sugrue M, Deane SA. Prospective evaluation of early missed injuries and the role of the tertiary trauma survey. *J Trauma* 1998 Jun;**44(6)**:1000–6; discussion 1006-7.

51. Nair AS, Naik VM, Rayani BK. FAST HUGS BID: Modified Mnemonic for Surgical Patient. *Indian J Crit Care Med*. 2017 Oct;**21(10)**:713–714. doi: 10.4103/ijccm.IJCCM_289_17.

Recommended Reading

Devlin JW, Skrobik Y, Gélinas C, Needham DM, Slooter A, Pandharipande PP, et al. Clinical Practice Guidelines for the Prevention and Management of Pain, Agitation/Sedation, Delirium, Immobility, and Sleep Disruption in Adult Patients in the ICU. *Crit Care Med*. 2018 Sept;**46(9)**:e825–73. doi: 10.1097/CCM.0000000000003299.

Devlin JW, Skrobik Y, Gélinas C, Needham DM, Slooter A, Pandharipande PP, et al. Executive Summary: Clinical Practice Guidelines for the Prevention and Management of Pain, Agitation/Sedation, Delirium, Immobility, and Sleep Disruption in Adult Patients in the ICU. *Crit Care Med*. 2018 Sept; **46(9)**:1532–48. doi: 10.1097/CCM.0000000000003259.

Eastern Association for the Surgery of Trauma. Practice Management Guidelines. Available from www.east.org (accessed online January 2019).

Gaarder C, Naess PA, Frischknecht CE, Hakala P, Handolin L, Heier HE, et al. Scandinavian Guidelines – "The massively bleeding patient". *Scand J Surg*. 2008;**97(1)**:15–36.

Marino PL. Ed The ICU Book. 4th Edn. Wolters Kluwer Health/Lippincott Williams and Wilkins. Philadelphia PA, USA. 2014.

Trauma Anaesthesia **18**

18.1 INTRODUCTION

Trauma anaesthesiologists are an essential part of the trauma team working in close collaboration with the surgeon. Trauma anaesthesia is involved in the entire chain of trauma care; from pre-hospital, to emergency room, often multiple operating room episodes, intensive care, and pain management. Strategies that work in elective cases may not be appropriate for trauma patients. The trauma anaesthesiologist participates in and contributes to the decision-making process during the initial resuscitation, and provides resuscitation and anaesthesia in the perioperative setting.

Because of this comprehensive involvement and the frequent multiple surgeries for some severely injured, trauma anaesthesiologists may be a consistent asset throughout the entire treatment process.

In this chapter, we will cover the aspects of trauma anaesthesia related to damage control in trauma. Anaesthetic involvement in specific situations, such as head trauma, is dealt with in the other relevant chapters in this volume. Special skills are also described in those chapters.

18.2 PLANNING AND COMMUNICATING

When the trauma patient enters the emergency room, the trauma anaesthesiologist should take charge of the airway, optimize oxygenation and resuscitation, while taking in to account the patient's neurological condition and temperature.

The trauma team should then decide the optimal process of care for that individual.

Pitfall

Interventions in the emergency room (ER) should be limited to those that are essential for survival. Ensuring adequate venous access and perhaps an extra-large bore IV cannula may make an important difference; an arterial line may not be worth the time.

The anaesthesiologist has a crucial role in optimizing the physiology to match the surgical strategies. Their assessment of ongoing dynamic changes and reaction to treatment is an essential contribution to the decision-making process.

The planned strategy for resuscitation and surgery should be communicated closely between the surgeon, anaesthesiologist and team, coordinated by the trauma team leader.

(See also Chapter 2.)

18.3 DAMAGE CONTROL RESUSCITATION[1]

Damage control includes damage control anaesthesia, damage control resuscitation (DCR), and damage control surgery, aiming to stop bleeding rapidly, restore blood volume, and aggressively preventing and correcting coagulopathy, hypothermia, and acidosis[2] (see Chapter 6).

Additional knowledge of damage control radiology is of great assistance.[3]

The five principal pillars of DCR are:

- Limiting or omitting fluid administration, early use of blood product.
- Permissive hypotension.
- Targeting coagulopathy.
- Prevent and treat hypothermia.
- Early use of tranexamic acid where indicated.

DCR aims to treat and prevent conditions that exacerbate haemorrhagic shock and the ensuing systemic inflammatory response. DCR addresses the pathophysiological consequences of tissue trauma and blood loss, and reduces the risks of overly aggressive fluid resuscitation, while targeting correction of metabolic derangements and coagulopathy. DCR supports the concept of limiting operative stress by delaying definitive repair until after control of haemorrhage and after the patient's physiology improves. The importance of an early transfer to an ICU for subsequent normalization of microcirculation, correction of coagulopathy, and re-warming is stressed.

With early haemorrhage control and optimal resuscitation, some patients may rapidly improve their haemodynamic state. Therefore, even if initially considered for the DCR pathway, they might now be suitable for definitive care. Constant re-assessment is crucial and the role of the anaesthesiologist in providing continued information about the patient's haemodynamic and organ perfusion is key for joint decision-making.

18.3.1 Limited Fluid Administration

Aggressive fluid resuscitation to restore normal circulatory function has long been the mainstay of the initial approach for haemorrhagic shock. In 2004, Moore et al.[2] coined the term 'bloody vicious cycle', showing that crystalloid administration leads to a transient rise in blood pressure, followed by increased haemorrhage, which requires further fluid administration, leading to the sequence of hypotension, fluid bolus, re-bleeding, and deeper hypotension. It is currently accepted that administration of high volumes of fluid before achieving definitive haemostasis increases the rate of bleeding by raising cardiac output, increased blood pressure counteracting local vasoconstriction and re-opening spontaneously clotted vessels. In addition to dilutional coagulopathy, large volumes of crystalloid fluids have deleterious effects on organ function, the endothelium, and immunological and inflammatory mediators. All of these are associated with poor outcomes. Recent studies have shown that high volumes of crystalloids increase reperfusion injury and leukocyte adhesion, resulting in an increased incidence of infectious complications and multiple organ failure (Table 18.1).

During ongoing surgical bleeding, clear fluids should be limited to minimal amounts or even omitted until definitive control of haemorrhage has been achieved. Early use of blood and blood products in this critically bleeding group of trauma patients reduces crystalloid administration and is the mainstay of resuscitation in damage control. Some even recommend limiting the use of crystalloids

Table 18.1 Consequences of Aggressive Crystalloid Resuscitation[4,5]

Respiratory	↑ Capillary permeability
	Pulmonary oedema, which also results in acute lung injury (ALI)/ acute respiratory distress syndrome (ARDS)
Gut	↑ Intestinal permeability
	Bacterial translocation
	Paralytic ileus
	Abdominal compartment syndrome (ACS)
	Anastomotic dehiscence
Heart	↓ Myocyte action potential
	Ventricular dysfunction
	Arrhythmia
	↓ Membrane polarization
	Disruption of phosphorylation
	Cellular oedema
	Apoptysis
Blood	Dilution of coagulation factors
	Increased blood loss
	Counteracting vasoconstriction
	↓ Oncotic pressure
Vessels	↓ Catecholamine release
	↑ Vascular resistance to catecholamines
Inflammatory Pathways	Activation of inflammation (TNFα, interleukins, SIRS)
	Early vasoplegia
Endothelium	Damage to endothelial integrity
	↑ Capillary leak

Source: Adapted from Cotton BA et al. *Shock.* 2006 August; 26(2):115–21.[4]; Kasotakis G et al. *J Trauma Acute Care Surg.* 2013 May;74(5):1215–21; discussion 1221–2.[5]; Kozer RA. *Anesth Analg.* 2011;112(6):1289–95.

in trauma related haemorrhagic shock to a function of carrier of drugs and to keep lines open between blood product administrations. Preferred types of crystalloids are balanced solutions such as Ringers lactate solution or Plasmalyte. Sodium chloride solution (0.9%, 'normal saline') can contribute to hyperchloraemic acidosis, which may have an adverse effect on renal function.

Limiting fluid administration raises the question of how to maintain blood pressure. The use of vasopressors for haemodynamic support during resuscitation after injury is controversial. While arginine vasopressin and phenylephrine have shown to provide some beneficial effects in patients with traumatic brain injury, lung contusion, or in animal models with haemorrhagic shock, a prospective multicentre study on blunt trauma patients has shown an increased mortality in patients with early vasopressors use.[7] Therefore, hypovolaemic shock should be treated primarily by volume replacement, but low doses of vasopressors might be useful to counteract the sympatholytic and cardiovascular depressant effect of anaesthetic agents.

Subsequently, the question around maintaining blood pressure is: what blood pressure goal should be aimed for during the acute resuscitation of the bleeding trauma patients?

18.3.2 Targeting Coagulopathy

Up to 30% of injured patients present with impaired coagulation on arrival at the care facility. The presence of trauma-related coagulopathy is a surrogate marker of the extent and severity of tissue trauma and shock and correlates with mortality. Coagulation abnormalities related to severe trauma have several causal factors including consumption of clotting factors and platelets, dilution after administration of fluids, fibrinolysis as well as hypothermia and acidosis. Early identification of patients with acute coagulopathy of trauma (ACoT) is crucial for timely initiation of haemostatic resuscitation.[8,9] Early blood gases are a quick and helpful tool to identify patients in shock. Base deficit or lactate has shown to provide a reliable correlation with the need for massive transfusion and risk of death. A base deficit of >2 mmol/L correlates with class two, and

BD >6 mmol/L with class three shock according to the ATLS definition.[10] In the absence of timely laboratory assessment, in patients with evidence of impaired end-organ perfusion and extensive tissue trauma, initiation of haemostatic resuscitation may be indicated even before biological or viscoelastic confirmation of ATC. Early administration of blood products raises logistical challenges. The implementation of a massive transfusion protocol (MTP) is recommended, which will allow the ready availability of blood products, guided by viscoelastic assays.[11]

Fibrinolysis is a key feature of the ATC. A bolus of 1 g of tranexamic acid, followed by an infusion of 1 g over 8 hours is used within many MTPs. It should be given as early as possible to bleeding trauma patients; if treatment is not given until 3 hours or later after injury, it is less effective and could even be harmful. In major haemorrhage, fibrinogen reaches critically low values earlier than other coagulation factors or platelets. The CRASH-2 Trial[12] showed a 15% mortality reduction after the administration of tranexamic acid in trauma patients at risk of significant haemorrhage *in the environments in which the trial took place*. Replacement is generally necessary to maintain a plasma concentration of 150–200 mg/dL and its early use (in the form of cryoprecipitate or fibrinogen concentrate) has been integrated in many MTPs, even though strong evidence supporting this is lacking. A recent study indicated that most severely injured patients have a fibrinolysis shutdown, and therefore, tranexamic acid may have no effect.[13]

Tranexamic acid is not widely used routinely outside of Europe, and despite the increased use of tranexamic acid, the gathering and validity of the data has been called into question in a major trauma centre environment.

18.3.3 Prevent and Treat Hypothermia

Hypothermia adversely affects coagulation as well as cardiac output and function in most bodily organs. Hypothermia and acidosis compromise thrombin generation kinetics via different mechanisms. Hypothermia primarily inhibits the initiation phase, whereas acidosis severely inhibits the propagation phase of thrombin generation. Similarly, hypothermia and acidosis affect fibrinogen metabolism differently. Hypothermia inhibits fibrinogen synthesis, whereas acidosis accelerates fibrinogen degradation, leading to a potential deficit in fibrinogen availability. Thus, the specific steps related to hypothermia prevention and treatment are:

- The operating room (OR) temperature should be warm (25°C or higher). Maintaining a warm OR on patient arrival helps keep patients warm.
- Have additional warming devices available, including a forced air device system, fluid warmers on the IV line, warm IV solutions, and warm blankets.
- Have a system to warm all solutions that are to be used in the surgical field.

KEY MESSAGES

- Assess arterial blood gases on every trauma patient to aid decision-making.
- Before surgical control of haemorrhage:
  - Limit crystalloid fluid resuscitation.
  - Do not use synthetic colloids.
  - Commence blood products and goal directed haemostatic resuscitation early.
  - Allow blood pressure to be below than normal during early haemorrhage control.
- Arrange early transfer to ICU and effective multidisciplinary communication.

18.4 DAMAGE CONTROL SURGERY

Damage control surgery (DCS) describes the strategy of limiting surgical intervention in haemodynamically compromised trauma patients by restricting procedures to early control of haemorrhage and contamination, and postponing the definitive anatomical repair until the patient is more stable.

18.4.1 Anaesthetic Procedures

Being able to predict situations is a key skill for the trauma anaesthesiologist and is derived from extensive experience. The anaesthesiologist should be able to predict how the patient physiology will evolve over a short period of time, and his response to treatment. The anaesthesiologist should anticipate the treatment the patient will receive and the route the patient will need to take to get to a stable state.

18.4.1.1 AIRWAY

In order to be able to correct hypoxia, manage CO_2, protect the airway, and facilitate interventions, most severe trauma patients will require intubation. Anaesthesiologists who deal with airway management daily are probably the best group to perform this task, but if other groups are to perform this, they should be trained to perform it to the same standards and quality. Intubation in patients with possible neck trauma is a recognized difficult airway management situation. There are difficult airway algorithms available to assist decision-making for situations. An oral tube may be impossible, a laryngeal mask not suitable, and a surgical airway the only and fastest option. This decision needs to be made before the patient decompensates, and it requires skills and experience to make the decision in a timely manner. The anaesthesiologist may need to rely on their own skills rather than wait for another individual. The skill of establishing a surgical airway needs to be taught and practised to be retained.

18.4.1.2 BREATHING

Mechanical ventilation is a life-saving treatment but also has increased dangers for trauma patients. Trauma patients are at increased risk of volume and barotrauma, and ARDS from mechanical ventilation, referred to as ventilator induced lung injury (VILI). The injured lung is more susceptible to maldistribution of pressure between healthy and injured parts, leading to collapse in some areas with overdistension in others even at lower tidal volumes. The anaesthesiologist needs to apply judicious amounts of positive end expiratory pressure (PEEP) and a ventilation strategy aimed at minimizing overdistension of the lung.

Damage to the thoracic wall and to the lung increase the risks of pneumothorax, air embolism, and VILI adding to the original acute lung injury. During ventilation, the anaesthesiologist needs to be aware of these potential complications and the options for treatment.

While ventilating the patient, the anaesthesiologist also needs to consider associated injuries and the influence of ventilation on injury. For example, PEEP, $PaCO_2$, and PaO_2 are important in traumatic brain injury treatment strategies. PEEP may reduce blood pressure, especially in the presence of hypovolaemia. Furthermore, PEEP at high levels (>12 mm Hg) may increase intracranial pressure (ICP). Nevertheless, it has also been demonstrated that in brain injured patients during mechanical ventilation, the application of moderate levels of PEEP (up to 8 cm H_2O) provided protection against the occurrence of lung injury, probably by restoring lung volume and reducing lung heterogeneity, that is atelectasis, airway closure, and tidal expiratory flow limitation. Mean arterial pressure (MAP) and ICP monitoring, and prevention of hypoxia are essential for prevention of secondary brain injury. $PaCO_2$ also affects ICP and the aim is to achieve normocarbia ($PaCO_2 = 35$–4.5 mm Hg/4.6–6 kPa). Hypocarbia increases cerebral vasoconstriction leading to decreased cerebral blood flow (CBF), which may decrease ICP but also cause ischaemia. Decreasing $PaCO_2$ (by hyperventilating the patient) is a treatment strategy that should be limited to short duration management of critically raised ICP, for example, en route to an intervention for reducing the ICP (e.g. surgery). Hypercarbia increases CBF by vasodilatation and increases ICP in severe brain injury with the risk of decreasing cerebral perfusion pressure and causing or worsening secondary brain injury.

18.4.1.3 CIRCULATION

Control of exsanguinating bleeding has taken priority over the Airway Breathing Circulation changing the ABC mnemonic to C(Control of Catastrophic Bleeding)-A-B-C, certainly in the prehospital and military setting.

18.4.1.4 VASCULAR ACCESS

Vascular access is required for the administration of resuscitation drugs and blood transfusion. The ATLS® approach calls for two large-bore intravenous (IV) cannulas. The rationale is not to put twice as much volume in (permissive hypotension) but to have redundancy and availability when required. With a second IV you can have a separate access for medication that cannot be mixed, and as backup if you have a dysfunctional line.

If one of the IVs is a small calibre one, there is the option to change it to a larger one using a wire Seldinger technique that will allow exchange for a rapid infusion catheter. Another way to gain better IV access is to apply a tourniquet above the small catheter, infuse 60 mL of IV fluid, and insert a larger bore IV catheter above the small catheter in the now distended vein.

If the need for a rapid infusor system is forseen, an at least 14 G catheter will be needed to allow high flow (500–800 mL/min). The IV lines used for the rapid infusor should not have one-way valves such as in use in intensive care unit (ICU) and only high flow three-way stopcocks if you really need them. Medication should have a separate line from the high flow system. A central venous line allows multiple ports, central venous

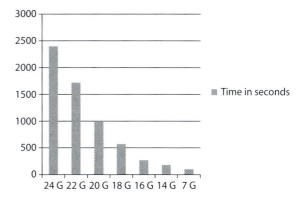

Figure 18.1 Time in seconds to infuse 1 L of clear fluids versus catheter gauge.

pressure measurement, and high flow fluid administration as well as venous blood gas measurements. A central venous line allows early intravenous feeding.

The larger the bore of the IV cannula, the greater the flow (Figure 18.1).

18.4.2 Monitoring

Besides the standard anaesthesia monitoring, a five-lead ECG in case of thoracic injury is advisable. Blunt cardiac injury can be detected by changes in ECG and treated with supportive therapy. Ventilation should be monitored with pulse oximetry for adequate oxygenation and end-tidal (ET) CO_2 for assuring adequate respiratory minute volume. $ETCO_2$ further informs us about cardiac output decreasing in case of circulatory collapse.

An arterial line provides the opportunity for beat-to-beat blood pressure monitoring, blood sampling and physiological status, but should not delay time to surgery or intervention. Arterial line insertion is first attempted peripherally (radial or brachial or dorsal foot arteries) secondarily moving proximally (femoral or axillary arteria) in difficult situations with massive bleeding.

In the OR, in due time and according to the clinical condition, haemodynamic status can be evaluated by accessing cardiac output. The purpose is to evaluate the status of the blood volume and cardiac function in order to secure normovolaemia and -perfusion meanwhile avoiding hypo- as well as hypervolaemia. In the early dramatic phase of DCR using pulse, BP, pulse oximetry, and ETCO2 can be the only possibilities, but when more control is achieved haemodynamic monitoring can be intensified according to the clinical condition.

Haemodynamic monitoring – means of cardiac output and volume estimation:

- Pulse and BP.
- Central venous pressure or central venous saturation ($S_{cv}O_2$) accessed via a central line.
- Transthoracic or transoesophageal echocardiogram – focus assessed transthoracic echocardiography (FATE).
- Mixed venous oxygen saturation via pulmonary artery catheter (rarely indicated in damage control).
- Minimally-invasive cardiac output estimation via arterial line.

Monitoring of a bispectral index (BIS) may prevent awareness during trauma anaesthesia, although BIS responses to ketamine administration are atypical and can be paradoxical.

Monitoring urine output may give some indication of the volume status. Due consideration should be given to insertion of a urine catheter in case of suspected urethra injury.

Temperature monitoring is essential in trauma management. Intra-operative normothermia is an important quality performance measure for patients undergoing surgery as it should be in trauma management. See also below.

18.5 ANAESTHESIA INDUCTION IN HYPOVOLAEMIC SHOCK

18.5.1 Introduction

Anaesthetizing a severely injured patient requires a thorough knowledge of the medications used and their altered pharmacokinetics and pharmacodynamics in the hypovolaemic, acidotic, and hypothermic trauma patient. The principal goal of anaesthesia for trauma patients is to provide analgesia, unconsciousness, and amnesia, and eventually muscle relaxation without further deteriorating the deranged physiology and hemodynamic situation. In traumatic brain injury, systolic blood pressure <90 mm Hg and PaO_2 <60 mm Hg are independently associated with increased morbidity and mortality.

The pharmacokinetics (absorption, distribution, metabolism, and elimination) change significantly with hypovolaemic shock. The severely injured patient is in a condition of increased sympathetic tone in attempts to redistribute the circulation to brain and heart. In shock,

the body becomes the equivalent of a single compartment model, a blood-brain circuit, at the expense of the perfusion of gut, liver, kidneys, and muscles. Intravenous drugs will be almost instantaneously distributed to heart and brain, resulting in a more rapid onset, higher brain concentrations, and more profound effects. Further, many anaesthesia induction agents show a high protein binding. Hence, in hypovolaemic shock and especially after fluid resuscitation, reduced plasma protein binding leads to increased availability of free drug with higher effect site concentration and concomitantly increased adverse haemodynamic effects.

Anaerobic metabolism and metabolic acidosis will alter the distribution of ionizable drugs, leading to an enhanced brain concentration. Furthermore, in shock, hepatic and renal blood flow is markedly decreased impairing the intrinsic metabolic capacity leading ultimately to an increase in the free fraction of drugs and prolonged action. Drugs with a high hepatic extraction rate, such as propofol, ketamine, and morphine and synthetic opioids, will show a prolonged duration of action.

18.5.2 Drugs for Anaesthesia Induction

The effect site equilibration constant, cited as ($t_{1/2}Ke^0$), represents the time necessary for the administered drug to reach an appropriate anaesthetic concentration in the brain. The longer the $t_{1/2}Ke^0$ of a drug, the higher the initial plasma concentration will be needed to achieve a rapid anaesthetic concentration. Hence, intravenous anaesthetic agents with the shortest $t_{1/2}Ke^0$ are generally best suited for a rapid induction in the severely injured, hypovolaemic patient (Table 18.1).

Commonly used anaesthetic drugs have a direct depressant effect on the cardiovascular system, inhibit compensatory mechanisms, and carry a high risk to further deteriorate the haemodynamic status of trauma patients. Subsequent positive pressure ventilation will impair venous return and contribute to further haemodynamic impairment. Recognition of masked hypovolaemia and an accurate estimation of its extent are crucial in the choice of type and dose of anaesthetic drugs.

For induction of general anaesthesia, the most commonly used drugs include ketamine, thiopental, etomidate, midazolam, and propofol. For the choice of the most suited induction agent, the patient's physiology, co-morbidities and the anaesthesiologist's experience should be taken into consideration. All anaesthetic induction agents can be vasodepressors and have potential to cause hypotension, therefore the skill and experience of the anaesthesiologist are the most important determinants for a good outcome. Short-term use of a vasopressor can reverse vasodepressor effects, but it must be emphasized that continued need for vasopressors in the trauma patient population is associated with poor outcomes.

18.5.2.1 PROPOFOL

Propofol has a long $t_{1/2}Ke^0$ of up to 20 minutes, indicating that for rapid induction a higher initial dose is required. However, in shocked patients, propofol shows an increased end-organ sensitivity (e.g. lower C50) and a slower intercompartmental clearance. Haemorrhagic shock has demonstrated to shift the concentration/effect relationship to the left, demonstrating a 2.7-fold decrease in the effect site concentration required to achieve 50% of the maximal effect in the BIS scale. In shock, potency of propofol is increased and the dose required to reach effect site concentration is 5.4-fold reduced. Therefore, rapid induction can be performed with propofol, but a high dose is required in patients exhibiting increased organ sensitivity. This, in the view of the important concomitant negative effects on haemodynamics, makes propofol a poor choice for the trauma setting, but if used, dose reduction to approximately 1/3 is highly recommended.

18.5.2.2 KETAMINE

Ketamine is a highly lipid soluble drug. At a physiologic pH, almost 50% is dissociated and only 12% is bound to plasma proteins. This ensures a rapid blood-brain equilibration and fast clinical onset.

Ketamine is the least likely agent to cause cardiovascular depressant effects. Its direct negative inotrope effect is counteracted by a stimulatory effect on the cardiovascular system, probably by a centrally mediated sympathetic response and inhibition of noradrenaline reuptake. In the severely shocked patient with a state of catecholamine exhaustion or resistance to further catecholamine effect, the direct effects of ketamine on myocardial depression may outweigh the indirect sympathetic effects and haemodynamic collapse may still occur. A reduction of the induction dose to 0.25–0.5 mg/kg IV may be indicated. Ketamine has further shown to provide anti-inflammatory proprieties; however, its clinical impact in trauma patients remains to be determined. Ketamine has reportedly both raised and lowered intracranial pressure. In traumatic brain injury, the cerebral autoregulation is impaired and the CBF is directly depending on the cerebral perfusion pressure. Maintenance of hemodynamic stability may therefore outweigh potential risks. Further, ketamine reduces cerebral oxygen consumption and the cerebral vasodilatation as observed in spontaneously breathing patients may be reduced by controlled ventilation.

18.5.2.3 ETOMIDATE

Haemorrhagic shock produces minimal changes in the pharmacokinetics and pharmacodynamics of etomidate. Etomidate preserves the pressor response to intubation and shock affects only minimally its ability to reach rapidly the effector site. Its central and peripheral volumes are only lightly decreased in acute hypovolaemia, increasing its blood levels by about 20%. Therefore, unlike other hypnotics, only minimal adjustments in induction dose are required to achieve the same drug effect in haemorrhagic shock. As compared to propofol, no increased drug sensitivity had been demonstrated for etomidate. These points provide etomidate with a good safety profile as an induction agent in trauma patients.

However, in many countries, etomidate has been withdrawn after studies showing that in septic patients, even a single dose may suppress the corticoadrenal axis for up to 67 hours. In the non-septic trauma patients, suppression of steroid synthesis does not seem to be associated with worse outcome as increased on mortality or prolonged length of stay.

18.5.2.4 THIOPENTAL

Thiopental exhibits several desirable properties in the shocked patient as a short $t_{1/2}Ke^0$ (1.5 minutes) and a tendency to preserve autonomic responsiveness as a reflex tachycardia or the pressor response to laryngoscopy. However, its usefulness in the setting of hypovolaemic shock is compromised by the important negative inotropy and arteriolar vasodilation, leading to severe hypotension in shocked patients. Doses must therefore be carefully adapted to values, if possible, below a range of 3 mg/kg.

18.5.2.5 MIDAZOLAM

Midazolam in induction dose has shown to significantly decrease plasma noradrenaline/norepinephrine concentration and alters baroreflex control of the heart rate. It also causes reduction of systemic vascular resistance and left ventricular stroke work index. Hence, in hypovolaemic patients, it may further decrease blood pressure and prevent compensatory tachycardia. Additionally, midazolam is highly protein bound inhibiting a rapid entry into the brain effector site. The half-life for closure of its imidazol-ring, which enhances lipid solubility and brain entry, is long (10 minutes), making this agent of little value for rapid sequence induction (RSI) (Table 18.2).

There is no hard outcome evidence supporting one agent over the other, but whatever agent is chosen, induction doses must be adapted and most often reduced to the patient's physiology. Many use a combination of induction drugs combining their different effects. Normalization of haemodynamic parameters with aggressive fluid resuscitation prior to induction has not proven to completely reverse the increase in induction drug potency.

Maintenance of anaesthesia during damage control procedures in the haemodynamically compromised patient needs a careful choice and titration of drugs. Perioperative awareness is well recognized during emergency anaesthesia, often because of dose reduction. A comparison of patients treated by ketamine induction and maintenance with volatiles versus no maintenance drug showed a perioperative awareness rate of 11% versus 43%. The choice of the optimal maintenance drug is influenced by the patient's physiology and their injury profile. For traumatic brain injury and trauma to the spinal cord, intravenous anaesthesia as with propofol is recommended while as in other settings, inhalational anaesthesia might be more suited. A BIS measure might be a valuable help in preventing awareness in the severely shocked patient with altered dose requirements.

Table 18.2 Effects of Anaesthetic Induction Agents			
Induction Agent	**Effector Site Equilibration ($t_{1/2}Ke^0$)**	**Haemodynamic Effects**	**Comments**
Propofol	≤20 minutes	↔ HR unchanged (↔)	Poorly suited for rapid induction in haemodynamic compromise. Potential increase in intracranial pressure outweighed maintenance of haemodynamics.
		↓ Cardiac output	
		↓ Blood Pressure	
		↓ Laryngeal reflexes	
		Vagotonic	
Ketamine	±2 minutes	↑ Heart rate	Minimal dose adjustment needed in hypovolaemic shock.
		↑ Cardiac output	
		↑ Blood pressure	
		Sympathomimetic	
Etomidate	±2.5 minutes	↔ Cardiac output	Possible adrenocortical suppression.
		↔ Blood pressure	
		↓ Steroid synthesis	
		↔ Heart rate	
		↓ Inotropy	
		↔ Laryngeal reflexes	
Thiopental	±1.5 minutes	Vasodilatation	Dose reduction required, ideally <3 mg/kg.
Benzodiazepines	±9 minutes	↓ Cardiac output	Time to reach effector site is slow.
		↓ SVR	
		↓ Sympathetic tone	

18.6 **BATTLEFIELD ANAESTHESIA (See also Chapters 21 and 22)**

Battlefield anaesthesia is both an anaesthetic as well as an operational problem. It is not an exclusive medical problem. It occurs in an environment that both provides the platform from which you treat and influences the decision making.

Battlefield anaesthesia presents many challenges; including the need to maintain airway control, hypothermia of the casualty, restricted drug availability, lack of supplementary oxygen, and the possible requirement for prolonged post-operative mechanical ventilation. Mass casualty situations are also a constant possibility in the military arena. Surgery requires both adequate analgesia and anaesthesia. No single agent can provide both an appropriate level of anaesthesia and analgesia, hence a combination of drugs and techniques is required. The choices of anaesthetic are narrowed in austere conditions; these are limited to general anaesthesia (either intravenous or inhalational), regional anaesthesia, or none at all. For surgical exploration of body cavities, general anaesthesia is most frequently chosen, while a regional anaesthetic may be more appropriate for injuries of the extremities or perineum. In the field, RSI is the norm, using fast-acting hypnotic and neuromuscular blocking agents to facilitate rapid airway control. In the absence or limitation of supplemental oxygen supplies, RSI becomes even more crucial as pre-oxygenation of the patient's lungs is often not possible. There are several RSI cocktails used in the pre-hospital setting, most using a combination of induction agent, paralysing agent, and analgesia. Sedation, amnesia, and analgesia can then be maintained with intravenous agents such as ketamine, benzodiazepines, and opiates.

For long procedures or surgical sites involving the abdomen or thorax, a combination anaesthetic that includes an inhalation agent such as isoflurane may be used. British surgical teams use a portable 'Tri-service Apparatus' that does not require a compressed gas source and have gained much experience with this technique of field anaesthesia. This 'draw-over' type vaporizer is currently also in use by several other countries in austere settings. The draw-over configuration places the ventilator distal to the vaporizer, entraining ambient air and vapour across the vaporizer in the same manner as the spontaneously breathing patient.

Regional anaesthesia remains an important option in battlefield anaesthesia, as it provides both patient comfort and surgical analgesia, while maintaining patient consciousness and spontaneous ventilation. With the relatively large number of extremity wounds in modern conflicts, and certainly in the mass casualty setting with a limited anaesthesia capability, regional aesthetic techniques should not be overlooked. Continuous infusion nerve blocks provide excellent analgesia for post-operative casualties during evacuation.

18.6.1 **Damage Control Anaesthesia in the Military Setting**

Anaesthesia for 'damage control' procedures and major cavity injury is really a fusion of continuing resuscitation and critical care. This requires optimization of haemodynamic status, re-warming of the casualty, and pain relief. One of the biggest challenges will be reversing the hypothermia that is almost universal in haemorrhagic patients in these conditions. As well as warming all intravenous fluids and ventilator circuits, an active re-warming device will be required. If a return to the operating theatre for more definitive surgery is not planned in the forward location, critical care must be maintained throughout the aeromedical evacuation.

18.6.2 **Battlefield Analgesia**

Relief of pain is an important consideration for both the wounded and the military care giver. Provision of effective analgesia is humane, but also attenuates the adverse pathophysiological responses to pain and is likely to aid evacuation from the battlefield and maintain morale. Analgesia may be given at self and buddy-aid levels; protocols to guide medical and paramedical staff in the provision of safe and effective analgesia are available.

Analgesia methods used in recent conflicts include:

- Simple non-pharmacological.
- Reassurance.
- Splinting of fractures.
- Cooling of burns.
- Oral analgesics:
  - Non-steroidal anti-inflammatory drugs.
  - Paracetamol.
- Nerve blocks and infiltration of local anaesthesia.
- Intramuscular and intravenous opiates.

- Fentanyl lollipops.
- Methods under development include intranasal ketamine, fentanyl and inhalation analgesics, for example, methoxyflurane inhalation.

REFERENCES

1. Holcomb JB, Jenkins D, Rhee P, Johannigman J, Mahoney P, Mehta S, Cox ED, Gehrke MJ, Beilman GJ, Schreiber M, et al. Damage control resuscitation: directly addressing the early coagulopathy of trauma. *J Trauma.* 2007;**62(2)**: 307–10.

2. Moore FA, McKinley BA, Moore EE. The next generation in shock resuscitation. *Lancet.* 2004;**363(9425)**:2088–96.

3. Chakraverty S, Zealley I, Kessel D. Damage control radiology in the severely injured patient: what the anaesthetist needs to know. *Brit J Anaesth.* 2014 Aug;**113(2)**:250–7. doi: 10.1093/bja/aeu203.

4. Cotton BA, Guy JS, Morris JA Jr., Abumrad NN. The cellular, metabolic, and systemic consequences of aggressive fluid resuscitation strategies. *Shock.* 2006 Aug;**26(2)**:115–21.

5. Kasotakis G, Sideris A, Yang Y, de Moya M, Alam H, King DR, et al. Inflammation, Host Response to Injury I: Aggressive early crystalloid resuscitation adversely affects outcomes in adult blunt trauma patients: an analysis of the Glue Grant database. *J Trauma. Acute Care Surg* 2013 May;**74(5)**:1215–21; discussion 1221–2. doi: 10.1097/TA. 0b013e3182826e13.

6. Zarychanski R, Abou-Setta AM, Turgeon AF, Houston BL, McIntyre L, Marshall JC, et al. Association of hydroxyethyl starch administration with mortality and acute kidney injury in critically ill patients requiring volume resuscitation: a systematic review and meta-analysis. JAMA: *J Amer Med Assoc.* 2013 Feb 20;**309(7)**:678–88. doi:10.1001/jama.2013.430.

7. Sperry JL, Minei JP, Frankel HL, West MA, Harbrecht BG, Moore EE, Maier RV, Nirula R. Early use of vasopressors after injury: caution before constriction. *J Trauma.* 2008 Jan;**64(1)**:9–14. doi: 10.1097/TA.0b013e31815dd029.

8. Brohi K, Singh J, Heron M, Coats T. Acute traumatic coagulopathy. *J Trauma.* 2003 Jun;**54(6)**:1127–30.

9. Brohi K, Cohen MJ, Ganter MT, Matthay MA, Mackersie RC, Pittet JF. Acute traumatic coagulopathy: initiated by hypoperfusion: modulated through the protein C pathway? *Ann Surg.* 2007 May;**245(5)**:812–18.

10. Mutschler M, Nienaber U, Brockamp T, Wafaisade A, Fabian T, Paffrath T, et al. TraumaRegister DGU®: Renaissance of base deficit for the initial assessment of trauma patients: a base deficit-based classification for hypovolemic shock developed on data from 16,305 patients derived from the TraumaRegister DGU®. *Crit Care.* 2013 Mar 6;**17(2)**:R42. doi: 10.1186/cc12555.

11. Stensballe J, strowski SR, Johansson PI. Viscoelastic guidance of resuscitation. *Curr Opin Anesthesiol.* 2014 Apr;**27(2)**:212–8. doi: 10.1097/ACO.0000000000000051. Review.

12. Shakur H, Roberts I, Bautista R, Caballero J, Coats T, Dewan Y, et al. Effects of tranexamic acid on death, vascular occlusive events, and blood transfusion in trauma patients with significant haemorrhage (CRASH-2): a randomised, placebo-controlled trial. *Lancet* 2010;**376(9734)**:23–32.

13. Moore HB, Moore EE, Gonzales E, Chapman MP, Chin TL, Silliman CC, et al. Hyprinofibrinolysis, physiologic fibrinolysis, and fibrinolysis shutdown: The spectrum of post injury fibrinolysis and relevance to antifibrinolytic therapy. *J Trauma. Acute Care Surg.* 2014 Dec;**77(6)**:811–7; discussion 817. doi: 10.1097/TA.0000000000000341.

Psychology of Trauma **19**

19.1 WHAT IS PSYCHOLOGICAL TRAUMA?

Psychological trauma can be defined as an incident or event involving a perceived or actual threat of harm, injury and/or death, which overwhelms an individual's coping resources. Traumatic events affect all those involved: this means not only the survivors, but also their relatives and friends, as well as rescue workers and medical staff.

19.2 REACTIONS TO TRAUMA

Within 24 hours of the event, patients may begin to experience a number of common reactions affecting their thoughts (cognitive), feelings (emotional), physical reactions, and behaviours. These vary in intensity and duration and are normal reactions to the abnormal event just experienced. Common reactions include:

- Difficulty concentrating/remembering things.
- Recurrent dreams, nightmares, or flashbacks.
- Mentally replaying/reconstructing the event.
- A sense of helplessness and/or hopelessness.
- Questioning beliefs, meaning.
- Feeling numb or disconnected.
- Low mood, anger, or irritability.
- Anhedonia (a psychological condition characterized by inability to experience pleasure in normally pleasurable acts).
- Irregularities in sleep and appetite or digestive problems.
- Hyper vigilance, startling easily.
- Avoidance of associations with the event.

If the trauma also involved loss, such as the death of a friend or loved one, or even the loss of a limb or mobility

(paraplegia or quadriplegia), the above reactions will also be accompanied by grief reactions.

Some people are at greater risk for developing sustained and long-term reactions to a traumatic event, developing post-traumatic stress disorder (PTSD), depression, and generalized anxiety. Factors that may contribute include:

- History of previous trauma. A traumatic event may activate unresolved fears or frightening memories.
- Premorbid chronic medical illness or psychological/psychiatric disorders.
- Multiple stressors prior to the incident.

19.3 POST-TRAUMATIC STRESS DISORDER

Post-traumatic stress disorder can be defined as a serious and potentially debilitating mental condition triggered by being exposed to a trauma. Symptoms are intense, invasive, and extreme and may include distress, physical reactions (nausea, sweating, heart racing), flashbacks, nightmares, anxiety, and depression.

PTSD is classically described as having four phases:

- Fear (am I/is s(he) going to survive?).
- Anger (why did this happen?).
- Frustration (why can't I do.../why can't I/they return to 'normal?').
- Resignation (life goes on...).

19.4 TRAUMA AND ICU

Patients who were injured through a traumatic event and are thus admitted to the intensive care unit (ICU) are not only experiencing psychological distress due to the initial event, but also from the treatment itself: procedures, sleep disturbance, delirium, pain, and the general ICU environment. This may occur weeks, months, or even years after discharge from the ICU.

The patients' psychological distress and frustration may be exacerbated by reduced physical functioning resulting from injuries, slow progress of healing, and the prospect of many months of recovery (see PTSD above), as well as the patients' inability to remember the events of the initial trauma owing to the injury, or the medication administered (sedatives and analgesia). Furthermore, the occurrence of bizarre hallucinations and delusions in ICU ('ICU psychosis') is terrifying and causes the patient to be extremely upset, aggressive, paranoid, and uncooperative.

19.5 THE CLINICAL PSYCHOLOGIST

19.5.1 The Role of the Clinical Psychologist

The clinical psychologist will assist in identifying, treating, and preventing the psychological aspects of trauma for the patient, family members, and medical team.

19.5.1.1 FOR THE PATIENT

- Establish method of communication if patient is still ventilated or unable to speak due to the nature of their injury.
- Identify/diagnose, treat, and potentially prevent psychological disorders.
- Identify other complications that may hinder the patient's ability to heal (substance abuse, family dynamics, personality traits, pre-existing psychiatric conditions).
- Offer psychological support (orientation, containment, acknowledgement, and normalization of situation).
- Debriefing of incident and ICU environment.
- Provide psycho-education on ICU process, trauma, recovery, mental/emotional/social aspects of experience.
- Teach and develop coping mechanisms/strategies to deal with shock of waking up in ICU, being ventilated, processing initial event, managing ongoing trauma in ICU and throughout recovery process even after patient is discharged from hospital/rehabilitation.
- Motivate patients to be compliant with other disciplines (physiotherapists, dietician, etc.).

- Help the patient to accept physical changes, process losses, and recover mentally and emotionally.
- Assist the patient to be able to contemplate their future and to reintegrate back into their life.
- Conduct grief counselling.

19.5.1.2 FOR THE FAMILY

For the family/support system (starts when patient is unconscious):

- Teach family-centred collaborative decision-making.
- Manage family dynamics.
- Debriefing of incident, ICU environment, and appearance of patient.
- Provide psycho-education on ICU process, trauma, patient recovery, mental/emotional/social aspects of experience.
- Teach and develop coping mechanisms to deal with the many facets of this experience.
- Teach family skills to support the patient mentally and emotionally.
- Assist family in taking care of themselves through the stressful event and after discharge.
- Conduct grief counselling.

Visitors are important for the patient's well-being, but at the same time they may have a negative influence. The patient's relatives have witnessed them so critically ill for days and even weeks in ICU; every day being an emotional struggle. Once the patient is awake, they can often be extremely overprotective or overbearing, as they are terrified by the possibility of a relapse. The patient's support system experiences symptoms of compassion fatigue, anxiety, depression, and PTSD.

19.5.1.3 FOR THE TEAM

- Promote development of skills so they can assist in the psychological well-being of the patient.
- Provide training.
- Encourage communication with patients and family members.
- Inspire a multidisciplinary approach to patient care.
- Offer debriefing, as team members are constantly exposed to trauma, death, and psychological stressors.
- Assist in helping them take care of themselves mentally/emotionally and socially.

19.5.2 **When to Call the Clinical Psychologist**

No matter what the physical injury, **every** patient admitted to the ICU should be referred to the clinical psychologist, who will determine the length of therapy and type of intervention, in consultation with the primary physician/surgeon. Some of the interventions will overlap with the trauma counsellors and the social worker, all of whom are trained to assist the patient and their family through the trauma experience.

Early intervention can assist the patient to recover more quickly, both physically and emotionally, as well as limit new psychological disorders: **patients should be referred within 48 hours of admission**.

For those patients who are ventilated and sedated, the clinical psychologist will begin working with the family. Once the patient's sedation is lifted, the clinical psychologist will begin assessing and subsequently treating the patient. It is not necessary to wait for the patient to be weaned from the ventilator, become distressed, or personally request psychological assistance before intervening.

All trauma patients can benefit from some form of psychological intervention. When patients and family members receive psychological intervention, they are more cooperative with other members of the team, and there are less family 'explosions', sabotage, and fighting with staff.

RECOMMENDED READING

American Psychological Association (APA) Handbooks in Psychology® Apr 17, 2017.

American Psychiatric Association (APA) Handbook of Trauma Psychology: Cook JM, Gold SN Eds. Volume 1. Foundations in Knowledge, Volume 2. Trauma Practice.

Diagnostic and Statistical Manual of Mental Disorders, 5th Edition: DSM. 2013.

The psychological aspects of intensive care units. Dannenfeldt G. *Curationis*. 1982 Sep;**5(3)**:27–31.

This two-volume handbook provides a survey of major areas and subtopics of empirical knowledge and practical applications in the field of trauma psychology.

Physical and Rehabilitation **20** Medicine P&RM

20.1 DEFINITION

This speciality is known as *physiatry* in the USA, or physical and rehabilitation medicine (P&RM) elsewhere. It is a medical speciality which treats the injured patient following acute trauma to restore function and work towards reintegration of the patient into all spheres of social and occupational life. The terms are often used to describe the whole medical team caring for the patient, not only the doctor.

20.2 THE REHABILITATION 'TEAM'

Just as the concept in trauma resuscitation of the 'team' is well established as per ATLS® principles, a similar concept applies to the rehabilitation process. The team members will include: doctor, physiotherapist, occupational therapist, speech therapist, social worker, dietician, psychologist, vocational therapist (a subspecialty of occupational therapy), and possibly a recreational therapist in developed countries. The type of therapy each patient receives is determined according to their injury and physical needs, and is a team decision following a full assessment.

20.3 REHABILITATION STARTS IN ICU

Ideally the rehabilitation of all trauma patients should commence in the intensive care unit (ICU), especially once the patient is reasonably physiologically stable. *Physiotherapy* is critical in the ICU setting for respiratory function as well as joint mobility to prevent contractures. *Occupational therapy*, particularly for hand and upper limb function, should also commence, and is essential in the management of burn patients. The *speech therapist* can assist in ICU if the patient is unable to swallow, and formally evaluate the swallowing, to advise, for example, whether a percutaneous gastrostomy (PEG) is required if swallowing is neurologically impaired. A video swallow examination is the ideal investigation in a cooperative patient to fully assess the swallowing function. The *dietician* can work closely with the speech therapist in advising the type of diet to maintain optimal nutrition during the ICU stay. Within a few days post-injury, a patient will develop malnutrition, requiring anticipation by the clinician, as this will impact on wound healing, raise the risk of pressure ulcers, and increase the risk of wound sepsis. Many trauma patients develop a paralytic ileus, and this will need prokinetics as well as careful nutritional support. *Social worker* intervention in ICU is invaluable to identify premorbid social issues and liaise with the *psychologist* to provide support and treatment for both the patient and the family members. Many patients benefit from early intervention with antidepressant medication commenced in intensive care. The role of the *doctor* is to minimize secondary disability and guide the trauma team regarding specific functional impairments such as bladder and bowel function (particularly in spinal cord injured patients). Acidification of the urine, using ascorbic acid (vitamin C) or cranberry juice, may be helpful in minimizing urinary tract infections. Urodynamic studies will only be performed after the 'spinal shock' phase of the injury, and guide on long-term management of bladder function. In the ICU, it is critical to ensure regular functioning of the bowel with use of laxatives, especially as higher spinal injuries (above T6) are prone to autonomic dysreflexia with constipation. Patients frequently arrive in the rehabilitation facility with the rectum loaded with faeces, or even impacted.

The doctor can advise as to where the patient should be transferred, post ICU to continue rehabilitation. Traumatic brain injury (TBI) patients who are unable to follow commands or respond to therapy may require initial treatment post-ICU in a sub-acute unit and continual assessment to evaluate their readiness for acute rehabilitation therapy. Medical stability is important, although the need for subsequent surgery, for example, orthopaedic or reconstructive plastic surgery, should not delay the process of commencing rehabilitation. It is essential that the acute care surgeons communicate their future surgical plans to allow for preparation of the patient whilst in a rehabilitation facility.

Specific issues that require resolution prior to transfer for acute rehabilitation include establishment of a colostomy, if required. If the patient is likely to be a long-term wheelchair user, consideration should include siting the colostomy higher up on the abdominal wall for ease of patient access and maintenance.

Nursing care in ICU to prevent pressure sores is critical, as pressure sores can delay the whole process of acute rehabilitation and result in extremely high costs for funders, patients, and their families.

A restless patient is not usually the one at high risk, but rather the immobilized patient who is, for example, in traction or on a ventilator. Occipital sores are a scar for life, with no hair growth.

Medical management in the ICU will directly impact on the medical care in the rehabilitation facility. For example, management of pain with drugs contacting codeine result in dependency and chronic constipation. The use of a pain scale when administering analgesia is essential in the cooperative patient. Poorly controlled pain will impact negatively and affect the ability of the patient to participate in the rehabilitation process. This includes post-concussion headaches, which cause significant morbidity in TBI patients. Spinal cord injury (SCI) patients and amputees experience neuropathic pain, and many centres have clear guidelines for treatment of this common complication. Treatment and education of both the patient and the family should commence as soon as the patient develops symptoms.

20.4 OUTCOMES-BASED REHABILITATION (OBR)

Outcomes-based rehabilitation is the common method for continual monitoring and assessment of the progress of the rehabilitation patient, and setting of individualized goals for various aspects of the therapy as well as social and psychological goals, which all aim to reintegrate the patient into their home, community, and work environment. The assessment covers physical as well as cognitive goals, and is based on the anticipated outcomes of all the rehabilitation therapies.[1] OBR uses a variety of standardized tools to achieve this.

20.4.1 FIM/FAM Assessment[2,3]

One of the most common tools used is the FIM/FAM assessment (Functional Independence Measure and Functional Assessment Measure).

20.4.2 Glasgow Outcome Scale[4]

Specific to TBI, is the 'Glasgow Outcome Score' (GOS). This divides patient into five categories and assists in the prediction of longer-term outcomes in rehabilitation (see Appendix B.5.1) (Table 20.1).

Table 20.1 Glasgow Outcome Score

Parameter	Response	Score
Eye opening	Nil	1
	To pain	2
	To speech	3
	Spontaneously	4
Motor response	Nil	1
	Extensor	2
	Flexor	3
	Withdrawal	4
	Localizing	5
	Obeys command	6
Verbal response	Nil	1
	Groans	2
	Words	3
	Confused	4
	Orientated	5

20.4.3 Rancho Los Amigos Scale[5]

The Rancho Los Amigos Scale of Cognitive Functioning,[4] developed in a rehabilitation centre of the same name in California, is a graded scale, assessing TBI patients with closed injury, on a score of 1–10, based on cognition and behaviour. This can be used in combination with the OBR assessment tools and assists the family members to understand the stages of recovery in TBI (Table 20.2).

Table 20.2 Ranchos Los Amigos Scale	
Level	
Level I	No Response: Total Assistance
Level II	Generalized Response: Total Assistance
Level III	Localized Response: Total Assistance
Level IV	Confused/Agitated: Maximal Assistance
Level V	Confused/Inappropriate Non-agitated: Maximal Assistance
Level VI	Confused/Appropriate: Moderate Assistance
Level VII	Automatic, Appropriate: Minimal Assistance for daily living skills
Level VIII	Purposeful, Appropriate: Stand-by Assistance
Level IX	Purposeful, Appropriate: Stand-by Assistance on Request
Level X	Purposeful, Appropriate: Modified Independent

20.5 SUMMARY

In general terms, following trauma, most patients admitted to an acute rehabilitation facility will be dependent for all or some of their needs. The goal of physical rehabilitation is to maximize independence for each patient in terms of activities of daily living (ADLs). Most acute rehabilitation facilities will accept patients with tracheostomy tubes, PEG tubes and IV lines. Tracheostomy patients should be carefully reviewed prior to transfer for rehabilitation, and efforts made to possibly replace with a fenestrated tube, to encourage communication. Ventilated patients are accepted by some units, however the ability of the patient to follow an intensive therapy programme may be curtailed if they are ventilator.

Recent technological developments for use in the rehabilitation of patients, such as the Lokomat® (Hocoma GmBH, Zurich, Switzerland) and Exoskeleton are becoming more widespread and available in rehabilitation

facilities, and are used in spinal cord injuries and traumatic brain injuries.

Rehabilitation in a dedicated and suitable facility with access to a variety of supplies and equipment is the continuation of the acute trauma care for the patient, and is essential for reintegration of each trauma patient into their home, community, and workplace.

Pitfalls

- Failure to refer early, before muscle wasting or contractures develop.
- Failure to communicate on weight bearing status.
- Early psychological counselling is an integral part of physical rehabilitation.
- Intensive care medication is not always congruent with good rehabilitation therapy.

REFERENCES AND RECOMMENDED READING

References

1. Landrum PK, Schmidt ND, McLean A. Outcome-Oriented Rehabilitation. Aspen Publishers Inc. Gaithersburg, Maryland, 1995.
2. Turner-Stokes L, Nyein K, Turner-Stokes T, Gatehouse C. The UK FIM+FAM Functional Assessment Measure. *Clin Rehabil.* 1999 Aug;**13(4)**:277–87.
3. Wright J. The Functional Assessment Measure. *The Center for Outcome Measurement in Brain Injury.* http://www.tbims.org/combi/FAM (accessed online December 2018).
4. Jennet B, Bond M. Assessment of outcome: a practical scale. *Lancet*; 1975 Mar;**i(9705)**:480–4.
5. Rancho Los Amigos National Rehabilitation Center (1 March 2011). The Rancho Levels of Cognitive Functioning. Available from http://www.neuroskills.com/resources/rancho-los-amigos-revised.php (accessed online January 2019).

Recommended Reading

Chhabra HS (Ed.) *ISCoS Textbook on Comprehensive management of Spinal Cord Injuries.* Wolters Kluwer, Philadelphia PA, USA, 2015.

Cifu DMD (Ed.) 2016. *Braddon's Physical Medicine and Rehabilitation.* 5th Edition. Elsevier

Frontera WR (Ed.) *De Lisa's Physical Medicine and Rehabilitation: Principles and Practice.* Lippincot Williams Wilkins/Wolters Kluwer, Philadelphia PA, USA, 2010.

Robinson LR. *Trauma Rehabilitation.* Lippincot Williams Wilkins/Wolters Kluwer, Philadelphia PA, USA, 2005.

WHO International Classification of Functioning Disability and Health (International Classification of Function ICF) May 2001. Available from https://www.who.int/classifications/icf/en/ (accessed online Jan 2019).

Austere Environments

21.1 DEFINITION

Austere: **Severely simple, morally strict, harsh.**

Harsh: **Unpleasantly rough or sharp, severe, cruel.**

Multiple casualties: **More than one patient, but can be dealt with within existing resources.**

Mass casualties: **Many patients with demands beyond the resources available.**

21.2 OVERVIEW

In certain situations, as for example, in the early aftermath of a major natural disaster or in war situations, limited care may have to be delivered owing to limited resources. However, these situations can be avoided by better preparedness and organization of medical/surgical teams and their equipment.

The need to improve and standardize the humanitarian medical and surgical care became obvious after the Haiti earthquake in 2010, when many medical teams and 44 field hospitals were delivered, all with different medical policies and capacities to fulfil their missions as needed. Concerns were raised about legal rights to deliver care, the lack of coordination, and professional standards, as well as the wrong type of care being offered. This led to relief expert meetings and the creation of the 'Forward Medical Team' (FMT) group. Under the auspices of the Global Health Cluster and the World Health Organisation, the document, 'Classification and Minimum Standards for Foreign Medical Teams in Sudden Onset Disasters'[1] was published in 2013, in order to limit situations where 'futile care in resources limited circumstances' would be delivered. A minimum of standards should always be met, and preparedness is key. Nevertheless, this chapter briefly touches on hospital/surgical minimum standards and solutions available when hospital system and equipment or logistical support fail for unexpected reasons.

The perspective of working in an austere environment is quite different from the training paradigm, an academic practice with multi-tiered care, or an elective private practice. Austere surgery requires a thoughtful approach to realistic surgical care within the context of the environment in which the surgical team must alter their perspective.

Humanitarian surgical care operates within the framework of a staged systematic approach to care. The role of the team is not to merely operate on the individual patient, but to make every attempt at preserving lives and returning the patient back to his/her home. This can only be realized within the framework of the environment and contingencies. In the response to a natural or a human-made disaster, this also implies that medical aid workers should protect their own life, health, and work stamina, and not to become casualties of austere circumstances themselves. This includes not only infrastructure, resources, sutures, and drugs, but sleep discipline and self-protection against sleep disturbances. Flexibility and capability beyond one's conventional speciality are also required: surgeons do not often service generators, and anaesthetists do not often sterilize water, but they may have to.

21.3 INFRASTRUCTURE

Infrastructure requirements include shelter, power for lighting and temperature control, and water for hygiene and cooking purposes. Waste needs to be disposed of properly, medical waste disposal (particularly sharps) always being problematic. Resources include medical gases, food, drugs, fluids, and other consumables such as gloves and gowns.

Following a natural disaster, or in a conflict or post-conflict environment, supply chains and systems will be disrupted and vulnerable. Lack of security may enable looting or vandalism of medical aid facilities. No delivery can ever be guaranteed, and the team may have only what they carried with them initially.

21.3.1 Location

The location of a field hospital should be in a 'safe place' where all parties in the conflict are aware of its purpose. It should be protected by walls, sandbags, adhesive plastic on glass windows, and so on, against damage from explosions. Security guards speaking the common language should check all people entering.

21.3.2 Hospital Structures

21.3.2.1 WATER SUPPLY

Trauma and surgical/obstetrical emergency care consume approximately 60–100 L minimum of water/patient/day and is therefore dependent on a continuous secured water supply. That supply is essential when the hospital location is decided. However, extra water storage facilities should be installed as it is difficult to supply water by others means, for example, with water trucks.

21.3.2.2 ENERGY

Electrical or energy support needs to be robust, which may necessitate parallel systems such as, for example, electricity from a local supplier, from fuel/kerosene generators, or back-up electricity from car batteries in operating rooms (ORs). A surgical hospital of 50 beds requires 100 KVA for OR lights, heating or air-conditioning, sterilization, x-ray, and refrigeration.

21.3.2.3 WASTE DISPOSAL

A waste disposal system needs an efficient incinerator for contaminated solid waste and a septic tank for the main sewage.

21.3.2.4 STERILIZATION DEPARTMENT

The sterilization department should be located close to the ORs and is divided into a 'dirty area' where used instruments are collected and washed, and a 'clean area' where the same instruments are packed before being sent to the 'sterilization area'. The autoclave system

needs to be robust and can depend on electric or gas-heated steam/pressure autoclaves, but the same type of steam/pressure autoclaves heated by open fire can be sufficient when energy supplies are unreliable.

21.3.2.5 SURGICAL EQUIPMENT

Surgical instruments are subject to wear and tear when specially used for severe injuries to the extremities, including bone. For example, Gigli saws do break, and in rare situations other sterilizable tools (e.g. a hacksaw, for amputations) bought from the market can be used. The main principle is to use tools/instruments that do not cause any further harm (e.g. to soft tissues during amputations).

21.3.2.6 BLOOD BANK

Set-up of a blood-bank takes time, demands special equipment, and trained laboratory technicians. It also needs established routines to find blood donors, to test and preserve the donated blood, etc. Autotransfusion may be the only alternative, and the technique of collecting non-contaminated blood from the chest and/or the abdomen, filtering, and intravenously re-infusing blood should be well known. New portable and user-friendly devices have been developed and should be in the equipment available. This, in addition to total focus on blood-sparing surgical techniques, may be life-saving.

21.3.3 Health Protection of the Deployed Surgical Team

Psychological and physical stamina are preconditions *sine qua non*: psychologically, some doctors do not work well out their normal hospital or workplace, and some cannot adapt easily. In addition, the availability of a volunteer does not imply the ability or even the affability required to work in a small team. All members of a surgical team need to understand this and have a realistic expectation of what they can – or cannot – provide in the situation in which they find themselves.

21.3.3.1 VECTOR-BORNE DISEASE

In 2003, in Liberia, nearly 20% of 225 deployed US marines developed malaria; it was subsequently found that only 10% of the population at risk had been compliant with chemoprophylaxis and none had slept under mosquito nets. Attention must be paid to the existing threats and simple measures are effective: anti-malarial prophylaxis, long-sleeves at dawn and dusk, repellent, sleeping under nets, and mosquito control measures.

21.3.3.2 ENTERIC ILLNESS

The incidence of diarrhoea among deployed military personnel from industrialized countries to lesser developed countries is typically 30% per month overall, with clinical incidence between 5 and 7 per 100 person-months. The risk appears to be higher early during deployment and is associated with poor hygiene conditions and contaminated food sources. Meticulous attention to hand-washing and food source management mitigates this risk.

21.3.3.3 ROAD TRAUMA

Globally, many road trauma deaths now occur in the developing world and 50% of these deaths occur among vulnerable road users, such as pedestrians, cyclists, or motorcyclists. The risk of speeding, weak adherence to seatbelt discipline, and cavalier driving is not only to the vehicle occupants, but also to host nation road users. A deployed Westerner causing injury or death to a local child would not only be a personal tragedy for the child, the family and the driver, but could also ruin a mission.

21.3.3.4 PHYSICAL, SEXUAL, AND MENTAL HEALTH

Surgeons wishing to deploy need to have high health status; diabetics, for example, are unlikely to do well without their cold-chain controlled insulin. An unfit surgeon could become a liability rather than an asset to the mission. Deployments away from home, time away from duty, availability of alcohol, interaction of deployed workers with the local population prepared to undertake transactional sex and the non-use of condoms increase the risks of sexually-transmitted infections.

21.4 SURGICAL TECHNIQUES TO HAVE IN MIND

21.4.1 Bleeding Control

All surgeons should be able to operate while limiting blood loss to a minimum, whether diathermy is available or not. Each millilitre of extra blood loss may be

difficult to replace. Early decision to perform laparotomy or thoracotomy for suspect bleeding is necessary, particularly for penetrating trauma (e.g. anterolateral thoracotomy when chest drains yields 1100 mL or more). Chest drains do not need to be connected to a three-bottle system and suction. A collecting bottle with a water seal, or, for example, even a closed urinary bag system may suffice.

Thorough control of haemostasis before closure or packing of an abdomen, chest, or a wound may take extra time, but is even more important when blood is missing. Ligation of a large vessel may be the only life-saving possibility when shunting or repair is unfeasible.

21.4.2 Control of Contamination

Bowel injuries should be treated according to damage control when indicated. Control of contamination needs to be followed by primary repair or restoration of bowel continuity as early as possible, because stomas are poorly tolerated in this setting.

21.4.3 Treatment of War Wounds

Thorough examination, and if needed, also cleaning and debridement of war wounds is important, as it reduces the number of re-operations (number of nil per os) and infectious complications. Remove all dead tissue and loose bone fragments that do not have any blood supply. Be conservative with skin removal and when amputations are needed; skin can be harvested from the amputated part and spared in refrigerators. The wounds should be left open for delayed closure. Only do packing of the wounds for haemostasis, but dressings of wounds should allow some drainage. Change of dressing can be performed every third to fourth day unless signs of infection force the patient back to Operating Theatre (OR) earlier.

21.4.4 Amputations

Never perform amputation without consent from the patient and/or family, and a second opinion is important when possible. Avoid guillotine amputations and aim for preserving length. Use a pneumatic tourniquet to avoid bleeding from vessels before they have been ligated. Leave the wound of the stump open for delayed closure.

21.4.5 Stabilization of Fractures

Stabilization of fractures can satisfactory be achieved with plaster of paris or if available, external fixators. When strict sterile conditions are questionable, internal – and sometimes also external – fixation should not be applied. Traction is an option for certain fractures of the femurs, although ideally only for a limited time while waiting for better surgical circumstances. For the upper limb, mobility is a priority over stability in opposition to the lower limb, where stability is a priority before mobility.

21.4.6 Obstetrics

Obstetrical problems are frequently encountered also in war situations and the knowledge of Caesarean section technique is mandatory. Listen to the midwife's suggestions if they are available and always prioritize the health of the mother.

21.4.7 Anaesthesia[2,3]

Anesthesia is always a significant medical intervention and the anesthetist must be a qualified, registered specialist. The drug of choice for major surgery is, for the International Committee of the Red Cross (ICRC) still ketamine as it is safe and possible to administer intravenously or intramuscularly. A draw-over apparatus for anesthesia is an important option when supply of compressed gases is unavailable. The use of regional or peripheral nerve blockade with ultrasound guidance can be of great value, although care needs to be taken not to mask signs of compartment syndrome.

21.5 POST-OPERATIVE CARE AND DOCUMENTATION

The field hospital level II (WHO classification) does not allow advanced post-operative care with ventilator support, which implicates that indications for surgery need to be adapted. Pain relief is based on paracetamol and anti-inflammatory medication, tramadol, and oral morphine if needed (i.v. should be avoided). A minimum pre- and post-operative standard includes pulse oximetry and post-operative care protocol. Patient documentation should include admission number and individual patient file on paper. In mass casualty situations and when hospitals are overloaded, patient reports stay short and can be completed by written information on bandages, for example, date for next change of dressing.

21.6 SUMMARY

Although futile care in resource limited circumstances should be avoided by good preparedness, all medical personnel may have to rapidly adapt when situations are extreme or deteriorate. Acceptable levels of care can still be preserved by remaining thorough and adapting equipment and surgical/anesthesiologic techniques to more basic levels.

Austerity is characterized by deficiency and inadequacy. Even within a developed world setting, a person can find themselves in an austere environment. For example, imagine the situation of a surgical trainee (resident) facing a ruptured abdominal aneurysm for the first time, and knowing that there is no help available for several hours. The inadequacy is in the trainee's lack of knowledge and experience, and the deficiency is in the absence of immediate senior backup.

Therefore, it is important to understand where deficiencies and inadequacies lie, and how to deal with them. The underpinning mantra needs to be, 'Improvise, adapt, overcome.'

When the surgical team is placed in a position where they are aware that they are likely to be challenged professionally, it is imperative that they take stock of what they, personally, are capable of in terms of expertise in surgical care. This requires a hard, honest look in the mirror, without pride or ego fogging the reflected image.

- 'Do I have what it takes to be working solo in a surgical team in the bush/on a rescue mission/at an earthquake site/in a war zone/where the nearest qualified help may be over 1000 km away/with no communication or re-supply for at least 10 days?' This list is clearly not exhaustive.
- If I have enough surgical skills to tackle most problems, will the situation allow it?
- Is there even a hospital? Has it been destroyed by tsunami, earthquake, bombing? What shelter will I have to work in – if any? What can I do on the floor of a school room with only a headlight and no anaesthetist?
- What equipment is available to me? Do I have any surgical instruments, or must I take my own? Are

there any disposables – sutures, syringes, needles, drugs, drapes, gowns, gloves, etc.? If not, how can I get around these problems? Is it possible to make up my own intravenous fluids – do I know how? Where can I get clean water from? What 'disposables' can I re-use?

- If I can deal with all these deficiencies, can I relate to those whom I will be working with and/or my patients? Can I speak the language – or one that will allow communication?
- What – if any – arrangements can be made for a higher level of care or transfer out of my working environment? How long could I reasonably manage a patient post-operatively – with or without ventilation?
- What drugs do I have for dealing with pain, infection, anaesthesia, intercurrent illnesses? What antiseptics do I have for cleaning wounds and surgical site preparation?

These uncomfortable questions often must be dealt with in a hurry, on the spot, and when we are least prepared for them. It is therefore vital that we have prepared ourselves as best we can by our training and having thought out beforehand just what we would need if asked to pick up a grab-bag and go to a remote and possibly dangerous spot, where little or no support will be on hand for several days.

Along with our professional armamentarium and competence, we will need good interpersonal skills to deal with the stresses of facing a scenario where others may also be finding themselves in an isolated position and well out of their comfort zones, both professionally and personally. Those we are asked to work with may have been significantly traumatized, both physically and emotionally, owing to loss of property and loved ones. They may not be seeing priorities in the same way, and their normal skill levels may be affected by grief and anger. It is important to recognize that their emotions are probably not directed at you, but their level of control over them in crisis is not normal.

It is not the purpose of this section to provide the surgical team with all the answers when exposed to an austere environment for the first time, but rather to make them think of what can go wrong.

'If it can go wrong, it will – and in the worst way possible'.

However, whatever does go wrong can usually be mitigated by prior preparation and imaginative thought. In these uncomfortable situations, it is important to realize and accept that you will not achieve the standard that your usual working environment allows you, such that sterilization of equipment may not be 100% certain, valves on cylinders of gases may malfunction or not work at all, washed bandages and gloves may have to be recycled after drying on a cactus or thorn bush, and water may have to be drawn from a well to scrub-up with, using a piece of soap that has been getting smaller and dirtier for a week. Instruments may have to be improvized or made up. Scissors and knives from a kitchen may need to be called into service, and wooden spoons cut to a curve to use as vascular clamps or occluders.

There are no easy answers to such working environments, but the challenges are as exciting as they are demanding. In such scenarios, no one will expect miracles (though they sometimes occur!) and you will have to accept at the outset that you will not be able to save all that you could in a more replete and protected setting, so blaming yourself when you have tried your best is not sensible or intelligent.

But giving up is not an option either.

REFERENCES AND RECOMMENDED READING

References

1. Norton I, Von Schreeb J, Aitken P, et al. Classification and minimum standards for foreign medical teams in sudden onset disasters. World Health Organisation, Geneva, 2013.
2. Merry AF, Cooper JB, Soyannwo O, Wilson IH, Eichhorn JH. International Standards for a Safe Practice of Anaesthesia. *Can J Anaesth.* 2010 Nov;**57(11)**:1027–34. doi: 10.1007/s12630-010-9381-6.
3. Mahoney PF, Jeyanathan J, Wood P, et al. Anaesthesia Handbook. International Committee of the Red Cross, February 2017. shop@icrc.org www.icrc.org.

Recommended Reading

Chackungal S, Nickerson JW, Knowlton LM, Black L, Burkle FM, Casey K, et al. Best Practice Guidelines on Surgical Response in Disasters and Humanitarian Emergencies: Report of the 2011 Humanitarian Action Summit Working Group on Surgical Issues within the Humanitarian Space. *Prehosp Disaster Med.* 2011 Dec;**26(6)**:429–37. doi: 10.1017/S1049023X12000064.

Chu K, Trelles M, Ford NP. Quality of Care in Humanitarian Surgery. *World J Surg.* 2011 Jun;**35(6)**:1169–72; discussion 1173-4. doi: 10.1007/s00268-011-1084-9.

Giannou C, Baldan M. War Surgery: Working with Limited Resources in Armed Conflict and Other Situations of Violence. *War Surgery Vol. 1 & 2.* ICRC Publication 2009 ref. 0973. International Committee of the Red Cross, Geneva.

Hayward-Karlsson J, Jeffery S, Kerr A, Schmidt H. Hospitals for War-Wounded, ICRC, Geneva, 2005, available at https://www.icrc.org/ eng/assets/files/other/icrc_002_0714.pdf.

Herard P, Boillot F. Amputation in emergency situations: indications, techniques and Médecins sans Frontiéres experience in Haiti. *International Orthopaedics* 2012:1–3.

Management of limb injuries during disasters and conflicts. World Health Organisation (WHO), International Committee of the Red Cross (ICRC) and AO Foundation. 2016. Available from: www.aofoundation.org/Structure/the-ao-foundation/StrategyFund/Project-Profiles/Pages/A-Field-Guide_Management-of-Limb-Injuries.aspx (accessed online January 2019).

World Health Organization. *The Clinical Use of Blood in Medicine, Obstetrics, Paediatrics, Surgery & Anaesthesia, Trauma & Burns*, WHO, Geneva. Available from: https://www.who.int/bloodsafety/clinical_use/en/Handbook_EN.pdf (accessed online January 2019).

Military Environments 22

22.1 INTRODUCTION

Military surgery operates within the framework of a staged or echeloned system of care. The role of the surgical team is not to merely operate on the individual patient, but to preserve the fighting force through good surgical care and decision-making such that individual servicemen and women can be restored to health as soon as possible. The deployed surgical team must understand their environment and contingencies.

Infrastructure requirements include shelter, power for lighting and temperature control, and water for hygiene and cooking purposes. Waste needs to be disposed of properly, medical waste disposal (particularly sharps), always being problematic. Resources include medical gases, food, drugs, fluids, and other consumables such as gloves and gowns. Fluids include blood and blood products, and these need a reliable and documented cold chain.

In the civilian setting, these materials and resources are provided by a series of complex supply chains that are carefully controlled and tracked, guaranteeing delivery within 24 hours anywhere in the world. To provide a similar standard of care in a deployed environment requires similar supply chains, which, in times of conflict, even the most advanced countries cannot always be achieved. Following a natural disaster, or in a conflict or post-conflict environment, supply chains and systems will be disrupted and vulnerable; in a conflict, they may be deliberately targeted. No delivery can ever be guaranteed, and the team may have only what they carried.

Modern militaries ensure that small surgical teams train together prior to deployment in order to prepare the team members for work that is well beyond normal civilian experience. Training permits assessment and refinement of interpersonal dynamics such that individuals are melded in to an effective team. It enables instillation of a thoughtful approach to realistic surgical care that acknowledges the context of the environment within which one works. The surgical team must alter their perspective from definitive management toward a staged approach of surgical care.

Military medical services have committed to delivering trauma care aligned to the principles of established civilian trauma systems approach, with a coherent chain of care from point of wounding, though trauma hospitals, to definitive specialist care and rehabilitation. This approach has borne fruit in recent conflicts in Iraq and Afghanistan, with reductions in mortality after combat injury to record low levels compared to historical conflicts. Small improvements in care at every point have translated into dramatic improvements in overall performance. In one study of critically-injured servicemen between 2003/4 and an injury-matched cohort in 2007/8, mortality was reduced from 47% to 20%.

22.2 INJURY PATTERNS

In the 19th century, warfare was infantry-based. In the 20th century, it became mechanized and airborne, and in the 21st century, combat is asymmetric, with possibly only one side in uniform. To quote General Sir Rupert Smith, author of *The Utility of Force*,[1] the modern battlefield is 'amongst the people'. Injuries sustained in contemporary combat operations are inflicted on combatant and non-combatant alike: in a recent review of activity at a coalition hospital in Afghanistan, 60% of casualties were local nationals, including women and children.

Similarly, in the urban setting of Somalia,[2] casualty distribution in military personnel was like that of the Vietnam War.[3] Eleven per cent died on the battlefield, 3% died after reaching a medical facility, 47% were evacuated, and 39% returned to duty. Over the past decade of conflict in Iraq and Afghanistan, US and coalition military casualties exceeded 4879 (Iraq) and 3540 (Afghanistan) totalling 8419 combat deaths.[4] There have been 1472 deaths due to disease, non-battle injury, and other causes, and over 52,000 troops wounded in action. Casualty rates in Iraq and Afghanistan have been considerably lower than during the Vietnam conflict, and a greater proportion of troops wounded have survived their wounds (<2% mortality). The leading causes of injury among casualties in the Afghanistan and the Iraq wars were explosive devices and gunshot wounds. Over 35% of those killed in action are instantaneous and the most common cause of death is torrential haemorrhage (>90%). It is estimated that more than one-third of these may be controlled in future, thus saving more soldiers on the battlefield from exsanguination.

The availability of personal protection devices to torso and head (ballistic vests, Kevlar helmet) has changed the wound and death spectrum significantly. In a review of coalition combat deaths up to the end of 2009, there had been >6000 allied military deaths in Iraq and Afghanistan. The leading cause of death was blast mechanisms followed by gunshot wounds. Chest or abdominal injury (40%) and traumatic brain injury (35%) were the main causes of death for soldiers killed in action. The case fatality rate in Iraq was approximately half as high as in the Vietnam War. In contrast, the amputation rate was twice as high. Approximately 8%–15% of the deaths appeared to be preventable.

The defining injury pattern in recent counter insurgency operations is that caused by improvised explosive devices (IEDs): the combination of bilateral lower limb amputation with pelvic fracture and perineal injury[1,2] has been described as the 'signature injury' of the conflicts in Afghanistan and Iraq.

In the UK Role 3 hospital in Afghanistan, the overall survival rate was 93.2% (see Table 22.1). The survival rate was influenced by the nationality of the patient, with the reduced rate amongst the Afghan population attributed to the lower use of personal protective equipment (PPE) and increased co-morbidities.

Table 22.1 Outcomes of Admissions to the UK Role 3 Hospital in Afghanistan

	Survivors	Deaths	Recovery Rate (%)
UK military	1906	58	97
Coalition military and entitled civilians	1206	42	97
Afghan	3250	367	90
Totals	6362	467	93

Wounding patterns are modified by the presence or absence of modern ballistic protection (armour) and the pre-hospital timeline. Many fatal penetrating injuries are likely to be caused by missiles entering through areas not protected by body armour, such as the face and junctional areas in the neck, groin, and buttocks. Injuries can be sustained by gunshot or the effect of conventional explosive munitions (air-delivered bombs, artillery shells, rocket-propelled grenades, or hand grenades). However, the defining injury pattern in recent counterinsurgency operations is that caused by IEDs, which cause a combination of blast and missile wounds in association with blunt injury.

One of the characteristics of military wounding is early lethality, with a high proportion of deaths occurring soon after injury. Of those who survive to reach hospital, the majority will have injury to the extremities. Protocols for casualty assessment, tourniquet application, the use of haemostatic wound dressings, and the direct transfer of casualties from ambulance to operating theatre are designed to recognize that exsanguination remains the main cause of preventable battlefield death. In a recent review of deaths of servicemen after combat injury, half of those that were potentially survivable were the result of intracavity haemorrhage.[5]

Military medical practitioners have been described as 'working at the interface of two dynamic technologies, warfare and trauma management'. In addition to the problems of dispersed battlefields, highly mobile front lines, extended lines of logistics, and a delay in evacuation, the modern military surgical team is likely to be called upon to treat civilians, including females (especially obstetric care) and children, as well as service personnel, with a requirement to offer immediate care well away from their speciality; problems in ophthalmology, maxillofacial surgery, ear, nose, and throat medicine, paediatrics, gynaecology, tropical medicine, or even public health will fall under the remit of the military surgeon. These challenges are magnified by the nature of modern surgical training, with its accent on early training in subspecialties, combined with the non-operative trends in the management of trauma surgery. Military surgical teams therefore must be trained in a variety of specialities and undergo multiple training courses (including team training) – before they deploy. Blended learning (digital interactive education, theoretical and skills training) before deployment has become increasingly important.

When it comes to providing care outside of one's specialty, a rational approach in the context of one's environment should prevail.

Everything should be as simple as possible...but not simpler.

Modern all-arms battle presents a vast array of potential wounding agents, from high-velocity military rifles, fragments from mortars or mines, blast from any explosive, and chemical, biological, and nuclear exposure (depleted uranium in shells), to motor vehicle crashes. The latter are often the most common cause of injury. As could be seen in Syria recently, it is imperative that military medical personnel become familiar with the medical consequences of toxin exposure, the illnesses caused by these agents, and the measures required to protect military healthcare providers themselves.

22.3 EMERGENCY MEDICAL SERVICES SYSTEMS

22.3.1 The Echelons of Medical Care

The patient presenting to the surgical team in a civilian hospital has already been part of a 'supply chain'. Considering the victim of a road traffic collision, summoning help requires the existence of an intact telephone or radio system, appropriately trained individuals arriving in suitably equipped vehicles, and an unimpeded journey, delivering an appropriately 'packaged' patient to the hospital. In the deployed environment, this pre-hospital chain is particularly vulnerable. Patients may experience delays of hours or days getting to care, which will in turn influence how they present to the surgical team. During such dynamic care, detailed pre-hospital protocols and training of their providers are critically important to optimize outcomes.

Deployed military medical systems usually consist of an echeloned series of levels (roles) of care in military medical treatment units, traditionally called medical treatment facilities (MTF), and divided by NATO into Role 1 to Role 4.

Close to the point of injury, a casualty either applies self-aid or receives 'buddy aid' (such as field dressing or tourniquet application).

22.3.1.1 ROLE 1

The next stage is care by a military paramedical provider, then by a doctor or nurse at an aid post (Role 1 facility). The Role 1 MTF provides primary healthcare, specialized first aid, triage, resuscitation, and stabilization.

Generally, Role 1 medical support must be readily and easily available to all force personnel.

22.3.1.2 ROLE 2

A Role 2 MTF is a structure capable of the reception and triage of casualties, as well as being able to perform resuscitation and treatment of shock to a higher level than Role 1. It will routinely include damage control surgery (DCS) and may include a limited holding facility for the short-term holding of casualties until they can be returned to duty or evacuated. It may be enhanced to provide basic secondary care including primary surgery, intensive care, and nursed beds. NATO countries felt the need to increase the clinical capability of their Role 2 MTFs. Therefore, Role 2 MTFs are now classified into Role 2 light manoeuvre (Role 2LM) and Role 2 enhanced (Role 2E).

22.3.1.3 ROLE 2 LIGHT MANOEUVRE

A Role 2LM MTF can conduct triage and advanced resuscitation procedures up to DCS. It will usually evacuate its post-surgical cases to Role 3 (or Role 2E) for stabilization and possible primary surgery before evacuation to Role 4.

22.3.1.4 ROLE 2 ENHANCED

Role 2E MTFs are effectively small field hospitals. They provide basic secondary healthcare, built around primary surgery, ICU, and nursed beds. A Role 2E MTF can stabilize post-surgical cases for evacuation to Role 4 without needing to put them through a Role 3 MTF first. Computed tomography (CT) scanning may be available.

22.3.1.5 ROLE 3

Role 3 MTFs are designed to provide combat theatre secondary health care. Role 3 medical support is deployed hospitalization and the elements required to support it. It basically includes surgical care at primary surgery level, ICU, nursed beds, and diagnostic support.

22.3.1.6 ROLE 4

Role 4 medical support provides definitive care of patients for whom the treatment required is longer than the theatre evacuation policy or for whom the capabilities usually found at Role 3 are inadequate. This would normally comprise specialist surgical and medical procedures, reconstruction, rehabilitation, and conva-lescence. This level of care is usually highly specialized, time consuming, and normally provided in the country of origin. Under unusual circumstances, this level of care may be established in a theatre of operations.

Pitfall

The situation becomes complicated when casualties move between systems (e.g. military to host nation, or non-governmental organization to military) having received surgery in the first system. Because standards of care can vary enormously between systems, these casualties need a thorough examination and re-evaluation. Soldiers have been trained and issued their equipment *before* the disaster or injury occurs, in order to perform immediate aid on themselves or each other. Civilians, however, have not. It is critically important that full documentation accompanies the patient in order to prevent overtreatment.

22.3.2 Incident Management and Multiple Casualties

At incidents in which bombs are involved or secondary devices are suspected, the '4 Cs' must be adopted (Table 22.2).

22.3.2.1 CONFIRM

Incident commanders must be clear about what is happening, and about the risk and position of further hazards. Factors that must be considered are clearance priorities, cordon locations, safe areas, access and egress routes, and rendezvous points.

22.3.2.2 CLEAR

The scene should be cleared to a safe distance. This distance will vary depending on the terrain. The method and urgency of clearance will depend on the incident.

Table 22.2 The Four Cs of Incident Management

- Confirm
- Clear
- Cordon
- Control

22.3.2.3 CORDON

Cordons establish the area in which the rescue effort is taking place, and define safe zones and tiers of command. An outer cordon should be established as a physical barrier preventing accidental or unauthorized access to the site. An inner cordon may be set up around wreckage, especially if hazards still exist.

22.3.2.4 CONTROL

Once cordons are set up, the control of the cordons and scene is maintained by clear rendezvous and access points.

Once the '4 Cs' have been established, medical management and support can begin (see Table 22.3).

22.3.2.5 COMMAND AND CONTROL

This is the paramount principle. If good command and control are not established, the initial chaos will continue, and the injured will suffer regardless of how well some individual casualties are treated. Command usually overrides control. Command implies the overall responsibility for the mission, whereas control implies the authority to modify procedures or actions by services.

22.3.2.6 SAFETY

Healthcare workers must remember that their own safety is paramount, and that they *must* not become casualties themselves. This may include infectious agents that may occur coincidently during a natural disaster.

22.3.2.7 COMMUNICATION

Communication is the transmission between a sender and a receiver, preferably such that the receiver is in no

Table 22.3 Medical Management and Support

- **Command and control**
- **Safety**
- **Communication**
- **Assessment**
- **Triage**
- **Treatment**
- **Transport**

doubt about the intent and need of the sender. Every major incident inquiry has identified failings in communications. Without good communication, command and control is impossible. When a formal medical record system may not exist, simply writing instructions over wound bandages may suffice.

22.3.2.8 ASSESSMENT

This is a constant process. Commanders should always consider the current situation; what resources are required and where these can be obtained.

22.3.2.9 TRIAGE

In any situation when there is more than one casualty, a system of triage must be used (see also Section 22.4). There are many different systems in use (Table 22.4).

22.3.2.10 TREATMENT

At the scene of any ballistic incident, treatment teams may be faced with casualties with multiple serious injuries. Treatment must follow the ⟨C⟩A-B-C paradigm:

- ⟨C⟩–Catastrophic Haemorrhage Control
- A–Airway
- B–Breathing
- C–Circulation

22.3.2.11 TRANSPORT

Not every patient needs to travel in an ambulance. Buses or other multi-passenger vehicles should be used to move the walking wounded. The judicious use of other resources, including armoured vehicles and aircraft, is essential.

Table 22.4 Triage Categories		
	Label Colour	**Description**
T1	Red	Immediate
T2	Yellow	Urgent
T3	Green	Delayed
Dead	White or black	Dead
T4	Blue (not standard)	Expectant

22.4 TRIAGE

22.4.1 Source and Aim of Triage

Effective triage is crucial in an efficient military healthcare system, and was first described by Napoleon's surgeon, Dominique Jean Larrey, who introduced a system of sorting casualties as they presented to field dressing stations. His priority, and the aim of the system, was to identify those soldiers who had minor wounds, and therefore could, with minor treatment, return to the battle. Although we might now call this reverse triage, he had introduced a formal system of prioritizing casualties. Triage remains a fundamental principle in modern military and disaster medicine. It is dynamic and can be applied at all levels of medical care, from the point of wounding to definitive surgical care.

The system for 'surgical triage' may be slightly different from the triage system used in resuscitation, but the same principles apply. Those requiring life-saving surgical intervention take priority over patients requiring limb-saving surgery in the forward locations, and considering all the other factors, the key question will be 'Do they need to go on the table at all?' Overtriage is a feature of all mass casualty situations; however, a rate of overtriage is acceptable to avoid missing patients who really did require an intervention. In a series of 1350 laparotomies from the Vietnam War, based on the clinical assessment of wounded soldiers, the rate of negative laparotomy was 19.2%. The philosophy of selective non-operative management (SNOM) was not available at that time. In a modern military setting, accurate screening tools (e.g. using CT or focused abdominal sonography for trauma (FAST) may aid SNOM; nevertheless, its time-consuming procedures may not be appropriate in busy surgical situations, where a quick laparotomy yields definite information.

Effective triage is crucial in an efficient military healthcare system. It is dynamic and can be applied at all levels of medical care, from the point of wounding to definitive surgical care. Triage should be repeated at every point of care, and at any point of deterioration. Patients compensate, change condition, and deteriorate without warning. In civilian practice, 'expectant' patients are rarely categorized because resources are relatively unlimited. In the military environment, care is often 'rationed'. The needs of the dying, who will require 50% of the resources of a surgical team to save them, need to be balanced against the needs of the next 10 patients who arrive and can be saved with the same effort. Table 22.5 summarizes the patterns of injury for non-survivors in a military or austere environment.

Table 22.5 Patterns of Injury for Non-Survivors in an Austere Environment

- Long bone amputations[a]
- Open skull fracture
- Full thickness burns >30%
- Inhalation injury
- Head injury with GCS <8
- Arrival in cardiac arrest

[a] Amputations with a reasonably long stump may be closed with a tourniquet if available, which can be left till further surgical capacity is available.

Table 22.6 Factors Affecting Triage

- Patient load and severity
- Medical capability and supply
- Local situation and safety
- Available evacuation assets and flight times
- Theatre medical assets

Triage itself depends on resources (Table 22.6).

Transfer time will also dictate who requires life-saving interventions at that point, and who can wait until they reach the next echelon of medical care. Equipment will always be in limited supply in these forward locations and must be used appropriately as resupply will take time. The flow of casualties in a fast-moving battle will also influence how many and what type of casualties should be operated on. The prospect of incoming serious casualties will change triage decisions for the wounded already at the medical facility. If there is only one surgical table available forward, 'Who goes on first?' and 'Do they need to go on at all?' may be simple questions to ask, but the answers are anything but straightforward.

The need for effective triage poses simple questions that are sometimes difficult to answer (see also Sections 22.4.2 and 22.4.3). A patient with extensive multiple injuries, who would get maximum effort and resources in a civilian trauma centre, may need to be labelled 'expectant' if several other patients face a better chance of survival given early access to the limited equipment and expertise available. Thus, an awareness of the overall tactical picture on the part of the senior surgeon is paramount. It may be wise to remember that triage, including surgical triage, means doing the 'best for the most', and expectant treatment for some may eventually benefit the 'most'.

22.4.2 **Forward Surgical Teams and Triage**

Forward surgical teams must be light, mobile, and rapidly deployable to allow them to respond in an uncertain battlefield (see also Section 22.6). Restrictions and constraints within these teams are many, and include limitations of space and equipment, poor lighting, and the need to achieve some degree of climate control for the human resources and, particularly, for blood and other products. Some re-sterilization of surgical tools may be possible, but disposable equipment, water, and especially oxygen will all be limited.

Human factors of physical and emotional fatigue will also affect how long the surgical team can endure the challenges of operating in austere and dangerous environments without reinforcement or resupply. The teams will often have to function independently, but may also deploy as augmentation of an existing medical facility during a casualty surge. Even in wartime, the best surgical teams could not operate for more than 19 hours at a time over a sustained period without breaking after 3 days.

There is a difference between a well-equipped relatively static 'field' (or combat support) hospital and a 'forward surgical team'. The *raison d'être* of the team is delivery of the life- and limb-saving surgery as far forward as possible without major evacuation delay, to a select group of potentially salvageable patients who would otherwise suffer owing to delays in evacuation from the battlefield. Without patient selection (by security perimeter or guard-force) a small team will not function.

Triage is challenging, it requires difficult decisions to be made, but it remains crucial to the effective use and efficiency of the forward surgical teams. If there is a choice, then the most senior surgeon should adopt this task.

22.4.3 **Forward Surgical Team Decision-Making**

Small surgical teams can be expected to work in tactical environments where insecure lines of evacuation, minimal diagnostic infrastructure, and very constrained patient-hold make clear decision-making on *who* to operate on and *what* operation to execute critical functions (see also Section 22.6). Surgical decision-makers must ensure that their choices do not unfairly reduce treatment options available for future patients and factor in likely predicted clinical states (and unlikely but impactful worst case states), plus the capacity of the echeloned care system. Critically, the surgeon must avoid a difficult decision by defaulting to judgements based purely on factors used in civilian practice that pay no heed to pressing operational realities. Whilst 'surgical' in nature, such decisions must be made in conjunction with other key stakeholders and operational, physiological, ethical, and resource issues must be considered.

The surgical team should understand available clinical and human resource. Stock-taking cannot be left to the medical storeman; the surgical team must know what the current supply state is of key consumables (kit, blood, oxygen) to anticipate shortage and develop a contingency plan.

22.4.4 Selection of Patients for Surgery

Role 2 patient-load consists of two categories: those who require damage control resuscitation/damage control surgery (DCR/DCS) and non-damage control cases. The former group require *immediate haemorrhage control*. The latter group are usually better served by rapid transport to a higher echelon of care for an operation *later*. The questions that the surgeon must ask of every patient who arrives in their small unit are therefore:

1. Does the patient need surgery?
2. Does this surgery need to be done here (*non-discretionary intervention*) or can the patient be transferred for surgery elsewhere (*discretionary non-intervention*)?

If the timelines to transfer a patient to Role 3 or Role 4 are prolonged – or the evacuation route becomes more tenuous – the surgeon may decide that the risk of in-flight deterioration justifies *discretionary intervention* and surgery. The surgeon must balance the risks of each strategy; that is, the excess individual patient morbidity incurred by a longer wait for surgery at a different location versus the impact on Role 2 capacity if a greater proportion of patients are triaged in to a *discretionary* pathway.

22.5 MASS CASUALTIES

One of the fundamental planning parameters for medical support is an estimate of the numbers and types of casualty expected. An estimate of the numbers and types of casualty, the resources required to deal with them per phase of battle, and their evacuation is the cornerstone of operational medical planning. Casualty estimates are major resource drivers and will determine what capabilities and what level of care is required. The medical support for a specific operation will therefore be planned considering the perceived threat.

Mass casualties, however, may occur for many reasons, and the cause of the major incident may not have been identified as one of the known 'threats'. The term 'mass casualty' is of course, relative, and for a small team, this number may be as low as three casualties. Multiple motor vehicle crashes, downed helicopters, floods, and even earthquakes have recently produced mass casualty situations or major incidents for military forces around the world. All these incidents have produced an unexpected surge in casualties, far greater than the casualty estimate that each operation had declared. The key in all these events was that the medical facilities were overwhelmed, and available resources could not meet the required demand.

When major incidents produce mass casualties in civilian situations, for example, from rail crashes or as a result of urban terrorism events, there are often several receiving hospitals to choose from, to spread the load of casualties. This luxury is rarely available in the military environment. In some situations, other nations' medical facilities may be available, but often the only available 'receiving hospital' will be the forward surgical team. Triage remains the key to effective medical management of a mass casualty event, especially when large numbers of wounded arrive at the location in a short space of time. Equipment, staff, and transport will be in short supply, so sound training and adherence to the principles of triage should ensure effective use of the limited resources available.

In civilian practice, advanced triage tools have been developed to predict workload capacity in mass casualties. Critically injured casualties exceeding more than one per hour, may rapidly exceed the capability of competent trauma teams. A good estimate to reliably predict patient volume after a mass casualty event is shown in Figure 22.1.

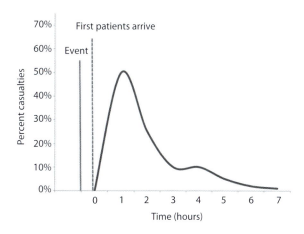

Figure 22.1 Percent casualties arriving to casualty reception.

Typically, 50% of total patient volume will occur by one hour of an incident. More than 75% of casualties will have arrived by the second hour. Therefore, total patient volume and requisite staffing may be somewhat predictable in an isolated mass casualty event.

After triage and treatment, transport remains the third key element of medical support in a mass casualty event. Unlike in a civilian environment, where there will be many options for both ground and air transport, transport is likely to be very limited in the military mass casualty situation. Regular and effective triage will determine who is transported first, and by what means, to ensure that the right patient arrives at the right time at the next level of medical care.

22.6 EVACUATION[4,5]

It is recognized that speed of evacuation from point of wounding to first surgical intervention is a critical determinant of outcome. The Korean War saw the introduction of helicopter evacuation of the wounded from the front line to mobile army surgical hospitals (MASH), with onward transport by fixed-wing aircraft to base hospitals. During the Vietnam conflict, the average pre-hospital time for combat casualties treated at a US Navy hospital was 80 minutes. Limited provision of aircraft in a combat setting has meant that medical evacuation has used assets earmarked for other purposes. During Operations Desert Shield/Desert Storm in 1991, many patients were successfully airlifted using converted cargo aircraft. This concept of using cargo aircraft was originally validated in World War II and is still current today. Dedicated aeromedical capability in the military now exists with two distinct models: the UK Medical Emergency Response Team (MERT) and the US Air Force helicopter rescue fleet known as PEDROs (named after the call sign of the first US Air Force HH-43 rescue helicopters in the Vietnam conflict). A landmark study documented prohibitively long pre-hospital times. Since the introduction of a dedicated air asset, pre-hospital times from wounding to point of care have fallen to approximately 45 minutes.

In Afghanistan, a successful international system of evacuation assets provides cover to the whole theatre of operations. The different evacuations provide different levels of care ranging from a flight medic to complex ICU capability. A recent study of more than 900 patients evacuated to a Role 4 facility demonstrated a <0.02% mortality with significantly injured soldiers (mean injury severity score of 23).[6]

Many military healthcare teams around the globe are now incorporating far forward resuscitative surgery capabilities into doctrine and mission planning. Although these forward surgical teams can provide trauma surgical capability for only a limited number of patients, they aim to provide life and limb saving surgery to the select group of potentially salvageable patients who would otherwise die or suffer permanent disability owing to delays in evacuation. However, such a surgical team will necessarily have a very limited scope of activity and require commitment of other military assets in order to protect the medical workforce.

These teams are designed to be capable of providing life-saving thoraco-abdominal haemorrhage control, control of contamination within body cavities, temporary limb or carotid revascularization, stabilization of fractures, and evacuation of major intracranial haematomas. Each nation has a slightly different balance and skill mix within their forward surgical capability, but most will normally provide the three main tenets of forward care: a resuscitation capability, one or more surgical tables, and a critical care capability. Most nations 'mission-tailor' their teams in size to the specific operational environment. As part of the casualty estimate, military planners need to decide on the number of surgical tables required and the speed at which they can safely transfer patients to the next echelon of care ('emptying the back door'). The size and sophistication of the attached critical care element will be determined by the capability of tactical aeromedical evacuation (TACEVAC). If there is no such facility, either in - or out-country, then the first few patients will fill a facility and render it completely ineffective.

22.7 RESUSCITATION

22.7.1 Overview

The treatment and resuscitation available will alter with each echelon of care; resources and complexity of care generally increase as the casualty moves away from the battlefield. Exsanguinating haemorrhage remains the commonest cause of death amongst those killed in action during military conflicts. Unlike in the urban setting, the military must consider weight and therefore quantity of supplies that can be transported into austere locations. Large volumes of fluids at any stage in the resuscitation process are therefore not a feasible option. More importantly, recent conflicts have demonstrated improved mortality with a balanced haemostatic resuscitation. Replacing crystalloid with early utilization of blood products, to include fresh whole blood, has even made its way to the far forward treatment station.[7] For patients with haemorrhagic shock in whom surgical intervention is not immediately available, the goal of maintaining a systolic arterial pressure of 70–80 mm Hg (palpable radial pulse) is now generally accepted (see Table 22.7).

22.7.2 **Damage Control Resuscitation[8]**

Approximately 90% of casualties are in a stable condition on arrival at hospital; however, about 10% of combat casualties will require massive transfusion and it is in these maximally injured patients that major improvements in care have been achieved. The concept of damage control resuscitation in

Table 22.7 Clinical Considerations in Penetrating Injury

Catastrophic Haemorrhage

- Penetrating wounds to the groin, axilla, and neck. Consider temporary packing.
- Penetrating wounds to major limb vessels/traumatic amputations. Consider early use of tourniquet.

Airway and C spine

Simple first: Jaw thrust, oral airway.
Airway at risk from:
- Burn injury.
- Disruption from fragments.
- Compression from penetrating vascular injury in the neck.

Consider early anaesthesia and intubation (aided by fibreoptic scopes and use of small diameter endotracheal tubes) or early surgical airway.
Cervical Collars: Limited role in pure penetrating injury and may conceal developing haematoma in the neck. Are needed in mixed injury as occurs in bombings.
Use of cervical collars is a balance of risk: protection of C spine versus concealing injury.

Breathing

- Needle decompression for tension pneumothorax.
- Manage sucking chest wounds with Asherman seals and then consider chest drainage.

Circulation

- Catastrophic bleeding should have been controlled early. Smaller external bleeds can be managed with simple first aid measures of compression and elevation. Ongoing internal bleeding from penetrating cavity injury needs to be suspected or recognized from history and clinical findings.
- Difficulty in obtaining vascular access can be experienced in austere conditions, when hypotension, low ambient temperature, and tactical considerations, such as the presence of mass casualties or operating light restriction can conspire to frustrate attempts at vascular access; intra-osseous access is an attractive option in these scenarios.

Deficit

The majority of casualties who sustain a high energy penetrating brain injury do not survive to medical care. Casualties who survive to care from penetrating injury are generally a preselected group and in the absence of obvious devastating injury should be resuscitated as above to minimize secondary injury. There is an obvious conflict between hypotensive resuscitation for cavity bleeding and the need to maintain cerebral perfusion and this becomes a judgement call at the time.

Environment

Hypothermia needs to be treated and managed with warm air blankets and environmental control. The temperature of any fluid given to trauma patients, particularly in a military or austere environment, is crucial. Any fluid used in resuscitation must be warmed to avoid further cooling of a haemorrhagic casualty. The actual process of warming the fluids remains a considerable challenge and in most cases requires improvization on behalf of the provider.

the field implies that rather that treat haemorrhage per se by replacement of fluid, efforts are primarily directed at stopping any bleeding, using local methods such as pressure, topical agents such as zeolite (QuikClot®), and chitosan (HemCon®), and regional haemostasis with the use of tourniquets. This is followed by rapid evacuation to a surgical facility where damage control surgery can take place. Resuscitation fluids are minimized where possible, and the early transfusion of blood and blood products where available is encouraged (see also Section 6.2).

In the severely injured casualty, DCR consists of two parts; first, pre-surgical fluid therapy is limited to keep blood pressure at approximately 90 mm Hg, preventing renewed bleeding from recently clotted vessels (in practice this means limiting crystalloid fluid infusion and using the level of consciousness and/or presence of a radial pulse as a guide). Second, intravascular volume restoration is accomplished by using thawed plasma as a primary resuscitation fluid in at least a 1:1 or 1:2 ratio with packed red cells and empiric transfusion with platelets. An example of this is the UK Damage Control Resuscitation protocol (Table 22.8).

Difficulty in obtaining vascular access can be experienced in austere conditions, when hypotension, low ambient temperature and tactical considerations, such as the presence of mass casualties or operating light restriction can conspire to frustrate attempts at vascular access; intraosseous access is an attractive option in these scenarios.[9]

Blood is the gold standard fluid of choice in such casualties, particularly for those in profound shock, and is now carried by many military resuscitation teams forward of the first surgical teams. However, in many military healthcare systems, blood will not be available and other fluids need to be carried. Options available to resuscitation teams include isotonic crystalloids, colloids, hypertonic saline, and hypertonic saline plus colloid. The choice of fluid remains unresolved and may in fact be less important that the quantity and rate of fluid infused in patients with uncontrolled haemorrhage.

The temperature of any fluid given to trauma patients, particularly in a military or austere environment, is crucial. Any fluid used in resuscitation must be warmed to avoid further cooling of a haemorrhagic casualty. The actual process of warming the fluids remains a considerable challenge and, in most cases, requires improvisation on behalf of the provider. Locally available re-warming/protective devices, such as plastic bags, use of hot car engines, and so on, may suffice.

22.7.3 Damage Control Surgery in the Military Setting[10–12]

The typical civilian damage control patient is likely to require the direct attention of at least two surgeons and one nurse during the first 6 hours, full invasive monitoring, multiple operations, massive transfusion of blood and products, and prolonged ICU stay, with a high mortality. The utility of this philosophy was even recently labelled as 'impractical for common use in a forward military unit during times of war'. However, experience in the current counterinsurgency conflicts has led to a widespread adoption of the philosophy of damage control surgery in the military context as 'minimally acceptable care' with rapid procedures and pragmatic objectives. Current military surgical efforts are framed within a 'damage control' mind-set, with temporary revascularization of limbs and damage control laparotomy providing good

	Table 22.8 UK Damage Control Resuscitation Protocol
1	For the first hour after injury, resuscitate to a palpable radial pulse, and after this (if not in surgery) resuscitate to a 'normal' blood pressure (an approach known as novel hybrid resuscitation and taught on the UK Battlefield Advanced Life Support course (BATLS™).
2	For severely injured casualties, recognize they are likely to be coagulopathic early – and resuscitate with blood, thawed plasma, and platelets (blood and plasma initially in a 1:1 ratio).
3	Balance the need for volume replacement against the risk of overtransfusion – reassess constantly.
4	Early use of tranexamic acid.
5	Monitoring of blood gases, lactate, calcium and potassium – with active management of falling calcium or rising potassium.
6	With blast casualties anticipate lung injury and ventilate using adult respiratory distress syndrome protocols.
7	The anaesthesia team and surgical team work closely together to ensure the correct sequencing of damage control procedures.

control to enable early transport as soon as the military situation allows (see also Section 6.3).

In the far forward, highly mobile, austere military environment, it is quite likely that the surgeon will not have the luxury of being able to perform definitive surgery on every casualty. Short, focused operative interventions can be used on peripheral vascular injuries, extensive bone and soft tissue injuries, and thoracoabdominal penetrations in patients with favourable physiology, instead of *definitive* surgery being provided for every injured soldier. This may conserve precious resources such as time, operating table space, and blood. Instead of applying these temporary abbreviated surgical control (TASC) manoeuvres to patients about to exhaust their physiological reserve, as in classic damage control, TASC is applied when the limitations of reserve exist outside the patient.

This philosophy relies heavily on the military medical system, with post-operative care and evacuation to the 'resource-replete environment' a priority. In the military, the key is triage (patient selection) and knowledge of own resources as well as tactical situation. The philosophy for the military surgical team exposed to numbers of casualties in the setting of limited resources remains to do the best for the most, rather than expend resources on limited numbers of critically wounded. As international laws and protective signs (Red Cross/Red Crescent, Geneva Convention) are respected less in current conflicts, forward surgical teams and patients cannot be risked being left behind in fast changing battlefields. Thus evacuation transport for every patient operated on is needed.

22.8 BLAST INJURY

Blast injury is the physiological and anatomical insult to the human body caused by the physical properties of an explosion. The shock wave that results from the explosion is referred to as the blast wave, its leading edge is the blast front, and the rush of air caused by the blast wave is the blast wind.

In open air, the force of a blast rapidly dissipates, but within confined spaces the blast wave is magnified by its reflection off walls, floors, and ceilings, increasing its destructive potential. Because water is less compressible than air, an underwater blast wave propagates at high speeds and loses energy less quickly over long distances, being approximately three times greater in strength than that which is detonated in the air.

Blast injuries have been classified into five specific and distinct categories that reflect the mechanism of tissue injury and physical tissue damage that occur as a result of blast phenomena:

- *Primary blast injury*: This refers to the effects of direct pressure (barotrauma) owing to either underpressurization or overpressurization relative to atmospheric pressure. Gas-enclosing organs, such as the lung, tympanic membrane (the most common injury), and bowel are the most vulnerable.
- *Secondary blast injury*: These are penetrating injuries caused by blast projectiles and debris. They are the leading cause of death and injury in both military and civilian terrorist attacks, except in cases of major building collapse.
- *Tertiary blast injury*: Displacement injuries result from persons or objects falling or being thrown because of the blast wave. Structural collapse or large airborne fragments lead to crush injury and extensive blunt trauma.
- *Quaternary blast injury*: This includes asphyxia, burns, and inhalation injuries.
- *Quinary blast injury*: This is an early hyperinflammatory state, thought to be due to exposure to unconventional materials used in the manufacture of the explosives.

22.8.1 Diagnosis and Management of Blast Injuries

22.8.1.1 RUPTURE OF THE TYMPANIC MEMBRANE

All explosion victims should be evaluated with an otoscopic examination. Small perforations typically heal within a few weeks, and treatment should be expectant, with topical antibiotics if the ear canal is full of debris. Some studies have reported a high (30%) incidence of permanent high-frequency hearing loss 1 year after injury.

22.8.1.2 BLAST LUNG INJURY (BLI)

This may be immediately lethal or present a pattern like blunt trauma, with pulmonary contusion, often without rib fractures or chest wall injury. The earliest sign of blast lung injury is systemic arterial oxygen desaturation, often in the absence of other symptoms.

Radiological features can range from a typical 'butterfly pattern' bihilar shadowing on the chest x-ray to a 'white-out'. Management is principally supportive. Mechanical ventilation and effective chest drainage form the mainstay of treatment. High-peak inspiratory pressures should be avoided to decrease the chance of iatrogenic pulmonary barotraumas.

22.8.1.3 INTRA-ABDOMINAL INJURIES

Primary blast injury to the gastrointestinal tract is rare. The characteristic bowel lesion is a mural haematoma, ranging in severity from a minor submucosal haemorrhage to full-thickness disruption and perforation. The ileocaecal junction and colon are the most commonly affected sites, and delayed perforation can occur. Pneumoperitoneum alone may be a non-specific sign only associated with bowel perforation in less than 50% of the patients.

Rupture of solid organs has been observed in the absence of other mechanisms of injury. Management should be in accordance with the principles of damage control. Diagnostic peritoneal lavage can be difficult to interpret because of the high incidence of retroperitoneal and mesenteric haematoma. Patients can also develop haematemesis or melena without obvious intraperitoneal involvement owing to mucosal and submucosal haemorrhage. Colonoscopy is not recommended because of the risk of perforation.

22.8.1.4 OTHER INJURIES

- Transfer of kinetic energy from the blast wave to the eye can result in rupture of the globe, serous retinitis, and hyphaema. Ophthalmology consultation should be obtained.
- The most common blast-induced arrhythmias, in addition to bradycardia, are premature ventricular contractions and asystole. The treating physician should be aware that haemorrhaging, explosion-injured patients may not have the expected compensatory tachycardia and may become hypotensive without rapid resuscitation.
- Traumatic amputations from primary blast injury are uncommon and controversial as to whether the blast wave alone is the cause.
- Primary blast injury can also result in cranial fractures around air-filled sinuses, and focal neurological deficits as a result of air embolism. There are data supporting the concept of blast-induced brain injury, with psychological as well as physical symptoms.

22.9 BATTLEFIELD ANALGESIA[13,14]

Relief of pain is an important consideration for both the wounded person and the military caregiver. Provision of effective analgesia is humane, but also attenuates the adverse pathophysiological responses to pain, and is likely to aid evacuation from the battlefield and maintain morale. Analgesia may be given at self- and buddy-aid levels; protocols to guide medical and paramedical staff in the provision of safe and effective analgesia are available.

Analgesia methods used in recent conflicts include:

- Simple non-pharmacological:
  - Reassurance.
  - Splinting of fractures.
  - Cooling of burns.
- Oral analgesics:
  - Non-steroidal anti-inflammatory drugs.
  - Paracetamol.
- Nerve blocks and infiltration of local anaesthesia.
- Intramuscular and intravenous opiates.
- Fentanyl 'lollipops'.

Methods under development include intranasal ketamine, fentanyl, and inhalational analgesics, such as methoxyflurane inhalation.

22.10 BATTLEFIELD ANAESTHESIA

Battlefield anaesthesia presents many challenges, including the need to maintain airway control, hypothermia of the casualty, restricted drug availability, lack of supplementary oxygen, and the possible requirement for prolonged post-operative mechanical ventilation. Mass casualty situations are also a constant possibility in the military arena.

Surgery requires both adequate analgesia and anaesthesia. No single agent can provide both an appropriate level of anaesthesia and analgesia; hence a combination of drugs and techniques is required. The choices of anaesthetic are narrowed in austere conditions, being limited to general anaesthesia (either intravenous or inhalational), regional anaesthesia, or none. For surgical exploration of body cavities, general anaesthesia is most frequently chosen, while a regional aesthetic may be more appropriate for injuries of the extremities or perineum.

In the field, rapid sequence induction (RSI) is the norm, using fast-acting hypnotic and neuromuscular blocking agents to facilitate rapid airway control. In the absence or limitation of supplemental oxygen supplies, RSI becomes even more crucial as pre-oxygenation of the patient's lungs is often not possible. There are several RSI cocktails used in the pre-hospital setting, most using a combination of an induction agent, a paralysing agent, and analgesia. Sedation, amnesia, and analgesia can then be maintained with intravenous agents such as ketamine, benzodiazepines, and opiates.

For long procedures or surgical sites involving the abdomen or thorax, a combination anaesthetic that includes an inhalational agent such as isoflurane may be used. British surgical teams use a portable 'Triservice apparatus' that does not require a compressed gas source and have gained much experience with this technique of field anaesthesia. This 'draw-over' type of vaporizer is currently also in use by US forces in austere settings.

Regional anaesthesia remains an important option in battlefield anaesthesia, as it provides both patient comfort and surgical analgesia, while maintaining patient consciousness and spontaneous ventilation. With the relatively large number of extremity wounds in modern conflicts, and certainly in the mass casualty setting with a limited anaesthesia capability, regional aesthetic techniques should not be overlooked. Continuous infusion nerve blocks provide excellent analgesia for post-operative casualties during evacuation.

The pragmatic approach is to build systems around managing the severely injured patient and then adapt them to other situations when necessary.

22.10.1 Induction of Anaesthesia

Rapid sequence induction of anaesthesia is the accepted standard for the trauma casualty. Indications for RSI in the emergency department include:

- Casualties requiring immediate airway protection or mechanical ventilation.
- Uncontrollable agitation or Glasgow Coma Score (GCS) <8.
- Severe uncontrollable pain.
- In cases of non-compressible haemorrhage such as intra-abdominal bleeding, RSI is usually more appropriately performed on the operating table with the casualty prepared for immediate surgery.

Prior to RSI, equipment and team preparation is paramount. A trained anaesthetic assistant should be available and ideally a second clinician whose role is to administer drugs and to monitor vital signs. A team member should be designated to perform thoracostomy should a tension pneumothorax become evident. In the event of cervical spine control being necessary, any cervical collar should be opened or removed and replaced with manual in-line stabilization by another team member. All equipment should be checked daily and again prior to casualty arrival. Minimum equipment immediately available includes:

- Self-inflating bag and correctly sized facemask.
- Two sizes of laryngoscope (MAC 3 and 4 for adults).
- Appropriately sized endotracheal tubes.
- Failed/difficult intubation equipment.
- Bougie.
- Oropharyngeal and nasopharyngeal airways.
- Laryngeal mask airway (ideally second generation e.g. ProSeal®, iGel®).
- Alternative laryngoscope (e.g. AirTraq®, Glidescope® if available).
- Surgical airway equipment.
- Working suction.
- Monitoring including end-tidal CO_2, ECG, non-invasive blood pressure (NIBP) and SpO_2.

Choice of induction agent(s) is not prescriptive. The aim is to preserve cardiac output as far as possible. For this reason, most military anaesthetists favour ketamine (1–2 mg/kg) in major trauma. In the most severely injured, a lower dose than that suggested may be required. The choice of muscle relaxant in RSI has long been suxamethonium (1.5 mg/kg), by virtue of its rapid onset and offset. An alternative to this is rocuronium (1.2 mg/kg), which provides good intubating conditions within 60 seconds. The much longer time to offset of neuromuscular blockade is argued as advantageous should the need for a surgical airway arise. Rocuronium is also the drug of choice for RSI in cases of hyperkalaemia, burns older than 24 hours, and spinal cord injuries older than 10 days. Immediate reversal is with sugammadex 16 mg/kg. This may not be available in the deployed environment.

Extreme care should be taken with RSI in hypovolaemic casualties. Severe hypovolaemia should be corrected prior to induction to avoid the risk of a pulseless electrical activity (PEA) cardiac arrest. The aim of resuscitation should be to achieve a normal blood pressure in controlled haemorrhage and a palpable radial pulse in uncontrolled haemorrhage. If immediate RSI is required, the dose of induction agent should be reduced accordingly. Ventilation should be established minimizing the respiratory rate (e.g. 6 bpm) and airway pressures (avoid PEEP).

22.10.2 Maintenance of Anaesthesia

Anaesthesia can be maintained initially by use of IV agents. This is particularly useful if induction has taken place in the emergency department and further imaging is needed or if there is a delay prior to transfer to the operating theatre.

Fentanyl (1–2 μg/kg initially) is used as an adjunct to blood product resuscitation by virtue of its effect as a sympatholytic countering the extreme vasoconstriction seen in extreme hypovolaemia. This permits further volume resuscitation and avoids rebound hypertension. Further doses are titrated during DCR/DCS up to 15 μg/kg.

Midazolam (0.02–0.05 mg/kg initially) can be used to maintain anaesthesia immediately following RSI in addition to fentanyl. Further boluses of 0.02 mg/kg can be titrated to anaesthetic effect. Anaesthesia for surgery is usually maintained with a volatile agent. In ongoing hypovolaemia, volatile use should be carefully titrated along with fentanyl according to physiological parameters. The Tri-Service Anaesthetic Apparatus (TSAA) (UK Defence Medical Services) can be used to administer a volatile anaesthetic without a supply of compressed gas. It can be used in conjunction with an oxygen concentrator that preserves supplies of cylinder oxygen. The US Defence Medical Services have 'draw-over' anaesthesia apparatus like the TSAA. An alternative to volatile anaesthesia is total intravenous anaesthesia (TIVA). In its simplest form, this could be bolus administration of ketamine for short cases. Syringe drivers are now in common use and allow for a variety of TIVA drugs to be used.

Epidural anaesthesia is usually not undertaken in the most austere environments. This is due to difficulty in ensuring a consistently sterile environment for safe catheter placement, as well as the requirement for specialist equipment and the need for trained staff to escort in evacuation. In the mature deployment with a robust logistical and evacuation chain, epidural placement may be considered.

Spinal anaesthesia is a common technique in developing countries where there may be a lack of trained anaesthesia practitioners; the risk of airway complications associated with general anaesthesia can thus be avoided. Placement of a spinal block in the shocked casualty leads

to catastrophic hypotension from loss of sympathetic tone. Spinal anaesthesia should be avoided in this situation. In patients where spinal anaesthesia may be appropriate, the risks of infection from placement in the field may outweigh any benefits.

22.11 CRITICAL CARE (See also Chapter 17)

If damage control is going to be the norm for the far-forward surgeon, a critical care capability must be a part of the forward surgical team structure. The priorities will be therefore be optimization of haemodynamic status, re-warming of the patient, control of coagulopathy, pain relief, and preparation for return to theatre or evacuation depending on the situation.

22.12 TRANSLATING MILITARY EXPERIENCE TO CIVILIAN TRAUMA CARE[15–17]

Six aspects of military trauma care have been identified as contributing to recent good outcomes for patients wounded in combat.

22.12.1 Leadership

Current military trauma care systems are delivered by consultants.

22.12.2 Front-End Processes

The treatment of patients wounded by military weapons is fundamentally geared towards the concept of damage control. Correction of a patient's deranged physiology is recognized as a greater priority than definitive anatomical repair. In addition, the key hospital infrastructure (emergency department, operating room, CT scanner, and ICU) is planned around the needs of the time-critical patient, ensuring that all key components are close to each other.

22.12.3 Common Training

It is considered that the common military training model (from first aid to multidisciplinary field hospital simulation) facilitates effective team working and delivery of appropriate human and other resources at the right time for wounded patients.

22.12.4 Governance

Military trauma systems operate a robust and diligent framework that, through a vigorous review of injury data, clinical processes and patients' outcomes, provides feedback to improve the system's performance.

22.12.5 Rehabilitation Services

Formal, dedicated rehabilitation specialists and facilities are recognized as being fundamental to favourable long-term outcomes.

22.12.6 Translational Research

Integrated basic and clinical research streams feed rapid improvements in all aspects of care to clinicians, which can then be introduced into clinical care.

22.13 SUMMARY

These are exciting times in which to be a military medical practitioner. Geopolitical shifts have re-focused the priorities for military planners, and surgical doctrines also must adapt to the emerging scenarios of future conflict. The latter include peer-on-peer conflict as well as asymmetric warfare set in low-density dispersed battlefields; highly mobile operations, extended lines of evacuation, and logistic supply; the prospects of large and untreated populations of civilian wounded and the possibility of chemical, biological, and nuclear attack. All of these necessitate the retention of surgical adaptability and resourcefulness, as well as technical skill.

In summary, in the operational setting, resources are more limited, and the word 'finite' should underpin all clinical decision-making. Triage and intervention may be modified by an open or closed back door, or by open skies. Environmental protection is minimal when compared with civilian structures. Surgery must be tailored taking into consideration operational realities. Procedures such as simple burr holes, evacuation of a retro-orbital haematoma (compressing the optic

nerve), damage control thoracotomy and laparotomy, shunting of vascular injuries, fasciotomies and, above all, the extent of debridement required must be readily executable.

Experience of war advances trauma care; the concentration of the severely wounded in the hands of well-resourced, motivated clinicians provides the impetus for advances in the surgical care of the wounded. This recent period of conflict has certainly provided opportunities for advancement on many levels. Each mission will bring a new set of technical and personal challenges.

REFERENCES AND RECOMMENDED READING

References

1. Smith R. *The Utility of Force: The Art of War in the Modern World*. Allen Lane, 2005.
2. Mabry RL, Holcomb JB, Baker AM, Cloonan CC, Uhorchak JM, Perkins DE, et al. United States Army Rangers in Somalia: an analysis of combat casualties on an urban battlefield. *J Trauma*. 2000 Sep;**49(3)**:515–28.
3. Hardaway RMIII. Vietnam wound analysis. *J Trauma*. 1978 Sept; **18(9)**:635–42.
4. iCasualties.org. Casualty Reports. Deaths in Iraq and Afghanistan. Available from: http://icasualties.org (accessed online January 2019).
5. Eastridge BJ, Mabry RL, Seguin P, Cantrell J, Tops T, Uribe P, et al. Death on the battlefield (2001-2011): implications for the future of combat casualty care. *J Trauma Acute Care Surg*. 2012 Dec;**73(6 Suppl 5)**:S431–7. doi: 10.1097/TA.0b013e3182755dcc.
6. Ingalls N, Zonies D, Bailey JA, et al. A review of the first 10 years of critical care aeromedical transport during operation Iraqi freedom and operation enduring freedom: the importance of evacuation timing. *JAMA Surg*. 2014;**149(8)**:807–813.
7. Cordova CB, Capp AP, Spinella PC. Fresh whole blood transfusion for a combat casualty in austere combat environment. *J Spec Oper Med*. 2014 Spring;**14(1)**:9–12.
8. Holcomb JB. Damage control resuscitation. *The Journal of Trauma*. 2007 Jun;**62(6 Suppl)**:S36–37.
9. Cooper BR, Mahoney PF, Hodgetts TJ, Mellor A. Intraosseous access (EZ-IO) for resuscitation: UK military combat experience. *J R Army Med Corps*. 2007 Dec;**153(4)**:314–6.
10. Holcomb JB, Helling TS, Hirshberg A. Military, civilian, and rural application of the damage control philosophy. *Mil Med*. 2001 Jun;**166(6)**:490–3.

11. Rotondo MF, Zonies DH. The damage control sequence and underlying logic. *Surg Clin North Am.* 1997 Aug;**77(4)**:761–77. Review

12. Granchi TS, Liscum KR. The logistics of damage control. *Surg Clin North Am.* 1997 Aug;**77(4)**:921–8.

13. Fisher AD, Rippee B, Shehan H, Conklin C, Mabry RL. Prehospital analgesia with ketamine for combat wounds: a case series. *J Spec Oper Med.* 2014 Winter;**14(4)**:11–7.

14. Clifford JL, Fowler M, Hansen JJ, Cheppudira B, Nyland JE, Salas MM, et al. State of the science review: Advances in pain management in wounded service members over a decade at war. *J Trauma Acute Care Surg.* 2014 Sep;**77(3 Suppl 2)**:S228–36. doi: 10.1097/TA.000000000 0000403.

15. Beekley AC, Starnes BW, Sebesta JA. Lessons learned from modern military surgery. *Surgical Clinics of North America.* 2007 Feb;**87(1)**:157–194, vii.

16. Caterson EJ, Carty MJ, Weaver MJ, Holt EF. Boston bombings: a surgical view of lessons learned from combat casualty care and the applicability to Boston's terrorist attack. *J Craniofac Surg.* 2013 Jul;**24(4)**:1061–7. doi: 10.1097/SCS.0b013e31829ff967.

17. Dubose J, Rodriguez C, Martin M, Nunez T, Dorlac W, King D, et al. Preparing the surgeon for war: present practices of US, UK, and Canadian militaries and future directions for the US military. *J Trauma Acute Care Surg.* 2012 Dec;**73(6 Suppl 5)**:S423–30. doi: 10.1097/TA.0b013e3182754636. Review.

Recommended Reading

BALLISTICS: HISTORY, MECHANISMS, BALLISTIC PROTECTION, AND CASUALTY MANAGEMENT

Mahoney PF, Ryan JM, Brooks AJ, Schwab CW. *Ballistic Trauma: A Practical Guide*, 2nd edn. Springer Verlag, London, 2005.

Ryan J. *Ballistic Trauma: Clinical Relevance in Peace and War.* Arnold, London, 1997.

Volgas DA, Stannard JP, Alonso JE. Ballistics: a primer for the surgeon. *Injury* 2005 Mar;**36(3)**:373–9. Review.

BLAST INJURY

Champion HR, Holcomb JB, Young LA. Injuries from explosions: physics, biophysics, pathology, and required research focus. *J Trauma.* 2009 May;**66(5)**:1468–77; discussion 1477. doi: 10.1097/TA.0b013e3181a27e7f. Review.

DePalma RG, Burris DG, Champion HR, Hodgson MJ. Blast injuries. *N Engl J Med.* 2005 Mar 31;**352(13)**:1335–42.

Neuhaus SJ, Sharwood PF, Rosenfeld JV. Terrorism and blast explosions: lessons for the Australian surgical community. *A NZ J Surg.* 2006 Jul;**76(7)**:637–644.

Ritenour AE, Baskin TW. Primary blast injury: update on diagnosis and treatment. *Crit Care Med.* 2008 Jul;**36(7 Suppl)**:S311–7. doi: 10.1097/CCM.0b013e31817e2a8c.

WAR SURGERY

Battlefield Advanced Trauma Life Support BATLS. *J R Army Med Corps* Available from https://jramc.bmj.com (accessed online January 2019).

Bono R, Thomas RW, Peacock T, Cubano M, Elster E, Gurney J, et al. Eds. *Emergency War Surgery* 5th Edn. U.S. Department of Defence, The Borden Institutem, 2018.

Butler FK Jr, Hagmann JH, Richards DT. Tactical management of urban warfare casualties in special operations. *Mil Med* 2000 Apr;**165(4 Suppl)**:1–48.

Calderbank P, Woolley T, Mercer S, et al. Doctor on board? What is the optimal skill-mix in military pre-hospital care? *Emerg Med J* 2011 Oct;**28(10)**:882–3. doi: 10.1136/emj.2010.097642.

Coupland RM. *War Wounds of Limbs: Surgical Management.* Butterworth Heinemann, Oxford, 2000.

Coupland R, Molde A, Navein J. *Care in the Field for Victims of Weapons of War.* International Committee of the Red Cross, Geneva, 2001.

Defence and Veterans Pain Management Initiative. *The Military Advanced Regional Anesthesia and Analgesia Handbook.* Available from www.arapmi.org.

Department of the Army. *War Surgery in Afghanistan and Iraq: A Series of Cases, 2003–2007.* Textbooks of Military Medicine, Department of the Army, Washington DC USA, 2008.

Dufour D, Kromann Jensen S, Owen-Smith M, et al. *Surgery for Victims of War*, 3rd edn. International Committee of the Red Cross, Geneva, 1998.

Giannou C, Baldan M. *War Surgery: Working with Limited Resources in Armed Conflict and Other Situations of Violence.* War Surgery Vol. 1 & 2. ICRC Publication 2009 ref. 0973. International Committee of the Red Cross, Geneva.

Greenfield RA, Brown BR, Hutchins JB, Iandolo JJ, Jackson R, Slater LN, et al. Microbiological, biological, and chemical weapons of warfare and terrorism. *Am J Med Sci.* 2002 Jun;**323(6)**:326–40. Review.

Holcomb J. Causes of death in US Special Operations Forces in the global war on terrorism: 2001-2004. *US Army Med Dep J.* 2007(Jan–Mar):24–37.

Husum H, Gilbert M, Wisborg T. *Save Lives, Save Limbs: Life Support for Victims of Mines, Wars and Accidents*. Third World Network, Penang, Malaysia, 2000.

International Committee of the Red Cross. *First Aid in Armed Conflict and Other Situations of Violence*. ICRC, Geneva, 2006.

Journal of the Royal Army Medical Corps. Wounds of Conflict (Vol. 147, No. 1, February 2001), Combat Casualty Care (Vol. 153, No. 4, December 2007), Wounds of Conflict II (Vol. 155, No. 4, December 2009). Available from www.ramcjournal.com (accessed online December 2010).

Lounsbury DE, Brengman M, Bellamy RF, eds. *Emergency War Surgery*, Third United States Revision. Borden Institute, Washington DC USA, 2004.

North Atlantic Treaty Organisation. *Allied Joint Medical Support Doctrine*. AJP-4.10(A). March 2006.

North Atlantic Treaty Organization. *Emergency War Surgery NSATO Handbook 2010*. The Borden Institute, Washington DC.

Roberts P, ed. *The British Military Surgery Pocket Book*. AC No. 12552. HMSO, London, 2004.

Santry HP, Alam HB. Fluid resuscitation: past, present, and the future. *Shock* 2010 Mar;**33(3)**:229–41. doi: 10.1097/SHK.0b013e3181c30f0c.

Willy C, Voelker HU, Steinmann R, Engelhardt M. Patterns of injury in a combat environment. 2007 update. *Chirurg* 2008 Jan;**79(1)**:66–76.

Appendix A
Trauma Systems

A.1 INTRODUCTION

Care of the injured patient has been fundamental to the practice of medicine since recorded history. The word 'trauma' derives from the Greek meaning 'bodily injury'. The first trauma centres were used to care for wounded soldiers in Napoleon's armies, and the first modern trauma centre was the Birmingham Accident Hospital in the United Kingdom, opened in 1944 in what was then the Queen's Hospital. It is most unfortunate that many trauma cases are still managed within non-existent or poorly organized trauma systems.

The lessons learned in successive military conflicts have advanced our knowledge of care of the injured patient. The Korean conflict and the Vietnam War established the concept of minimizing the time from injury to definitive care. The extension of this concept to the management of civilian trauma led to the evolution of today's trauma systems from the 1970s onwards. The Middle East and Afghan conflicts in the last decade resulted in massive progress in the sphere of military trauma care, with significant enhancement in civilian care as well. For the first time, prospective high quality research has taken place in the conflict situation.

A.2 THE INCLUSIVE TRAUMA SYSTEM

In principle, a hospital that provides acute care for the severely injured patient (a trauma centre) should be a key component of a system that encompasses all aspects and phases of care, from prevention and education to pre-hospital care, to acute care, and through to rehabilitation (Figure A.1). The initial trauma systems did not consider the non-trauma centre hospitals, even though they cared for most patients and those who were less severely injured. Instead, these trauma systems were driven by the major or severely injured trauma patient who required immediate treatment, optimally at a trauma centre.

A system must be fully integrated into the emergency medical services (EMS) system and must meet the needs of all the patients requiring acute care for injury, regardless of severity of injury, geographical location, and population density. The trauma centre remains an essential component, but the system recognizes the necessity for other healthcare facilities.

The goal of the most cost-effective trauma care is to match the facility's resources with the needs of the patient.

The goal of the system is to match the regional needs and facilities, with the resources and patient care loads required.

A.3 COMPONENTS OF AN INCLUSIVE TRAUMA SYSTEM

The structure of a trauma care system involves several components and providers, each of which must be adapted to a specific environment. These components and providers, graphically represented in Figure A.2, are:

- **Administrative components:**
  - Leadership.
  - System development.
  - Legislation.
  - Finances.
- **Operational and clinical components.**
- **Injury prevention and control.**
- **Human resources – workforce resources.**
- **Education.**
- **Pre-hospital care – EMS system.**
- **Ambulance and non-transporting guidelines:**
  - Communications systems.
  - Emergency disaster preparedness plan.
- **Definitive care facilities:**
  - Trauma care facilities.
  - Interfacility transfer.
  - Medical rehabilitation.

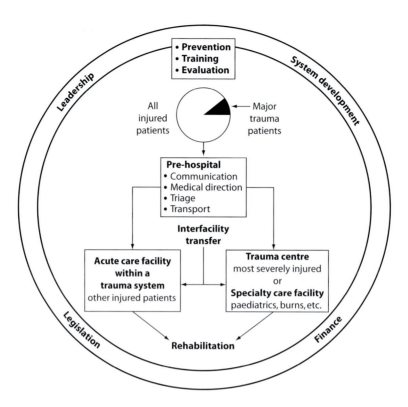

Figure A.1 The inclusive trauma system.

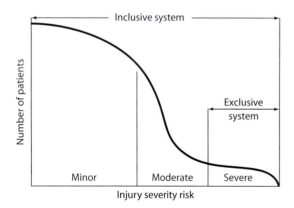

Figure A.2 The components of an inclusive trauma system.

- **Information systems.**
- **Evaluation.**
- **Research.**

A.3.1 **Administration**

The system requires administrative leadership, authority, planning and development, legislation, and finances.

Together, these components form an outer sphere of stability that is vital for the continuation of activities directly related to patient care. The diversity of the population, as defined by the environment (urban or rural) or by special segments of the population (the young or the elderly), must be addressed by the system.

A.3.2 **Prevention**

Prevention reduces the actual incidence of injury and is cost-efficient for the system and for society. Injury prevention is achieved through public education, legislation, and environmental modification.

A.3.3 **Public Education**

Public education leads to a change in behaviour, and thus minimizes injury exposure. Education includes the proper recognition of injury, and efficient access to the EMS system. These components stimulate the necessary political and legislative activity to establish legal authority, leadership, and system changes.

The development of a system is a major challenge for any community. The concept of centralizing trauma care creates potential political and economic problems, since the normal flow of patients might be altered by trauma triage protocols. Trauma systems, by their nature, will direct the care of the most critically injured patients to a limited number of designated 'trauma centres'. The trauma system will only succeed if all parties are involved in the initial planning, development, and implementation.

It is crucial that doctors, especially surgeons and anaesthesiologists, are involved in the system-planning process. They should help to establish standards of care for all clinical components, and participate in planning, verification, performance improvement, and system evaluation.

A.4 MANAGEMENT OF THE INJURED PATIENT WITHIN A SYSTEM

Once the injury has been identified, the system must ensure easy access and an appropriate response at the scene of injury. The system must assign responsibility and authority for care and triage decisions made prior to trauma centre access. Triage guidelines must be accepted by all providers and used to determine which patients require access to trauma centre care. This coordination requires direct communication between pre-hospital care providers, medical direction, and the trauma facility. Protocols at primary care level should focus or early detection of severe injuries, initiation of resuscitation, and prompt transfer to appropriate facility.

The trauma centre, which serves as the definitive specialized care facility, is a key component of the system, and is different from other hospitals within the system in that it guarantees immediate availability of *all* the specialities necessary for the assessment and management of the patient with multiple injuries. These centres need to be integrated into the other components of the system to allow the best match of resources with the patients' needs. The system coordinates care between all levels of the facility, so that prompt and efficient integration of hospital and resources can take place according to patient need.

Access to rehabilitation services, first in the acute care hospital and then in more specialized rehabilitation facilities, is an integral part of the total management of the patient. It is important that the patients be returned to their communities when appropriate.

A.5 STEPS IN ORGANIZING A SYSTEM

A.5.1 Public Support

Public support is necessary for the enabling and necessary legislation to take place. The process takes place as follows:

- Identification of the need.
- Establishment of a patient database to assist with need and resource assessment.
- Analysis to determine the resources available.
- Resource assessment, formulated to identify the current capabilities of the system.
- Highlighting of deficiencies, and formulation of solutions.

A.5.2 Legal Authority

This is established once the need for a system has been demonstrated. Legislation will be required to establish a lead agency with a strong oversight, or an advisory body composed of healthcare, public and medical representatives. This agency will develop the criteria for the system, regulate and direct pre-hospital care, establish pre-hospital triage, ensure medical direction, designate the proper facilities to render care, establish a trauma registry and establish performance improvement programmes.

A.5.3 Establish Criteria for Optimal Care

These must be established by the lead authority in conjunction with health and medical professionals. The adoption of system-wide standards is integral to the success of any system.

A.5.4 Designation of Trauma Centres

This takes place through a public process directed by the lead agency. Consideration must be given to the role of all acute care facilities within the region. Representatives from all these facilities must be involved in the planning process.

The number of trauma centres should be limited to the number required (based on the established need) for the patient population at risk of major injury. Having too many trauma centres may weaken the system by diluting the workload, thus reducing the experience for training, and will unnecessarily consume resources that are not fully utilized.

Development of a system requires that all the principal players be involved from the beginning. There must be agreement about the minimal data that will be contributed by *all* acute care facilities. Without the data from the hospitals managing the less severely injured, the data will be incomplete, and skewed towards major injury.

A.5.5 System Evaluation

Trauma systems are complex organizational structures with evolving methods and standards of care. It is necessary to have a mechanism for ongoing evaluation, based on:

- Self-monitoring.
- External evaluation.

A.6 RESULTS AND STUDIES

The Skamania Conference was held in July 1998, with the purpose of evaluating the evidence regarding the efficacy of trauma systems. During the conference, the evidence was divided into three categories: that resulting from panel studies, registry comparisons, and population-based research.

A.6.1 Panel Review

An overview of panel studies was presented at the Skamania Conference. The critique of panel reviews is that they vary widely, and interrater reliability has been very low in some studies. Furthermore, autopsy results alone are inadequate, and panel studies vary regarding the process of review and the rules used to come to a final judgement. In general, all panel studies were classified as weak class III evidence. Nevertheless, MacKenzie concluded that when all panel studies are considered collectively, they do provide some face validity and support of the hypothesis that treatment at a trauma centre versus a non-trauma centre is associated with fewer inappropriate deaths and possibly disabilities.

A.6.2 Registry Study

Jurkovich and Mock reported on the evidence provided by trauma registries in assessing overall effectiveness. They concluded that this was not class I evidence, but that it was probably better than a panel study. Their critique of trauma registries included the following six items: data are often missing, mis-codings occur, there may be inter-rater reliability factors, the national norms are not population-based, there is less detail about the causes of death, and they do not consider pre-hospital deaths. A consensus of the participants at the Skamania Conference concluded that registry studies were better than panel studies, but not as good as population studies.

A.6.3 Population-Based Studies

Populated-based studies probably also fall into class II evidence. They are not prospective randomized trials, but, because of nature of the population-based evidence, they cover all aspects of trauma care, including pre-hospital, hospital, and rehabilitative. A critique of the population-based studies pointed out that there are a limited number of clinical variables, and it is difficult to adjust for severity of injury and physiological dysfunction. There are other problems, although these probably apply to all studies, including secular trends, observational issues, and problems with longitudinal population mortality studies.

A.7 SUMMARY

Although there are difficulties with all three types of study, each may also offer advantages to various communities and regions. All three types may also influence health policy, and all can be used pre- and post-trauma system start-up. There was consensus at the Skamania Conference that the evaluation of trauma systems should be extended to include an economic evaluation and assessment of quality-adjusted-life-years.

RECOMMENDED READING

American College of Emergency Physicians: Guidelines for Trauma Care Systems. Available from https://www.acep.org/globalassets/new-pdfs/policy-statements/trauma-care-systems.pdf (accessed online December 2018).

American College of Surgeons. Regional Trauma System: Optimal elements, Integration, and Assessment. In: Committee on Trauma. *Resources for Optimal Care of the Injured Patient 2015.* Chicago: American College of Surgeons, (Orange

Book) 2015. Sixth Edition. Available online: www.facs.org (accessed online December 2018).

Ciesla DJ, Kerwin AZ, Tepasa JJ III. Trauma Systems, Triage, and Transport. In: Moore EE, Mattox KL, Feliciano DV, Eds. *Trauma* 8th Ed. New York, NY. McGraw Hill Education; 2017. 54–76.

Jurkovich GJ, Mock C. Systematic review of trauma system effectiveness based on registry comparisons. *J Trauma*. 1999 Sep;**47(3 Suppl)**:S46–55. Review.

MacKenzie EJ, Rivara FP, Jurkovich GJ, Nathens AB, Frey KP, Egleston BL, et al. A national evaluation of the effect of trauma-center care on mortality. *N Engl J Med*. 2006 Jan;**354(4)**:366–378.

MacKenzie EJ, Weir S, Rivara FP, Jurkovich GJ, Nathens AB, Wang W, et al. The value of trauma center care. *J Trauma*. 2010 Jul;**69(1)**:1–10. doi: 10.1097/TA.0b013e3181e03a21.

Appendix B
Trauma Scores and Scoring Systems

B.1 INTRODUCTION

Estimates of the severity of injury or illness are fundamental to the practice of medicine. The earliest known medical text, the Smith Papyrus, classified injuries into three grades: treatable, contentious, and untreatable.

Modern trauma scoring methodology uses a combination of an assessment of the severity of anatomical injury with a quantification of the degree of physiological derangement to arrive at scores that correlate with clinical outcomes.

Trauma scoring systems facilitate pre-hospital triage, identify trauma patients suitable for quality assurance audit, allow an accurate comparison of different trauma populations, and organize and improve trauma systems.

In principle, scoring systems can be divided into:

- Physiological scoring systems, based on the body's response to injury.
- Anatomical scoring systems, based on the physical injury that has occurred.
- Scoring systems based on both anatomical injury description and physiological response.
- Outcome analysis systems based on the result after recovery.

B.2 PHYSIOLOGICAL SCORING SYSTEMS

B.2.1 Glasgow Coma Scale[1]

The Glasgow Coma Scale (GCS),[1] devised in 1974, was one of the first numerical scoring systems (Table B.1). The GCS has been incorporated into many later scoring

Table B.1 Glasgow Coma Scale

Parameter	Response	Score
Eye-opening	Nil	1
	To pain	2
	To speech	3
	Spontaneously	4
Motor response	Nil	1
	Extensor	2
	Flexor	3
	Withdrawal	4
	Localizing	5
	Obeys command	6
Verbal response	Nil	1
	Groans	2
	Words	3
	Confused	4
	Orientated	5

systems, emphasizing the importance of head injury as a triage and prognostic indicator.

B.2.2 Paediatric Trauma Score[2]

The Paediatric Trauma Score (PTS; Table B.2) has been designed to facilitate triage of children. The PTS is the sum of six scores, and values range from –6 to +12, with a PTS of 8 or less being recommended as the trigger to send the child to a trauma centre. The PTS has been shown to accurately predict risk for severe injury or mortality but is not significantly more accurate than the RTS and is a great deal more difficult to measure.

Table B.2 Paediatric Trauma Score (PTS)

Clinical Parameter	Category	Score
Size (kg)	>20	2
	10–20	1
	<10	−1
Airway	Normal	2
	Maintainable	1
	Unmaintainable	−1
Systolic blood pressure (mm Hg)	>90	2
	50–90	1
	<50	−1
Central nervous system	Awake	2
	Obtunded/decreased LOC	1
	Coma/decerebrate	−1
Open wound	None	2
	Minor	1
	Major/penetrating	
Skeletal	None	2
	Closed fracture	1
	Open/multiple fractures	−1

Note: The values for the six parameters are summed to give the overall PTS.
Abbreviation: LOC, level of consciousness.

B.2.3 Revised Trauma Score[3]

Introduced by Champion et al., the Revised Trauma Score (RTS) evaluates blood pressure, the GCS and the respiratory rate to provide a scored physiological assessment of the patient.

The RTS can be used for field triage and enables pre-hospital and emergency care personnel to decide which patients should receive the specialized care of a trauma unit. An RTS score of 11 or less is suggested as the triage point for patients requiring at least level 2 trauma centre status (surgical facilities, 24-hour x-ray, etc.). An RTS of 10 or less carries a mortality of up to 30%, and these patients should be moved to a level 1 institution.

The difference between RTS on arrival and best RTS after resuscitation will give a reasonably clear picture of the prognosis. By convention, the RTS on admission is the one documented.

Table B.3 Revised Trauma Score (RTS)

Clinical Parameter	Category	Score	× Weight
Respiratory rate (breaths per minute)	10–29	4	0.2908
	>29	3	
	6–9	2	
	1–5	1	
	0	0	
Systolic blood pressure	>89	4	0.7326
	76–89	3	
	50–75	2	
	1–49	1	
	0	0	
Glasgow Coma Scale score	13–15	4	0.9368
	9–12	3	
	6–8	2	
	4–5	1	
	3	0	

Note: The values for the three parameters are summed to give the triage-RTS. Weighted values are summed for the RTS.

The RTS (non-triage) is designed for retrospective outcome analysis. Weighted co-efficients are used, which are derived from trauma patient populations, and provide a more accurate outcome prediction than the raw RTS (Table B.3). Since a severe head injury carries a poorer prognosis than a severe respiratory injury, the weighting is therefore heavier. The RTS thus varies from 0 (worst) to 7.8408 (best). The RTS is the most widely used physiological scoring system in the trauma literature.

B.2.4 Acute Physiologic and Chronic Health Evaluation II[4]

The Acute Physiologic and Chronic Health Evaluation II (APACHE II) score is used to evaluate mortality, and prognosis in ICU patients.

Calculation is based on several physiological and clinical comorbidity parameters, as well as age.[5] Each parameter can score 0 points, considered as normal physiology, to a maximum of 4 points (Table B.4).

Mortality interpretation is based on overall score (Table B.5).

Table B.4 APACHE II Score

Input	Measured	Measured	Points
Temperature (°C)	36–38°		0
	34.0–35.9°	38–38.5°	1
	32–33.9°	38.5–39°	2
	30–31.9°	39–40.9 °	3
	≤29.9°	≥41°	4
Heart rate	70–109		0
	–	–	1
	55–69	110–139	2
	40–54	140–179	3
	<40	≥180	4
Mean arterial pressure (mm Hg)	70–109		0
			1
	50–69	110–129	2
		130–159	3
	≤49	≥159	4
Respiratory rate (b.p.m.)	12–24		0
	10–11	25–34	1
	6–9	35–49	2
	–		3
	≤5	≥50	4
A-aPO$_2$ (FiO$_2$ >50%) or PaO$_2$ (FiO$_2$ <50%) (mm Hg)	<200 or PaO$_2$ > 70		0
	–	PaO$_2$ 61–70	1
	200–349	–	2
	350–499	PaO$_2$ 55–60	3
	>500	PaO$_2$ < 55	4
Arterial pH or HCO$_3$ (mmol/L)	7.33–7.49/22–31.9		0
	–	7.5–7.59/32–40.9	1
	7.25–7.32/18–21.9	–	2
	7.15–7.24/15–17.9	7.6–7.69/41–51.9	3
	<7.15/<15	≥7.7/>52	4
Serum Na$^+$ (mmol/L)	130–149		0
	–	150–154	1
	120–129	155–159	2
	111–119	160–179	3
	<110	>180	4

(Continued)

Table B.4 (*Continued*) APACHE II Score

Input	Measured	Measured	Points
Serum K$^+$ (mmol/L)	3.5–5.4		0
	3–3.4	5.5–5.9	1
	2.5–2.9	–	2
	–	6–6.9	3
	<2.5	≥7	4
Haematocrit (%)	30–45.9		0
	–	46–49.9	1
	20–29.9	50–59.9	2
	–	–	3
	<20	>60	4
White cell count (x10^3 cells/ mm^3)	3–14.9		0
	–	15–19.9	1
	1–2.9	20–39.9	2
	–	–	3
	<1	40	4
Glasgow Coma Scale	15		0
	Subtract actual GCS from 15 e.g. GCS 9/15 = 6 points		0–15
Age (years)	≤44 years		0
	45–54		1
	55–64		2
	65–74		3
	≥75		4
			5
			6
Chronic health problems	None		0
	Acute renal failure		1
	Yes + elective Surgery		+2
	Yes, but not post-operative		+5
	Yes + emergency surgery		+6

B.3 ANATOMICAL SCORING SYSTEMS

B.3.1 Abbreviated Injury Scale[6]

The Abbreviated Injury Scale (AIS) is an anatomically based, consensus-derived, global severity-based scoring system that classifies each injury by body region according to its relative importance on six-point ordinal scale.

Table B.5 Mortality-Based on APACHE II Scores

APACHE II Score: Approximate Mortality Interpretation		
Score	**Non-Operative**	**Post-Operative**
0–4	4%	1%
5–9	8%	3%
10–14	15%	7%
15–19	24%	12%
20–24	40%	30%
25–29	55%	35%
30–34	73%	73%
35–100	85%	88%

Table B.6 Injury Severity Score

Number	Region
1	Head and neck
2	Face
3	Thorax
4	Abdomen/pelvic contents
5	Extremities
6	External/skin/general

The AIS was developed in 1971 as a system to describe the severity of injury throughout the body. The 2015 Revision is currently used.

In AIS 2015, each injury is assigned a six-digit unique numerical identifier, to the left of the decimal point. This in known as the 'pre-dot' code, and is based on:

- Body region (first digit).
- Type of anatomical structure (second digit).
- Nature of injury (third and fourth digits).
- Level (fifth and sixth digits).
- There is an additional single digit to the right of the code (the 'post-dot' code), which is the AIS severity code. The AIS grades each injury by severity from 1 (least severe) to 5 (critical: survival uncertain). A score is 6 is given to certain injuries termed 'maximal (currently untreatable/unsurvivable)'.

The AIS manual is divided, for ease of reference, into nine different sections based on anatomy. All injuries therefore carry a unique code that can be used for classification, for indexing in trauma registry data bases and for severity.

B.3.2 **The Injury Severity Score[7]**

In 1974, Baker et al. created the Injury Severity Score (ISS) to relate AIS scores to patient outcomes. ISS body regions are listed in Table B.6.

The ISS is calculated by summing the square of the highest AIS scores in the three most severely injured regions. ISS scores range from 1 to 75 (since the highest AIS score for any region is 5). By convention, an AIS score of 6 (defined as a non-survivable injury) for any region becomes an ISS of 75.

The ISS only considers the single most serious injury in each region, ignoring the contribution of injury to other organs within the same region. Diverse injuries may have identical ISS scores but markedly different survival probabilities (an ISS of 25 may be obtained with isolated severe head injury or by a combination of lesser injuries across different regions). In addition, the ISS does not have the power to discriminate between the impact of similarly scored injuries to different organs, and therefore cannot identify, for example, the different impact of cerebral injury over injury to other organ systems.

B.3.3 **The New Injury Severity Score[8]**

In response to these limitations, the ISS was modified in 1997 to become the New Injury Severity Score (NISS).[8] NISS is calculated in the same way as ISS but takes the three most severe injuries (i.e. the three highest AIS scores regardless of body region). The NISS is then the simple sum of the squares of these three body regions.

The NISS can predict survival outcomes better than the ISS. In a separate study, the NISS yielded better separation between patients with and without multiple organ failure and showed that the NISS is superior to the ISS in the prediction of multiple organ failure.[9] Although the proponents of the NISS proclaim its superiority, its use is not yet widespread.

B.3.4 **Anatomic Profile Score[10]**

The Anatomic Profile Score (APS) was introduced in 1990 to overcome some of the limitations of the ISS. In contrast to ISS, the APS allows the inclusion of more than one serious body injury per region and considers the primacy of central nervous system and torso injury over other injuries. AIS scoring is used, but four values are used for injury characterization, roughly weighting the body regions. Serious trauma to the brain and spinal cord, anterior neck and chest, and all remaining injuries constitute three of the four values. The fourth value is a summary of all the remaining non-serious injuries. The APS score is the square root of the sum of the squares of all the AIS scores in a region, thus enabling the impact of multiple injuries within that region to be recognized. Component values for the four regions are summed to constitute the APS score.

A modified APS (mAPS) has recently been introduced, which is a four-number characterization of injury. The four component scores are the maximum AIS score and the square root of the sum of the squares of all AIS values for serious injury (AIS $\geq$3) in specified body regions (Table B.7). This leads to an Anatomic Profile Score, the weighted sum of the four mAPS components. The coefficients are derived from logistic regression analysis of admissions to four level 1 trauma centres (the 'controlled sites') in the Major Trauma Outcome Study.

A limitation of the use of AIS-derived scores is their cost. International Classification of Disease (ICD) taxonomy is a standard used by most hospitals and other healthcare providers to classify clinical diagnoses. Computerized mapping of ICD-9CM rubrics into AIS body regions and severity values has been used to compute ISS, AP, and NISS scores. Despite limitations, ICD–AIS conversion has been useful in population-based evaluation when AIS scoring from medical records is not possible. Outside North America, the ICD-10 is most commonly used.

Table B.7 Anatomic Profile Score

Component	Body Region	Abbreviated Injury Scale Severity
mA	Head/brain	3–6
	Spinal cord	3–6
mB	Thorax	3–6
	Front of neck	3–6
mC	All other	3–6

Note: mA, mB and mC scores are derived by taking the square root of the sum of the squares for all injuries defined by each component.

B.3.5 ICD-based Injury Severity Score[11]

Severity scoring systems also have been directly derived from ICD-coded discharge diagnoses. Most recently, the ICD-9 Severity Score (ICISS) has been proposed, which is derived by multiplying survival risk ratios associated with individual ICD diagnoses. Neural networking has been employed to further improve ICISS accuracy. ICISS has been shown to be better than ISS and to outperform the Trauma and Injury Severity Score (TRISS) in identifying outcomes and resource utilization. However, modified-AP scores, AP, and NISS appear to outperform ICISS in predicting hospital mortality.

There is some confusion over which anatomical scoring system should be used; however, currently, NISS probably should be the system of choice for AIS-based scoring.

B.3.6 Organ Injury Scaling System[12]

Organ Injury Scaling (OIS) is a scale of anatomical injury within an organ system or body structure. The goal of OIS is to provide a common language between trauma surgeons and to facilitate research and continuing quality improvement. It is not designed to correlate with patient outcomes. The OIS tables can be found on the American Association for the Surgery of Trauma (AAST) website[12] or at the end of this chapter.

B.3.7 Penetrating Abdominal Trauma Index[13]

Moore and colleagues facilitated the identification of the patient at high risk of post-operative complications when they developed the Penetrating Abdominal Trauma Index (PATI) scoring system for patients whose only source of injury was penetrating abdominal trauma. A complication risk factor was assigned to each organ system involved, and then multiplied by a severity of injury estimate. Each factor was given a value ranging from 1 to 5. The complication risk designation for each organ was based on the reported incidence of post-operative morbidity associated with that injury.

The severity of injury was estimated by a simple modification to the AIS, ranging from 1 = minimal injury to 5 = maximal injury. The sum of the individual organ score times the risk factor comprised the final PATI score. If the PATI score is 25 or less, the risk of complications is reduced (and where it is 10 or less, there are no complications), whereas if it is greater than 25, the risks are much higher.

In a group of 114 patients with gunshot wounds to the abdomen Moore et al.,[13] showed that a PATI score of more than 25 dramatically increased the risk of postoperative complications (46% of patients with a PATI score of over 25 developed serious postoperative complications, compared with 7% of patients with a PATI of less than 25). Further studies have validated the PATI scoring system.

B.3.8 Revised Injury Severity Classification II[14,15]

The first version of the Revised Injury Severity Classification (RISC) score was derived from the German Trauma Registry DGU (TR-DGU®) in 2003,[14] and has recently updated in 2014 to RISC II.[15]

The first version was developed and validated on 2000 patients documented between 1993 and 2000 in the TR-DGU. Eleven different data points were required from a trauma patient: new ISS, head injury, pelvic injury, age, GCS, coagulation, base deficit, haemoglobin, cardiac arrest, shock, and mass transfusion. Similar to the TRISS, the calculated score is transformed into a probability of survival P(s) by the logistic function $P(s) = 1/(1 + e^{-X})$. Comparative analyses showed that the predictive performance of the RISC was better than TRISS since it contained additional predictive variables, such as initial laboratory values on admission. The RISC has been used by the TR-DGU for outcome adjustment in inter-hospital comparisons and scientific analyses since 2003.

However, the original RISC also had some limitations. Missing values were partly replaced by a specific algorithm, but the number of patients who did not receive a RISC prognosis increased to more than 15% in the registry. Furthermore, observed mortality was about 2% lower than the predicted RISC prognosis. Finally, additional prognostic factors had been proposed, based on recent database analyses. Thus, in 2013, an enhanced version of the RISC was developed.[15]

The RISC II includes some well-known prognostic factors, like age and blood pressure, some variables already used in the original RISC (such as base deficit, haemoglobin, cardiac arrest) but also new variables like gender, pre-injury ASA, and pupil size and

reactivity. It is also interesting to mention that the overall injury severity is no longer described as ISS or NISS, but as AIS severity level of the worst and the second worst injury (plus head injury). This also allows differentiation between isolated and multiple injuries. If the injury is an isolated one, the AIS level of the second worst injury is zero, which means that outcome prediction improves (the respective coefficient for the second worst injury is +0.2).

RISC II attempts a new concept of treating missing values, in that there is no attempt to impute a missing value; however, the values are included in the model. Thus, if a certain value is missing it will not have any influence on the outcome prediction. This is seen in Table B.8 where all categories for missing values (indicated by '???') receive 0 points in the score. No missing values will be accepted for the variables which describe the injury pattern and age, because these elements were considered essential for any outcome estimation. Both variables (age and list of injuries as AIS codes) are also compulsory variables in the TR-DGU, which means that a prognostic score could be calculated for all patients in the registry.

The RISC II is based on data of 30,000 trauma cases documented in 2010 and 2011. Data from 2012 were used to validate the score. It is applied to patients with an injury of at least OIS grade 2 (thus the ISS is at least 4 points). The components of the RISC II are listed in Table B.8.

Validation results and comparisons with existing scores (ISS, TRISS, RISC) showed that RISC II not only could be applied to more patients but also has an improved discrimination (area under the ROS curve), precision (the predicted mortality better fits the observed one), and calibration (Hosmer-Lemeshow goodness-of-fit).[15]

B.4 COMORBIDITY SCORING SYSTEMS

There are several co-morbidities, which are known to affect trauma outcomes:

- Liver cirrhosis.
- Chronic obstructive pulmonary disease.
- Congenital coagulopathy.
- Diabetes.
- Congenital heart disease.
- Morbid obesity.

Table B.8 Components of RISC II

Variable	Value	Coefficient	Variable	Value	Coefficient
Worst injury	AIS 3	−0.5	Sex	Female	+0.2
	AIS 4	−1.3		Male/???	0
	AIS 5	−1.7	ASA pre-trauma	1–2	+0.3
	AIS 6	−2.9		3/???	0
Second worst injury	AIS 0–2	+0.2		4	−0.3
	AIS 3	0	Mechanism	Blunt/???	0
	AIS 4	−0.6		Penetrating	−0.6
	AIS 5	−1.4	GCS Motor function	Normal	+0.6
Head injury	AIS 0–2	0		Localizes/???	0
	AIS 3–4	−0.1		No localizing	−0.4
	AIS 5–6	−0.8		None	−0.8
Age	1–5	+1.4	Systolic BP on admission	<90	−0.7
	6–10	+0.6		90–110/???	0
	11–54	0		111–50	+0.3
	55–59	−0.5		>150	0
	60–64	−0.8	CPR	No	0
	65–69	−0.9		Yes	−1.8
	70–74	−1.2	Coagulation (INR)	<1.2	+0.6
	75–79	−1.9		1.2–1.4	+0.2
	80–84	−2.4		1.4–2.4/???	0
	85+	−2.7		>2.4	−0.4
Pupil reactivity	Brisk	+0.2	Blood haemoglobin (g/dL)	7.0–11.9/???	0
	Sluggish/???	0		<7.0	−0.5
	Fixed	−1.0	Acidosis (base deficit)	<6	+0.3
Pupil size	Normal	+0.2		6–9/???	0
	Unequal	0		9–15	−0.4
	Bilat dilated	−0.5		>15	−1.5

Note: *Coefficients of the RISC II score.* Starting with the constant value of 3.6, specific values (the coefficients) were added or subtracted, based on the observed findings, to finally give the score value. This value is then transformed into a probability of survival using the logistic function. Positive coefficients refer to an improved prognosis while negative ones worsen the prognosis.

Specific co-morbidity weighting is used in other discipline (including the APACHE II); however, their use in trauma so far has not been validated:

- Charlson comorbidity index[16]: generally used in medical disciplines.
- TRISSCOM[17]: This adjusts the TRISS score with an age factor of 65, rather than the more common 55 years, and includes eight comorbidities.

B.5 OUTCOME ANALYSIS

B.5.1 Functional Independence Measure and Functional Assessment Measure[18,19]

The Functional Independence Measure (FIM) is an 18-item global measure of disability, and can be scored alone, or with the additional 12 that formulate the Functional Assessment Measure (FAM). The FIM + FAM is designed to measure disability in the brain injured population. It has ordinal scoring system for all 30 items from 1–7, where 1 is complete dependence, to 7, complete independence. Scoring is completed at two time points, the first 7–10 days after admission (admission score), and the second within 7 days of discharge (discharge score).

B.5.2 Glasgow Outcome Scale[20]

For head-injured patients, the level of coma on admission or within 24 hours expressed by the GCS was found to correlate with outcome. The Glasgow Outcome Scale (GOS) was an attempt to quantify the outcome parameters for head-injured patients. A five-point scale was described (Table B.9).

Duration as well as intensity of disability should be included in an index of ill-health; this applies particularly after head injury, because many disabled survivors are young (Table B.10).

The grading of depth of coma and neurological signs was found to correlate strongly with outcome, but the low accuracy of individual signs limits their use in predicting outcomes for individuals.

B.5.3 Major Trauma Outcome Study

In 1982, the American College of Surgeons Committee on Trauma began the ongoing Major Trauma Outcome

Table B.9 Glasgow Outcome Scale

Outcome Parameters		
Low disability (good recovery)	GR	Light damage with minor neurological and psychological deficits.
Moderate disability	MD	No need for assistance in everyday life, employment is possible but may require special equipment.
Severe disability	SD	Severe injury with permanent help with daily living.
Persistent vegetative state	PVS	Severe damage with prolonged state of unresponsiveness and a lack of higher mental functions.
Death	D	Severe injury or death without recovery of consciousness.

Table B.10 Outcome Related to Signs

	Dead or Vegetative (%)	Moderate Disability or Good Recovery (%)
Pupils		
Reacting	39	50
Non-reacting	91	4
Eye movements		
Intact	33	56
Absent/bad	90	5
Motor response		
Normal	36	54
Abnormal	74	16

Study (MTOS), a retrospective, multicentre study of trauma epidemiology and outcomes.

The MTOS uses the TRISS methodology[21] to estimate the probability of survival, or P(s), for a given trauma patient. P(s) is derived according to the formula:

$$P(s) = 1/(1 + e^{-b})$$

where e is Euler's constant (approximately 2.718282) and $b = b_0 + b_1(RTS) + b_2(ISS) + b_3(age > 55)$. The b coefficients are derived by regression analysis from the MTOS database (Table B.11).

Table B.11 Coefficients from the Major Trauma Outcome Study Database

Blunt	Penetrating
$b_0 = -1.2470$	-0.6029
$b_1 = 0.9544$	1.1430
$b_2 = -0.0768$	-0.1516
$b_3 = -1.9052$	-2.6676

The P(s) values range from zero (survival not expected) to 1.000 for a patient with a 100% expectation of survival. Each patient's values can be plotted on a graph with ISS and RTS axes (Figure B.1).

The sloping line in Figure B.1 represents patients with a probability of survival of 50%; these PRE-charts (from PREliminary) are provided for those with blunt versus penetrating injury, and for those above versus below 55 years of age. Survivors whose coordinates are above the P(s)50 isobar and non-survivors below the P(s)50 isobar are considered atypical (statistically unexpected), and such cases are suitable for focused audit.

In addition to analysing individual patient outcomes, TRISS allows a comparison of a study population with the huge MTOS database. The 'Z-statistic' identifies whether study group outcomes are significantly different from expected outcomes as predicted from the MTOS. Z

is the ratio $(A - E)/S$, where $A =$ actual number of survivors, $E =$ expected number of survivors, and $S =$ scale factor, to transform the value into a standard normal distribution. Z may be positive or negative, depending on whether the survival rate is greater or less than predicted by TRISS. Z values of greater than 1.96 or less than –0.96 describe statistically significant deviation from prognosis (P < 0.05).

The so-called M-statistic is an injury severity match allowing a comparison of the range of injury severity in the sample population with that of the main database (i.e. the baseline group). The closer M is to 1, the better the match; the greater the disparity, the more biased Z will be. This bias can be misleading; for example, an institution with many patients with low-severity injuries can falsely appear to provide a better standard of care than another institution that treats a higher number of more severely injured patients.

The 'W-statistic', or Relative Outcome Score, calculates the actual numbers of survivors greater (or fewer) than predicted by the MTOS, per 100 trauma patients treated. The Relative Outcome Score can be used to compare W-values against a 'perfect outcome' of 100% survival. Thus, W could also be interpreted as the percentage of survivors above or below prediction The Relative Outcome Score may then be used to monitor improvements in trauma care delivery over time.

TRISS has been used in numerous studies. Its value as a predictor of survival or death has been shown to be

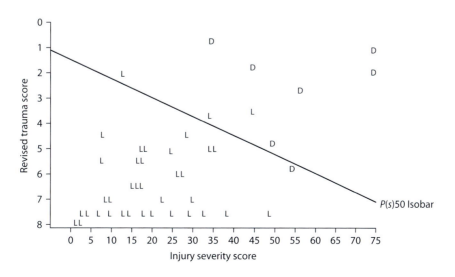

Figure B.1 PRE chart (D, dead; L, live).

Table B.12 Coefficients Derived from Major Trauma Outcome Study Data for the ASCOT Probability of Survival, P(s)

K-Coefficients	Type of Injury	
	Blunt	Penetrating
K_1	−1.157	−1.135
K_2 (RTS GCS value)	0.7705	1.0626
K_3 (RTS SBP value)	0.6583	0.3638
K_4 (RTS RR value)	0.281	0.3332
K_5 (AP head region value)	−0.3002	−0.3702
K_6 (AP thoracic region value)	−0.1961	−0.2053
K_7 (AP other serious injury value)	−0.2086	−0.3188
K_8 (age factor)	−0.6355	−0.8365

Abbreviations: APS, Anatomic Profile Score; ASCOT, A Severity Characterization of Trauma; GCS, Glasgow Coma Scale; RR, Respiratory rate; RTS, Revised Trauma Score; SBP, Systolic blood pressure.

from 75%–90% as good as a perfect index, depending on the patient data set used.

B.5.4 A Severity Characterization of Trauma[22,23]

A Severity Characterization of Trauma (ASCOT), introduced by Champion et al. in 1990, is a scoring system that uses the APS to characterize injury in place of the ISS. Different coefficients are used for blunt and penetrating injury, and the ASCOT score is derived from the formula: $P(s) = 1/(1 + e^{-k})$. The ASCOT model coefficients are shown in Table B.12. ASCOT has been shown to outperform TRISS, particularly for penetrating injury (Table B.12).

B.6 COMPARISON OF TRAUMA SCORING SYSTEMS

Table B.13 presents a comparison of trauma scoring systems.

B.7 SCALING SYSTEM FOR ORGAN SPECIFIC INJURIES[12,26–32]

Tables B.14 through B.45 present scaling systems for organ-specific injuries.

Table B.14 Cervical vascular organ injury scale
Table B.15 Chest wall injury scale
Table B.16 Heart injury scale
Table B.17 Lung injury scale
Table B.18 Thoracic vascular injury scale
Table B.19 Diaphragm injury scale
Table B.20 Spleen injury scale
Table B.21 Liver injury scale
Table B.22 Extrahepatic biliary tree injury scale
Table B.23 Pancreas injury scale
Table B.24 Oesophagus injury scale
Table B.25 Stomach injury scale
Table B.26 Duodenum injury scale
Table B.27 Small bowel injury scale
Table B.28 Colon injury scale
Table B.29 Rectum injury scale
Table B.30 Abdominal vascular injury scale
Table B.31 Adrenal organ injury scale
Table B.32 Kidney injury scale
Table B.33 Ureter injury scale
Table B.34 Bladder injury scale
Table B.35 Urethra injury scale
Table B.36 Uterus (non-pregnant) injury scale
Table B.37 Uterus (pregnant) injury scale
Table B.38 Fallopian tube injury scale
Table B.39 Ovary injury scale
Table B.40 Vagina injury scale
Table B.41 Vulva injury scale
Table B.42 Testis injury scale
Table B.43 Scrotum injury scale
Table B.44 Penis injury scale
Table B.45 Peripheral vascular organ injury scale

In all the tables in this section, ICD refers to the International Classification of Diseases (ICD9-CM[24] and ICD-10, 2015 edition[25]), and AIS to the Abbreviated Injury Scale 2015 of the American Association for the Advancement of Automotive Medicine.[6]

ICD-11 was released in June 2018, to be implemented in January 2022.[25]

Where necessary, in the ICD-10 system, a *fifth* digit is used as follows:

- Closed injury: 0
- Open injury: 1

Table B.13 Comparison of Trauma Scoring Systems

Scoring System	Year	Predicts What?	How Calculated?	Score Range/ Interpretation	Benefits	Limitations
Physiological Scoring Systems						
GCS	1977	Brain function patient survival.	Based on higher cerebral response to stimulation (eyes, motor, and verbal).	Range from 3/15 (no or minimal neurological function) to 15/15 (normal or near normal neurological function).	Simple and easy to calculate.	The best available score needs to be used, otherwise scale is inaccurate.
PTS	1988	Facilitates triage Measure of mortality risk.	Sum of six physiological scores.	Range from 2 (best) to −1 (worst).	Used as a trigger to refer a child to a trauma centre.	Not widely used.
RTS	1989	Patient survival.		Range from 0 (severe physiological derangement) to 7.84 (no physiological derangement).	Provides physiological assessment of the patient, high association with mortality. Superior to TRISS and ISS are predicting mortality in the ICU.	Incubation and sedation prior to arrival alter accuracy.
APACHE-II	1985	Patient survival and disease severity.	Based on the worst 12 routine physiological measurements, in the first 24 hours of ICU admission, as well as age and chronic health conditions.	Range from 0 (very low risk of mortality) to 71 (very high risk of mortality). Scores of greater than 15 are considered moderate to severe risk.	Superior to TRISS and ISS in predicting mortality in the ICU. Generally, now web-based entry and calculation.	ICU specific. Use limited by missing data. Time-consuming and complex to calculate.
Anatomical Scoring Systems						
AIS	1971	Patient survival			Developed to classify severity of injury, but validated to measure probability of death.	Does not predict functional impairment.

(Continued)

Table B.13 *(Continued)* Comparison of Trauma Scoring Systems

Scoring System	Year	Predicts What?	How Calculated?	Score Range/ Interpretation	Benefits	Limitations
ISS	1974	Patient survival	Body divided into six anatomical regions, each of which is given a score. Highest three scores are squared and summed.	44 possible scores, ranging from one (less severe) to 75 (unsurvivable).	Most widely used trauma severity score. Relates AIS to patient outcomes.	No physiological predictors. Does not account for more than one injury in the same region. Complex.
NISS	1997	Patient survival	Sum of the squares of the three most severe AIS severities, regardless of body region.	As for ISS.	Addresses multiple occurrence of serious injury within body region. Slight predictive advantage over ISS and ICISS.	Not widely used. Complex.
APS	1990	Patient survival	Three "modified components" are scored based on AIS and waited to form a single APS.	Range varies. Higher numbers have worse prognosis.	Based on location and severity of trauma.	Not widely used. Complex.
ICISS	1996	Patient survival	Computed directly from ICD-9 codes into a survival risk ratio (SRR).	Range from 0 (unsurvivable) to 1 (high chance of survival).	Not based on AIS/ISS no specialized training required. Outperforms ISS.	Not widely used. Based on ICD-9 codes only. May reflect hospital rather than injury survival.
ICDMAP-90	1997	Injury severity	Translates ICD-9 discharge diagnosis codes into an ISS, ISS and APS.	Variability in ICD/AIS scores.	Like ICISS. Conservative estimates of injury severity.	Not widely used. Based on ICD-9 codes only.
TRAIS	2003	Patient survival	Same as ICISS, but uses AIS descriptor codes.	Range from 0 (unsurvivable) to 1 (high chance of survival).	Like ICISS. Outpredicts ISS, NISS, and APS.	Not widely used.
OIS	1987	Anatomic injury	Anatomic injury.	Ranges from grade 1 (minor injury), to grade 5 (major injury), and grade 6 (fatal injury).	Standardised severity of injury. Widely used.	No predictability of mortality when used in isolation.

(Continued)

Table B.13 (*Continued*) Comparison of Trauma Scoring Systems

Scoring System	Year	Predicts What?	How Calculated?	Score Range/ Interpretation	Benefits	Limitations
RISC II	2014	Patient survival	German Trauma Registry based.	Uses multiple coefficients based on injury, age, and physiology.	Validation results and comparisons with existing scores showed that RISC II had improved discrimination, predicted mortality, and calibration.	Not widely used outside the Federal Republic of Germany.
Comorbidity Scoring Systems						
Charlson	1987	Patient survival	Score consists of 19 possible co-morbid conditions, each allocated a weight of 1–6 based on the relative risk of 1-year mortality. Values are summed.	Range from 0 (low chance of death) to 37 (high chance of death).	Validated in internal medicine patients only.	Not trauma specific, and not generally used for the trauma patient. Adapted for ICD-9 codes only.
TRISSCOM	2004	Patient survival	Like TRISS with adjustments for age (dichotomised to 65 rather than 55) and with the addition of 8 co-morbidity variables.	Scores range from 0 (unsurvivable) to 1 (high likelihood of survival).	Reflects the ageing population.	Not widely used. No severity weighting on comorbidities.
Combination Scoring Systems						
TRISS	1987	Patient survival	Combines ISS, RTS, and age; regression coefficients derived from MTOS database.	Scores run from 0 (unsurvivable) to 1 (high likelihood of survival).	Separate coefficients/ probabilities for patients with blunt and penetrating injuries.	Requires multiple variables.
ASCOT	1990	Patient survival	Uses APS to define injury severity.	Range varies.	As for TRISS with better predictive values for penetrating trauma.	Requires multiple variables.

(Continued)

Table B.13 (*Continued*) Comparison of Trauma Scoring Systems

Scoring System	Year	Predicts What?	How Calculated?	Score Range/ Interpretation	Benefits	Limitations
Outcome Based Analysis						
FIM/FAM	2000	Outcome following brain injury	Two scores – an admission score and a discharge score.	30 data points, each of which can be score from 1 (fully dependent) to 7 (fully independent).	Allows objective assessment to assess recovery, and the setting of goals.	Proprietary score therefore expensive. Widely used in rehabilitation centres.
GOS	1975	For outcome following head injury	The level of coma on admission correlates with outcome. The GOS attempts to quantify this.	Grading is made between a good recovery to death.	Grading of coma correlates strongly with outcome.	Low accuracy of individual signs.
MTOS	1982	Probability of survival	ISS methodology for a given trauma patient using coefficients representing RTS, ISS, and age.	The predictability of survival can be calculated.	Allows a comparison of the study population by a huge database, with individuals or hospitals.	Complex to calculate.

Source: Table modified from Champion H, Moore L, Vickers R. Injury Severity Scoring and Outcomes Research. In: Moore EE, Feliciano DV, Mattox KL, (Eds.) *Trauma*, 8th ed. McGraw Hill Education, New York, NY, 2017: 75–7.

Abbreviations: AIS, Abbreviated Injury score; APACHE-II, Acute Physiologic and Chronic Health Evaluation II; APS, Anatomic Profile Score; ASCOT, A Severity Characterisation of Trauma; Charlson, Charlson Comorbidity Index (CCI); FIM, Functional Independence Measure; FAM, Functional Assessment Measure; GCS, Glasgow Coma Scale; GOS, Glasgow Outcome Scale; ICDMAP-90, International Classification of Disease "map" – 1990; ICISS, International Classification of Disease Injury Severity Score; ISS, Injury Severity Score; MTOS, Major Trauma Outcome Study; NISS, New Injury Severity Score; OIS, American Association for the Surgery of Trauma Organ Injury Scale; PTS, Paediatric Trauma Score; RISC II, Revised Injury Severity Classification II; RTS, Revised Trauma Score; TRAIS, Trauma Registry Abbreviated Injury Score; TRISS, Trauma and injury Severity Score; TRISSCOM, Trauma and Injury Severity Score Comorbidity.

Table B.14 Cervical Vascular Organ Injury Scale

Grade[a]	Description of Injury	ICD-9	ICD-10	AIS-2005
I	Thyroid vein	900.8	S15.8	
	Common facial vein	900.8	S15.8	
	External jugular vein	900.81	S15.2	1–3
	Non-named arterial/venous branches	900.9	S15.9	
II	External carotid arterial branches (ascending pharyngeal, superior thyroid, lingual, facial, maxillary, occipital, posterior auricular)	900.8	S15.0	1–3
	Thyrocervical trunk or primary branches	900.8	S15.8	1–3
	Internal jugular vein	900.1	S15.3	1–3
III	External carotid artery	900.02	S15.0	2–3
	Subclavian vein	901.3	S25.3	3–4
	Vertebral artery	900.8	S15.1	2–4
IV	Common carotid artery	900.01	S15.0	3–5
	Subclavian artery	901.1	S25.1	3–4
V	Internal carotid artery (extracranial)	900.03	S15.0	3–5

Source: Moore EE et al. *J Trauma.* 1996 September;41(3):523–4.[26]

[a] Increase one grade for multiple grade III or IV injuries involving more than 50% of the vessel circumference. Decrease one grade for less than 25% vessel circumference disruption for grade IV or V.

Table B.15 Chest Wall Injury Scale

Grade[a]	Injury Type	Description of Injury	ICD-9	ICD-10	AIS-2005
I	Contusion	Any size	911.0/922.1	S20.2	1
	Laceration	Skin and subcutaneous	875.0	S20.4	1
	Fracture	<3 ribs, closed;	807.01/807.02	S22.3	1–2
		non-displaced, clavicle closed	810.00/810.03	S42.0	2
II	Laceration	Skin, subcutaneous and muscle	875.1	S20.4	2
	Fracture	≥3 adjacent ribs, closed	807.03/807.08	S22.4	1
		Open or displaced clavicle	810.10/810.13	S42.0	2–3
		Non-displaced sternum, closed	807.2	S22.2	2
		Scapular body, open or closed	811.00/811.18	S42.1	2
III	Laceration	Full thickness including pleural penetration – front	862.29	S21.1	2
		Full thickness including pleural penetration – back	862.29	S21.2	2
	Fracture	Open or displaced sternum	807.2	S22.2	2
		Flail sternum	807.3	S22.2	2
		Unilateral flail segment (<3 ribs)	807.4	S22.5	3–4
IV	Laceration	Avulsion of chest wall tissues with underlying rib fractures	807.10/807.18	S22.8	4
	Fracture	Unilateral flail chest (≥3 ribs)	807.4	S22.5	3–4
V	Fracture	Bilateral flail chest (≥3 ribs on both sides)	807.4	S22.5	5

Source: Moore EE et al. *J Trauma.* 1992 September;33(3):337–8.[27]

Note: This scale is confined to the chest wall alone and does not reflect associated internal or abdominal injuries. Therefore, further delineation of upper versus lower or anterior versus posterior chest wall was not considered, and a grade VI was not warranted. Specifically, thoracic crush was not used as a descriptive term; instead, the geography and extent of fractures and soft tissue injury were used to define the grade.

[a] Upgrade by one grade for bilateral injuries.

Table B.16 Heart Injury Scale				
Grade[a]	Description of Injury	ICD-9	ICD-10	AIS-2005
I	Blunt cardiac injury with minor ECG abnormality (non-specific ST or T wave changes, premature arterial or ventricular contraction or persistent sinus tachycardia).	861.01	S26.0	3
	Blunt or penetrating pericardial wound without cardiac injury, cardiac tamponade or cardiac herniation.			
II	Blunt cardiac injury with heart block (right or left bundle branch, left anterior fascicular or atrioventricular) or ischaemic changes (ST depression or T wave inversion) without cardiac failure.	861.01	S26.0	3
	Penetrating tangential myocardial wound up to, but not extending through, endocardium, without tamponade.	861.12	S26.0	3
III	Blunt cardiac injury with sustained ($\geq$6 beats/min) or multifocal ventricular contractions.	861.01	S26.0	3–4
	Blunt or penetrating cardiac injury with septal rupture, pulmonary or tricuspid valvular incompetence, papillary muscle dysfunction or distal coronary arterial occlusion without cardiac failure.	861.01	S26.0	3–4
	Blunt pericardial laceration with cardiac herniation.	861.01	S26.0	3–4
	Blunt cardiac injury with cardiac failure.	861.01	S26.0	3–4
	Penetrating tangential myocardial wound up to, but extending through, endocardium, with tamponade.	861.12	S26.0	3
IV	Blunt or penetrating cardiac injury with septal rupture, pulmonary or tricuspid valvular incompetence, papillary muscle dysfunction or distal coronary arterial occlusion producing cardiac failure.	861.12	S26.0	3
	Blunt or penetrating cardiac injury with aortic mitral valve incompetence.	861.03	S26.0	5
	Blunt or penetrating cardiac injury of the right ventricle, right atrium or left atrium.	861.03	S26.0	5
V	Blunt or penetrating cardiac injury with proximal coronary arterial occlusion.	861.03	S26.0	5
	Blunt or penetrating left ventricular perforation.	861.13	S26.0	5
	Stellate wound with <50% tissue loss of the right ventricle, right atrium or left atrium.	861.03	S26.0	5
VI	Blunt avulsion of the heart; penetrating wound producing >50% tissue loss of a chamber.	861.13	S26.0	6

Source: Moore EE et al. *J Trauma.* 1994 March;36(3):299–300.[28]
Note: With ICD-10, use supplementary character: 0 = without an open wound into the thoracic cavity; 1 = with an open wound into the thoracic cavity.
[a] Advance one grade for multiple wounds to a single chamber or multiple chamber involvement.

Table B.17 Lung Injury Scale

Gradeᵃ	Injury Type	Description of Injury	ICD-9	ICD-10	AIS-2005
I	Contusion	Unilateral, <1 lobe	861.12/861.31	S27.3	3
II	Contusion	Unilateral, single lobe	861.20/861.30	S27.3	3
	Laceration	Simple pneumothorax	860.0/1/4/5	S27.0	3–5
III	Contusion	Unilateral, >1 lobe	861.20/861.30	S27.3	3
	Laceration	Persistent (>72-hour) air leak from distal airway	860.0/1/4/5	S27.3	3–4
	Haematoma	Non-expanding intraparenchymal	862.0/861.30	S27.3	
IV	Laceration	Major (segmental or lobar) air leak	862.21/861.31	S27.4	4–5
	Haematoma	Expanding intraparenchymal		S25.4	
	Vascular	Primary branch intrapulmonary vessel disruption	901.40	S25.4	3–5
V	Vascular	Hilar vessel disruption	901.41/901.42	S25.4	4
VI	Vascular	Total uncontained transection of pulmonary hilum	901.41/901.42	S25.4	4

Source: Moore EE et al. *J Trauma.* 1994 March;36(3):299–300.[28]
Note: Haemothorax is scored under the thoracic vascular injury scale. With ICD-10, use supplementary character: 0 = without an open wound into the thoracic cavity; 1 = with an open wound into the thoracic cavity.
ᵃ Advance one grade for bilateral injuries up to grade III.

Table B.18 Thoracic Vascular Injury Scale

Gradeᵃ	Description of Injury	ICD-9	ICD-10	AIS-2005
I	Intercostal artery/vein	901.81	S25.5	2–3
	Internal mammary artery/vein	901.82	S25.8	2–3
	Bronchial artery/vein	901.89	S25.4	1–3
	Oesophageal artery/vein	901.9	S25.8	2–3
	Hemiazygos vein	901.89	S25.8	2–3
	Unnamed artery/vein	901.9	S25.9	2–3
II	Azygos vein	901.89	S25.8	2–3
	Internal jugular vein	900.1	S15.3	2–3
	Subclavian vein	901.3	S25.3	3–4
	Innominate vein	901.3	S25.3	3–4
III	Carotid artery	900.01	S15.0	3–5
	Innominate artery	901.1	S25.1	3–4
	Subclavian artery	901.1	S25.1	3–4
IV	Thoracic aorta, descending	901.0	S25.0	4–5
	Inferior vena cava (intrathoracic)	902.10	S35.1	3–4
	Pulmonary artery, primary intraparenchymal branch	901.41	S25.4	3
	Pulmonary vein, primary intraparenchymal branch	901.42	S25.4	3
V	Thoracic aorta, ascending and arch	901.0	S25.0	5
	Superior vena cava	901.2	S25.2	3–4
	Pulmonary artery, main trunk	901.41	S25.4	4
	Pulmonary vein, main trunk	901.42	S25.4	4
VI	Uncontained total transection of thoracic aorta or pulmonary hilum	901.0	S25.0	5
	Uncontained total transection of pulmonary hilum	901.41/901.42	S25.4	5

Source: Moore EE et al. *J Trauma.* 1994 March;36(3):299–300.[28]
ᵃ Increase one grade for multiple grade III or IV injuries if more than 50% of the circumference. Decrease one grade for grade IV injuries if less than 25% of the circumference.

Table B.19 Diaphragm Injury Scale

Grade[a]	Description of Injury	ICD-9	ICD-10	AIS-2005
I	Contusion	862.0	S27.8	2
II	Laceration <2 cm	862.1	S27.8	3
III	Laceration 2–10 cm	862.1	S27.8	3
IV	Laceration >10 cm with tissue loss ≤25 cm^2	862.1	S27.8	3
V	Laceration with tissue loss >25 cm^2	862.1	S27.8	3

Source: Moore EE et al. *J Trauma*. 1994 March;36(3):299–300.[28]
[a] Advance one grade for bilateral injuries up to grade III.

Table B.20 Spleen Injury Scale (1994 Revision)

Grade[a]	Injury Type	Description of Injury	ICD-9	ICD-10	AIS-2005
I	Haematoma	Subcapsular, <10% surface area	865-01/865.11	S36.0	2
	Laceration	Capsular tear, <1 cm parenchymal depth	865.02/865.12	S36.0	2
II	Haematoma	Subcapsular, 10%–50% surface area; intraparenchymal, <5 cm in diameter	865.01/865.11	S36.0	2
	Laceration	Capsular tear, 1–3 cm parenchymal depth that does not involve a trabecular vessel	865.02/865.12	S36.0	2
III	Haematoma	Subcapsular, >50% surface area or expanding; ruptured subcapsular or parenchymal haematoma; intraparenchymal haematoma ≥5 cm or expanding	865.03	S36.0	3
	Laceration	>3 cm parenchymal depth or involving trabecular vessels	865.03	S36.0	3
IV	Laceration	Laceration involving segmental or hilar vessels producing major devascularization (>25% of spleen)	865.13	S36.0	4
V	Laceration	Completely shattered spleen	865.04	S36.0	5
	Vascular	Hilar vascular injury with devascularized spleen	865.14	S36.0	5

Source: Moore EE et al. *J Trauma*. 1995 December;39(6):1069–70.[29]
Note: With ICD-10, use supplementary character: 0 = without an open wound into the abdominal cavity; 1 = with an open wound into the abdominal cavity.
[a] Advance one grade for multiple injuries up to grade III.

Table B.21 Liver Injury Scale (1994 Revision)

Grade[a]	Type of Injury	Description of Injury	ICD-9	ICD-10	AIS-2005
I	Haematoma	Subcapsular, <10% surface area	864.01/864.11	S36.1	2
	Laceration	Capsular tear, <1 cm parenchymal depth	864.02/864.12	S36.1	2
II	Haematoma	Subcapsular, 10%–50% surface area: intraparenchymal <10 cm in diameter	864.01/864.11	S36.1	2
	Laceration	Capsular tear 1–3 cm, parenchymal depth, <10 cm in length	864.03/864.13	S36.1	2
III	Haematoma	Subcapsular, >50% surface area or ruptured subcapsular or parenchymal haematoma; intraparenchymal haematoma >10 cm or expanding	864.04/864.14	S36.1	3
	Laceration	3 cm parenchymal depth	864.04/864.14	S36.1	3
IV	Laceration	Parenchymal disruption involving 25%–75% hepatic lobe or 1–3 Couinaud's segments within a single lobe	864.04/864.14	S36.1	4
V	Laceration	Parenchymal disruption involving >75% of hepatic lobe or >3 Couinaud's segments within a single lobe	864.04/864.14	S36.1	5
	Vascular	Juxtahepatic venous injuries; i.e. retrohepatic vena cava/central major hepatic veins	864.04/864.14	S36.1	5
VI	Vascular	Hepatic avulsion	864.04/864.14	S36.1	5

Source: Moore EE et al. *J Trauma*. 1995 December;39(6):1069–70.[29]
Note: With ICD-10, use supplementary character: 0 = without an open wound into the abdominal cavity; 1 = with an open wound into the abdominal cavity.
[a] Advance one grade for multiple injuries up to grade III.

Table B.22 Extrahepatic Biliary Tree Injury Scale

Grade[a]	Description of Injury	ICD-9	ICD-10	AIS-2005
I	Gallbladder contusion/haematoma	868.02	S36.1	2
	Portal triad contusion	868.02	S36.1	2
II	Partial gallbladder avulsion from liver bed; cystic duct intact	868.02	S36.1	2
	Laceration or perforation of the gallbladder	868.12	S36.1	2
III	Complete gallbladder avulsion from liver bed	868.02	S36.1	3
	Cystic duct laceration	868.12	S36.1	3
IV	Partial or complete right hepatic duct laceration	868.12	S36.1	3
	Partial or complete left hepatic duct laceration	868.12	S36.1	3
	Partial common hepatic duct laceration (<50%)	868.12	S36.1	3
	Partial common bile duct laceration (<50%)	868.12	S36.1	3
V	>50% transection of common hepatic duct	868.12	S36.1	3–4
	>50% transection of common bile duct	868.12	S36.1	3–4
	Combined right and left hepatic duct injuries	868.12	S36.1	3–4
	Intraduodenal or intrapancreatic bile duct injuries	868.12	S36.1	3–4

Source: Moore EE et al. *J Trauma*. 1990 November;30(11):1427–9.[30]
Note: With ICD-10, use supplementary character: 0 = without an open wound into the abdominal cavity; 1 = with an open wound into the abdominal cavity.
[a] Advance one grade for multiple injuries up to grade III.

Table B.23 Pancreas Injury Scale

Grade[a]	Type of Injury	Description of Injury	ICD-9	ICD-10	AIS-2005
I	Haematoma	Minor contusion without duct injury	863.81/863.84	S36.2	2
	Laceration	Superficial laceration without duct injury		S36.2	2
II	Haematoma	Major contusion without duct injury or tissue loss	863.81/863.84	S36.2	2
	Laceration	Major laceration without duct injury or tissue loss	863.81/863.84	S36.2	3
III	Laceration	Distal transection or parenchymal injury with duct injury	863.92/863.94	S36.2	3
IV	Laceration	Proximal transection or parenchymal injury involving ampulla	863.91	S36.2	4
V	Laceration	Massive disruption of pancreatic head	863.91	S36.2	5

Source: From Moore EE et al. *J Trauma.* 1990 November;30(11):1427–9.[31]
Note: With ICD-10, use supplementary character: 0 = without an open wound into the abdominal cavity; 1 = with an open wound into the abdominal cavity. 863.51,863.91: head; 863.99,862.92: body; 863.83,863.93: tail. The proximal pancreas is to the patients' right of the superior mesenteric vein.
[a] Advance one grade for multiple injuries up to grade III.

Table B.24 Oesophagus Injury Scale

Grade[a]	Type of Injury	Description of Injury	ICD-9	ICD-10	AIS-2005
I	Contusion	Contusion/haematoma (cervical oesophagus)	862.22/826.32	S10.0	2
		Contusion/haematoma (thoracic oesophagus)	862.22/826.32	S27.8	3
		Contusion/haematoma (abdominal oesophagus)	862.22/862.32	S36.8	3
II	Laceration	Partial thickness laceration	862.22/826.32	S10.0/S27.8/S36.8	4
III	Laceration	Laceration <50% circumference	862.22/826.32	S10.0/S27.8/S36.8	4
IV	Laceration	Laceration >50% circumference	862.22/826.32	S10.0/S27.8/S36.8	5
V	Tissue loss	Segmental loss or devascularization <2 cm	862.22/826.32	S10.0/S27.8/S36.8	5
	Tissue loss	Segmental loss or devascularization >2 cm	862.22/826.32	S10.0/S27.8/S36.8	

Source: Moore EE et al. *J Trauma.* 1990 November;30(11):1427–9.[30]
Note: With ICD-10, use fifth character supplementary character: 0 = without an open wound into the abdominal or thoracic cavity; 1 = with an open wound into the abdominal or thoracic cavity.
Abbreviation: S10.0: cervical oesophagus; S27.8: thoracic oesophagus; S36.8: abdominal oesophagus.
[a] Advance one grade for multiple lesions up to grade III.

Table B.25 Stomach Injury Scale

Grade[a]	Type of Injury	Description of Injury	ICD-9	ICD-10	AIS-2005
I	Contusion	Contusion/haematoma	863.0/863.1	S36.3	2
	Laceration	Partial thickness laceration	863.0/863.1	S36.3	2
II	Laceration	<2 cm in gastro-oesophageal junction or pylorus	863.0/863.1	S36.3	3
		<5 cm in proximal 1/3 stomach	863.0/863.1	S36.3	3
		<10 cm in distal 2/3 stomach	863.0/863.1	S36.3	3
III	Laceration	>2 cm in gastro-oesophageal junction or pylorus	863.0/863.1	S36.3	3
		>5 cm in proximal 1/3 stomach	863.0/863.1	S36.3	3
		>10 cm in distal 2/3 stomach	863.0/863.1	S36.3	3
IV	Tissue loss	Tissue loss or devascularization <2/3 stomach	863.0/863.1	S36.3	4
V	Tissue loss	Tissue loss or devascularization >2/3 stomach	863.0/863.1	S36.3	4

Source: Moore EE et al. *J Trauma.* 1990 November;30(11):1427–9.[30]
Note: With ICD-10, use supplementary character: 0 = without an open wound into the abdominal cavity; 1 = with an open wound into the abdominal cavity.
[a] Advance one grade for multiple lesions up to grade III.

Table B.26 Duodenum Injury Scale

Grade[a]	Type of Injury	Description of Injury	ICD-9	ICD-10	AIS-2005
I	Haematoma	Involving single portion of duodenum	863.21	S36.4	2
	Laceration	Partial thickness, no perforation	863.21	S36.4	3
II	Haematoma	Involving more than one portion	863.21	S36.4	2
	Laceration	Disruption <50% of circumference	863.31	S36.4	3
III	Laceration	Disruption 50%–75% of circumference of D2	863.31	S36.4	4
		Disruption 50%–100% of circumference of D1, D3, or D4	863.31	S36.4	4
IV	Laceration	Disruption >75% of circumference of D2	863.31	S36.4	5
		Involving ampulla or distal common bile duct	863.31	S36.4	5
V	Laceration	Massive disruption of duodenopancreatic complex	863.31	S36.4	5
	Vascular	Devascularization of duodenum	863.31	S36.4	5

Source: From Moore EE et al. *J Trauma.* 1990 November;30(11):1427–9.[31]
Note: With ICD-10, use supplementary character: 0 = without an open wound into the abdominal cavity; 1 = with an open wound into the abdominal cavity.
Abbreviation: D1, first portion of duodenum; D2, second portion of duodenum; D3, third portion of duodenum; D4, fourth portion of duodenum.
[a] Advance one grade for multiple injuries up to grade III.

Table B.27 Small Bowel Injury Scale

Grade[a]	Type of Injury	Description of Injury	ICD-9	ICD-10	AIS-2005
I	Haematoma	Contusion or haematoma without devascularization	863.20	S36.4	2
	Laceration	Partial thickness, no perforation	863.20	S36.4	2
II	Laceration	Laceration <50% of circumference	863.30	S36.4	3
III	Laceration	Laceration ≥50% of circumference without transection	863.30	S36.4	3
IV	Laceration	Transection of the small bowel	863.30	S36.4	4
V	Laceration	Transection of the small bowel with segmental tissue loss	863.30	S36.4	4
	Vascular	Devascularized segment	863.30	S36.4	4

Source: Moore EE et al. *J Trauma*. 1990 November;30(11):1427–9.[31]
Note: With ICD-10, use supplementary character: 0 = without an open wound into the abdominal cavity; 1 = with an open wound into the abdominal cavity.
[a] Advance one grade for multiple injuries up to grade III.

Table B.28 Colon Injury Scale

Grade[a]	Type of Injury	Description of Injury	ICD-9	ICD-10	AIS-2005
I	Haematoma	Contusion or haematoma without devascularization	863.40–863.44	S36.5	2
	Laceration	Partial thickness, no perforation	863.40–863.44	S36.5	2
II	Laceration	Laceration <50% of circumference	863.50–863.54	S36.5	3
III	Laceration	Laceration ≥50% of circumference without transection	863.50–863.54	S36.5	3
IV	Laceration	Transection of the colon	863.50–863.54	S36.5	4
V	Laceration	Transection of the colon with segmental tissue loss	863.50–863.54	S36.5	4

Source: Moore EE et al. *J Trauma*. 1990 November;30(11):1427–9.[31]
Note: With ICD-9, 863.40/863.50 = non-specific site in colon; 863.41/863.51 = ascending colon; 863.42/863.52 = transverse colon; 863.43/863.53 = descending colon; 863.44/863.54 = sigmoid colon.
With ICD-10, use supplementary character: 0 = without an open wound into the abdominal cavity; 1 = with an open wound into the abdominal cavity.
[a] Advance one grade for multiple injuries up to grade III.

Table 29 Rectum Injury Scale

Grade[a]	Type of Injury	Description of Injury	ICD-9	ICD-10	AIS-2005
I	Haematoma	Contusion or haematoma without devascularization	863.45	S36.6	2
	Laceration	Partial-thickness laceration	863.45	S36.6	2
II	Laceration	Laceration <50% of circumference	863.55	S36.6	3
III	Laceration	Laceration ≥50% of circumference	863.55	S36.6	4
IV	Laceration	Full-thickness laceration with extension into the perineum	863.55	S36.6	5
V	Vascular	Devascularized segment	863.55	S36.6	5

Source: Moore EE et al. *J Trauma*. 1990 November;30(11):1427–9.[31]
Note: With ICD-10, use supplementary character: 0 = without an open wound into the abdominal cavity; 1 = with an open wound into the abdominal cavity.
[a] Advance one grade for multiple injuries up to grade III.

Table B.30 Abdominal Vascular Injury Scale

Grade[a]	Description of Injury	ICD-9	ICD-10	AIS-2005
I	Non-named superior mesenteric artery or superior mesenteric vein branches	902.20/39	S35.2	NS
	Non-named inferior mesenteric artery or inferior mesenteric vein branches	902.27/.32	S35.2	NS
	Phrenic artery or vein	902.89	S35.8	NS
	Lumbar artery or vein	902.89	S35.8	NS
	Gonadal artery or vein	902.89	S35.8	NS
	Ovarian artery or vein	902.81/902.82	S35.8	NS
	Other non-named small arterial or venous structures requiring ligation	902.80	S35.9	NS
II	Right, left or common hepatic artery	902.22	S35.2	3
	Splenic artery or vein	902.23/902.34	S35.2	3
	Right or left gastric arteries	902.21	S35.2	3
	Gastroduodenal artery	902.24	S35.2	3
	Inferior mesenteric artery/trunk or inferior mesenteric vein/trunk	902.27/902.32	S35.2	3
	Primary named branches of mesenteric artery (e.g. ileocolic artery) or mesenteric vein	902.26/902.31	S35.2	3
	Other named abdominal vessels requiring ligation or repair	902.89	S35.8	3
III	Superior mesenteric vein, trunk and primary subdivisions	902.31	S35.3	3
	Renal artery or vein	902.41/902.42	S35.4	3
	Iliac artery or vein	902.53/902.54	S35.5	3
	Hypogastric artery or vein	902.51/902.52	S35.5	3
	Vena cava, infrarenal	902.10	S35.1	3
IV	Superior mesenteric artery, trunk	902.25	S35.2	3
	Coeliac axis proper	902.24	S35.2	3
	Vena cava, suprarenal and infrahepatic	902.10	S35.1	3
	Aorta, infrarenal	902.00	S35.0	4
V	Portal vein	902.33	S35.3	3
	Extraparenchymal hepatic vein only	902.11	S35.1	3
	Extraparenchymal hepatic veins + liver	902.11	S35.1	5
	Vena cava, retrohepatic or suprahepatic	902.19	S35.1	5
	Aorta suprarenal, subdiaphragmatic	902.00	S35.0	4

Source: Moore EE et al. *J Trauma*. 1992 September;33(3):337–8.[27]
Note: With ICD-10, use supplementary character: 0 = without an open wound into the abdominal cavity; 1 = with an open wound into the abdominal cavity.
Abbreviation: NS, not scored.
[a] This classification system is applicable to extraparenchymal vascular injuries. If the vessel injury is within 2 cm of the organ parenchyma, refer to the specific organ injury scale. Increase one grade for multiple grade III or IV injuries involving >50% of the vessel circumference. Downgrade one grade if <25% of the vessel circumference laceration for grades IV or V.

Table B.31 Adrenal Organ Injury Scale

Grade[a]	Description of Injury	ICD-9	ICD-10	AIS-2005
I	Contusion	868.01/.11	S37.9	1
II	Laceration involving only cortex (<2 cm)	868.01/.11	S37.8	1
III	Laceration extending into medulla (≥2 cm)	868.01/.11	S37.8	2
IV	>50% parenchymal destruction	868.01/.11	S37.8	2
V	Total parenchymal destruction (including massive intraparenchymal haemorrhage) Avulsion from blood supply	868.01/.11	S37.8	3

Source: Moore EE et al. *J Trauma.* 1989 December;29(12):1664–6.[31]
Note: With ICD-10, use supplementary character: 0 = without an open wound into the abdominal cavity; 1 = with an open wound into the abdominal cavity.
[a] Advance one grade for bilateral lesions up to grade V.

Table B.32 Kidney Injury Scale

Grade[a]	Type of Injury	Description of Injury	ICD-9	ICD-10	AIS-2005
I	Contusion	Microscopic or gross haematuria, urological studies normal	866.00/866.01	S37.0	2
	Haematoma	Subcapsular, non-expanding without parenchymal laceration	866.01	S37.0	2
II	Haematoma	Non-expanding perirenal haematoma confined to renal retroperitoneum	866.01	S37.0	2
	Laceration	<1.0 cm parenchymal depth of renal cortex without urinary extravasation	866.11	S37.0	2
III	Laceration	>1.0 cm parenchymal depth of renal cortex without collecting system rupture or urinary extravasation	866.11	S37.0	3
IV	Laceration	Parenchymal laceration extending through renal cortex, medulla and collecting system	866.02/866.12	S37.0	4
	Vascular	Main renal artery or vein injury with contained haemorrhage	866.03/866.11	S37.0	4
V	Laceration	Completely shattered kidney	866.04/866.14	S37.0	5
	Vascular	Avulsion of renal hilum that devascularizes kidney	866.13	S37.0	5

Source: Moore EE et al. *J Trauma.* 1989 December;29(12):1664–6.[32]
Note: With ICD-10, use supplementary character: 0 = without an open wound into the abdominal cavity; 1 = with an open wound into the abdominal cavity.
[a] Advance one grade for bilateral injuries up to grade III.

Table B.33 Ureter Injury Scale

Grade[a]	Type of Injury	Description of Injury	ICD-9	ICD-10	AIS-2005
I	Haematoma	Contusion or haematoma without devascularization	867.2/867.3	S37.1	2
II	Laceration	<50% transection	867.2/867.3	S37.1	2
III	Laceration	≥50% transection	867.2/867.3	S37.1	3
IV	Laceration	Complete transection with <2 cm devascularization	867.2/867.3	S37.1	3
V	Laceration	Avulsion with >2 cm devascularization	867.2/867.3	S37.1	3

Source: Moore EE et al. *J Trauma.* 1992 September;33(3):337–8.[27]
Note: With ICD-10, use supplementary character: 0 = without an open wound into the abdominal cavity; 1 = with an open wound into the abdominal cavity.
[a] Advance one grade for bilateral up to grade III.

Table B.34 Bladder Injury Scale

Grade[a]	Injury Type	Description of Injury	ICD-9	ICD-10	AIS-2005
I	Haematoma	Contusion, intramural haematoma	867.0/867.1	S37.2	2
	Laceration	Partial thickness	867.0/867.1	S37.2	3
II	Laceration	Extraperitoneal bladder wall laceration <2 cm	867.0/867.1	S37.2	4
III	Laceration	Extraperitoneal (≥2 cm) or intraperitoneal (<2 cm) bladder wall laceration	867.0/867.1	S37.2	4
IV	Laceration	Intraperitoneal bladder wall laceration ≥2 cm	867.0/867.1	S37.2	4
V	Laceration	Intraperitoneal or extraperitoneal bladder wall laceration extending into the bladder neck or ureteral orifice (trigone)	867.0/867.1	S37.2	4

Source: Moore EE et al. *J Trauma.* 1992 September;33(3):337–8.[27]
Note: With ICD-10, use supplementary character: 0 = without an open wound into the pelvic cavity; 1 = with an open wound into the pelvic cavity.
[a] Advance one grade for multiple lesions up to grade III.

Table B.35 Urethra Injury Scale

Grade[a]	Injury Type	Description of Injury	ICD-9	ICD-10	AIS-2005
I	Contusion	Blood at urethral meatus; urethrography normal	867.0/867.1	S37.3	2
II	Stretch injury	Elongation of urethra without extravasation on urethrography	867.0/867.1	S37.3	2
III	Partial disruption	Extravasation of urethrography contrast at injury site with visualization in the bladder	867.0/867.1	S37.3	2
IV	Complete disruption	Extravasation of urethrography contrast at injury site without visualization in the bladder; <2 cm of urethra separation	867.0/867.1	S37.3	3
V	Complete disruption	Complete transection with ≥2 cm urethral separation, or extension into the prostate or vagina	867.0/867.1	S37.3	4

Source: Moore EE et al. *J Trauma.* 1992 September;33(3):337–8.[27]
Note: With ICD-10, use supplementary character: 0 = without an open wound into the pelvic cavity; 1 = with an open wound into the pelvic cavity.
[a] Advance one grade for bilateral injuries up to grade III.

Table B.36 Uterus (Non-Pregnant) Injury Scale

Grade[a]	Description of Injury	ICD-9	ICD-10	AIS-2005
I	Contusion/haematoma	867.4/867.5	S37.6	2
II	Superficial laceration (<1 cm)	867.4/867.5	S37.6	2
III	Deep laceration (≥1 cm)	867.4/867.5	S37.6	3
IV	Laceration involving the uterine artery	902.55	S37.6	3
V	Avulsion/devascularization	867.4/867.5	S37.6	3

Source: Moore EE et al. *J Trauma.* 1990 November;30(11):1427–9.[30]
Note: With ICD-10, use supplementary character: 0 = without an open wound into the pelvic cavity; 1 = with an open wound into the pelvic cavity.
[a] Advance one grade for multiple injuries up to grade III.

Table B.37 Uterus (Pregnant) Injury Scale

Grade[a]	Description of Injury	ICD-9	ICD-10	AIS-2005
I	Contusion or haematoma (without placental abruption)	867.4/867.5	S37.6	2
II	Superficial laceration (<1 cm) or partial placental abruption <25%	867.4/867.5	S37.6	3
III	Deep laceration (≥1 cm) occurring in second trimester or placental abruption >25% but <50%	867.4/867.5	S37.6	3
	Deep laceration (≥1 cm) in third trimester	867.4/867.5	S37.6	4
IV	Laceration involving uterine artery	902.55	S37.6	4
	Deep laceration (≥1 cm) with >50% placental abruption	867.4/867.5	S37.6	4
V	Uterine rupture			
	Second trimester	867.4/867.5	S37.6	4
	Third trimester	867.4/867.5	S37.6	5
	Complete placental abruption	867.4/867.5	S37.6	4–5

Source: Moore EE et al. *J Trauma.* 1990 November;30(11):1427–9.[30]
Note: With ICD-10, use supplementary character: 0 = without an open wound into the pelvic cavity; 1 = with an open wound into the pelvic cavity.
[a] Advance one grade for multiple injuries up to grade III.

Table B.38 Fallopian Tube Injury Scale

Grade[a]	Description of Injury	ICD-9	ICD-10	AIS-2005
I	Haematoma or contusion	867.6/867.7	S37.5	2
II	Laceration <50% circumference	867.6/867.7	S37.5	2
III	Laceration ≥50% circumference	867.6/867.7	S37.5	2
IV	Transection	867.6/867.7	S37.5	2
V	Vascular injury; devascularized segment	902.89	S35.8	2

Source: Moore EE et al. *J Trauma.* 1990 November;30(11):1427–9.[30]
Note: With ICD-10, use supplementary character: 0 = without an open wound into the abdominal or pelvic cavity; 1 = with an open wound into the abdominal or pelvic cavity.
[a] Advance one grade for bilateral injuries up to grade III.

Table B.39 Ovary Injury Scale

Grade[a]	Description of Injury	ICD-9	ICD-10	AIS-2005
I	Contusion or haematoma	867.6/867.7	S37.4	1
II	Superficial laceration (depth <0.5 cm)	867.6/867.7	S37.4	2
III	Deep laceration (depth ≥0.5 cm)	867.8/867.7	S37.4	3
IV	Partial disruption or blood supply	902.81	S35.8	3
V	Avulsion or complete parenchymal destruction	902.81	S37.4	3

Source: Moore EE et al. *J Trauma*. 1990 November;30(11):1427–9.[30]
Note: With ICD-10, use supplementary character: 0 = without an open wound into the abdominal or pelvic cavity; 1 = with an open wound into the abdominal or pelvic cavity.
[a] Advance one grade for bilateral injuries up to grade III.

Table B.40 Vagina Injury Scale

Grade[a]	Description of Injury	ICD-9	ICD-10	AIS-2005
I	Contusion or haematoma	922.4	S30.2	1
II	Laceration, superficial (mucosa only)	878.6	S31.4	1
III	Laceration, deep into fat or muscle	878.6	S31.4	2
IV	Laceration, complex, into cervix or peritoneum	868.7	S31.4	3
V	Injury into adjacent organs (anus, rectum, urethra, bladder)	878.7	S39.7	3

Source: Moore EE et al. *J Trauma*. 1990 November;30(11):1427–9.[30]
Note: With ICD-10, use supplementary character: 0 = without an open wound into the abdominal or pelvic cavity; 1 = with an open wound into the abdominal or pelvic cavity.
[a] Advance one grade for multiple injuries up to grade III.

Table B.41 Vulva Injury Scale

Grade[a]	Description of Injury	ICD-9	ICD-10	AIS-2005
I	Contusion or haematoma	922.4	S30.2	1
II	Laceration, superficial (skin only)	878.4	S31.4	1
III	Laceration, deep (into fat or muscle)	878.4	S31.4	2
IV	Avulsion; skin, fat or muscle	878.5	S38.2	3
V	Injury into adjacent organs (anus, rectum, urethra, bladder)	878.5	S39.7	3

Source: Moore EE et al. *J Trauma*. 1990 November;30(11):1427–9.[30]
[a] Advance one grade for multiple injuries up to grade III.

Table B.42 Testis Injury Scale

Grade[a]	Description of Injury	ICD-9	ICD-10	AIS-2005
I	Contusion/haematoma	911.0–922.4	S30.2	1
II	Subclinical laceration of tunica albuginea	922.4	S31.3	1
III	Laceration of tunica albuginea with <50% parenchymal loss	878.2	S31.3	2
IV	Major laceration of tunica albuginea with ≥50% parenchymal loss	878.3	S31.3	2
V	Total testicular destruction or avulsion	878.3	S38.2	2

Source: Moore EE et al. J Trauma. 1996 September;41(3):523–4.[26]
[a] Advance one grade for bilateral lesions up to grade V.

Table B.43 Scrotum Injury Scale

Grade	Description of Injury	ICD-9	ICD-10	AIS-2005
I	Contusion	922.4	S30.2	1
II	Laceration <25% of scrotal diameter	878.2	S31.2	1
III	Laceration ≥25% of scrotal diameter	878.3	S31.3	2
IV	Avulsion <50%	878.3	S38.2	2
V	Avulsion ≥50%	878.3	S38.2	2

Source: Moore EE et al. J Trauma. 1996 September;41(3):523–4.[26]

Table B.44 Penis Injury Scale

Grade[a]	Description of Injury	ICD-9	ICD-10	AIS-2005
I	Cutaneous laceration/contusion	911.0/922.4	S30.2/31/2	1
II	Buck's fascia (cavernosum) laceration without tissue loss	878.0	S37.8	1
III	Cutaneous avulsion	878.1	S38.2	3
	Laceration through glans/meatus			
	Cavernosal or urethral defect <2 cm			
IV	Partial penectomy	878.1	S38.2	3
	Cavernosal or urethral defect ≥2 cm			
V	Total penectomy	876.1	S38.2	3

Source: Moore EE et al. J Trauma. 1996 September;41(3):523–4.[26]
[a] Advance one grade for multiple injuries up to grade III.

Table B.45 Peripheral Vascular Organ Injury Scale

Grade[a]	Description of Injury	ICD-9	ICD-10	AIS-2005
I	Digital artery/vein	903.5	S65.5	1–3
	Palmar artery/vein	903.4	S65.3	1–3
	Deep palmar artery/vein	904.6	S65.3	1–3
	Dorsalis pedis artery	904.7	S95.0	1–3
	Plantar artery/vein	904.5	S95.1	1–3
	Non-named arterial/venous branches	903.8/904.7	S55.9/S85.9	1–3
II	Basilic/cephalic vein	903.8	S45.8/S55.8	1–3
	Saphenous vein	904.3	S75.2	1–3
	Radial artery	903.2	S55.1	1–3
	Ulnar artery	903.3	S55.0	1–3
III	Axillary vein	903.02	S45.1	2–3
	Superficial/deep femoral vein	903.02	S75.1	2–3
	Popliteal vein	904.42	S85.5	2–3
	Brachial artery	903.1	S45.1	2–3
	Anterior tibial artery	904.51/904.52	S85.1	1–3
	Posterior tibial artery	904.53/904.54	S85.1	1–3
	Peroneal artery	904.7	S85.2	1–3
	Tibioperoneal trunk	904.7	S85.2	2–3
IV	Superficial/deep femoral artery	904.1/904.7	S75.0	3–4
	Popliteal artery	904.41	S85.0	2–3
V	Axillary artery	903.01	S45.0	2–3
	Common femoral artery	904.0	S75.0	3–4

Source: Moore EE et al. *J Trauma*. 1996 September;41(3):523–4.[26]

[a] Increase one grade for multiple grade III or IV injuries involving >50% of the vessel circumference. Decrease one grade for <25% disruption of the vessel circumference for grades IV or V.

B.8 SUMMARY

Trauma scoring systems are designed to facilitate prehospital triage, identify trauma patients whose outcomes are statistically unexpected for quality assurance analysis, allow an accurate comparison of different trauma populations, and organize and improve trauma systems. They are vital for the scientific study of the epidemiology and the treatment of trauma and may even be used to define resource allocation and reimbursement in the future.

Trauma scoring systems that measure outcome solely in terms of death or survival are at best blunt instruments. Despite the existence of several scales (Quality of Well-being Scale, Sickness Impact Profile, etc.), further efforts are needed to develop outcome measures that evaluate the multiplicity of outcomes across the full range of diverse trauma populations.

Despite the profusion of acronyms, scoring systems are a vital component of trauma care delivery systems. The effectiveness of well-organized, centralized, multidisciplinary trauma centres in reducing the mortality and morbidity of injured patients is well documented, trauma scoring systems play a central role in the provision of trauma care today and for the future.

REFERENCES

1. Teasdale G, Jennet B. Assessment of coma and impaired consciousness: a practical scale. *Lancet.* 1974;**ii**:81–4.
2. Tepas JJ 3rd, Ramenofsky ML, Mollitt DL, Gans BM, DiScala C. The Paediatric Trauma Score as a predictor of injury severity: an objective assessment. *J Trauma.* 1988 April;**28(4)**:425–9.
3. Champion HR, Sacco WJ, Copes WS, Gann DS, Gennarelli TA, Flanagan ME. A revision of the Trauma Score. *J Trauma.* 1989 May;**29(5)**:623–9.
4. Knaus WA, Draper EA, Wagner DP, Zimmerman JE. APACHE II: A severity of disease classification system. *Crit Care Med.* 1985 Oct;**13(10)**:818–29.
5. Calculation of the APACHE II Score. Available from: https://www.mdcalc.com/apache-ii-score (accessed online December 2018).
6. American Association for the Advancement of Automotive Medicine. *The Abbreviated Injury Scale: 2015 Revison.* Chicago, IL: AAAM, 2015. Available from: www.AAAM.org.
7. Baker SP, O'Neill B, Haddon W, Long WB. The Injury Severity Score: a method for describing patients with multiple injuries and evaluating emergency care. *J Trauma.* 1974 Mar;**14(3)**:187–96.
8. Osler T, Baker SP, Long W. A modification of the Injury Severity Score that both improves accuracy and simplifies scoring. *J Trauma.* 1997 Dec;**43(6)**:922–5; discussion 925-6.
9. Balogh Z, Offner PJ, Moore EE, Biffl WL. NISS predicts postinjury Multiple Organ Failure better than the ISS. *J Trauma.* 2000 Apr;**48(4)**:624–7; discussion 627-8.
10. Copes WS, Champion HR, Sacco WJ, Lawnick MM, Gann DS, Gennarelli T, et al. Progress in characterising anatomical injury. *J Trauma.* 1990 Oct;**30(10)**:1200–7.
11. Osler T, Rutledge R, Deis J, Bedrick E. ICISS: An International Classification of Disease-9 based injury severity score. *J Trauma.* 1997 Sep;**41(3)**:380–6; discussion 386-8.
12. Organ Injury Scale of the American Association for the Surgery of Trauma (OIS-AAST). Available from: www.aast.org (accessed online December 2018).
13. Moore EE, Dunn EL, Moore JB, Thompson JS. Penetrating Abdominal Trauma Index. *J Trauma.* 1981 Jun;**21(6)**:439–45.
14. Lefering R. Development and validation of the Revised Injury Severity Classification (RISC) score for severely injured patients. *Europ Trauma Emerg Surg.* 2009 Oct;**35(5)**:437–47. doi: 10.1007/s00068-009-9122-0.
15. Lefering R, Huber-Wagner S, Nienaber U, Maegele M, Bouillon B. Update of the trauma risk adjustment model of the Trauma Register DGU: The Revised Injury Severity Classification, version II. *Crit Care.* 2014 Sep;**18(5)**:476. doi: 10.1186/s13054-014-0476-2.
16. Gabbe BJ, Magtengaard K, Hannaford AP, Cameron PA. Is the Charlson Comorbidity Index (CCI) useful for predicting trauma outcomes? *Acad Emerg Med.* 2005;**12(4)**;318–21.
17. Bergeron E, Rossignol M, Osler T, Clas D, Lavoie A. Improving the TRISS methodology by restructuring age categories and adding comorbidities. *J Trauma.* 2004 April;**56(4)**:760–67.
18. Turner-Stokes L, Nyein K, Turner-Stokes, Gatehouse C. The UK FIM+FAM Functional Assessment Measure. *Clin Rehabil.* 1999 Aug;**13(4)**:277–87.
19. Wright J. The Functional Assessment Measure. *The Center for Outcome Measurement in Brain Injury.* http://www.tbims.org/combi/FAM (accessed online December 2018).
20. Jennet B, Bond M. Assessment of outcome: a practical scale. *Lancet.* 1975 Mar;**i(9705)**:480–4.
21. Boyd CR, Tolson MA, Copes WS. Evaluating trauma care: the TRISS model. *J Trauma.* 1987 April;**27(4)**:370–8.
22. Champion HR, Copes WS, Sacco WJ, Lawnick MM, Bain LW, Gann DS, et al. A new characterisation of injury severity. *J Trauma.* 1990 May;**30(5)**:539–46.
23. Champion HR, Copes WS, Sacco WJ, Frey CF, Holcroft JW, Hoyt DB, et al. Improved predictions from A Severity Characterization of Trauma (ASCOT) over Trauma and Injury Severity Score (TRISS): results of an independent evaluation. *J Trauma.* 1996 Jan;**40(1)**:42–8; discussion 48-9.
24. World Health Organization. ICD-9CM. *International Classification of Diseases, Ninth Revision, Clinical Modification.* Center for Diseases Control and Prevention, Hyattsville MD. Available from: https://www.cdc.gov/nchs/icd/index.htm (accessed online December 2018).
25. World Health Organization. *ICD-10 Codes.* 2015 version online. Available from: www.who.int/classifications/icd/en/ (accessed online December 2018).
26. Moore EE, Malangoni MA, Cogbill TH, Peterson NE, Champion HR, Shackford SR. Organ injury scaling VII: cervical vascular, peripheral vascular, adrenal, penis, testis and scrotum. *J Trauma.* 1996 Sept;**41(3)**:523–4.
27. Moore EE, Cogbill TH, Jurkovich GJ. Organ injury scaling III: chest wall, abdominal vascular, ureter, bladder and urethra. *J Trauma.* 1992 Sept;**33(3)**:337–8.

28. Moore EE, Malangoni MA, Cogbill TH, Shackford SR, Champion HR, Jurkovich GJ, et al. Organ injury scaling IV: thoracic, vascular, lung, cardiac and diaphragm. *J Trauma*. 1994 Mar;**36(3)**:299–300.

29. Moore EE, Cogbill TH, Jurkovich GJ, Shackford SR, Malangoni MA, Champion HR. Organ injury scaling: spleen and liver (1994 Revision). *J Trauma*. 1995 Mar;**38(3)**:323–4.

30. Moore EE, Jurkovich GJ, Knudson MM, Cogbill TH, Malangoni MA, Champion HR, et al. Organ injury scaling VI: extrahepatic biliary, oesophagus, stomach, vulva, vagina, uterus (non-pregnant), uterus (pregnant), fallopian tube, and ovary. *J Trauma*. 1995 Dec;**39(6)**:1069–70.

31. Moore EE, Cogbill TH, Malangoni MA, Jurkovich GJ, Champion HR, Gennarelli TA, et al. Organ injury scaling II: pancreas, duodenum, small bowel, colon and rectum. *J Trauma*. 1990 Nov;**30(11)**:1427–9.

32. Moore EE, Shackford SR, Pachter HL, McAninch JW, Browner BD, Champion HR, et al. Organ injury scaling: spleen, liver and kidney. *J Trauma*. 1989 Dec;**29(12)**:1664–6.

Appendix C
The Definitive Surgical Trauma Care Course: The Definitive Anaesthetic Trauma Care Course: Course Requirements And Syllabus

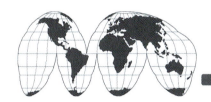

International Association for Trauma Surgery and Intensive Care

IATSIC Secretariat

International Society of Surgery

Seefeldstrasse

CH-8008 Zurich

Switzerland

Phone: +41 44 533 76 50

Fax: +41 44 533 76 59

E-mail: Iatsic@iss-sic.com

URL: http://www.iatsic.org

C.1 BACKGROUND

Injury (trauma) remains a major healthcare problem throughout the world. In addition to improving awareness of trauma prevention and management, improved application of surgical skills is expected to save further lives and contribute to minimizing disability. It is widely recognized that training of surgeons and anaesthesiologists in the management of trauma is substantially deficient because of:

- Limited exposure within individual training programmes to the types of patient required to develop the appropriate level of skills, and
- Traditional trauma training, which has been organ-specific.

Consequently, surgeons can finish their training with suboptimal skills in this field, where there is often little time to contemplate an appropriate course of action.

Through the early 1990s, it became apparent to several surgeons familiar with trauma management around the world that there was a specific need for surgical training in the technical aspects of the operative care of trauma patient, with emphasis on those who were close to completing, or had recently completed, their training. This course had its origins during a meeting in October 1993 between Howard Champion (USA), David Mulder

(Canada), Donald Trunkey (USA), Stephen Deane (Australia), and Abe Fingerhut (France).

This postgraduate surgical course, developed in collaboration with professional educators, assumes competence with assessment and resuscitative measures that have become standardized through the Advanced Trauma Life Support® (ATLS) course of the American College of Surgeons. It draws on the specialist training of all course participants, and reviews, strengthens, and organizes the performance of established and new procedures specially required in trauma surgery. The course has special relevance for surgeons and anaesthesiologists in countries where major trauma rates are high. It is also likely to be valuable in developing countries where education and physical resources are limited, and particularly in those countries with humanitarian or military peacekeeping roles, where use is made of healthcare professionals who have limited experience in trauma.

C.2 COURSE DEVELOPMENT AND TESTING

There have been many attempts to test the concept:

- There was a Swedish Trauma Surgery Course, which Drs Trunkey, Fingerhut, and Champion attended in Sweden in November 1994. This was run by Dr Sten Lennquist. The course was four days of didactic teaching and one day of practical work.
- In Sydney in May 1996, a very successful pilot course was organized at Prince Henry Hospital. The international faculty at that course included Don Trunkey, Abe Fingerhut, and Howard Champion. The course was a tremendous success, and successful courses have since been held worldwide.
- From 1999, following courses in Australia, Austria, and South Africa, a standardized manual and slide set were developed.
- The course is revised every four years, with updated material, in order to stay current and to recognize the rapid improvements in trauma care globally.

C.3 COURSE DETAILS

C.3.1 Ownership

The Definitive Surgical Trauma Care™ (DSTC™) and Definitive Anaesthetic Trauma Care™ (DATC™)

course is a registered trademark of the International Association for Trauma Surgery and Intensive Care (IATSIC). IATSIC is an Integrated Society of the International Society of Surgery/Société Internationale de Chirugie (ISS–SIC) based in Zurich, Switzerland. Only courses recognized by IATSIC may be called DSTC courses.

C.3.2 Mission Statement

The course is designed to train participants in the techniques required for the care of the surgical trauma patient. This is done by a combination of lectures, demonstrations, case discussions, and practical sessions, utilizing live tissue and human (cadaver or prosected) tissue if available.

C.3.3 Application to Hold a Course

Application can be made to IATSIC for recognition of a course. Provided the minimum requirements for the course have been met, as laid down below, IATSIC will recognize the course, which will then be entitled to be called a DSTC™ course and carry the IATSIC logo. DATC™ is a specific module within the DSTC™ course. The initial course to be presented will be the course prescribed by IATSIC, and no changes may be made to the course material or syllabus.

C.3.4 Eligibility to Present

C.3.4.1 LOCAL ORGANIZATIONS

The DSTC course can be presented by any tertiary academic institution or recognized surgical organization.

C.3.4.2 NATIONAL ORGANIZATIONS

National organizations can present the course in their own country on behalf of IATSIC. A memorandum of understanding will be signed with IATSIC. Following the presentation of the first two courses, the national organization shall have the right to modify the course to enhance its relevance to local conditions, although still respecting the core curriculum.

C.3.5 **Course Materials and Overview**

The course takes place over three days with the following course materials:

- The administrative details of running the course are contained in the Course Director's Manual, available from the IATSIC office.
- The content of the course will, as a minimum, contain the core curriculum, as laid down in the IATSIC DSTC™ manual (see Appendix D). Additional material and modules may be included at the discretion of the local organizers, provided such material is not in conflict with the core curriculum.
- Additional 'add-on' modules may be presented at the discretion of the local organizers.
- The course will use a specific set of slides and the DSTC course manual.
- IATSIC is able to furnish the IATSIC DSTC course manual, and course materials (including slides on PowerPoint) if requested, at a substantial discount. However, provided the minimum core syllabus is adhered to, a local course manual and material can be used.

C.3.6 **Course Director**

In addition to the requirements below, the course director must be a full, current member of IATSIC. For an inaugural course, the course director must be a member of the IATSIC Executive Committee.

C.3.7 **Course Faculty**

- Course faculty will be divided into:
  - Local faculty.
  - International faculty.
  - Guest lecturers.
- Course faculty members must have themselves attended a DSTC course.
- Course faculty members must have completed an ATLS Instructor course, Royal College of Surgeons 'Train the Trainers' course, or an equivalent instructor training course.
- Course International faculty must be members of IATSIC.
- Additional guest lecturers with particular expertise in a subject are permitted.

- Details of all faculty members with confirmation of the above, and full Ethics Committee approval, must be lodged with IATSIC at least three months prior to the prior to commencement of the course.
- The recommended student:instructor ratio should ideally be 4:1, not including the course director.

C.3.8 **Course Participants**

- All course participants must be licensed medical practitioners.
- Attendance at the entire course is mandatory.
- The level of applicants can be decided locally, provided that the participants are licensed medical practitioners, and are ***actively involved in the surgical decision-making and surgical care*** of the trauma patient.
- An entrance examination can be used if needed. An exit examination is not mandatory.

C.3.9 **Practical Skill Stations**

Practical skills may take place on different material, depending on the local constraints. The practical component of the course *must* include a live tissue training laboratory. However, the use of cadavers is optional and dependent on local conditions. Full local ethical committee certificates of approval for all animal and other tissue work, and any other legal necessary approvals, *must* be obtained and must be submitted to IATSIC *before* a course can be approved or held.

C.3.10 **Course Syllabus**

In order for IATSIC to recognize the course as a valid DSTC course, the course must meet or exceed the minimum requirements of the core curriculum. The core curriculum and 'modules' are contained in this manual and the course consists of:

- Core knowledge.
- Surgical skills (see Appendix D).
- Additional modules, which may be added as required, at the discretion of the local organizing committee and as required for local needs.
- Where human material is available for dissection, the course is often enhanced by presentation in

association with the American College of Surgeons (ACS), of the ACS Course in Advanced Surgical Skills for Exposure in Trauma (ASSET).

C.3.11 **Course Certification**

- Participants are required to attend the entire course.
- Certification of attendance and completion of the course can be issued.
- The certificates of the courses will be numbered.
- Details of the course, final faculty and participants, as well as a course evaluation, must be submitted to IATSIC after the course.

C.4 **IATSIC RECOGNITION**

Application for recognition of individual courses should be made to IATSIC. IATSIC recognized courses may carry the endorsement logos of IATSIC and the ISS-SIC, and will be entitled be called DSTC courses.

The DSTC course is the intellectual property and a registered trademark of IATSIC, and IATSIC is an Integrated Society of the ISS-SIC based in Zurich, Switzerland. Although it may carry the endorsement (support) of other bodies, this does not imply that other organizations may operate or control the DSTC course in any way.

The DSTC course is designed to train medical practitioners in the techniques required for the definitive surgical care of the trauma patient. This is done by a combination of lectures, demonstrations, case discussions, and practical sessions.

The registration and control of the DSTC courses will be controlled by the DSTC Sub-Committee on behalf of IATSIC. While it is desirable that national courses be controlled by a national organization, there will be no restriction on local courses provided that international DSTC criteria are met. Application to hold a course must be made through IATSIC.

Only courses recognized by IATSIC may be called DSTC courses.

C.5 **COURSE INFORMATION**

Course information is obtainable from IATSIC.

Appendix D
Definitive Surgical Trauma Care™ Course – Core Surgical Skills

D.1 THE NECK

D.1.1. Standard Neck (Pre-Sternomastoid) Incision
D.1.2. Control and Repair of the Carotid Vessels
    D.1.2.1. Zone II
    D.1.2.2. Extension into Zone III
    D.1.2.3. Division of the Digastric Muscle and Subluxation or Division of the Mandible
    D.1.2.4. Extension into Zone I
D.1.3. Extension by Supraclavicular Incision
    D.1.3.1. Ligation of the Proximal Internal Carotid Artery
    D.1.3.2. Repair with a Divided External Carotid Artery
D.1.4. Access to, Control of and Ligation of the Internal Jugular Vein
D.1.5. Access to and Repair of the Trachea
D.1.6. Access to and Repair of the Cervical Oesophagus

D.2 THE CHEST

D.2.1. Incisions
    D.2.1.1. Anterolateral Thoracotomy
    D.2.1.2. Sternotomy
    D.2.1.3. 'Clamshell' Bilateral Thoracotomy Incision
D.2.2. Thoracotomy
    D.2.2.1. Exploration of the Thorax
    D.2.2.2. Ligation of the Intercostal and Internal Mammary Vessels
    D.2.2.3. Emergency Department (Resuscitative) Thoracotomy
        D.2.2.3.1. Supradiaphragmatic Control of the Aorta
        D.2.2.3.2. Control of the Pulmonary Hilum
        D.2.2.3.3. Internal Cardiac Massage

D.2.3. Pericardiotomy
    D.2.3.1. Preservation of the Phrenic Nerve
    D.2.3.2. Access to the Pulmonary Veins
D.2.4. Access to and Repair of the Thoracic Aorta
    D.2.4.1. Cross Clamping of the Aorta
D.2.5. Lung Wounds
    D.2.5.1. Oversewing
    D.2.5.2. Stapling
    D.2.5.3. Partial Lung Resection
    D.2.5.4. Tractectomy
    D.2.5.5. Lobectomy
D.2.6. Access to and Repair of the Thoracic Oesophagus
D.2.7. Access to and Repair of the Diaphragm
D.2.8. Compression of the Left Subclavian Vessels from Below
D.2.9. Left Anterior Thoracotomy
    D.2.9.1. Visualization of the Supra-Aortic Vessels
D.2.10. Heart Repair
    D.2.10.1. Finger Control
    D.2.10.2. Involvement of the Coronary Vessels
D.2.11. Insertion of a Shunt

D.3 THE ABDOMINAL CAVITY

D.3.1. Midline Laparotomy
    D.3.1.1. How to Explore (Priorities)
    D.3.1.2. Packing
    D.3.1.3. Localization of Retroperitoneal Haematomas – When to Explore?
    D.3.1.4. Damage Control
        D.3.1.4.1. Techniques
        D.3.1.4.2. Abdominal Closure
    D.3.1.5. Extension of Laparotomy Incision
        D.3.1.5.1. Lateral Extension
        D.3.1.5.2. Sternotomy

D.3.1.6. Cross-Clamping of the Aorta at the Diaphragm (Division at the Left Crus)

D.3.2. Left Visceral Medial Rotation

　D.3.2.1. Reflection of the Left (Descending) Colon Medially

　D.3.2.2. Reflection of the Pancreas and Spleen Towards the Midline

D.3.3. Right Visceral Medial Rotation

　D.3.3.1. Kocher's Manoeuvre

　D.3.3.2. Reflection of the Right (Ascending) Colon Medially

D.3.4. Abdominal Oesophagus

　D.3.4.1. Mobilization

　D.3.4.2. Repair

　　D.3.4.2.1. Simple

　　D.3.4.2.2. Mobilization of the Fundus to Reinforce Sutures

D.3.5. Stomach

　D.3.5.1. Mobilization

　D.3.5.2. Access to Vascular Control

　D.3.5.3. Repair of Anterior and Posterior Wounds

D.3.6. Bowel

　D.3.6.1. Resection

　D.3.6.2. Small and Large Bowel Anastomosis

　D.3.6.3. Staple Colostomy

　D.3.6.4. Ileostomy Technique

D.4 **THE LIVER**

D.4.1. Mobilization (Falciform, Suspensory, Triangular And Coronary Ligaments)

D.4.2. Liver Packing

D.4.3. Hepatic Isolation

　D.4.3.1. Control the of Infrahepatic Inferior Vena Cava

　D.4.3.2. Control of the Suprahepatic Superior Vena Cava

　D.4.3.3. Pringle's Manoeuvre

D.4.4. Repair of Parenchymal Laceration

D.4.5. Technique of Finger Fracture

D.4.6. Tractotomy

D.4.7. Packing for Injury to Hepatic Veins

D.4.8. Hepatic Resection

D.4.9. Non-Anatomical Partial Resection

D.4.10. Use of Tissue Adhesives

D.4.11. Tamponade for Penetrating Injury (Foley/Penrose Drains, Sengstaken Tube)

D.5 **THE SPLEEN**

D.5.1. Mobilization

D.5.2. Suture

D.5.3. Use of Tissue Adhesives

D.5.4. Partial Splenectomy

　D.5.4.1. Sutures

　D.5.4.2. Staples

D.5.5. Total splenectomy

D.6 **THE PANCREAS**

D.6.1. Mobilization of the Tail of the Pancreas

D.6.2. Mobilization of the Head of the Pancreas

D.6.3. Localization of the Main Duct and its Repair

D.6.4. Distal Pancreatic Resection

　D.6.4.1. Stapler

　D.6.4.2. Oversewing

D.6.5. Use of Tissue Adhesives

D.6.6. Access to the Mesenteric Vessels (Division of the Pancreas)

D.7 **THE DUODENUM**

D.7.1. Mobilization of the Duodenum

　D.7.1.1. Kocher's Manoeuvre (Rotation of the Duodenum)

　D.7.1.2. Division of the Ligament of Treitz

　D.7.1.3. Repair of the Duodenum

D.8 **THE GENITOURINARY SYSTEM**

D.8.1. Kidney

　D.8.1.1. Mobilization

　D.8.1.2. Vascular control

　D.8.1.3. Repair

　D.8.1.4. Partial Nephrectomy

　D.8.1.5. Nephrectomy

D.8.2. Ureter

　D.8.2.1. Mobilization

　D.8.2.2. Stenting

　D.8.2.3. Repair

D.8.3. Bladder

　D.8.3.1. Repair of Intraperitoneal Rupture

　D.8.3.2. Repair of Extraperitoneal Rupture

D.9 **ABDOMINAL VASCULAR INJURIES**

D.9.1. Exposure and Control
  D.9.1.1. Aorta and its Branches
    D.9.1.1.1. Exposure
    D.9.1.1.2. Repair
    D.9.1.1.3. Shunt
  D.9.1.2. Inferior Vena Cava
    D.9.1.2.1. Suprahepatic Inferior Vena Cava
    D.9.1.2.2. Infrahepatic Inferior Vena Cava
    D.9.1.2.3. Control of Haemorrhage with Swabs
    D.9.1.2.4. Repair both Anteriorly and Posteriorly, through an Anterior Wound
    D.9.1.2.5. Shunting
D.9.2. Pelvis
  D.9.2.1. Control of the Pelvic Vessels
    D.9.2.1.1. Extraperitoneal Packing
    D.9.2.1.2. Suture of Artery and Vein
    D.9.2.1.3. Ligation of Artery and Vein
    D.9.2.1.4. Packing/anchor Ligation of the Sacral Vessels

D.10 **PERIPHERAL VASCULAR INJURIES**

D.10.1. Extremities: Vascular Access
  D.10.1.1. Axillary
  D.10.1.2. Brachial
  D.10.1.3. Femoral
  D.10.1.4. Popliteal
D.10.2. Fasciotomy
  D.10.2.1. Upper Limb
  D.10.2.2. Lower Limb

D.11 **INSERTION OF RESUSCITATIVE BALLOON OCCLUSION OF THE AORTA (REBOA) CATHETER**

D.11.1. Groin Insertion, using Ultrasound

Appendix E
Briefing for Operating Room Scrub Nurses

E.1 INTRODUCTION

Damage control techniques for the management of the major trauma patient are now accepted concepts, and include temporizing measures to prevent a cold, acidotic, and coagulopathic patient from further deterioration and eventual death. Some personnel working in the operation room/theatre (OR/OT) environment may not have had previous exposure to these techniques, especially in countries where trauma volumes are limited, and major trauma is a stressful rarity. This appendix is intended to help prepare the team for the imminent arrival and intraoperative management of the major trauma patient. Good communication is the key to success. Anticipate and think laterally. (Refer also to Chapter 9.1.)

The aspects of care referred to in this section are as follows:

- Preparation.
- Cleaning and draping.
- Instruments and issues of technique.
- Special tools and equipment – including improvised gadgets.
- Medico-legal aspects.
- Communication.

E.2 PREPARING THE OPERATING ROOM

Patients with major trauma are complex; they have deranged physiology and may have complex injuries with competing priorities for treatment. Optimizing the OR before the patient arrives and planning for every eventuality is what will make the difference between a stressful, chaotic experience for all concerned, and a planned environment where every member of the team has a role and acknowledges the strength of all the members of the team.

E.2.1 Environment

Because of the underlying coagulopathy and hypothermia, the patient needs to be prevented from further heat loss at all costs to maximize haemostasis.

- The internal temperature of the operating room/theatre (OR/OT) should be set to at least 27°C and maintained at this level.[1]
- Fluid and blood should be warmed before and during administration, using devices such as a Level 1® (Smiths Medical, St Paul, MN, USA) or Ranger® (3M Medical, St Paul, MN, USA) device, which allow for rapid infusion without sacrificing adequate heat transmission to the fluid. Ideally, the temperature should be set at 41°C.
- Patient warming devices should be present and readied for use. These can include a circulating warm fluid underlay or warm air circulation device (e.g. Bair Hugger® (3M Medical, St Paul, MN, USA), which must be directly in contact with the skin and not over a bed sheet.

E.2.2 Blood Loss

Because of the propensity for massive blood loss, one should consider activating and priming a cell-saving device of some description. Blood from the chest drain need not be washed and can be autotransfused directly provided that normal saline (0.9%) has been used in the collection device (plus 1000 I.U. of calcium heparin) and not water.

E.2.3 Instruments

- Now is the time to request extra instrument packs and obtain packs of sponges/swabs as these will be rapidly required in large numbers.
- A trolley with multiple drawers with pre-packed equipment may be a useful option.[2]
- Equipment for thoracotomy and vascular access/ repair should be mandatory and a large selection of sutures, staplers, and drains should be available including items for unusual uses, such as a Sengstaken-Blakemore tube.

E.2.4 Cleaning

With damage control surgery, there is less time than usual to provide a truly sterile field, and alternate methods should be used to achieve the same result. It is often said that 'sterility is a luxury in trauma'.

- Typically, either an iodophore- or a chlorhexidine-based skin preparation is utilized, and this applies equally to the trauma patient. One should not use both types as they may inactivate each other. Chlorhexidine-based solutions are the current solution of choice.[3]
- The method of application may, however, vary. One option, utilized in several prominent North American centres, is the use of a spray bottle to apply the preparation solution. This has been shown to be as effective as traditional circular sponging techniques.[3,4]
- Cleaning should be extended widely beyond the expected bounds of the operative field, and the recommendation is to clean from neck to knees, as this allows for extension from abdomen to chest or for vein harvest from the saphenous veins.
  - Laparotomy cleaning should extended to the chest and the knees to allow for extension into the chest or control of vessels in the thigh.
  - Cleaning the chest for vascular injury to the subclavian or axillary injury must extent into free draping of the affected limb and the thigh for possible saphenous vein harvesting.
  - Laparotomy cleaning should be extended as laterally as possible to accommodate drains.

E.2.5 Draping

Draping is also along unconventional lines, and this ensures that the surgeons can have ready access to more than just the area of single focus, which is usual for when elective surgery is performed.

- Drape widely using drapes that attach to the skin, or fix them with skin staples, laterally from the neck, lateral to the chest at the mid-axillary lines and along the same plane to the knees. The genitalia are covered with a small drape or an opened swab (Figure E.1).
- Prevent further heat loss by covering the areas not initially needed for surgical access with sterile drapes. For example, if the abdomen is the default operation, cover the chest and legs with drapes that are easily removed if access to those regions is required.

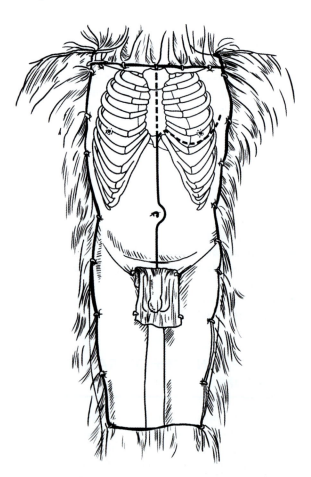

Figure E.1 Draping required for a trauma laparotomy.

E.2.6 **Adjuncts**

As far as pre-planning for the actual procedure is concerned, one can only recommend that the OR team 'anticipate' all eventualities. Remember, too, that as there is little time to spare, the risk of injury to operative team members is high, and that all precautions should be taken to ensure maximal protection.

Meticulous sharps handling is required in this relatively uncontrolled situation. NEVER hand or receive sharps, except in a bowl.

- Although there is no good evidence that masks, overshoes, and caps protect the patient from infection during surgery, standard precautions should be maintained to protect the team members. The OR nurse should ensure that all staff in the 'sterile area' are appropriately attired.
- Place the scalpel in a receiver (kidney bowl) for the surgeon to take and replace. The body cavities should be opened primarily with a scalpel and heavy (Mayo) scissors.
- Have 20–30 large *dry* swabs or sponges ready for the surgeon to perform rapid packing. These are best passed 'folded' initially, unless the surgeon specifies otherwise, as for definitive packing, swabs should be used *folded* in layers.
- Do NOT use wet swabs. They rapidly become cold wet swabs!
- The suction devices should be ready and should preferably be routed to the cell-saver device. It is useful for there to be *two* suction devices at the table.
- An electrocautery machine should be available, but there is no time for small vessel haemostasis at this point, and this will most likely be used later.

E.3 **SURGICAL PROCEDURE**

E.3.1 **Instruments**

The instrument sets one should have at the ready are as follows:

- A thoracotomy tray ready in the room, but not open unless the chest is the primary operative focus. A sternal saw or Lebsche knife should also be available.
- A standard laparotomy set open and ready, including a bowel resection set.

- Vascular instruments, including large aortic clamps (Crawford and Satinsky) open on the set-up trolley.
- Extra small, medium and large crushing clamps (e.g. Halstead, Crile, Roberts and mosquito) as there may be many bleeding vessels to clamp.
- Several Babcock forceps for holding or marking a bowel injury.
- A right-angled dissecting forceps such as is used for bile ducts (Lahey, Heiss, Mixter, etc.).
- A full selection of retractors (e.g. Morris, Army-Navy, Langenbeck, Deaver, and copper malleables), as well as some form of a self-retaining system such as a Bookwalter, Omni-Tract, or Gray system.
- At least one pair of forceps should be rubber-shod, as retrieval of a bullet will otherwise result in scratching the round, rendering it inadmissible for forensic evidence, should the case come to court.

Since most major trauma (especially penetrating trauma) affects the abdomen, one must prepare for bowel and solid organ injury.

- Skin staplers can temporise small holes from bullets and lacerations in the stomach (and may be useful on the heart).
- GI-type linear cutting staplers are handy for the rapid closure of bowel ends during non-reconstructive resection of small bowel or colon.
- TA-type non-cutting staplers can be used to fashion a pyloric exclusion, or for distal pancreas resection when the need for rapid resection is present.
- Umbilical tapes or the tapes on large sponges can be used to ligate segments of bowel to control effluent.
- Ligaclips can be useful for controlling bleeding vessels on the liver or spleen or in the mesentery.
- It is useful to keep handy a Sengstaken–Blakemore tube for placing in a bleeding hepatic tract to attempt to tamponade the deep bleeding. A Penrose drain inflated over a 16G nasogastric tube, can achieve a similar effect.
- For suspected vascular injury or to control bleeding from non-ligatable vessels, various forms of temporary arterial shunt and similar devices are required.
- The Rumel tourniquet is a useful device made by simply placing a cylindrical plastic tube over a vascular loop and using this to compress a friable vessel once it has been isolated and looped. It may also be used to hold a shunt in place proximally and distally in an injured artery. The tourniquets can be kept in place with either Ligaclips or small artery clamps.

- Proprietary shunts (such as Javid or Barker shunts) should be available; alternatively, one can manufacture them using intravenous tubing, nasogastric tubing, or chest drain tubing, depending on the vessel size.
- A selection of vascular grafts should be close at hand. A selection or plastic drapes for damage control closure:
  - Opsite® (Smith and Nephew, London, UK)
  - Ioban® or Steridrape® (3M Medical, St. Paul, MN, USA).
- Proprietary Vacuum closures:
  - V.A.C.® Kinetic Concepts Inc. (KCI) San Antonio, TX, USA.
- Renasys® (Smith and Nephew, London, UK).

E.3.2 Special Instruments and Improvised Gadgets

The first goal of the damage control procedure is to stop the bleeding and then control contamination, while maintaining tissue perfusion. This may require the use of other specific instruments and some improvised or 'home-made' gadgets to achieve the desired result. Again, a useful option is to have this equipment 'pre-selected' and placed for use in a dedicated mobile, multiple-drawer trolley.

A suitable damage control surgery storage cupboard will contain a selection, such as is shown Table E.1 and Figure E.2.

E.4 ABDOMINAL CLOSURE

Closure of the abdomen may be final and definitive, but more likely will involve some form of temporary closure device. The options include a vacuum-assisted closure (VAC) sandwich (best), plastic silo bags sutured to the skin (Bogota bag), or towel-clip closures (neither of the latter being recommended). Equipment for the vacuum-sandwich is described below. The commercial vacuum dressings are not appropriate until definitive closure.

- One sterile adhesive drape (Opsite or Ioban) is placed sticky side up, and one or two sterile towels or swabs are placed on the sticky surface. Note that only one side of the swab is covered in plastic membrane. Placing plastic on *both* sides, allows the drape to slide somewhat inside the abdomen, and prevents the gauze swabs from effectively 'wicking' any

Table E.1 Damage Control Equipment	
Top	**Sutures**
Tray 1	**Surgical drapes**
Tray 2	**Disposable gowns**
Tray 3	**Universal instrument set: Babcocks**
	Right angle forceps, Satinsky clamp
Tray 4	**Thoracic instrument set**
Tray 5	**Abdominal instrument set**
Tray 6	**Vascular instrument set**
Tray 7	**Disinfection material**
	Drapes (Steridrape®, Opsite®, Ioban®)
Tray 8	**Large gauze, abdominal swabs**
Tray 9	**Mesh grafts, pledgets**
	Shunts: carotid, Javed
	Tubes: nasogastric, urinary, chest
	Silicon loops, Rumel tourniquets
Tray 10	**Staplers: Skin stapler/GIA/TA/vascular**
Side	**Fogarty catheters**
	List of contents

intra-abdominal fluid away into the suction drains, but traps the fluid inside the abdominal cavity.
  - Do NOT make slits in the plastic.
  - Do NOT have suction of greater than 24 mm Hg, as this predisposes to fistulae in the hypotensive, cold, damage control patient.
- This is tucked under the fascia over the bowel, with the smooth plastic protecting the bowel, while the sponges/swabs prevent evisceration by adhering to the parietal peritoneal surface.
- Two large drains or nasogastric tubes are laid inside the gap between the sheath and the skin and are tunnelled cranially for about 5–8 cm under the skin to enable an adequate seal of the other adhesive drape over the entire abdomen.
- A second large sterile adhesive drape is then used to close the wound.
- The drains are connected with a Y-connector and may be placed on *low-pressure* wall suction (maximum suction <25 mm Hg). This controls effluent and creates a good seal. It is also easiest to nurse in the ward or intensive care unit.

A commercial VAC device is available, but owing to expense, and often, the higher suction used, it is NOT

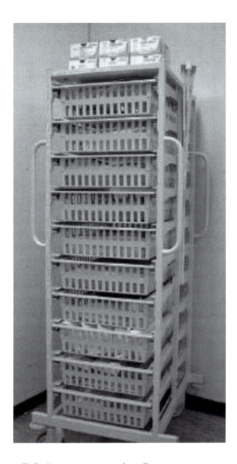

Figure E.2 Damage control trolley.

recommended for *initial* closure. It is, however, the device of choice for subsequent wound management of the open abdomen.

E.5 INSTRUMENT AND SWAB COUNT

As usual, counts are performed before closure.

However, after *damage control*, a second count is performed *after* the abdominal vacuum dressing has been completed. This allows a count of how many swabs have been left in the abdomen. (Don't forget to count the swabs in the vacuum sandwich!)

An accurate record should be kept of any retained instruments and swabs, as there may be a different scrub team at the time of the re-look laparotomy.

An abdominal x-ray before final closure is advisable, as an extra safeguard to avoid retained swabs or instruments.

E.6 MEDICO-LEGAL ASPECTS AND COMMUNICATION SKILLS

- Failing to plan and failing to communicate efficiently are the two major instigators of error and error avoidance is an important aspect of medicine. The common medicolegal areas of dispute in trauma relate to aspects of consent and management of foreign bodies.
- Consent in emergency in most countries is based on the clinician doing what is in the best interest of the patient and as such the surgery to save a life takes precedence over a piece of paper. Family assent is useful and is of importance with small children, but must not influence against needed surgery unless there is an advanced directive. Surgical checklists are also of benefit in reducing error prior to surgery.
- Foreign bodies are often present in penetrating trauma. There is a need to remove these and the local procedure for forensic analysis should be well-known to the operation suite staff. Bullets should be removed without metal-to-metal instrument contact, to prevent damage to the markings used for identification of the bullet. Rubber- or plastic-shod instruments should be used for removal if they are removed at all, as there are clear indications to leave alone those that are unlikely to cause further harm.[5]
- Forensic evidence is also essential in cases of major trauma due to sexual and paediatric abuse. Try to preserve all the evidence as best as possible. Never handle bullets or metal fragments with metal instruments. Use mosquito forceps, the jaws of which are plastic or rubber covered. Wrap the fragment in gauze. Place each fragment in a separate container, marked with the exact site of removal.
- Communication is enhanced by all the members of the trauma team addressing the following aspects:
  - Information-sharing allows for optimal preparation.
  - Assign roles to each member and ensure each prepares their aspect of the care pathway.
  - Thinking ahead to ensure all possible equipment and patient care aspects are addressed.
  - Closed-loop communication with feedback to the initial person asking the question/giving the instruction and assignment of actions to named persons reduces risk of error (see also Chapter 2).

E.7 **CRITICAL INCIDENT STRESS ISSUES**

The trauma environment is stressful for all concerned, and time is of the essence – tempers often flare, and one must not take the issues personally.

Occasionally, the patient will not survive, and the risk is that staff may develop post-traumatic stress disorder, especially if major trauma is a rare occurrence for them. The best method for dealing with this situation is via a debriefing session as soon as everyone has cleaned up or first thing the next morning (see also Chapter 22).

E.8 **CONCLUSION**

The success of trauma surgery depends on a team performing at its peak with effective communication, willing to work outside of the traditional norms and yet with maximal concern for patient safety.

REFERENCES AND RECOMMENDED READING

References

1. Hardcastle TC, M Stander, N Kalafatis, E Hodgson, D Gopalan. External patient temperature control in emergency centres, trauma centres, intensive care units and operating theatres: A multi-society literature review. *S Afr Med J.* 2013 Aug;**103(9)**:609–11. doi: 10.7196/samj.7327.
2. Goslings JC, Haverlag R, Ponsen KJ, Luitse JSK. Facilitating damage control surgery with a dedicated DCS equipment trolley. *Injury.* 2006 May;**37(5)**:466–7.
3. Woodhead K, Taylor EW, Bannister G, Chesworth T, Hoffman P, Humphreys H. Behaviours and Rituals in the Operating Theatre: A report from the Hospital Infection Society Working Group on Infection Control in the Operating Theatres (published 2002). Available from: http://www.his.org.uk/_db/_documents/Rituals-02.doc (accessed online December 2010).
4. Ritter MA, French ML, Eitzen HE, Gioe TJ. The antimicrobial effectiveness of operative-site preparative agents: a microbiological and clinical study. *J Bone Joint Surg Am.* 1980;**62**:826–8.
5. Dienstknecht T, Horst K, Sellei R, Berner A, Nerlich N, Hardcastle T. Indications for bullet removal: A literature overview and clinical practice guideline for European Trauma Surgeons. *Eur J Trauma and Emerg Surg.* 2012,**38(2)**:89–93.

Recommended Reading

Emergency Exploratory Laparotomy. In: *Berry and Kohn's Operating Room Technique*, 11th ed. Phillips N. (Ed.) Mosby, St. Louis, MO, 2007.
Goldman MA. In: *Pocket Guide to the Operating Room*, 3rd Ed. FA Davis. Philadelphia, PA, 2008.
Saullo DC. Trauma Surgery. In: Rothrock JC. (Ed.) *Alexander's Care of the Patient in Surgery*, 14th ed. Mosby, St Louis, 2003:1182–223.

Index

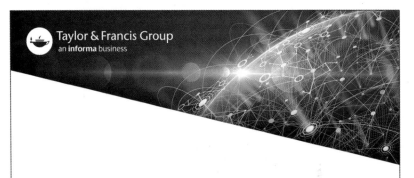